Oncodermatology

Cristina Martinez Zugaib Abdalla
José Antonio Sanches
Rodrigo Ramella Munhoz
Francisco Aparecido Belfort
Editors

Oncodermatology

An Evidence-Based, Multidisciplinary Approach to Best Practices

Springer

Editors
Cristina Martinez Zugaib Abdalla
Dermatology
Hospital Sírio-Libanês
São Paulo, São Paulo, Brazil

Rodrigo Ramella Munhoz
Oncology
Hospital Sírio-Libanês
São Paulo, São Paulo, Brazil

José Antonio Sanches
Dermatology
Faculdade de Medicina da Universidade de São Paulo
São Paulo, São Paulo, Brazil

Francisco Aparecido Belfort
Cutaneous Oncology and Sarcomas Center
Hospital Sírio-Libanês
São Paulo, São Paulo, Brazil

ISBN 978-3-031-29279-8 ISBN 978-3-031-29277-4 (eBook)
https://doi.org/10.1007/978-3-031-29277-4

This Springer imprint is published by the registered company Springer Nature Switzerland AG
The registered company address is: Gewerbestrasse 11, 6330 Cham, Switzerland

Contents

Contributors

Beatrice Martinez Zugaib Abdalla Hospital Sírio-Libanês, São Paulo, Brazil

Cristina Martinez Zugaib Abdalla Hospital Sírio-Libanês, São Paulo, São Paulo, Brazil

Núcleo de Oncodermatologia Hospital Sírio-Libanês, São Paulo, São Paulo, Brazil

Eduardo Hiroshi Akaishi Sarcoma and Melanoma Group, Instituto do Câncer do Estado de São Paulo—ICESP, São Paulo, SP, Brazil

Cutaneous Oncology and Sarcomas Center, Hospital Sírio-Libanês, São Paulo, SP, Brazil

Marcelo Neira Ave Sírio-Libanês Hospital, São Paulo, Brazil

Beatriz Mendes Awni Oncology Center, Hospital Sírio-Libanês, São Paulo, SP, Brazil

Renato Marchiori Bakos Department of Dermatology, Hospital de Clínicas de Porto Alegre, Porto Alegre, Brazil

Carlos Barcauí School of Medical Sciences, State University of Rio de Janeiro, Rio de Janeiro, Brazil

Francisco Aparecido Belfort Hospital Sírio-Libanês, São Paulo, São Paulo, Brazil

NOCS - Hospital Sírio-Libanês, São Paulo, Brazil

Brazilian Melanoma Group, São Paulo, SP, Brazil

Eduardo Bertolli Cutaneous Oncology and Sarcoma Group, Hospital Sírio-Libanês, São Paulo, Brazil

Skin Cancer Department, AC Camargo Cancer Center, São Paulo, Brazil

Melanoma and Sarcoma Group, Beneficência Portuguesa de São Paulos, São Paulo, Brazil

Tatiana Cristina Moraes Pinto Blumetti AC Camargo Cancer Center, São Paulo, Brazil

Juliana Casagrande Tavoloni Braga AC Camargo Cancer Center, São Paulo, Brazil

Flavio Cavarsan Brazilian Melanoma Group, São Paulo, SP, Brazil

Intensive Training in Mohs Surgery (TIMOS), São Paulo, SP, Brazil

Cutaneous Oncology of Honcord Clinic, Goiânia, GO, Brazil

María Catalina Gavilanes Coloma Hospital Sírio-Libanês, São Paulo, Brazil

Paula Yume Sato Serzedello Correa Dermatology, Faculdade de Medicina da Universidade de Sao Paulo, São Paulo, Brazil

Erico Tosoni Costa Laboratory of Tumor Cell Biology of the Molecular Oncology Center, Hospital Sírio-Libanês, São Paulo, SP, Brazil

Jade Cury-Martins Hospital das Clínicas, Faculdade de Medicina da Universidade de São Paulo, São Paulo, Brazil

Dermatology, Faculdade de Medicina da Universidade de São Paulo, São Paulo, São Paulo, Brazil

Instituto do Cancer do Estado de São Paulo—ICESP, São Paulo, São Paulo, Brazil

Carolina Atallah Pontes da Silva Sírio-Libanês Hospital, São Paulo, Brazil

João Luis Fernandes da Silva Radiation Oncology Department, Hospital Sírio-Libanês, São Paulo, Brazil

Elisabeth de Albuquerque Cavalcanti Callegaro Hospital Sírio-Libanês, São Paulo, Brazil

Fernando Augusto de Almeida Hospital Sírio-Libanês, São Paulo, Brazil

Vera Maria Bacelar de Barros NOCS, Sírio-Libanês Hospital, São Paulo, Brazil

Letícia Hernandes de Brito Radiation Oncology Medical Residency Program, Hospital Sírio-Libanês, São Paulo, Brazil

Ana Cristina Pugliese de Castro Hospital Sírio-Libanês, São Paulo, Brazil

André Luis de Freitas Perina NOCS - Hospital Sírio-Libanês, São Paulo, São Paulo, Brazil

Laryssa Gonçalves de Gouvea Faiçal AMO Clinic, Salvador, Bahia, Brazil

Luiz Guilherme Cernaglia Aureliano de Lima Oncology Center, Hospital Sírio-Libanês, São Paulo, Brazil

Instituto do Cancer do Estado de Sao Paulo, São Paulo, São Paulo, Brazil

NOCS - Hospital Sírio-Libanês, São Paulo, Brazil

Mariana Petaccia de Macedo Laboratory of Pathology, Hospital Sírio-Libanês, São Paulo, São Paulo, Brazil

Andreia Cristina de Melo Division of Clinical Research and Technological Development, Brazilian National Cancer Institute, INCA, Rio de Janeiro, Brazil

Priscila Muniz Gonçalves de Moraes Oncology Center, Hospital Sírio-Libanês, São Paulo, Brazil

Fabio de Oliveira Ferreira General Surgery, Faculdade de Medicina da Universidade de São Paulo, São Paulo, SP, Brazil

Sarcoma and Melanoma Group, Instituto do Câncer do Estado de São Paulo—ICESP, São Paulo, SP, Brazil

Cutaneous Oncology and Sarcomas Center, Hospital Sírio-Libanês de São Paulo—HSL/SP, São Paulo, SP, Brazil

High-Risk Clinic of the Oncogenetics Service, Hospital Beneficência Portuguesa de São Paulo, São Paulo, SP, Brazil

Oncology Center, Hospital Sírio-Libanês, São Paulo, São Paulo, Brazil

Cláudia Regina Cardin Mendes de Oliveira Hospital Sírio-Libanês, São Paulo, São Paulo, Brazil

Walmar Roncalli Pereira de Oliveira Dermatology, Faculdade de Medicina da Universidade de Sao Paulo, São Paulo, Brazil

Bianca Costa Soares de Sá AC Camargo Cancer Center, São Paulo, Brazil

Ana Paula de Souza Borges Hospital Sírio-Libanês, São Paulo, Brazil

Alice Roxo Nobre de Souza e Silva Radiation Oncology Department, Hospital Sírio-Libanês, São Paulo, Brazil

Maria Isabel Achatz Centro de Oncologia, Hospital Sírio-Libanês, São Paulo, Brazil

Isabela dos Santos Alves Department of Radiology, Hospital Sírio-Libanês, São Paulo, SP, Brazil

Gustavo dos Santos Fernandes DASA Oncology, Brasília, DF, Brazil

Suzy Maria Rabello Ferrer Hospital Sírio-Libanês, São Paulo, SP, Brazil

Reinaldo Tovo Filho Hospital Sírio-Libanês, São Paulo, Brazil

Naiara A. Fraga Braghiroli Miami Cancer Institute, Miami, FL, USA

Elimar Elias Gomes BP—A Beneficiência Portuguesa de São Paulo, São Paulo, Brazil

Samir Abdallah Hanna Radiation Oncology Department, Hospital Sírio-Libanês, São Paulo, Brazil

Radiation Oncology Medical Residency Program, Hospital Sírio-Libanês, São Paulo, Brazil

Maria Fernanda Vianna Hunziker Hospital Sírio-Libanês, São Paulo, SP, Brazil

João Paulo Junqueira Hospital Sírio-Libanês, São Paulo, Brazil

Caio Lamounier Instituto do Cancer do Estado de São Paulo, São Paulo, São Paulo, Brazil

Melissa Fugimori Lissae Hospital Sírio-Libanês, São Paulo, Brazil

Department of Pathology, Hospital Sírio Libanês, São Paulo, Brazil

Carlos Diego Holanda Lopes Oncology Center, Hospital Sírio-Libanês, São Paulo, São Paulo, Brazil

Antônio Sérgio Zafred Marcelino Department of Radiology, Hospital Sírio-Libanês, São Paulo, SP, Brazil

Jade Cury Martins Dermatology, Faculdade de Medicina da Universidade de São Paulo, São Paulo, São Paulo, Brazil

Instituto do Cancer do Estado de São Paulo—ICESP, São Paulo, São Paulo, Brazil

Isadora Zago Miotto Dermatology, Medicina da Universidade de São Paulo, São Paulo, Brazil

Ana Carolina Souza Porto Mitsunaga AC Camargo Cancer Center, São Paulo, Brazil

Denis Miyashiro Dermatology, Faculdade de Medicina da Universidade de São Paulo, São Paulo, São Paulo, Brazil

Hospital das Clínicas da Faculdade de Medicina da Universidade de São Paulo, Instituto do Câncer do Estado de São Paulo, São Paulo, Brazil

André Sapata Molina Hospital Sírio-Libanês, São Paulo, Brazil

Rodrigo Ramella Munhoz Cutaneous Oncology and Sarcoma Group, Hospital Sírio-Libanês, São Paulo, Brazil

Oncology Center, Hospital Sírio-Libanês, São Paulo, Brazil

Juliana Pereira Division of Hematology, Faculdade de Medicina da Universidade de São Paulo, São Paulo, São Paulo, Brazil

Marcela Soares Pincelli Dermatology, University of São Paulo Medical School, São Paulo, Brazil

Juan Manuel Piñeiro-Maceira Universidade do Estado do Rio de Janeiro, Rio de Janeiro, Brazil

Dermoscopy and Confocal Microscopy Section, Pedro Ernesto University Hospital-UERJ, Rio de Janeiro, Brazil

Marcello Moro Queiroz Oncology Center, Hospital Sírio-Libanês, São Paulo, SP, Brazil

Marcelo Araújo Queiroz Department of Radiology, Hospital Sírio-Libanês, São Paulo, SP, Brazil

Mauricio Fernando Silva Almeida Ribeiro Oncology Center, Hospital Sírio-Libanês, São Paulo, SP, Brazil

Division of Medical Oncology and Hematology, Princess Margaret Cancer Center - University of Toronto, Toronto, Canada

Lílian Kelly Faria Licarião Rocha Hospital das Clínicas de São Paulo, São Paulo, Brazil

Marina Sahade Hospital Sírio-Libanês, São Paulo, Brazil

Alessandra Corte Real Salgues Oncology Center, Hospital Sírio-Libanês, São Paulo, São Paulo, Brazil

José Antonio Sanches Faculdade de Medicina da Universidade de São Paulo, São Paulo, Brazil

Hospital Sírio-Libanês, São Paulo, Brazil

Dermatology, Faculdade de Medicina da Universidade de São Paulo, São Paulo, São Paulo, Brazil

Faculdade de Medicina da Universidade de São Paulo, Instituto do Câncer do Estado de São Paulo, São Paulo, Brazil

Ana Maria Fagundes Sortino Hospital Sírio-Libanês, São Paulo, SP, Brazil

Frederico José Ribeiro Teixeira Junior Teixeira Surgical Oncology, General Surgery Service, Hospital das Clínicas, Faculdade de Medicina da Universidade de São Paulo, São Paulo, São Paulo, Brazil

Camila Cristina Tormena Hospital das Clínicas, Faculdade de Medicina da Universidade de São Paulo, Instituto do Câncer do Estado de São Paulo, São Paulo, Brazil

Luis Fernando Tovo Hospital Sírio-Libanês, São Paulo, Brazil

Fernanda Hayashida Yoshimoto Radiation Oncology Medical Residency Program, Hospital Sírio-Libanês, São Paulo, Brazil

Luciana Carmen Zattar Department of Radiology, Hospital Sírio-Libanês, São Paulo, SP, Brazil

Chapter 1
Diagnosing and Management of Skin Cancer: A Multidisciplinary Approach

José Antonio Sanches, Cristina Martinez Zugaib Abdalla, Rodrigo Ramella Munhoz, and Francisco Aparecido Belfort

Key Points
- Management of cancer patients is becoming a worldwide challenge.
- Skin cancer is an extremely heterogeneous group of neoplasms.
- The ideal multidisciplinary oncologic team should have the participation of several specialists.
- The main goals of this approach are the improvement of diagnosis, treatment, and outcomes.
- Dermatologists, pathologists, surgeons, radiation oncologists, among others, have a fundamental role in this team.

Introduction

Management of cancer patients is becoming a worldwide challenge, due to rapidly changing evidence, new drugs approval, and scientific guideline updates in diagnosis, staging procedures, therapeutics, and follow-up [1].

Skin cancer is an extremely heterogeneous group of neoplasms, including tumors of the epidermis (basal cell carcinoma, squamous cell carcinoma), tumors of the dermal adnexa (adnexal carcinomas), tumors of melanocytes (cutaneous melanoma), tumors of soft tissue (angiosarcoma and other sarcomas), and tumors of

J. A. Sanches (✉)
Faculdade de Medicina da Universidade de São Paulo, São Paulo, Brazil

Hospital Sírio-Libanês, São Paulo, Brazil

C. M. Z. Abdalla · R. R. Munhoz · F. A. Belfort
Hospital Sírio-Libanês, São Paulo, Brazil

C. M. Z. Abdalla et al. (eds.), *Oncodermatology*,
https://doi.org/10.1007/978-3-031-29277-4_1

neuroendocrine cells (Merkel cell carcinoma). Despite the better knowledge of its pathological and molecular features, skin cancer is a clinical challenge with relevant consequences in terms of morbidity and mortality. Indeed, skin cancer, including cutaneous melanoma and non-melanoma skin cancer, is the most common cancer worldwide [2].

The introduction of the multidisciplinary approach to skin cancer care has helped clinicians meet the growing needs of patients with improvement in management and outcomes. The central function of this approach is to bring together a group of healthcare professionals from different fields to determine optimal patients' treatment plans [2, 3].

The Team

The ideal multidisciplinary oncologic team should have a core team comprised of dermatologists, pathologists, radiologists, surgeons, clinical oncologists, hematologists, other internists, and radiation oncologists. No less important is a non-core team comprised of interventional radiologists, nuclear medicine specialists, geneticists, psychologists, palliative care physicians, dietitians, specialized nurses, and social workers, among others [1, 3].

Dermatologists, in the care of cancer patients, have a fundamental role. In relation to those patients with skin cancer, they are fundamental in the diagnostic suspicion, in the sampling of tumors for biopsy and histopathological examination, as well as in the execution of certain auxiliary diagnostic procedures and even in the execution of many treatments aimed at the primary tumor. In the care of patients with cancer in general, they are the fundamental specialists in the suspicion and proof of neoplastic dissemination to the skin, as well as of the changes related to cutaneous paraneoplastic syndromes. Adverse skin reactions to antineoplastic treatments are extremely common and its multidisciplinary approach led by the dermatologist is essential.

The Goals

The main goals of this approach are the improvement of the adherence to clinical guidelines, management of rare tumors, and/or, with clinical guidelines lacking, improvement of ability to reach decisions, quality of information presentation and quality of teamwork, improvement of patient's outcomes, changes in diagnostic or treatment plans, improvement in follow-up accuracy, and improvement in clinical trial screening and patient recruitment [1–5].

The multidisciplinary approach obviously brings additional financial costs, direct and indirect, for the patient and for the health systems. However, the benefits arising from this approach in proposing better care and quality of life for patients at all stages of the disease are indisputable and essential in the current scenario of skin cancer [1–5].

References

1. Berardi R, Morgese F, Rinaldi S, et al. Benefits and limitations of a multidisciplinary approach in cancer patient management. Cancer Manag Res. 2020;12:9363–74.
2. Ronchi A, Argenziano G, Brancaccio G, et al. Editorial: Multidisciplinary approach to the diagnosis and therapy of skin neoplasms. Front Oncol. 2022;12:939200.
3. Clifford K, Chaudhry S. The need for a multidisciplinary approach to cancer care. J Surg Res. 2002;105:53–7.
4. Taberna M, Moncayo FG, Jané-Salas E, et al. The multidisciplinary team (MDT) approach and quality of care. Front Oncol. 2020;10:85.
5. Haddad R, Annino D, Tishler RB. Multidisciplinary approach to cancer treatment: focus on head and neck cancer. Dent Clin. 2008;52:1–7.

Chapter 2
Basic Concepts of Carcinogenesis and Immunopathology

Suzy Maria Rabello Ferrer and Erico Tosoni Costa

Key Points

- This chapter provides an overview of fundamental cellular and molecular principles associated with tumor biology.
- In the era of molecular medicine and next-generation sequencing (NGS), we see a new form of management and treatment of skin neoplasms.
- The structure and function of normal skin are reviewed, as the relation between the sun and *p53* protection.
- Which is the mechanism of TMB? Looking for identifying which mutations are drivers and contribute to cancer development is a key step in understanding tumor biology and developing targeted therapies.
- Mechanisms of metastasis are analyzed and identified.
- Understanding the cell-intrinsic barrier mediated by p53 tumor suppressor and cell-extrinsic barrier mediated by both the skin architecture and the immune system are the mainlines of defense of our skin against tumorigenesis.

S. M. R. Ferrer
Hospital Sírio-Libanês, São Paulo, SP, Brazil

E. T. Costa (✉)
Laboratory of Tumor Cell Biology of the Molecular Oncology Center, Hospital Sírio-Libanês, São Paulo, SP, Brazil
e-mail: ecosta@mochsl.org.br

C. M. Z. Abdalla et al. (eds.), *Oncodermatology*,
https://doi.org/10.1007/978-3-031-29277-4_2

The Structure and Function of Normal Skin

Our skin is the outermost interface between the internal and external environments. It is a physical barrier to prevent the invasion of foreign pathogens, against ultraviolet (UV) rays, chemicals, and mechanical injury. It is also home to about 10^{12} microorganisms, including bacteria, fungi, and viruses (our skin microbiota) that live in complete harmony with the immune system and contribute to the epithelial barrier reinforcement. To exert normal function, human skin is constituted by three main layers, which are anatomically and biochemically distinct: epidermis, dermis, and hypodermis [1–3]. These compartments contain their own pool of lineage-restricted stem cells (SC) that maintain their homeostasis. The epidermis and dermis are separated by the basement membrane (BM), a thin and highly specialized collagen-rich barrier that has gate-keeping functions, limiting cell traffic and diffusion of bioactive molecules in both directions [4].

Above the BM, the interfollicular epidermis consists of over 90% keratinocytes (an epithelial cell that produces keratin) organized in four layers of cells with different levels of differentiation. From deep to superficial, these layers are the stratum basale, stratum spinosum, stratum granulosum, and stratum corneum, each of which is characterized by a specific expression pattern of matrix proteins. There are also three main types of keratinocytes organized there: the resident SC, transit-amplifying, and the committed keratinocytes. SC keratinocytes have a high proliferative potential, dividing asymmetrically to self-renew or to replace dying cells of the supra basal layers above. The transit-amplifying cells are destined to undergo terminal differentiation after a few rounds of division, and the committed cells, which are enucleated keratinocytes (also known as squames), are chemically cross-linked to fortify the barrier of the skin, and are continually shed to the environment. There exist other epidermis-resident cell types including melanocytes, Langerhans cells (LC), and Merkel cells, which equally contribute to ensuring skin homeostasis [5–7].

Let us look a little more closely at the stratum basale (or basal layer). SC keratinocytes reside in a deepest epidermal microenvironment called stem-cell niche. They are protected from apoptosis, are highly proliferative, and are long resident in the adult epidermis. This renders them more prone to be the origin of basal (BCC) and squamous cell carcinoma (SCC). This layer also contains a minority cell population of melanocytes (at the ratio of 1 melanocyte:10 keratinocytes); they are fusiform, smaller than SC keratinocytes, and divide infrequently (less than twice a year). SC of the melanocyte lineage can be identified in the lower portion of hair follicles of human skin, being immature cells, slow cycling, self-maintaining, and more prone to be the origin of melanomas. A mature melanocyte, identified by the expression of specific proteins, such as tyrosinase (TYR) and microphthalmia-associated transcription factor (MITF), synthesize melanin within melanosomes, and transfer them to about 40 keratinocytes and one LC, as a part of an epidermal melanin unit, involved in photo-protection and the maintenance of skin homeostasis. In turn, epidermal keratinocytes and LC use this melanin to shield their nucleus, reducing the amount of damage the ultraviolet radiation (UVR) does to DNA, which can lead to cancer [8–10].

Damaged DNA in keratinocytes indirectly controls the intensity of melanin produced by melanocytes. Molecularly, DNA damage in keratinocytes up-regulates the expression of the pro-opiomelanocortin (*POMC*) gene, which encodes the production, and secretion of melanocyte-stimulating hormone (α-MSH) genein, a *p53* gene-dependent manner. α-MSH activates melanocortin 1 receptor (MC1R) expressed on the surface of melanocytes. α-MSH/MC1R transduces extracellular signals to downstream effectors including MITF, to regulate melanin production. MITF is a fate regulator of the melanocyte lineage, which is a target of the MAPKpathway. MITF expression directly enhances melanin production by raising levels of TYR, which is the rate-limiting enzyme of melanin production [11–13]. Tan is a sign of skin DNA damage [14, 15]. The risk of skin cancer is heavily influenced by UVR exposure, genetic factors, and skin pigmentation. In the next sections, we will focus our attention on the nuclei of cells, more specifically where all cancers begin: errors in their genome.

The Dark Side of the Sun and the p53 Protection

Solar emissions include visible light, heat, and ultraviolet radiation (UVR). UVR is considered a complete carcinogen, for its ability to damage genomic DNA through both direct and indirect means. Owing to changes in lifestyle and the environment, the incidence of sunburn-associated melanomas and non-melanoma skin cancers (NMSC) has been steadily increasing, being recognized as a primary risk factor for skin cancer development [16]. BCC and SCC account for about 99% of all NMSCs. Other NMSCs include Merkel cell carcinoma, adnexal cutaneous tumors, and other rare tumors [17].

UVR reaches our skin in the form of two main wavelengths, ultraviolet A (UVA) (315–400 nm) and UVB (280–315 nm). UVC (100–280 nm) is the most damaging type of UVR, however it is completely absorbed by the atmosphere. UVA is particularly dangerous in certain unnatural situations, such as the frequent use of indoor tanning beds [18]. Acute effects include photodamage, erythema, mutation, immunosuppression, synthesis of vitamin D, and tanning. Chronic responses to UVR include photoaging and photo carcinogenesis, which is induced by DNA mutation and immunosuppression. Some cutaneous tumors, like melanoma, can be broadly categorized by their origins from the skin that is or is not chronically sun-damaged. Others, like SCC, the majority of mutations contain an UVA-mediated genomic toxicity origin.

Molecularly, excessive exposure to UVA and UVB can be seriously harmful to biomolecules such as proteins, lipids, RNA, and especially DNA. UVR causes two classes of DNA lesions or photoproducts: cyclobutane pyrimidine dimers (CPD), and pyrimidine-6-4-pyrimidinone (6-4PP), both of them distort DNA's natural structure, introducing bends and facilitating breakages. These photoproducts create a specific pattern of mutations in DNA, which are unique to UVR, called the UV-signature. A confirmed UV-signature was characterized by more than 60% of mutations are C→T, with more than 5% of CC→TT [19–21].

To counteract the genotoxic effects of UVR, CPDs and 6-4PPs are both repaired by different protective cell-intrinsic molecular mechanisms, named base and nucleotide excision repair (BER and NER) and mismatch repair (MMR) pathways. At this phase, molecular repair mechanisms activate DNA damage checkpoint and increase the expression of tumor suppressor genes, such as the *p53* gene, to stall the proliferative cycle of skin cells for DNA repair [22, 23]. Normally, there is little p53 protein in the cell, but in response to UV damage, high levels of p53 are induced, allowing the cellular BER, NER, and MMR pathways to remove DNA lesions before mitosis. But if the damage in the genome is too severe, the molecular machinery can trigger a natural cell "suicide" program, called apoptosis, through both p53-dependent and p53-independent routes. In striking contrast with accidental cell death (e.g., burned or wounded skin), apoptosis is a cell-intrinsic program that specifically induces cell death to highly mutated and potentially dangerous cells. In some circumstances, total removal of dead body cells is not an advantage and apoptosis results in the accumulation of a "shield" of cell corpses, as when they fulfill a specific function of the skin barrier [24, 25]. So, trigger *p53* is a kind of "first line of defense" against mutationally corrupted cancer (stem) cells. Not surprisingly, corruption of the machinery that senses DNA damage or implements apoptosis greatly predisposes to skin cancers.

Are a Few Specific Wrong Letters Enough to Trigger Cancer?

Any somatic normal cell in the human body, including keratinocytes and melanocytes, contains a total of 3000 Mb (megabases) or 3 billion DNA base pairs ("letters") in their genome. Despite their chromosome structures are relatively well preserved, single base substitutions—a type of point mutation; or small insertions or deletions (indels)—can occur in physiologically normal skin more often than we suppose. Owing to their long lifetime of exposure to physical (e.g., sun rays), chemical (e.g., tobacco), and biological (microbes and virus) damages, cells of skin frequently accumulate chemical errors, known as "mutations," in their DNA. Specific combinations of these mutations may modulate many skin physio pathological processes, including photoaging and photocarcinogenesis. Accordingly, cancers associated with mutagens, such as lung (tobacco) and skin cancers (sun rays), had the highest relative mutation number/Mb of DNA than any other cancer type.

Biopsies of sun-exposed but physiologically normal skin from healthy individual exhibited a surprisingly high burden of DNA mutations (2–6 mutations/Mb), higher than that of many types of human neoplasms. Not surprisingly, NMSC is the most common malignancy affecting humans worldwide: SC cells are highly proliferative and their genome is highly mutated. Many of these mutations that are known to drive the growth of cutaneous cancers, like single mutations of *BRAF*, *NRAS*, or *PTCH1* or gene fusions with the kinase domains of *NTRK* or *MET*, are also present in benign nevi or actinic keratosis and were already under strong positive selection in normal skin. More dramatic is the observation that more than 25% of skin cells carried a single-driver mutation, and every square centimeter of skin contained hundreds of mutant clones [26, 27].

So, how the skin can harbor mutant, potentially malignant cells without developing cancer? Central to this idea is that a specific combination and not the number of mutations defines skin tumorigenesis. By definition, tumor formation and development are accelerated by the accumulation of driver mutations in two different categories of cancer genes: proto-oncogenes (e.g., *NRAS* and *BRAF*) and tumor suppressor genes (e.g., *p53* and *PTEN*). The gain-of-function convert proto-oncogenes into oncogenes together with the loss-of-function of tumor suppressors determine the processes that control cancer development. Moreover, a significant component of cancer etiology is profoundly determined by the interplay of these genes and the (micro)environment, like the individual lifestyle and their status of immunologic defenses [28–32]. For example, an oncogenic *BRAF* mutation in melanocyte reliably produces benign nevi, but may not contribute to the development of melanoma. The reasons nevi stop growing are attributed to a cell-autonomous process called "oncogene-induced senescence," or cell-extrinsic process, such as immune surveillance, and/or physical and mechanical restraint imposed by healthy skin architecture. However, $BRAF^{mut}$ accompanying mutations in tumor suppressor genes, like *p53*, are commonly indispensable leading to the progression of malignant neoplasia [33].

In the next section, we will show that mutations in the skin DNA are a part of life. We will discuss how sunlight may have several deleterious consequences to our genetic code and show that there are different systems of defense to guarantee a minimum of DNA integrity.

"Cancer Was Not Disorganized Chromosomal Chaos. It Was Organized Chromosomal Chaos"

The first basic information from Mukherjee's quote above is that cancer is a disease with a strong genetic component. The second is that the accumulation of driver mutations needs to happen in a "permissive order" for which chromosomal or nucleotide sequence variations can diverge from the normal karyotype and cancer cells survive [34].

Epithelial cells in healthy skin usually maintained normal karyotypes (46, XY). When skin architecture is disrupted, cells lose the extracellular cues that influence intrinsic features such as cell polarity and shape, leading to chromosome segregation errors [35]. Accordingly, genetic instability and chromosomal aberrations are considered hallmarks of cancers. Highly aberrant karyotypes are seen in melanoma,

SCC, solar keratosis, and Merkel cell carcinoma, with relatively more stable karyotypes seen in BCC and cutaneous lymphomas [36, 37].

Not all errors in DNA are gross chromosomal aberrations. Owing to their limited resolution, standard karyotyping techniques cannot be used to accurately identify more discrete genomic changes or alterations at the single-base level. More recently, the next-generation sequencing (NGS) has enough sensibility to detect all kinds of DNA mutations in detail in a tumor biopsy and helps inform therapy decisions.

The total number of mutations per coding area of a tumor cell genome is quantified and commonly referred to as the "**tumor mutation burden**" (**TMB**). The TMB was highly variable between and within cancer classes, ranging from about 0.001 mutations/Mb in certain childhood cancers to more than 400 mutations/Mb in cancers related to chronic mutagenic exposures such as lung (tobacco) and sun-exposed skin tumors [38]. On average, TMB in skin tumors range from ~4 mutations/Mb in Merkel cell carcinoma and adnexal carcinomas to 14 mutations/Mb in sun-exposed melanomas, and 50 mutations/Mb in sun-exposed SCC [39, 40]. As a rule, the higher the degree of cumulative sun damage (CSD) the higher the TMB: 30 mutations/Mb in high-CSD melanoma; 15 mutations/Mb in low-CSD melanoma. Desmoplastic melanoma is a subtype of high-CSD characterized by a particularly high TMB of 62 mutations/Mb on average. Interestingly, non-sun exposed tumors, such as eye intraocular melanoma or anus SCC have the lowest TMB (1 and 5 mutations/Mb, respectively), denoting that many of the mutations detected in TMB-high skin tumors have been directly attributed by UVR [41, 42].

Before we go any further, understand that the vast majority of mutations in a cancer genome are not directly involved in cancer initiation and/or progression. Cancer-causing mutations (called "**driver mutations"**) are only a tiny fraction of the whole genetic modifications, most of which are "bystander" or "**passenger mutations**." But this does not mean that passenger mutations are useless or uninformative. These mutations can be recognized and attacked by the immune system or can be used by scientists to provide insight into the history of the tumor or to classify them (as we will see below), and is also of interest for the upcoming "liquid biopsy" diagnostic approaches [38, 43]. Only driver mutations in proto-oncogenes and tumor suppressor genes provide a real selective growth advantage and thus promote tumorigenesis, such as *BRAF* or *NRAS* in melanomas, *NOTCH1* and *CDKN2A* in SCC or the aberrant activation of the Hh pathway, induced by *PTCH1* inactivating mutations or *SMO* activating mutations in BCCs. Thus, identifying which mutations are drivers and contribute to cancer development is a key step in understanding tumor biology and developing targeted therapies [40, 44].

So, next we will present a brief description of the most recurrent somatic mutations in skin tumors, and a new proposal for genomic classification of melanomas into four genomic subtypes based on mutational status. Due to the page limitations, the detailed biology of these genes, their pathways, and products is beyond the scope of this chapter.

Receptor Tyrosine Kinases (RTK)

RTKs are a group of transmembrane receptors that bind and respond to growth factors (GF), cytokines, and hormones, including epidermal growth factor receptor (EGFR), keratinocyte growth factor (KGF), c-KIT, fibroblast growth factor receptor (FGFR) families, and others. RTKs play a crucial role in mediating melanogenesis, proliferative and migratory programs of keratinocytes during homeostasis, and wound re-epithelization. The binding of GF to the cognate RTK activates the receptor and transmits signals from the microenvironment to internal signaling pathways, such as mitogen-activated protein kinase (MAPK) and phosphoInositide 3-kinase (PI3K) pathways. Benign hyperproliferative lesions, including psoriatic plaques, seborrheic keratoses, as also skin malignancies, have been found to have UV-specific mutations or aberrant expression in *EGFR* [45–49]. *EGFR* gene has shown the highest frequency of genomic amplification, with a higher rate in metastatic melanomas compared to primary melanomas. Chromosomal amplifications or somatic mutations occur repeatedly in *c-Kit* and *EGFR* in both melanomas and SCCs [50–53].

In the human skin, the c-Kit, also called stem cell growth factor receptor (SCFR), is an RTK mainly expressed in melanocytes and it is essential for melanogenesis. In skin tumors, gain-of-function mutations in c-Kit are relatively common in acrallentiginous and mucosal melanomas and have also been associated with worse survival as compared with c-Kit wild-type melanomas [54–58]. During cancer progression, the SCF/c-Kit sustained activation induces the expression of the transcription factor Slug, which is involved in epithelial–mesenchymal transition (EMT), a first obligatory step for the metastatic disease [59]. C-Kit signal transduction can be shut off through a variety of mechanisms. Among them, neurofibromin (NF1) acts as a physiological negative regulator of SCF/c-Kit signaling. Accordingly, melanocytes bearing deleterious mutations in NF1 display a hyperactive c-Kit-mediated response to SCF [60].

Neurofibromin (NF1)

NF1 is one of the key drivers of melanoma, typically seen defective in 10–15% of cases, occurring on chronically sun-exposed skin, in older patients, in melanomas wild-type for *BRAF* and *NRAS*, or in the desmoplastic melanoma. NF1 loss-of-function induces the hyperactivation of NRAS protein, and thus, the activation of MAPK signaling pathway [61].

MAPK Pathway

Hyper-activation of the MAPK pathway (RAS → RAF → MEK → ERK cascade) is found in over 4% of BCC, 31% of SCC, and 90% of melanomas [62–64]. Driver mutations in MAPK pathways are frequently mostly affecting RAS and *BRAF*. About half of all melanomas have mutations in the *BRAF* gene.V600E is a hot-spot mutation of the *BRAF* in which valine (V) is substituted by glutamic acid (E) at amino acid position 600 (*BRAF*^{V600E}) and represents 85% of all *BRAF* mutations [33, 65]. The second most common driver mutation that leads MAPK pathway overactivation is *NRAS*. Among 15–30% of all melanomas harbor activating mutations in *NRAS*, rarely found in SCC and less than 4% in BCC. These mutations found at codon 61, prevent efficient GTP hydrolysis, rendering *NRAS* in a constitutive active state. In this conformation, *NRAS* can bind and activate their effectors including Raf [66]. Since the activation of MAPK pathway is often due to mutations in the *BRAF* or *NRAS* genes in these cancers, mutation testing for these genes has become a standard procedure to guide the oncologist's therapeutic choice and predict the course of therapy. Only patients with V600 mutations are expected to benefit from targeted therapies with *BRAF* inhibitors, while patients with a less common mutation (*BRAF*^{K601E}) respond only to specific mitogen-activated extracellular signal-regulated kinase (MEK) inhibitors [67]. For instance, two distinct approaches exist today to target the RAS pathways: targeting the EGFR family or RAS effector pathways, namely MAPK and PI3K. In contrast to cutaneous melanoma, uveal melanoma tends to develop from different mutations along the MAPK pathway. The most common mutations are mutually exclusive in GNAQ or GNA11 genes and are detected in approximately 90% of cases of uveal melanoma. Hyper-activation of the MAPK pathway can trigger MITF activation. MITF regulates the expression of genes controlling differentiation (e.g., *TYR*), proliferation (e.g., *CDK2*), and survival (e.g., *BCL2*, *BCL2A1*) and induces melanocyte proliferation [68, 69].

PI3K/AKT/MTOR Pathway

The mammalian target of rapamycin (mTOR) and associated phosphatidyl-inositol 3-kinase (PI3K)/protein kinase B (AKT) (or PI3K/Akt/mTOR) pathway is activated by multiple ways. It is mostly activated in keratinocytes, following their exposure to UVR or to cytokines aberrantly produced by activated immune cells. Skin hyperproliferative disorders, such as psoriasis and atopic dermatitis, in which epidermal keratinocytes respond to T-cell-derived cytokines (e.g., IL-17A, IL-22, TNF-α, and IFN-γ) upregulate PI3K/AKT/mTOR pathway. In turn, it controls secretion of pro-inflammatory mediators by keratinocytes, enhances proliferation, and impairs keratinocyte differentiation [70]. Loss of epidermal mTOR signaling attenuated keratinocyte proliferation and abrogated the epidermal stratification program that are both essential for proper skin morphogenesis and for the development of a protective epidermal barrier [71]. In contrast, hyperactivation of PI3K/Akt/mTOR pathway contributes to cutaneous cancers, implicated in hyperproliferation, and tumorigenesis, as well as in resistance to apoptosis. The two most common activating mutations ofPI3K/Akt/mTOR pathway in skin cancers are the oncogene *NRAS* and loss-of-function of the Phosphatase and Tensin Homolog (*PTEN*) [70].

Phosphatase and Tensin Homolog (PTEN)

PTEN is a well-characterized tumor suppressor gene, a key negative regulator of the PI3K/Akt/mTOR signaling pathway an effector of apoptosis. The loss-of-function of *PTEN* has been implicated in the pathogenesis of multiple skin cancers, leading to reduced apoptosis along with increased cell survival and associated with immune evasion in melanomas. Somatic *PTEN* alterations have been identified in nearly 50% of *BRAF*-mutated melanomas in contrast to 4% of *NRAS*-mutated melanomas or even in 6% of SCC. Additionally, loss of *PTEN* may be critical for BCC genesis through PI3K/AKT-dependent activation of Hedgehog (Hh) signaling. Defective *PTEN* correlates strongly with depth of invasion and risk of metastatic disease and has been motivated clinical trials of PI3K inhibitors in combination with immunotherapy [64, 72–75].

Hh Signaling Pathway

At least 90% of sporadic BCCs are driven by aberrant activation of the Hedgehog (Hh) pathway. Thus targeted inhibition of Hh pathway may be effective in treatment of BCC. The majority of BCCs have "UV-signature" mutations inducing loss-of-function in the Patched1 (*PTCH1*) gene (70–90%), preventing repression of the pathway, or have gain-of-function mutations in Smoothened (*SMO*) gene (10–20%), leading to overactivation of the Hh cascade resulting in dysregulated downstream *GLI* family of transcription factors. Once activated, *GLI* factors translocate into the nucleus and induce Hh target genes including growth factors or growth factor receptors, such as IGF-2, VEGF, and PDGFRα [44, 51, 76, 77]. Despite no mutations in Hh pathway, genes have been found in melanomas; aberrant expression of *GLI2* regulates invasion and metastasis in melanoma cells, which metastasize to bone more readily than cells with low *GLI2* expression.

P53

The first UV-specific driver mutation found in NMSC was the *p53* tumor suppressor gene described in 1993, which has been named "guardian of the genome." *P53* is mostly activated in responses to genotoxic injury, including exposure to UVR. In this context, once activated, p53 is a decision-making agent that selectively activates hundreds of genes that are involved in DNA damage repair, proliferation arrest, apoptosis, and cell senescence. Thousands of p53-mutant cell clones are found in sun-exposed normal skin from healthy individuals. There is a high frequency of p53 mutations reported in actinic keratosis and Bowen's disease. The p53-mutated keratinocytes acquire selective advantages by retaining defective forms of the p53, which radically subvert the normal function of the UV-induced apoptotic pathway by promoting metabolic plasticity, invasion, and chemoresistance. In p53-mutated benign lesions we found precancerous cells that escaped from the protective role of p53 on genomic integrity [78, 79]. UV-specific p53mutations are found in 20% of metastatic melanomas, in70% of BCC, and more than 90% of malignant SCCs [80–83].

CDKs and CDKs-Inhibitors

Other genes that can regulate proliferation rate of the epidermal cells include cyclins, cyclin-dependent kinases (*CDK*), CDK-inhibitors (such as *p16INK4A*, *p14ARF*, *p19ARF*, encoded by the *CDKN2A*, and *p21CP1/WAF1* and *p27Kip1* encoded by CDKN2B locus), and the retinoblastoma (pRb) family of proteins. Several skin diseases, including cancer, atopic dermatitis, and ichthyosis vulgaris, disrupt the balance between the proliferation, differentiation, and death of keratinocytes and result in abnormal skin. Mutations in these genes by UVR are frequently found in BCCs and SCCs. For example, inactivation of the inhibitor of cell cycle, *CDKN2A*, via allelic loss and/or UV-induced mutation was found in approximately 50% of primary melanomas, in over 75% of metastatic melanomas, 30–76% of SCCSs, and 3.5% of BCCs [84, 85].

TERT Activation

Cell immortality leads to macroscopic tumors, metastatic spread, and tumor relapse. This phenotype is correlated with a strong resistance to induction of both senescence and apoptosis, two distinct barriers against proliferation. The telomerase reverse transcriptase (*TERT*) gene, encodes the catalytic subunit of the enzyme telomerase that adds protective repeat nucleotide sequences at the both ends of each chromosome (called telomeres). The most prominent of a diverse series of TERT functions include cell immortalization and permitting excessive cell replication, a feature of virtually all solid malignancies. *TERT* promoter mutations exhibit UV-signature and were observed in a significant proportion of dysplastic nevi, in around 50% of BCCs and SCCs, and in above 75% of *BRAF*, *NRAS*, or *NF1* mutated melanomas but in only 7% of melanomas with wild-type (WT) versions of these three proto-oncogenes (triple-WT), suggesting an alternative mechanism of *TERT* activation in these tumors [86, 87].

Putting it all together, the Cancer Genome Atlas Network (TCGA) consortium interpreted the complex mutational data of melanomas and provided a molecular classification framework that can segregate malignant melanomas into four subtypes, designated: mutant *BRAF*, mutant RAS, mutant NF1, and Triple-WT, which can guide clinical decision-making for target therapies. Additional analysis reveals enrichment of KIT mutations and complex DNA structural rearrangements as genetic features of the Triple-WT subtype. Although this knowledge has contributed significantly to molecular classification of these tumors and stratification of patients, a substantial portion of patients do not benefit in a durable fashion from these new therapies because of the high plasticity of melanoma cells [87].

Mechanisms of Metastasis: Where No Tumor Cell Has Gone Before

In this section we will focus our attention on the most basic and aggressive functional unit of cancers: the metastatic cancer cell. These emigrant cells represent a minor subpopulation of tumor cells with a marked potential to convert a curable lesion into a deadly disease. After primary melanoma excision, more than 30% of the patients were diagnosed with metastatic lesions regionally or promiscuously throughout the body. On the contrary, NMSC rarely metastasize (nearly 4% for patients with SCC, and 0.003–0.55% for BCC). In general, and independently of the skin tumor, metastasis is a particularly threatening sign; when metastasis is clinically evident, prognosis is very poor [88–90].

Biologically, metastasis involves a series of steps, jointly called "metastatic cascade," which must be all completed before the emergence of clinical metastatic disease. These steps are: (1) local invasion, once tumor cells move away from the avascular epithelial layer and acquire the ability to degrade the BM and penetrate the dermis; (2) intravasation (or entry) into the blood vessels at the dermis; (3) survival in the circulation. At this point, tumor cells flowing through the body are called "circulating tumor cells" (CTCs); (4) extravasation or exit from vasculature. The elite of cells that survive at secondary organs is referred to as "disseminated tumor cells" (DTC). Finally, (5) the colonization step. Recent studies have shown that secondary organs, which are typically resistant to these malignant intruders, do not receive DTCs passively [91, 92]. DTCs can be eliminated or remain in secondary sites subclinically, in a dormant equilibrium for decades (called micrometastasis) or even consolidate the metastatic disease with the ability to perpetuate into these tissues, causing finally organ dysfunction and patient death (macrometastasis).

The multi-step nature of metastatic cascade is depicted as a "3S" process: sequential, selective with stochastic elements. The 3S concept helps to understand why metastasis is generally considered to be a succession of unlikely events rendering a highly inefficient process: each of these steps imposes distinctive and harsh conditions for the cancer cells. So, the accomplishment of metastasisis widely considered one of the most difficult events in the world of cells.

Curiously, skin cancers are invariably heterogeneous and cooperative partnerships may exist between cellular clones with different mutational profiles and behaviors. Distinct subclones of melanoma cells can cooperate to promote metastatic progression. This variability is called **intratumoral heterogeneity (ITH)**.

ITH provides tumors with significant phenotypic plasticity and it is one of the prominent determinants of therapeutic resistance and metastatic potential [93–95].

So, during progression from carcinoma in situ to an invasive tumor, a specific type of genetic program called **epithelial-mesenchymal transition (EMT)** has a central role in cancer invasiveness. EMT describes a transient genetic reprogramming in epithelial cells, mediated by key transcription factors, including SLUG, and SNAIL, that induces loss of many of their epithelial characteristics (e.g., strong cell-to-cell contacts with their neighbors, apical–basolateral polarization) and takes on properties that are typical of mesenchymal cells (e.g., loss of polarity and fibroblastic morphology), inducing complex changes in cell behavior, as such increased invasiveness. EMT contributes physiologically to re-epithelialization of wounded skin and it is initiated by signaling pathways that respond to extracellular cues [96–98]. Gene expression data of melanoma cells in the invasive front can be seen to have undergone an EMT, suggesting that these cancer cells are subject to microenvironmental stimuli distinct from those received by melanoma cells located in the core of the same lesions. Among these, interleukins and transforming growth factor-β (TGFβ) family signaling have predominant roles.

For DTC to survive at the secondary organs these organs must be selectively primed for tumor engraftment even before DTCs arrival. These primed microenvironments are termed **"pre-metastatic niches" (PMNs)**. So, PMNs refer to "fertilized" secondary niches that are the result of the combined systemic effects of tumor-secreted factors that promote a linear sequence of events during the "fertilization" of these niches. Vascular leakiness is the earliest event in this sequence, followed by the immunosuppression, and organotropism by the recruitment of non-resident cells, such as bone marrow-derived cells (BMDCs), subsequently attracting CTCs that are qualified cells to "hijacking" different types of immune cells that otherwise would be resistant to these malignant intruders [99, 100].

Immunology of Skin Tumors

Our skin is an arena where immune system acts daily as a second line of defense against external (e.g., pathogens) and internal intruders (e.g., precancerous lesions). Considering that skin accumulated a surprisingly high burden of DNA mutations, this tissue is continuously scanned by the immune system, so that immunogenic and suspicious-looking skin cells can be recognized and eradicated by the immune system before they manifest clinically as tumors.

The skin immune system is triggered when specific skin-resident immune cells are alerted about the presence of a neo antigen (Ag), a foreign or non-self molecule capable of inducing an immune response. From an immunological perspective, tumor-specific Ags can be considered truly suspicious proteins and entirely absent from normal human tissues. Moreover, to build an effective immune response against a cancer cell is crucial not only how immunogenic the Ags are, but also how abundantly they are expressed (a wild-type, but overexpressed protein may be considered a tumor Ag). Accordingly, the high TMB sets the background for a large number of potential Ags that can be recognized by the immune system. Indeed, high TMB level is a biomarker of sensitivity to immune checkpoint inhibitors (e.g., PD-1 and PD-L1 blockade immunotherapy) in different human cancers, including melanomas and unresectable SCC [101–103].

Due to their peculiarly high immunogenicity precancerous cutaneous lesions can evoke strong and effective immune protection in our skin. This is especially evident in immunosuppressed individuals with evidence in organ transplant recipients (OTRs) of a more than 100-fold increased risk of developing SCC and a ten-fold increased incidence of BCC [104, 105]. SCCs are also more aggressive in OTRs, with a metastasis rate increased in 30-fold compared to the general population [106]. Another example is the well-recognized association between chronic lymphocytic leukemia (CLL) and skin cancers. CLL B cells produce systemic immunosuppressive factors and several skin cancers, such as BCC, SCC, cutaneous melanoma, and Merkel cell carcinoma, which develop with increased frequency and with a heightened aggressive nature among CLL's patients [107–109]. Interestingly, UVR is also an immune suppressor. UVR stimulates keratinocytes and macrophages to produce cytokines such as IL-10, which is important for systemic immunosuppression. Moreover, UVR directly damages epidermal LCs, which are the only professional antigen-presenting cells (APC) that reside in the epidermis [110, 111].

Overall, once triggered, the skin immune system exert protective effects in three ways: (1) protecting against oncovirus (by eliminating viral infections that may cause aggressive forms of cancer, e.g., Merkel cell polyomavirus); (2) protecting against pathogens (by eliminating pathogens and prompt resolution of chronic inflammation, that otherwise predisposes to the development of cancer), and (3) promoting the "sterile inflammation," where the immune system can specifically identify cancerous or precancerous cells on the basis of their expression of tumor-specific Ags and eliminate them before they become clinically apparent. The third process is referred to as **tumor immune surveillance** [112, 113].

Tumor Immune Surveillance

Immune surveillance is the recognition and eradication of cancerous or precancerous cells by professional immune cells, which act as sentinels. The traditional classification divide immune surveillance system into two arms, called the "innate" and the "adaptive" immunity. Innate immunity form rapid, but nonspecific, responses against foreign Ags (e.g., oncoviral proteins) and self-Ags (e.g., point mutations). Contrarily, adaptive immune arm forms slower, but intruder-specific responses through an antibody-produced response. When the efforts from the innate immunity are insufficient to clear off an intruder, the adaptive immune system is activated [114].

Innate Immune Surveillance Cells: The Sentinels for Danger

The skin harbors basically two groups of innate immune cells: the "amateurs" and the "professionals." The "amateur" term used here should not be interpreted with a negative connotation, but rather, as a non-professional function of some skin cells that usually play non-immunological roles, such as the keratinocytes, melanocytes, and the fibroblasts. Skin professionals' innate immune cells include the skin-resident LCs in the epidermis, as well as mast cells, dendritic cells (DCs), and macrophages in the dermis.

The first sentinels of the skin are the keratinocytes and LCs. They act as sensors of early danger through alert systems such as the inflammasome and produce large quantities of interleukin-1 (IL-1) and tumor-necrosis factor (TNF) in response to various stimuli, including pathogens and UVR. LCs represent only 3% of the epidermal cell population but are in intimate association with keratinocytes through dendritic processes that radiate throughout the entire epidermis. Keratinocytes represent 90% of epidermal cells and are often under-appreciated players in immunology, but actually exert primary roles in the innate immunity by recognizing Ags via an especial receptor family expressed on their surfaces, called Toll-like receptors (TLRs). As a response to Ag/TLR stimulation, these sentinels can produce variable amounts of chemokines (CXCL-8, IP-10), growth factors (IL-6, granulocyte-macrophage colony-stimulating factor or GM-CSF, and TGF-α), and other immunoregulatory cytokines, (IL-1α, TNF-α, IL-6, TGF-β, and IL-10). These molecules have several effects on other cells in the dermis, such as DCs and macrophages, resulting in the expression of additional pro-inflammatory mediators and recruitment of other immune cells from the blood that lead to a predominant antitumoral T_H1-type immune response [115, 116].

At this point, immune system addresses the logistical challenge in getting the right innate immune cell to the right place in order to call the cavalry: the adaptive immune cells. Both innate and adaptive responses are linked and coordinated by APCs. Although keratinocytes and melanocytes may also be capable of acting as APCs, LCs are the main APC subset in the epidermis. To solve the logistical challenge, immunity incorporates the strategy for constant grouping activated APCs and naïve lymphocytes together in the lymph nodes for the activation of the adaptive immune responses. In other words, activated epidermal APCs (i.e., LCs carrying Ag bound to major histocompatibility complex (MHC) proteins on their surface) invade the dermis, emigrate from the skin to the skin-draining lymph nodes to present Ags to naïve T cells to undergo maturation and clonal expansion.

Adaptive Immune Response

The adaptive immune response is a system based on the function and activation of T and B lymphocytes (T and B cells). These are the only cells in the human body able to respond specifically to each Ag, through specific receptors recognition:

T-cell receptors (TCR) and B-cell receptors (BCR), respectively. Basically, the B cells are responsible for producing antibodies (Abs) while T cells recognize a specific Ag as long as it is presented by an activated and mature APC. In the case of T cells, the ultimate amplitude and quality of the response is regulated by a balance between co-stimulatory and inhibitory signals (i.e., immune checkpoints). The naïve T-cell that enter the skin-draining lymph nodes is activated, resulting in the self differentiation into effector Tcell that emigrate back to the site of the initial danger alert. Skin-homing effector Tcell will encounter a range of inflammatory mediators triggered by innate cells, which can present Ag and provide co-stimulatory signals [116, 117].

Tumor-infiltrating T cells (TILs) have been the major focus of efforts to therapeutically manipulate endogenous antitumor immunity owing to three reasons: (1) their capacity for the selective recognition of Ag-expressing cells; (2) their capacity to directly kill these cells (by CD8+ effector Tcells; also known as cytotoxic T lymphocytes); and (3) their ability to integrate adaptive and innate effector mechanisms (by CD4+ T helper (T_h) cells). Clinically, TILs have been associated with favorable prognosis in primary melanoma, sometimes resulting in partial tumor destruction [118]. Clonal expansion of T cells occurs in regressing primary melanoma, and lymphocytes explanted from such lesions are cytotoxic in vitro to autologous melanoma cells. Although TILs in the invasive melanoma occurs less frequently, this is correlated with prolonged survival and a reduced incidence of metastatic disease [116].

However, during tumor progression, cancer cells show resistance to the immune system, thus expanding and escaping the immune surveillance. The way in which cancer cells modify the immune system has been called immune editing.

A Paradox Lies at the Heart of Cancer Immunology

If the "intruder" is not completely eliminated, an equilibrium phase can develop in which the immune system and the intruder cells interact to yield alterations in both cell populations. In other words, during immune edition, the host immune system shapes the precancerous lesion. At this phase precancerous cells become progressively less immunogenic, adapt to evade the immune response, and/or actively immunosuppress the host. Next, cancerous lesion evolves and continues to grow despite the presence of an immune response. This tumor-associated chronic inflammation can also be pro-tumoral, inducing EMT and metastasis in cancer cells both by action of soluble mediators of cancer-associated inflammation (TGF-β, TNF-α, IL-1β, IL-6, IL-8, CCL2, among others) and by the action of various types of pro-tumoral immune cells, including T_H2-type immune cells (which usually suppress antitumoral T_H1-typeresponses). This situation implies that growing tumors and TILs coexist and rendered unresponsive to the tumor, despite being activated. Actually, it is now well recognized that these TILs within progressing cancers are "exhausted" or anergic. Exhausting markers include co-inhibitory receptors; such as programmed cell death-1 (PD1), cytotoxic T-lymphocyte- associated protein 4 (CTLA-4, referred as the "godfather of checkpoints"), and Lymphocyte activation gene 3 protein (LAG3). These molecules are also called checkpoint molecules. Under normal physiological conditions, checkpoint molecules are critical for the maintenance of self-tolerance (i.e., the prevention of autoimmunity diseases) and also to protect healthy tissues from damage when the immune system is responding to pathogenic infection [119–122].

One important mechanism by which cancer cells hinder antitumoral TILs responses is the direct activation of co-inhibitory molecules expressed at the surface of T cells. A co-inhibitory molecule is defined as a surface receptor that is able to negatively modulate outcome of TCR signaling, suppressing T-cell function, and thereby making the TILs dysfunctional. Two co-inhibitory receptors that have been most actively studied in the context of clinical cancer immunotherapy are the CTLA4 and PD1. CTLA4 predominantly regulates T-cell activation at the time of their initial response to Ags within the lymph nodes, whereas PD1 predominantly regulates inflammatory responses in tissues and tumors by effector T cells recognizing Ags in site of the initial danger alert or peripheral tissues. When PD1or CTLA4 binds to their specific ligands (PD-L1 and PD-L2 or CD80/CD86, respectively) on tumors, they form a "safeguard" protection on tumor cells, preventing from being destroyed by the immune system and causing effector T-cell exhaustion.

Knowledge of these two checkpoint inhibitors has emerged as successful new antitumoral treatment options, such as the use of monoclonal antibodies that block the aforementioned interactions (anti-PD1, anti-PD-L1, or anti-CTLA- 4). These antibodies interfere with the "safeguard" protection of the tumor. Finally, it is important to emphasize that multiple additional immune checkpoints (e.g., LAG3, B7-H3, B7-H4, and TIM3) represent promising targets for therapeutic blockade based on initial experiments, and inhibitors for many of these are under active development [123, 124].

Final Remarks

Paraphrasing the quote that starts this chapter: *To counteract the advanced skin cancers; it therefore becomes necessary to know the molecular nature of such affections*, it becomes clear that the advance of molecular medicine changed how greatly we can understand the nature of such affections and, consequently, changed the way we use this molecular data to counteract the disease. Cell-intrinsic barrier mediated by *p53* tumor suppressor and cell-extrinsic barrier mediated by both the skin architecture and the immune system are the mainlines of defense of our skin against tumorigenesis. Only those skin cells which overlapped these barriers have the opportunity to develop into tumors. Fortunately, the majority of these cases may be cured in a dermatologist's office with a small surgery and, therefore, preventing them to gradually evolve into cancers. However, for advanced cases or high-risk diseases, it is always possible to leave behind a group of invasive cells or DTCs.

In these cases, the rapid advances in NGS technologies enabled tremendous opportunities to gain insight into the landscape of genomic alterations of cancers in a systematic and unbiased approach. Accordingly, molecular phenotype is replacing the traditional "clinical phenotype" (such as tumor size, stage, and grade), characterizing the presence of druggable or actionable mutations in multiple driver genes. For example, the combination of mutant *BRAF* and/or MEK inhibitors with immune checkpoint blockade is a further option that has been proven to improve therapeutic response and overall survival. Before 2010, only one fourth of patients with metastatic disease were alive at 1 year. To date, about half of the patients with advanced melanoma are indeed alive at 5 years [125, 126].

Putting it all together, we see that, in pursuit of molecular understanding of the neoplastic disease, medicine is intelligently advancing along molecular routes. Understanding this complexity at the molecular level is what is expected of good physicians and oncologists.Conflict of InterestThe authors have no conflict of interest to declare.

References

1. Byrd A, Belkaid Y, Segre J. The human skin microbiome. Nat Rev Microbiol. 2018;16: 143–55. https://doi.org/10.1038/nrmicro.2017.157.
2. Abdallah F, Mijouin L, Pichon C. Skin immune landscape: inside and outside the organism. Mediat Inflamm. 2017;2017:5095293. https://doi.org/10.1155/2017/5095293.
3. Watt FM. Mammalian skin cell biology: at the interface between laboratory and clinic. Science. 2014;346:937–40. https://doi.org/10.1126/science.1253734.
4. Chang J, Chaudhuri O. Beyond proteases: basement membrane mechanics and cancer invasion. J Cell Biol. 2019;218(8):2456–69. https://doi.org/10.1083/jcb.201903066.
5. Yousef H, Alhajj M, Sharma S. Anatomy, skin (integument), epidermis. In: StatPearls. Treasure Island, FL: StatPearls; 2021. https://www.ncbi.nlm.nih.gov/books/NBK470464/.
6. Deckers J, Hammad H, Hoste E. Langerhans cells: sensing the environment in health and disease. Front Immunol. 2018;9:93.
7. Cichorek M, et al. Skin melanocytes: biology and development. Postepy Dermatol Alergol. 2013;30(1):30–41. https://doi.org/10.5114/pdia.2013.33376.
8. Pincelli C, Marconi A. Keratinocyte stem cells: friends and foes. J Cell Physiol. 2010;225(2):310–5. https://doi.org/10.1002/jcp.22275.
9. Jimbow K, Roth SI, Fitzpatrick TB, Szabo G. Mitotic activity in non-neoplastic melanocytes in vivo as determined by histochemical, autoradiographic, and electron microscope studies. J Cell Biol. 1975;66(3):663–70. https://doi.org/10.1083/jcb.66.3.663.
10. Fitzpatrick TB, Breathnach AS. The epidermal melanin unit system. Dermatol Wochenschr. 1963;147:481–9.
11. Sun X, et al. Ultraviolet radiation and melanomagenesis: from mechanism to immunotherapy. Front Oncol. 2020;10:951. https://doi.org/10.3389/fonc.2020.00951.
12. Cichorek M, et al. Skin melanocytes: biology and development. Postepy Dermatol Alergol. 2013;1:30–41. https://doi.org/10.5114/pdia.2013.33376.
13. Cui R, Widlund HR, Feige E, Lin JY, Wilensky DL, Igras VE, et al. Central role of p53 in the suntan response and pathologic hyperpigmentation. Cell. 2007;128:853–64.
14. Alexandrov LB, Kim J, Haradhvala NJ, et al. The repertoire of mutational signatures in human cancer. Nature. 2020;578:94–101. https://doi.org/10.1038/s41586-020-1943-3.

15. Li Y, Roberts ND, Wala JA, et al. Patterns of somatic structural variation in human cancer genomes. Nature. 2020;578:112–21. https://doi.org/10.1038/s41586-019-1913-9.
16. Fisher DE. James WD indoor tanning–science, behavior, and policy. N Engl J Med. 2010;363:901.
17. Ciążyńska M, Kamińska-Winciorek G, Lange D, et al. The incidence and clinical analysis of non-melanoma skin cancer. Sci Rep. 2021;11:4337. https://doi.org/10.1038/s41598-021-83502-8.
18. Sample A, He YY. Mechanisms and prevention of UVinduced melanoma. Photodermatol Photoimmunol Photomed. 2018;34(1):13–24.
19. Brash DE. UV signature mutations. Photochem Photobiol. 2015;91:15–26. https://doi.org/10.1111/php.12377.
20. Bissonauth V, Drouin R, Mitchell DL, Rhainds M, Claveau J, Rouabhia M. The efficacy of a broad-spectrum sunscreen to protect engineered human skin from tissue and DNA damage induced by solar ultraviolet exposure. Clin Cancer Res. 2000;6:4128–35.
21. Ikehata H, Ono T. The mechanisms of UV mutagenesis. J Radiat Res. 2011;52(2):115–25. https://doi.org/10.1269/jrr.10175.
22. Kumar N, et al. Cooperation and interplay between base and nucleotide excision repair pathways: from DNA lesions to proteins. Genet Mol Biol. 2020;43(1 Suppl 1) https://doi.org/10.1590/1678-4685-GMB-2019-0104. Epub 2 Mar 2020.
23. Rastogi RP, Richa, Kumar A, Tyagi MB, Sinha RP. Molecular mechanisms of ultraviolet radiation-induced DNA damage and repair. J Nucleic Acids. 2010;2010:1.
24. Huang R, Zhou PK. DNA damage repair: historical perspectives, mechanistic pathways and clinical translation for targeted cancer therapy. Sig Transduct Target Ther. 2021;6:254. https://doi.org/10.1038/s41392-021-00648-7.
25. Lippens S, Denecker G, Ovaere P, et al. Death penalty for keratinocytes: apoptosis versus cornification. Cell Death Differ. 2005;12:1497–508. https://doi.org/10.1038/sj.cdd.4401722.
26. Martincorena I, Roshan A, Gerstung M, Ellis P, Van Loo P, McLaren S, et al. Tumor evolution. High burden and pervasive positive selection of somatic mutations in normal human skin. Science. 2015;348(6237):880–6. https://doi.org/10.1126/science.aaa6806.
27. Shain AH, Yeh I, Kovalyshyn I, Sriharan A, Talevich E, Gagnon A, et al. The genetic evolution of melanoma from precursor lesions. N Engl J Med. 2015;373:1926–36. https://doi.org/10.1056/NEJMoa1502583.
28. Fusco MJ, West H, Walko CM. Tumor mutation burden and cancer treatment. JAMA Oncol. 2021;7(2):316. https://doi.org/10.1001/jamaoncol.2020.6371.
29. Ashford NA, et al. Cancer risk: role of environment. Science. 2015;347:727.
30. Wild C, et al. Cancer risk: role of chance overstated. Science. 2015;347:728.
31. Potter JD, Prentice RL. Cancer risk: tumors excluded. Science. 2015;347:727.
32. Song MY, Giovannucci EL. Cancer risk: many factors contribute. Science. 2015;347:728–9.
33. Cheng L, Lopez-Beltran A, Massari F, MacLennan GT, Montironi R. Molecular testing for BRAF mutations to inform melanoma treatment decisions: a move toward precision medicine. Mod Pathol. 2018;31:24–38.
34. Mukherjee S. The emperor of all maladies: a biography of cancer. Waterville, Me., Thorndike Press, 2010.
35. Knouse KA, Lopez KE, Bachofner M, Amon A. Chromosome segregation Fidelity in epithelia requires tissue architecture. Cell. 2018;175:200. https://doi.org/10.1016/j.cell.2018.07.042.
36. Hanahan D, Weinberg RA. Hallmarks of cancer: the next generation. Cell. 2011;144(5):646–74. https://doi.org/10.1016/j.cell.2011.02.013.
37. Carless MA, Griffiths LR. Cytogenetics of melanoma and nonmelanoma skin cancer. Adv Exp Med Biol. 2008;624:227–40. https://doi.org/10.1007/978-0-387-77574-6_18.
38. Alexandrov LB, Nik-Zainal S, Wedge DC, Aparicio SA, Behjati S, Biankin AV, Bignell GR, Bolli N, et al. Signatures of mutational processes in human cancer. Nature. 2013;500(7463):415–21. https://doi.org/10.1038/nature12477.

39. Chalmers ZR, Connelly CF, Fabrizio D, et al. Analysis of 100,000 human cancer genomes reveals the landscape of tumor mutational burden. Genome Med. 2017;9:34. https://doi.org/10.1186/s13073-017-0424-2.
40. Inman GJ, Wang J, Nagano A, et al. The genomic landscape of cutaneous SCC reveals drivers and a novel azathioprine associated mutational signature. Nat Commun. 2018;9:3667. https://doi.org/10.1038/s41467-018-06027-1.
41. Krauthammer M, Kong Y, Bacchiocchi A, Evans P, Pomputtapong N, Wu C, et al. Exome sequencing identifies recurrent mutations in NF1 and RASopathy genes in Sun-exposed melanomas. Nat Genet. 2015;47:996–1002. https://doi.org/10.1038/ng.3361.
42. Shain AH, Garrido M, Botton T, Talevich E, Yeh I, Sanborn IZ, et al. Exome sequencing of desmoplastic melanoma identifies recurrent NFKBIE promoter mutations and diverse activating mutations in the MAPK pathway. Nat Genet. 2015;47:1194–9.
43. Salvadores M, Mas-Ponte D, Supek F. Passenger mutations accurately classify human tumors. PLoS Comput Biol. 2019;15(4):e1006953. https://doi.org/10.1371/journal.pcbi.1006953.
44. Pellegrini C, et al. Understanding the molecular genetics of basal cell carcinoma. Int J Mol Sci. 2017;18:2485.
45. Easty DJ, Gray SG, O'Byrne KJ, O'Donnell D, Bennett DC. Receptor tyrosine kinases and their activation in melanoma. Pigment Cell Melanoma Res. 2011;24(3):446–61. https://doi.org/10.1111/j.1755-148X.2011.00836.x. Epub 2011.
46. Pastore S, Mascia F, Mariani V, Girolomoni G. The epidermal growth factor receptor system in skin repair and inflammation. J Invest Dermatol. 2008;128(6):1365–74. https://doi.org/10.1038/sj.jid.5701184. Epub 2007.
47. Wang Z, Wang Y, Bradbury N, et al. Skin wound closure delay in metabolic syndrome correlates with SCF deficiency in keratinocytes. Sci Rep. 2020;10:21732. https://doi.org/10.1038/s41598-020-78244-y.
48. Carvajal RD, Antonescu CR, Wolchok JD, Chapman PB, Roman RA, Teitcher J, et al. KIT as a therapeutic target in metastatic melanoma. JAMA. 2011;305:2327–34.
49. Holcmann M, Sibilia M. Mechanisms underlying skin disorders induced by EGFR inhibitors. Mol Cell Oncol. 2015;2(4):e1004969. https://doi.org/10.1080/23723556.2015.1004969.
50. Sánchez-Danés A, Blanpain C. Deciphering the cells of origin of squamous cell carcinomas. Nat Rev Cancer. 2018;18(9):549–61. https://doi.org/10.1038/s41568-018-0024-5.
51. Bonilla X, Parmentier L, King B, Bezrukov F, Kaya G, Zoete V, et al. Genomic analysis identifies new drivers and progression pathways in skin basal cell carcinoma. Nat Genet. 2016;48:398–406.
52. Ozanne B, Richards CS, Hendlen R, Bums D, Gusterson B. Overexpression of the EGF receptor is a hallmark of squamous cell carcinomas. J Pathol. 1986;149:9–14.
53. Sini MC, Doneddu V, Paliogiannis P, Casula M, Colombino M, Manca A, et al. Genetic alterations in main candidate genes during melanoma progression. Oncotarget. 2018;9(9):8531–41. https://doi.org/10.18632/oncotarget.23989.
54. Went PT, Dirnhofer S, Bundi M, et al. Prevalence of KIT expression in human tumors. J Clin Oncol. 2004;22:4514–22. https://doi.org/10.1200/JCO.2004.10.125.
55. Winship I, Young K, Martell R, Ramesar R, Curtis D, Beighton P. Piebaldism: an autonomous autosomal dominant entity. Clin Genet. 1991;39:330–7.
56. Matsuda R, Takahashi T, Nakamura S, et al. Expression of the c-kit protein in human solid tumors and in corresponding fetal and adult normal tissues. Am J Pathol. 1993;142:339–46.
57. Curtin JA, Fridlyand J, Kageshita T, Patel HN, Busam KJ, Kutzner H, et al. Distinct sets of genetic alterations in melanoma. N Engl J Med. 2005;353:2135–47.
58. Ma X, Wu Y, Zhang T, Song H, Jv H, Guo W, Ren G. The clinical significance of C-kit mutations in metastatic oral mucosal melanoma in China. Oncotarget. 2017;8:82661–73.
59. Perez-Losada J, Sanchez-Martin M, Rodriguez-Garcia A, Sanchez ML, Orfao A, Flores T, et al. Zinc-finger transcription factor slug contributes to the function of the stem cell factor c-kit signaling pathway. Blood. 2002;100:1274–86.

60. Ingram DA, Yang FC, Travers JB, Wenning MJ, Hiatt K, New S, et al. Genetic and biochemical evidence that haploinsufficiency of the Nf1 tumor suppressor gene modulates melanocyte and mast cell fates in vivo. J Exp Med. 2000;191:181–8.
61. Davis EJ, Johnson DB, Sosman JA, Chandra S. Melanoma: what do all the mutations mean? Cancer. 2018;124(17):3490–9. https://doi.org/10.1002/cncr.31345.
62. Dhillon AS, Hagan S, Rath O, Kolch W. MAPK kinase signaling pathways in cancer. Oncogene. 2007;26:3279–90. https://doi.org/10.1038/sj.onc.1210421.
63. Kilgour JM, Jia JL, Sarin KY. Review of the molecular genetics of basal cell carcinoma; inherited susceptibility, somatic mutations, and targeted therapeutics. Cancers (Basel). 2021;13(15):3870. https://doi.org/10.3390/cancers13153870.
64. Chang D, Shain AH. The landscape of driver mutations in cutaneous squamous cell carcinoma. npj Genom Med. 2021;6:61. https://doi.org/10.1038/s41525-021-00226-4.
65. Thomas NE, Berwick M, Cordeiro-Stone M. Could BRAF mutations in melanocytic lesions arise from DNA damage induced by ultraviolet radiation? J Invest Dermatol. 2006;126:1693–6.
66. Muñoz-Couselo E, Zamora AE, Ortiz C, Soberino García J, Perez-Garcia J. NRAS-mutant melanoma: current challenges and future prospect. Onco Targets Ther. 2017;10:3941–7.
67. Marconcini R, et al. Metastatic BRAF K601E-mutated melanoma reaches complete response to MEK inhibitor trametinib administered for over 36 months. Exp Hematol Oncol. 2017;6:6. https://doi.org/10.1186/s40164-017-0067-4.
68. Moore AR, Rosenberg SC, McCormick F, et al. RAS-targeted therapies: is the undruggable drugged? Nat Rev Drug Discov. 2020;19:533–52. https://doi.org/10.1038/s41573-020-0068-6.
69. Hemesath TJ, Price ER, Takemoto C, Badalian T, Fisher DE. MAP kinase links the transcription factor Microphthalmia to c-kit signalling in melanocytes. Nature. 1998;391:298–301. https://doi.org/10.1038/34681.
70. Mercurio L, Albanesi C, Madonna S. Recent updates on the involvement of PI3K/AKT/mTOR molecular cascade in the pathogenesis of Hyperproliferative skin disorders. Front Med (Lausanne). 2021;8:665647. https://doi.org/10.3389/fmed.2021.665647.
71. Ding X, Bloch W, Iden S, et al. mTORC1 and mTORC2 regulate skin morphogenesis and epidermal barrier formation. Nat Commun. 2016;7:13226. https://doi.org/10.1038/ncomms13226.
72. Cabrita R, et al. The role of PTEN loss in immune escape, melanoma prognosis and therapy response. Cancers. 2020;12(3):742. https://doi.org/10.3390/cancers12030742.
73. Hodis E, Watson IR, Kryukov GV, Arold ST, Imielinski M, et al. A landscape of driver mutations in melanoma. Cell. 2012;150:251–63.
74. Riobo NA, Lu K, Ai X, Haines GM, Emerson CP Jr. Phosphoinositide 3- kinase and Akt are essential for Sonic Hedgehog signaling. Proc Natl Acad Sci USA. 2006;103:4505–10.
75. Kubo Y, Urano Y, Hida Y, Arase S. Lack of somatic mutation in the PTEN gene in squamous cell carcinomas of human skin. J Dermatol Sci. 1999;19:199–201.
76. Kilgour JM, Jia JL, Sarin KY. Review of the molecular genetics of basal cell carcinoma; inherited susceptibility, somatic mutations, and targeted therapeutics. Cancers. 2021;13:3870. https://doi.org/10.3390/cancers13153870.
77. Xie J. Implications of hedgehog signaling antagonists for cancer therapy. Acta Biochim Biophys Sin (Shanghai). 2008;40:670–80.
78. Hafner A, Bulyk ML, Jambhekar A, et al. The multiple mechanisms that regulate p53 activity and cell fate. Nat Rev Mol Cell Biol. 2019;20:199–210. https://doi.org/10.1038/s41580-019-0110-x.
79. Mantovani F, Collavin L, Del Sal G. Mutant p53 as a guardian of the cancer cell. Cell Death Differ. 2019;26:199–212. https://doi.org/10.1038/s41418-018-0246-9.
80. Shain AH, Bastian BC. From melanocytes to melanomas. Nat Rev Cancer. 2016;16(6):345–58. https://doi.org/10.1038/nrc.2016.37.
81. Ziegler A, et al. Mutation hot spots due to sunlight in the p53 gene of nonmelanoma skin cancers. Proc Natl Acad Sci U S A. 1993;90:4216–20.

82. Ziegler A, Jonason AS, Leffell AD, et al. Sunburn and p53 in the onset of skin cancer. Nature. 1994;372:773.
83. Reifenberger J, Wolter M, Knobbe CB, et al. Somatic mutations in the PTCH, SMOH, SUFUH and TP53 genes in sporadic basal cell carcinomas. Br J Dermatol. 2005;152:43.
84. Ming Z, Lim SY, Rizos H. Genetic alterations in the INK4a/ARF locus: effects on melanoma development and progression. Biomol Ther. 2020;10(10):1447. https://doi.org/10.3390/biom10101447.
85. Brown VL, Harwood CA, Crook T, Cronin JG, Kelsell DP, Proby CM. p16INK4a and p14ARF tumor suppressor genes are commonly inactivated in cutaneous squamous cell carcinoma. J Invest Dermatol. 2004;122(5):1284–92. https://doi.org/10.1111/j.0022-202X.2004.22501.x.
86. Griewank KG, et al. TERT promoter mutations are frequent in cutaneous basal cell carcinoma and squamous cell carcinoma. PLoS One. 2013;8:e80354.
87. Cancer Genome Atlas Network. Genomic classification of cutaneous melanoma. Cell. 2015;161(7):1681–96. https://doi.org/10.1016/j.cell.2015.05.044.
88. Sandru A, Voinea S, Panaitescu E, Blidaru A. Survival rates of patients with metastatic malignant melanoma. J Med Life. 2014;7(4):572–6.
89. Ting PT, Kasper R, Arlette JP. Metastatic basal cell carcinoma: report of two cases and literature review. J Cutan Med Surg. 2005;9:10–5.
90. Alam M, Ratner D. Cutaneous squamous-cell carcinoma. N Engl J Med. 2001;344:975–83.
91. Talmadge JE, Fidler IJ. AACR centennial series: the biology of cancer metastasis: historical perspective. Cancer Res. 2010;70(14):5649–69. https://doi.org/10.1158/0008-5472.CAN-10-1040.
92. Nguyen TH. Mechanisms of metastasis. ClinDermatol. 2004;22(3):209–16. https://doi.org/10.1016/j.clindermatol.2003.12.007.
93. Costa E, Barnabé G, Li M, et al. Intratumoral heterogeneity of ADAM23 promotes tumor growth and metastasis through LGI4 and nitric oxide signals. Oncogene. 2015;34:1270–9. https://doi.org/10.1038/onc.2014.70.
94. Ramón y Cajal S, Sesé M, Capdevila C, et al. Clinical implications of intratumor heterogeneity: challenges and opportunities. J Mol Med. 2020;98:161–77. https://doi.org/10.1007/s00109-020-01874-2.
95. Luzzi KJ, MacDonald IC, Schmidt EE, et al. Multistep nature of metastatic inefficiency: dormancy of solitary cells after successful extravasation and limited survival of early micrometastases. Am J Pathol. 1998;153(3):865–73. https://doi.org/10.1016/S0002-9440(10)65628-3.
96. Thiery J, Sleeman J. Complex networks orchestrate epithelial–mesenchymal transitions. Nat Rev Mol Cell Biol. 2006;7:131–42. https://doi.org/10.1038/nrm1835.
97. Martin P. Wound healing—aiming for perfect skin regeneration. Science. 1997;276:75–81.
98. Savagner P, et al. Developmental transcription factor slug is required for effective re-epithelialization by adult keratinocytes. J Cell Physiol. 2005;202:858–66.
99. Peinado H, et al. Pre-metastatic niches: organ-specific homes for metastases. Nat Rev Cancer. 2017;17:302–17.
100. Fares J, Fares MY, Khachfe HH, et al. Molecular principles of metastasis: a hallmark of cancer revisited. Sig Transduct Target Ther. 2020;5:28. https://doi.org/10.1038/s41392-020-0134-x.
101. Choucair K, Morand S, Stanbery L, et al. TMB: a promising immune-response biomarker, and potential spearhead in advancing targeted therapy trials. Cancer Gene Ther. 2020;27:841–53. https://doi.org/10.1038/s41417-020-0174-y.
102. Eroglu Z, Zaretsky JM, Hu-Lieskovan S, et al. High response rate to PD-1 blockade in desmoplastic melanomas. Nature. 2018;553:347–50.
103. Yarchoan M, Hopkins A, Jaffee EM. Tumor mutational burden and response rate to PD-1 inhibition. N Engl J Med. 2017;377(25):2500–1. https://doi.org/10.1056/NEJMc1713444.
104. Harwood CA, et al. A surveillance model for skin cancer in organ transplant recipients: a 22-year prospective study in an ethnically diverse population. Am J Transplant. 2013;13:119–29.

105. Berg D, Otley CC. Skin cancer in organ transplant recipients: epidemiology, pathogenesis, and management. J Am Acad Dermatol. 2002;47(1):1–17. https://doi.org/10.1067/mjd.2002.125579.
106. Wells JL 3rd, Shirai K. Systemic therapy for squamous cell carcinoma of the skin in organ transplant recipients. Am J Clin Oncol. 2012;35(5):498–503. https://doi.org/10.1097/COC.0b013e318201a3ef.
107. Mehrany K, Weenig RH, Pittelkow MR, Roenigk RK, Otley CC. High recurrence rates of basal cell carcinoma after Mohs surgery in patients with chronic lymphocytic leukemia. Arch Dermatol. 2004;140(8):985–8.
108. Khezri F, Brewer JD, Weaver AL. Merkel cell carcinoma in the setting of chronic lymphocytic leukemia. Dermatol Surg. 2011;37(8):1100–5.
109. Velez NF, Karia PS, Vartanov AR, Davids MS, Brown JR, Schmults CD. Association of advanced leukemic stage and skin cancer tumor stage with poor skin cancer outcomes in patients with chronic lymphocytic leukemia. JAMA Dermatol. 2014;150(3):280–7. https://doi.org/10.1001/jamadermatol.2013.6249.
110. Granstein RD, Matsui MS. UV radiation-induced immunosuppression and skin cancer. Cutis. 2004;74:4–9.
111. Loser K, Beissert S. Regulation of cutaneous immunity by the environment: an important role for UV irradiation and vitamin D. Int Immunopharmacol. 2009;9(5):587–9. https://doi.org/10.1016/j.intimp.2009.01.024.
112. Feng H, Shuda M, Chang Y, Moore PS. Clonal integration of a polyomavirus in human Merkel cell carcinoma. Science. 2008;319:1096–100.
113. Swann JB, Smyth MJ. Immune surveillance of tumors. J Clin Invest. 2007;117(5):1137–46. https://doi.org/10.1172/JCI31405.
114. Chang RB, Beatty GL. The interplay between innate and adaptive immunity in cancer shapes the productivity of cancer immunosurveillance. J Leukoc Biol. 2020;108(1):363–76. https://doi.org/10.1002/JLB.3MIR0320-475R.
115. Richmond JM, Harris JE. Immunology and skin in health and disease. Cold Spring Harb Perspect Med. 2014;4(12):a015339. Published 2014 Dec 1. https://doi.org/10.1101/cshperspect.a015339.
116. Kupper TS, Fuhlbrigge RC. Immune surveillance in the skin: mechanisms and clinical consequences. Nat Rev Immunol. 2004;4(3):211–22. https://doi.org/10.1038/nri1310.
117. Abdallah F, et al. Skin immune landscape: inside and outside the organism. Mediat Inflamm. 2017;2017:5095293. https://doi.org/10.1155/2017/5095293.
118. Azimi F, Scolyer RA, Rumcheva P, Moncrieff M, Murali R, McCarthy SW, Saw RP, Thompson JF. Tumor-infiltrating lymphocyte grade is an independent predictor of sentinel lymph node status and survival in patients with cutaneous melanoma. J Clin Oncol. 2012;30:2678–83.
119. Suarez-Carmona M, Lesage J, Cataldo D, Gilles C. EMT and inflammation: inseparable actors of cancer progression. Mol Oncol. 2017;11:805–23.
120. Rangwala S, Tsai KY. Roles of the immune system in skin cancer. Br J Dermatol. 2011;165(5):953–65. https://doi.org/10.1111/j.1365-2133.2011.10507.x.
121. Boldajipour B, et al. Tumor-infiltrating lymphocytes are dynamically desensitized to antigen but are maintained by homeostatic cytokine. JCI Insight. 2016;1(20):e89289. https://doi.org/10.1172/jci.insight.89289.
122. Pardoll DM. The blockade of immune checkpoints in cancer immunotherapy. Nat Rev Cancer. 2012;12(4):252–64. https://doi.org/10.1038/nrc3239.
123. Chen L, Flies DB. Molecular mechanisms of T cell co-stimulation and co-inhibition. Nat Rev Immunol. 2013;13:227–42.
124. Schnell A, Bod L, Madi A, et al. The yin and yang of co-inhibitory receptors: toward antitumor immunity without autoimmunity. Cell Res. 2020;30:285–99. https://doi.org/10.1038/s41422-020-0277-x.
125. Korn EL, Liu PY, Lee SJ, Chapman JA, Niedzwiecki D, Suman VJ, et al. Meta-analysis of phase II cooperative group trials in metastatic stage IV melanoma to determine

progression-free and overall survival benchmarks for future phase II trials. J Clin Oncol. 2008;26(4):527–34. https://doi.org/10.1200/JCO.2007.12.7837.
126. Curti BD, Faries MB. Recent advances in the treatment of melanoma. N Engl J Med. 2021;384(23):2229–40. https://doi.org/10.1056/NEJMra2034861.
127. Alsaidan M, Simmons BJ, Bray FN, Falto-Aizpurua LA, Griffith RD, Nouri K. Hippocrates' contributions to dermatology revealed. JAMA Dermatol. 2015;151(6):658. https://doi.org/10.1001/jamadermatol.2015.
128. Liddell K. Choosing a dermatological hero for the millennium: Hippocrates of Cos (460-377 BC). Clin Exp Dermatol. 2000;25(1):86–8.
129. LeBlanc VG, Marra MA. NGS approaches in cancer: where have they brought us and where will they take us? Cancers. 2015;7(3):1925–58. https://doi.org/10.3390/cancers7030869.

Chapter 3
Epidemiology of Skin Cancer

Beatrice Martinez Zugaib Abdalla and Cristina Martinez Zugaib Abdalla

Key Points
- Skin cancer is the most common malignance worldwide.
- Non-melanoma skin cancer (NMSC) and melanoma incidence has increased in recent decades.
- Basal cell carcinoma and squamous cell carcinoma account for 99% of NMSC, with low mortality rates.
- Melanoma accounts for 1% of skin cancer but with higher mortality rates.
- Some risk factors include ultraviolet exposure, age, gender, history of skin malignancy, and immunosuppression.

Introduction

The cancer of the skin represents the most common worldwide malignancy [1]. One in every three diagnosed cancers is a skin cancer [2]. The overall incidence and prevalence of melanoma and non-melanoma skin cancer (NMSC), which include basal cell carcinomas (BCC) and squamous cell carcinomas (SCC), have increased in recent decades, and have a profound impact on public health [3, 4]. This increase may be due to ultraviolet (UV) exposure behavior, an increase in the aging population, and improved skin cancer detection [5].

The main types of NMSC, BCC, and SCC, account for about 99% of all NMSCs. Other NMSCs include Merkel cell carcinoma, sebaceous carcinoma, apocrine adenocarcinoma, and other rare tumors. The actual number of NMSC is underestimated because NMSCs are not required to be reported in the United States [1, 3] and European registries do not record individual types of NMSC [6].

B. M. Z. Abdalla (✉) · C. M. Z. Abdalla
Hospital Sírio-Libanês, São Paulo, Brazil

C. M. Z. Abdalla et al. (eds.), *Oncodermatology*,
https://doi.org/10.1007/978-3-031-29277-4_3

The incidence of melanoma has increased by 4–6% annually and 132,000 new cases were reported in 2020. It is the fifth and sixth most common new cancer diagnosis in men and women, respectively [2, 4]. Even though incidence rates have been increasing, 5-year survival suggests that early detection and treatment may play a role in increased melanoma survival rates [4]. Among the different types of skin cancers, BCC, accounting for 75% of cases in Caucasians, mainly affects the elderly population [3] and melanoma accounts for only about 1% of skin cancers but invasive melanoma is responsible for 80% of skin cancer deaths [7, 8].

The pathogenesis of skin cancer is multifactorial. UV radiation from sunlight is the main etiological agent in the development of melanoma and NMSC. Skin neoplasms are more frequent in the elderly, demonstrating the influence of cumulative exposure to the sun on the development of skin cancer [1].

NMSC is more associated with cumulative sun exposure and melanoma more related to intense sun exposure that leads to sunburn. Melanoma on the trunk and legs has been linked to frequent sunburns especially during childhood years, suggesting that melanomas that start in these areas are different from those that start on the face, neck, and arms, where sun exposure is more constant. On the other hand, acral lentiginous melanomas (palms, soles, and nail bed) are not related to sun exposure [9, 10].

Other risk factors include immunosuppression, as evidenced by the increased incidence of SCC in organ transplant recipients, hematological malignancies, and HIV/AIDS patients [4, 11].

The incidence of melanoma is much lower compared with NMSC but has been rising in fair-skinned populations. The annual increase has been estimated to be between 3% and 7%, with mortality rates increasing less quickly [11].

Melanoma mortality rates have shown stabilization. The reason being related to intervention strategies, early detection of suspected lesions which lead to a constant decrease of tumor thickness at the time of diagnosis, and overdiagnosis from increased biopsies, reclassification of non-malignant diagnoses as melanoma, and the increased sensitivity of diagnostics of imaging techniques [4, 11].

NMSCs are highly treatable if detected early and treated properly. The 5-year survival rate for melanoma with non-lymph node involvement is 99%. The 5-year survival rate for melanoma lymph node involvement is 66%. The 5-year survival rate for metastatic melanoma is 27% [9, 10, 12, 13].

Despite the high number of cases and psychosocial and economic burden of more advanced disease, early detection, and prompt treatment, usually has a good prognosis [4].

Non-melanoma Skin Cancer

It is estimated that 5.4 million cases of BCC and SCC are diagnosed annually in the United States among 3.3 million people. Some people are diagnosed with more than one skin cancer [9, 10]. In Brazil the statistics are underestimated because report is not required. There were 176,930 new cases reported in 2020, 83,770 men and 93,160 women [14]. There were 2616 deaths, 1488 men and 1128 women [15].

NMSC is by far the most frequent cancer in fair-skinned populations and 80% are BCC. Numerous studies have shown that incidence rates of NMSC are increasing worldwide. BCC is the most common malignant skin cancer and occurs four times more frequently than SCC [4]. Women had a greater incidence than men for both types of NMSC, as well as BCC on the trunk [16]. Sun exposure behavior could have been a reason for this increased incidence, as presented in studies that showed extensive use of sunbeds in women under 40 years old, around 20 years ago. However, more recent studies present greater recreational sun exposure regardless of gender, possibly stabilizing the difference in sex ratio, as well as, decreasing numbers due to prevention programs [16].

SCC is mostly associated with an advancing age especially in males [11]. SCC causes more deaths and is responsible for approximately 2500 deaths per year in the United States. Compared with the incidence, the mortality of NMSC is quite low. Non-genital SCC and BCC death rates have declined, and mortality due to genital carcinoma was about half of total NMSC deaths [11].

Risk Factors

- Ultraviolet (UV) light exposure: sun exposure and tanning beds are implicated in the pathogenesis of skin cancer. Researchers estimate that indoor tanning may cause upward of 400.000 cases of skin cancer in the United States each year [17]. UVB radiation is the most important environmental cause of SCC and intense and intermittent sun exposure with sunburn, and childhood exposure is the most important risk for both BCC and melanoma [18].
- Skin-type: fair-skinned population in the United States has been estimated to be as high as 150 and 360 per 100,000 individuals, respectively, the incidence in dark-skinned individuals is estimated to be 3 per 100,000. In individuals with highly pigmented skin, cutaneous SCC tends to arise on non-sun-exposed areas and is frequently associated with chronic inflammation, chronic wounds, or scarring [19].
- Age: the incidence of cutaneous SCC increases with age, mostly older than 50 years.
- Gender: men are more likely than women to get NMSC probably due to more sun exposure [20].
- Chemicals and radiation: arsenic increases the risk naturally found in some areas or from pesticides. Exposure to coal tar, paraffin, and certain types of petroleum products may also have an increased risk of skin cancer. Ionizing radiation, (environmental, therapeutic, and diagnosis) is a risk factor for NMSC [21–24].
- Previous history of skin cancer increases the incidence of developing another one.
- Cutaneous inflammation: there is a small risk of developing SCC on scars from burns, serious infections, and skin diseases as cutaneous lupus are more

likely to develop skin cancers. Psoriasis treatment with psoralens and ultraviolet light (PUVA) can increase the risk of developing SCC and other skin cancers [25].

- Inherited diseases [26, 27]:
  - Xeroderma pigmentosum (XP) is a condition that reduces the DNA repair to UV exposure. People with this disorder often develop many skin cancers, starting in childhood.
  - Basal cell nevus syndrome (Gorlin-Goltz syndrome) is an autosomal dominant disease characterized by the development of basal cell carcinomas, associated with other changes in multiple systems, which present with clinical and radiological changes and patients develop many basal cell cancers over their lifetime.
  - Other rare inherited diseases as Rombo, Bazex-Dupré-Christol, and epidermolysis bullosa, albinism, dyskeratosis congenita could develop NMSC.
- Immunosuppression: organ transplants, large doses of corticosteroids and other immunosuppressants, and biologic drugs for treatment of arthritis, psoriasis, and AIDS patients have an increased risk for BCC and SCC [28].
- Human papillomavirus (HPV) infection: HPV genital infection and anal areas and around the fingernails seem to be related to SCC in these areas [26].
- Smoking increases the risk of SCC on the lips [26].

Melanoma

The American Cancer Society's estimates that in the United States there were 106,110 new melanomas cases, 62,260 in men and 43,850 in women in 2021. About 7180 people are expected to die of melanoma (about 4600 men and 2580 women). Melanoma is the fifth most common cancer among men and women. It is more than 20 times more common in whites than in African Americans. The lifetime risk of getting melanoma is about 2.6% for whites, 0.1% for blacks, and 0.6% (1 in 167) for Hispanic population as per data from American Cancer Society [9, 10]. In Brazil there were 8450, 4200 men and 4250 women [14]. In 2019, the mortality was 1978, 1159 in men and 819 in woman [15].

Melanoma incidence has increased among older age groups (80+) and begun to decline in adolescents and adults, ages 30 and younger. Before age 50, rates are higher in women compared to men. After age 50 men have higher rates. The development of melanoma is more common as people grow older. But it also develops in younger people, including those younger than 30 years old [9, 10]. It is one of the most common cancers diagnosed in young adults, particularly in women. In 2020, about 2400 cases of melanoma were estimated to be diagnosed in people aged 15–29 [7].

Risk Factors

- Ultraviolet (UV) light exposure is a major risk factor for most melanomas. Sunlight is the main source of UV rays but tanning beds and sun lamps are also sources of UV rays. The pattern and timing of the UV exposure may play a role in melanoma development. For example, melanoma on the trunk (chest and back) and legs has been linked to frequent sunburns (especially in childhood). This might also have something to do with the fact that these areas are not constantly exposed to UV light. Some evidence suggests that melanomas that start in these areas are different from those that start on the face, neck, and arms, where the sun exposure is more constant. And different from either of these are melanomas on the palms of the hands, soles of the feet, or under the nails (known as acral lentiginous melanomas), or on internal surfaces such as the mouth and vagina (mucosal melanomas), where there has been little or no sun exposure [9, 10].
- Skin-type: fair-skinned population is much higher for whites than for African Americans. Whites with red or blond hair, blue or green eyes, or fair skin that freckles or burns easily are at increased risk.
- Age: melanoma is more likely to occur in older people, but it is also found in younger people. In fact, melanoma is one of the most common cancers in people younger than 30 (especially younger women). Melanoma that runs in families may occur at a younger age.
- Gender: men have a higher rate of melanoma than women, although this varies by age. Before age 50, the risk is higher for women; after age 50 the risk is higher in men.
- Dysplastic nevus syndrome (atypical mole syndrome, familial atypical multiple mole and melanoma syndrome, or FAMMM) has a very high lifetime risk of melanoma, proximally 500-fold increase in malignant melanoma risk. One risk factor specifically for malignant melanoma is the presence of atypical or numerous moles (more than 50). Families with multiple cases of malignant melanoma often exhibit the dysplastic nevus syndrome [1].
- Congenital melanocytic nevi: The lifetime risk of melanoma developing in congenital melanocytic nevi is estimated to be between 0% and 5%, depending on the size of the nevus.
- Family/personal history of melanoma: first-degree relatives (parents, brothers, sisters, or children) have had melanoma. Around 10% of all people with melanoma have a family history of the disease. A person who has already had melanoma has a higher risk of getting melanoma again. People who have had BCC or SCC cancers are also at increased risk of getting melanoma.
- Inherited disease: xeroderma pigmentosum (XP) is a rare, inherited condition that affects skin cells' ability to repair damage to their DNA. People with XP have a high risk of developing melanoma and other skin cancers when they are young, especially on sun-exposed areas of their skin.

References

1. Gordon R. Skin cancer: an overview of epidemiology and risk factors. Semin Oncol Nurs. 2013;29(3):160–9. https://doi.org/10.1016/j.soncn.2013.06.002.
2. Skin cancers. World Health Organization. Available at: https://www.who.int/uv/faq/skincancer/en/index1.html. Accessed 22 Apr 2020.
3. Urban K, Mehrmal S, Uppal P, Giesey RL, Delost GR. The global burden of skin cancer: a longitudinal analysis from the Global Burden of Disease Study, 1990-2017. JAAD Int. 2021;2:98–108. https://doi.org/10.1016/j.jdin.2020.10.013.
4. Gandhi SA, Kampp J. Skin cancer epidemiology, detection, and management. Med Clin North Am. 2015;99(6):1323–35. https://doi.org/10.1016/j.mcna.2015.06.002. Epub 2015 Sept 2.
5. Marks R. The epidemiology of non-melanoma skin cancer: who, why and what can we do about it. J Dermatol. 1995;22:853.
6. Ciążyńska M, Kamińska-Winciorek G, Lange D, et al. The incidence and clinical analysis of non-melanoma skin cancer. Sci Rep. 2021;11:4337. https://doi.org/10.1038/s41598-021-83502-8.
7. SEER Cancer Stat Facts: Melanoma of the skin. Bethesda, MD: National Cancer Institute; http://seer.cancer.gov/statfacts/html/melan.html.
8. Paulson KG, Gupta D, Kim TS. Age-specific incidence of melanoma in the United States. JAMA Dermatol. 2020;156(1):57–64. https://doi.org/10.1001/jamadermatol.2019.3353.
9. Mitchell TC, Karakousis G, Schuchter L. Chapter 66: Melanoma. In: Niederhuber JE, Armitage JO, Doroshow JH, Kastan MB, Tepper JE, editors. Abeloff's clinical oncology. 6th ed. Philadelphia, PA: Elsevier; 2020.
10. Ribas A, Read P, Slingluff CL. Chapter 92: Cutaneous melanoma. In: DeVita VT, Lawrence TS, Rosenberg SA, editors. DeVita, Hellman, and Rosenberg's cancer: principles and practice of oncology. 11th ed. Philadelphia, PA: Lippincott Williams & Wilkins; 2019.
11. Leiter U, Eigentler T, Garbe C. Epidemiology of skin cancer. In: Sunlight, vitamin D and skin cancer. New York: Springer; 2014. https://doi.org/10.1007/978-1-4939-0437-2_7.
12. Siegel RL, Miller KD, Fuchs H, Jemal A. Cancer statistics, 2021. CA Cancer J Clin. 2021;71:7–33. https://doi.org/10.3322/caac.21654.
13. Neville JA, Welch E, Leffell DJ. Management of nonmelanoma skin cancer in 2007. Nat Clin Pract Oncol. 2007;4(8):462–9. https://doi.org/10.1038/ncponc0883.
14. https://www.inca.gov.br/estimativa/taxas-ajustadas/melanoma-maligno-da-pele.
15. BRASIL. Ministério da Saúde. SIM: Sistema de informações sobre mortalidade. Brasília, DF: Ministério da Saúde; 2008. Available from: http://www.datasus.gov.br. Accessed 5 Sept 2019.
16. Muzic JG, Schmitt AR, Wright AC, Alniemi DT, Zubair AS, Olazagasti Lourido JM, Sosa Seda IM, Weaver AL, Baum CL. Incidence and trends of basal cell carcinoma and cutaneous squamous cell carcinoma: a population-based study in Olmsted County, Minnesota, 2000 to 2010. Mayo Clin Proc. 2017;92(6):890–8. https://doi.org/10.1016/j.mayocp.2017.02.015. Epub 2017 May 15.
17. Wehner MR, Chren MM, Nameth D, Choudhry A, Gaskins M, Nead KT, Boscardin WJ, Linos E. International prevalence of indoor tanning: a systematic review and meta-analysis. JAMA Dermatol. 2014;150(4):390–400. https://doi.org/10.1001/jamadermatol.2013.6896. Erratum in: JAMA Dermatol. 2014 May;150(5):577.
18. Armstrong BK, Kricker A. The epidemiology of UV induced skin cancer. J Photochem Photobiol B. 2001;63(1–3):8–18. https://doi.org/10.1016/s1011-1344(01)00198-1.
19. Gloster HM Jr, Neal K. Skin cancer in skin of color. J Am Acad Dermatol. 2006;55(5):741–60; quiz 761–4. https://doi.org/10.1016/j.jaad.2005.08.063.
20. Christensen SR, Wilson LD, Leffell DJ. Chapter 90: Cancer of the skin. In: DeVita VT, Lawrence TS, Rosenberg SA, editors. DeVita, Hellman, and Rosenberg's cancer: principles and practice of oncology. 11th ed. Philadelphia, PA: Lippincott Williams & Wilkins; 2019.

21. Lichter MD, Karagas MR, Mott LA, et al. Therapeutic ionizing radiation and the incidence of basal cell carcinoma and squamous cell carcinoma. The New Hampshire Skin Cancer Study Group. Arch Dermatol. 2000;136:1007.
22. Azizova TV, Bannikova MV, Grigoryeva ES, Rybkina VL. Risk of malignant skin neoplasms in a cohort of workers occupationally exposed to ionizing radiation at low dose rates. PLoS One. 2018;13:e0205060.
23. Gallagher RP, Bajdik CD, Fincham S, et al. Chemical exposures, medical history, and risk of squamous and basal cell carcinoma of the skin. Cancer Epidemiol Biomark Prev. 1996;5:419.
24. Huang HW, Lee CH, Yu HS. Arsenic-induced carcinogenesis and immune dysregulation. Int J Environ Res Public Health. 2019;16:2746.
25. Stern RS, PUVA Follow-Up Study. The risk of squamous cell and basal cell cancer associated with psoralen and ultraviolet A therapy: a 30-year prospective study. J Am Acad Dermatol. 2012;66:553.
26. Lim JL, Asgari M. Cutaneous squamous cell carcinoma: epidemiology, risk factors, and molecular pathogenesis. In: Post TW, editor. UpToDate. Waltham, MA: UpToDate. Accessed 5 Jan 2022.
27. Wu PA. Epidemiology, pathogenesis, and clinical features of basal cell carcinoma. In: Post TW, editor. UpToDate. Waltham, MA: UpToDate. Accessed 5 Jan 2022.
28. Liu R, Wan Q, Zhao R, et al. Risk of non-melanoma skin cancer with biological therapy in common inflammatory diseases: a systemic review and meta-analysis. Cancer Cell Int. 2021;21:614. https://doi.org/10.1186/s12935-021-02325-9.

Chapter 4
Risk Factors for Skin Cancer

Maria Isabel Achatz, María Catalina Gavilanes Coloma, and Elisabeth de Albuquerque Cavalcanti Callegaro

Key Points

- The acknowledgment of the environmental risk factors, as well as the cancer predisposition syndromes permits more accurate diagnosis, leads to adequate measures of care and prevention for skin cancer and internal malignancies.
- Environmental risk factors such as ultraviolet radiation (UV radiation), immunosuppression, viral infections and radiotherapy among others have been described.
- Physical and chemical risk factors are analyzed (UV radiation, sun exposure, skin types, radon and arsenic exposures) and correlated with skin cancer as NMSC and melanoma.
- Melanoma and non-melanoma skin cancer linked to hereditary cancer syndromes are discussed.
- Guidelines on genetic counseling and risk assessment in cancer predisposition syndromes.

Introduction

The causes of skin cancer including non-melanoma skin cancer (NMSC) and melanoma are influenced by risk factors related to the environment and to genetic syndromes. Environmental risk factors such as ultraviolet radiation (UV radiation),

M. I. Achatz (✉)
Centro de Oncologia, Hospital Sírio-Libanês, São Paulo, Brazil

M. C. G. Coloma · E. de Albuquerque Cavalcanti Callegaro
Hospital Sírio-Libanês, São Paulo, Brazil

C. M. Z. Abdalla et al. (eds.), *Oncodermatology*,
https://doi.org/10.1007/978-3-031-29277-4_4

immunosuppression, viral infections and radiotherapy among others have been described [1, 2]. Hereditary cancer predisposition syndromes present with mutations that interfere in molecular pathways involved in the pathogenesis of both NMSC and melanoma [1]. These syndromes are characterized by multiple family members carrying the same mutation and manifesting similar clinical features, although de novo mutations can also occur [3]. It is estimated that 7–15% of all melanomas occur in individuals with a family history [4, 5]. Due to its aggressive behavior, early diagnosis is very important to the prognosis especially in patients with hereditary cancer predisposition syndromes in which skin symptoms are often easier identified compared to visceral malignancies [3].

Environmental Risk Factors for Skin Cancer

Physical Environmental Risk Factors

Ultraviolet Radiation

Ultraviolet radiation (UV radiation) has beneficial effects in humans since it is responsible for the synthesis of vitamin D and endorphins. Nonetheless, it is known as the main environmental risk factor for skin cancer. UV radiation acts as a complete carcinogen since it acts as a mutagen as well as a non-specific damaging agent and has combined tumor initiator and tumor promoter properties [6].

Sun Exposure Pattern

The way of exposure to UV radiation influences in the development of the different kinds of skin cancer. Chronic cumulative sun exposure is more often related to the development of Cutaneous Squamous Cell Carcinoma (cSCC) but an association with melanomas located in the head, neck and arms has also been described. On the other hand, intermittent intense sun exposure is related to the development of BCC and non-acral cutaneous melanomas [7, 8]. Chronic cumulative sun exposure is especially seen in those who have outdoor occupations and intermittent intense sun exposure in those with a history of sunburns. In the latter, the risk for developing melanoma is doubled. Some studies reported that this occurs in patients with a history of five sunburns, regardless of if these occurred prior to or after the age of 15. Nonetheless, the highest risk has been described in people with sunburns that occur during childhood [8–10].

It is to note that given the rare occurrence of melanoma in absolute terms, it is difficult to perform a prospective study. Most of the data have been taken from retrospective studies, and as such, it is exceedingly difficult to characterize the pattern of sun exposure that places patients at greatest risk of developing melanoma through majority of the data [9].

Skin Types

In relation to skin types, the highest risk for developing skin cancer is seen in skin types I and II (Fitzpatrick). This is likely related to the higher sensitivity of these skin types to sun exposure [8].

Sociodemographic Characteristics

According to sociodemographic studies, higher risk of skin cancer is shown in populations that live in proximity to the equator and at higher altitudes. Studies of immigrant populations in Australia revealed that the risk of melanoma is proportional to the length of stay and inversely to age at arrival. In the North America, rates of early-stage and late-stage melanoma demonstrated to be significantly higher in high solar UV counties [10–12].

Indoor Tanning (Tanning Bed/Sunbed)

Indoor tanning devices primarily emit UVA radiation reaching values 10–15 times higher than that emitted by the summer noontime sun at intermediate latitudes [11]. Indoor tanning is associated with significantly increased risk of both NMSC and melanoma, being substantially higher when exposed for longer times and with earlier age at exposure [7, 13, 14].

Other Conditions

The relationship between UV radiation and the development of skin cancer has also been proven by the higher risk for developing melanoma seen in the sun-exposed skin of patients with xeroderma pigmentosum and in psoriasis patients who have received UV-A radiation photochemotherapy as a treatment. Some studies showed that psoriasis patients who received more than 450 PUVA treatments have a 35-fold increase in the rate of developing cSCC [7, 11].

Ionizing Radiation

Ionizing radiation (environmental, therapeutic and diagnostic radiation) is a well-known risk factor for NMSC [15]. Higher doses of ionizing radiation lead to a higher risk. This risk is higher in places with the most sun exposure and in those with lighter skin types. Most of the studies demonstrate a higher risk for cSCC but risk for BCC has also been described [7, 15].

Chemical Risk Factors

Arsenic Exposure

Consumption of contaminated water and occupational exposure are associated with both cSCC and BCC [7].

Radon Exposure

Environmental radon exposure may be a risk factor for cSCC as suggested in a study done in southwest England. Further research needs to be done in order to elucidate this relationship [7, 16].

Medications

Several observational studies have found modest increases in risk for cSCC among patients with a history of use of photosensitizing medications predominantly concerning thiazide diuretics. Other examples include azathioprine and voriconazole. Additional to the selective UVA photosensitizer effects of azathioprine, it also has mutagenic effects in the skin [7]. The association between voriconazole and cSCC was reported when used as a long-term therapy in immunosuppressed patients, including children. Even though it is known to cause cutaneous photosensitivity, the mechanism through which it influences to the occurrence of cSCC is unknown [7].

The use of BRAF inhibitors vemurafenib and dabrafenib in patients with metastatic melanoma has revealed frequent development of cSCC or keratoacanthomas being present in 15–30% of these patients [17]. The mechanism is related to paradoxical activation of the mitogen-activated protein kinase (MAPK) pathway in cells harboring pre-existing RAS or receptor tyrosine kinase mutations. This may contribute to the proliferation and survival of cancerous cells [17].

Immunosuppression

Patients with solid organ transplantation are at greater risk for both NMSC and melanoma. Between the two, the risk for NMSC is particularly higher. Compared to non-immunosuppressed patients, their risk for cSCC is 50–250 times, for BCC, 10 times and for melanoma 2–8 times. The latter can be 17.2 times higher in the African-American population [18].

Patients with hematopoietic cell transplantation and with HIV/AIDS also have a higher risk for melanoma [9, 11].

In a population of patients with intestinal bowel disease (IBD), a cohort nested study found a higher risk for melanoma and NMSC. While the risk of melanoma increased with the use of biologics, the risk of NMSC increased by use of thiopurines [19].

Biological Agents (Virus)

Multiple studies have reported indirect evidence supporting an etiologic relationship between human papillomavirus (HPV) and cSCC. HPV can lead to cSCC in genetically predisposed individuals (e.g., epidermodysplasia verruciformis) and verrucous carcinoma of the penis (Buschke-Löwenstein tumor) but its relationship in the general population is still unclear [7]. A type-specific analysis showed a significant association between types 5, 8, 15, 17, 20, 24, 36 and 38 and risk of cSCC [7].

A population-based study found no significant difference in HPV prevalence between cSCC and BCC, but cSCC lesions were significantly more infected with beta HPV than were BCC [20].

In a Taiwan nationwide cohort study, there was a 2.45-fold increased risk of developing new-onset skin cancers for patients with incident HPV. A prominent risk of skin cancers was found within the first 5 years after the index date and the risk was noticeably significant among patients aged >40 years [20].

Other Risk Factors

The influence of diet, alcohol consumption, cigarette smoking and the development of NMSC has also been investigated. However, the individual contribution of each factor is not clear, and data on interactions between sun exposure, host factors and other potential risk factors for NMSC are limited [21].

The environmental risk factors for skin cancer are summarized in Fig. 4.1.

Key Message

- UV radiation is the most recognized risk factor for NMSC and melanoma.
- Chronic cumulative sun exposure is more related to the development of cSCC but melanomas located in the head, neck and arms have also shown an association.
- Intermittent intense sun exposure is related to the development of BCC and non-acral cutaneous melanomas.
- Ionizing radiation is a known risk factor for NMSC, predominantly cSCC.
- Arsenic exposure is related to NMSC.

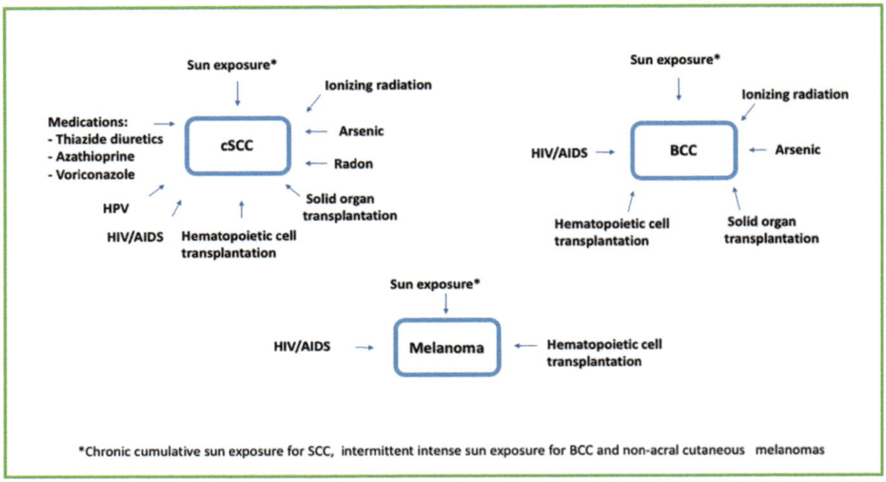

Fig. 4.1 Environmental risk factors for skin cancer and its association with cSCC, BCC and melanoma

- Medications, mainly thiazide diuretics, increase the risk of cSCC; azathioprine and voriconazole are also related.
- Solid organ transplantation patients have a higher risk of developing NMSC. Risk for melanoma has also been described in patients with hematopoietic cell transplantation and in patients with HIV/AIDS.
- HPV has shown indirect evidence supporting an etiologic relationship with cSCC.

Hereditary Cancer Predisposition Syndrome Predisposing to Non-melanoma Skin Cancer

Gorlin Syndrome (Basal Cell Nevus Syndrome, Gorlin-Goltz Syndrome or Nevoid BCC)

Inheritance: Autosomal dominant disorder with complete penetrance [3]. Incomplete penetrance is found in SUFU variant carriers [22].

Molecular genetics and pathophysiology: Mutation in the *PTCH1* gene on chromosome 9q22, the *PTCH2* gene on chromosome 1p32, or the *SUFU* gene on chromosome 10q24-q25 that plays a role in the hedgehog signaling pathway, controlling growth and tissue development [3].

Clinical features: This syndrome has to be suspected in individuals with clinical features, which are based on major and minor diagnostic criteria [22].

Diagnosis is done with the presence of two major and one minor criteria or one major and three minor criteria as described in Table 4.1. When clinical criteria

Table 4.1 Clinical criteria for Gorlin syndrome

Major criteria	Minor criteria
– Lamellar (sheet-like) calcification of the falx or clear evidence of calcification in an individual younger than age 20 years	– Vertebral/rib anomalies observed on chest X-ray and/or spinal X-ray (bifid/splayed/ extra ribs; bifid vertebrae)
– Jaw keratocyst. Odontogenic keratocyst histologically	– Macrocephaly (OFC >97th centile)
– Palmar/plantar pits (≥2)	– Cleft lip/palate
– Multiple BCCs (>5 in a lifetime) or a BCC before age 30 years	– Lympho-mesenteric or pleural cysts – Ocular anomalies
– First-degree relative with Gorlin syndrome	– Preaxial or postaxial polydactyly – Ovarian/cardiac fibromas

are inconclusive, the syndrome is confirmed by the presence of a heterozygous germline *PTCH1* or *SUFU* pathogenic variant on genetic test [22].

The main characteristic of this syndrome is the presence of multiple BCCs [1]. Some patients develop more than 1000 BCCs during life and rare are patients who do not develop any [1]. The median number of BCCs in these patients is eight and usually are present in the first years of life [1]. The median age of development is around 20 years [1]. Some affected individuals are radiosensitive, with lesions of BCCs in previous radiation areas [22].

Diagnosis

Two major and one minor criteria

OR

One major and three minor criteria

Key Message

- Autosomal dominant disorder.
- Pathogenic variants in the *PTCH1*, *PTHC2* and *SUFU* genes.
- Diagnosis: Two major diagnostic criteria and one minor diagnostic criteria or one major and three minor diagnostic criteria.
- BCC in a young age.

Bazex-Dupre-Christol Syndrome (Follicular Atrophoderma with BCC)

Inheritance: X-linked dominant disorder [23].

Molecular genetics and pathophysiology: Mutations in the *ARCT1* gene resulting in an activation of the Hedgehog signaling pathway [3].

Clinical features: This syndrome is known by the triad of hypotrichosis, follicular atrophoderma and BCCs [1]. These lesions don't appear simultaneously and they can be observed during the disease, usually by early childhood [1, 23]. The first sign that appears, shortly after birth, is hypotrichosis that tends to be diffuse [1]. Other less common features are trichoepitheliomas, milia cysts, facial hyperpigmentation and hypohidrosis [1]. BCC is very common in these patients and frequently develops around the second decade of life, although there are some cases reported in children [1, 3]. Tumors develop mainly in sun-exposed areas, especially the face and neck, and usually don't present the typical clinical presentation [1]. The tumors can be found in areas of follicular atrophoderma, in comedones and underneath milium cysts [1].

Key Message
- X-linked dominant disorder.
- Mutations in the *ARCT1* gene.
- Triad: hypotrichosis, follicular atrophoderma and BCC.
- Other features: trichoepitheliomas, milia cysts, facial hyperpigmentation and hypohidrosis.
- BCC in a young age.

Xeroderma Pigmentosum

Inheritance: Autosomal recessive disorder [3].

Molecular genetics and pathophysiology: Mutations in two groups of the *XP* genes: *XPA–XPG* and *XP* variant. The first seven genes (*XPA–XPG*) are associated with nucleotide excision repair whereas *XP* variant acts on replication of damaged DNA on the leading strand [24]. Individuals with mutations in one of these genes cannot repair the DNA after UV radiation exposure which predisposes these patients to skin cancer and ocular and/or neurological anomalies [24].

Clinical features: Patients with *XP* have an increased risk of developing NMSC before 9 years old and melanoma before 22 years old, probably due to UV radiation exposure during infancy [24, 25].

Other clinical features presented in these patients are photosensitivity, sunburn, skin aging, lentiginous pigmentation and photophobia [24, 25].

During the diagnosis, it is important to refer the patients to specialized investigation as they have an increased risk of ocular and neurological anomalies [3].

Key Message
- Autosomal recessive disorder.
- *XP* genes (*XPA–XPG*, *XP* variant).
- Photosensitivity, premature skin aging, melanoma and NMSC in early life, photophobia and pigmentary changes.
- Ocular and neurological anomalies.

Rothmund-Thomson Syndrome

Inheritance: Autosomal recessive disorder [26].

Molecular genetics and pathophysiology: Mutations in *RECQL4* gene. This gene is responsible for DNA replication, correcting double-stranded DNA breaks [3, 26]. Mutation in this gene leads to an accumulation of unrepaired DNA damage [3].

Clinical features: The main characteristic of this syndrome is the presence of facial erythema during childhood which spreads to extremities and buttocks without compromising the trunk [26]. This erythema progresses to poikiloderma during lifetime [26]. Patients can develop melanoma and NMSC being skin cancer the second most common cancer after osteossarcoma [26]. These malignancies occur at young age [26].

Key Message
- Autosomal recessive disorder.
- Defect in *RECQL4* gene.
- Consider this diagnostic in patients with poikiloderma, osteosarcoma and melanoma and/or NMSC.

Muir-Torre Syndrome

Inheritance: Autosomal dominant disorder with high penetrance and variable expression [3].

Molecular genetics and pathophysiology: The most frequent genes involved are *MLH1*, *MSH2*, *MSH6* and *PMS2*. Less frequent mutations can affect the *MLH3* and the non-MMR gene *EBCAM*, which epigenetically silences the closely linked *MSH2* gene [27]. It is caused by mutations in DNA mismatch repair genes (*MMR*) which disturb diving cells especially in viscera and skin [3].

Clinical features: Patients present with sebaceous neoplasms including adenomas, epitheliomas and carcinomas that can be aggressive because of local invasion and metastases [3]. Patients with multiple keratoacanthomas should rise suspicious for this syndrome and further investigation is recommended [3].

Even though colorectal cancer is the most common associated visceral cancer, other malignancies can be found. These include gastric and small bowel tumors, endometrial carcinoma, transitional cell carcinoma (ureter and renal pelvis) and ovarian and pancreatic tumors [27].

Key Message
- Autosomal dominant disorder.
- *MLH1*, *MSH2*, *MSH6*, *PMS2*, *MLH3* and *EBCAM* genes.
- Consider this diagnostic in a patient with sebaceous neoplasms, multiple keratoacanthomas and colorectal cancer.

Hereditary Cancer Predisposition Syndromes Predisposing to Melanoma

Melanoma is a complex disease associated with genetic, environmental and phenotypic characteristics that can be lethal if diagnosed in advanced stages [28, 29]. Presence of multiple nevi, atypical nevi as well as personal or family history of melanoma is an important risk factor [29]. About 7–15% of melanoma cases occur in patients with a family history of melanoma [28]. In cancer predisposition syndromes predisposing to melanoma patients usually present with early onset melanomas, multiple primary melanomas (MPM), family history and other internal organ malignancy [30]. The main associated mutation involves the *CDKN2A* gene and less frequently the *CDK4* gene [31].

Hereditary Melanoma Syndrome Related to CDKN2A *Gene*

Inheritance: Autosomal dominant disorder with high penetrance [32].

Molecular genetics and pathophysiology: Mutation in *CDKN2A* gene on chromosome 9p21.3 which encodes two different proteins: p16INK4a and p14ARF. These proteins play a role in cell cycle regulation [28, 33]. In cases of sporadic melanomas, *CDKN2A* can be somatically mutated [5].

Clinical features: *CDKN2A* is the most frequently mutated gene in hereditary melanoma and can be found in approximately 40% of familial melanoma cases [5, 33]. *CDKN2A* can also be found in approximately 10–15% of patients with previous melanoma and no family history [33].

The familial atypical mole and melanoma syndrome (FAMMM) is associated with *CDKN2A* mutation and, less common to CDK4 mutation [31]. Patients present with multiple atypical nevi, higher risk for multiple melanomas and pancreatic cancer [33]. The diagnostic criteria of FAMM includes malignant melanoma in one or more first- or second-degree relatives, more than 50 atypical melanocytic nevi and nevus with certain atypical characteristic in histopathology. To establish the diagnosis the presence of these three criteria is mandatory. An atypical nevus is characterized by the presence of one or more of the following: size >5 mm in diameter, border irregularity, color variegation or asymmetry [34]. Patients with nevi on the buttocks or dorsal feet are known to have the highest risk of being mutation carriers [5]. Mutation carriers tend to develop melanoma 15 years earlier (between 33 and 45 years old) when compared to the general population (53 and 61 years old). Superficial spreading melanoma is most common in *CDKN2A* mutation carriers, especially on the head and neck regions [5]. Clinically the melanomas tend to be thinner. This may be explained because these patients have a more committed skin check-up than the general population [5].

In families with mutation of the *CDKN2A* gene some have multiple melanomas as the predominant primary tumor type while others have early or late onset pancreatic cancer as the predominant primary tumor type [33]. Patients with CDKN2A mutation who develop pancreatic cancer have a worse prognosis compared to the general population [5]. Additionally, *CDKN2A* mutation carriers have an increased risk of other cancers including upper digestive cancer and cancers involving the respiratory tract, especially in ever-smokers [5]. This suggests that *CDKN2A* increases sensitivity to carcinogens in tobacco [5].

Key Message
- Autosomal dominant disorder.
- Most commonly mutated gene associated to hereditary melanoma.
- Associated with the familial atypical mole and melanoma (FAMMM syndrome).
- Individuals are at a higher risk of developing both multiple melanomas and pancreatic cancer.

Hereditary Melanoma Syndrome Related to CDKN2A *Mutations Affecting p14ARF Transcript*

Inheritance: Autosomal dominant disorder with high penetrance [32].
Molecular genetics and pathophysiology: Loss of p14 function [28].
Clinical features: This mutation causes melanoma-astrocytoma syndrome (MAS) that is a variant of FAMMM [28]. Patients develop tumors of the central nervous system, including astrocytoma, and nerve sheath tumors, including neurofibromas and schwannomas in addition to melanoma [5].

Key Message
- Autosomal dominant disorder.
- Melanoma-astrocytoma syndrome: Melanoma and tumors of the central nervous system.

Hereditary Melanoma Syndrome Related to CDK4 *Gene*

Inheritance: Autosomal dominant disorder with high penetrance [32].
Molecular genetics and pathophysiology: Mutation in the *CDK4* gene. This mutation inhibits binding of p16INK4 to *CDK4*, resulting in altered cell cycle regulation [5].

Clinical features: Very rare syndrome. Less than 20 families have been reported in the literature [5]. The clinical features are similar to *CDKN2A* mutation carriers and include the presence of atypical nevi, early onset of melanoma and MPM [5, 32]. Other cancers present in these patients are breast, pancreatic, ovarian, as well as cervical and gastric cancer [5].

Key Message

- Rare.
- Autosomal dominant disorder.
- Early-onset of cutaneous melanoma, development of MPM and presence of atypical nevi.
- Higher risk of developing non-melanoma skin cancers, and other cancers like breast, pancreatic, ovarian, cervical, gastric, among others.

Hereditary Melanoma Syndrome Related to TERT

Inheritance: Autosomal dominant disorder with high penetrance [32]. Somatic mutations have been described in sporadic cases of melanoma [30].

Molecular genetics and pathophysiology: Mutation in *TERT* gene. *TERT* gene regulates telomerase, responsible for the maintenance of telomere length. Mutation in *TERT* gene results in an increased expression of telomerase triggering replication in cancer cells [32, 34].

Clinical features: Besides melanoma, other cancers are related with *TERT* mutations including gliomas, breast, ovarian, prostate, bladder and hepatocellular carcinoma as well as hematological malignances [33]. Acral lentiginous melanomas are frequently related to *TERT* amplification [35].

Another syndrome caused by *TERT* mutation is dyskeratosis congenita (DC). This syndrome may present with mutations in ten different genes that can be X linked, autosomal dominant or recessive. It is characterized by nail dystrophy, reticulated pigmentation, leukoplakia and a higher risk of mucosal and cSCC [1].

Key Message

- Autosomal dominant disorder.
- Higher risk of developing melanoma, hematological malignancies, gliomas, lung cancer, keratinocyte carcinomas, pancreatic, prostate, breast, ovarian, bladder and hepatocellular carcinoma.

Hereditary Melanoma Syndrome Related to Shelterin Complex Genes: POT1, ACD *and* TERF2IP

Inheritance: Autosomal dominant disorder with incomplete penetrance [33].

Molecular genetics and pathophysiology: The shelterin family of genes, *ACD*, *TERF2IP*, *TERF1*, *TERF2*, *TINF2* and *POT1*, regulate telomere processing and stability [5].

Clinical features: Families with *POT1*, *ACD* and *TERF2IP* mutations present with MPM and melanoma at a young age [32]. When *ACD* and *TERFI2P* are mutated some other cancers may develop including lymphoma, leukemia, breast, ovarian, cervical, uterine, thyroid, colon, lung, renal, urinary, prostate and esophageal cancers [5]. *POT1* mutation carriers may manifest brain tumors, especially gliomas. Small cell lung cancer, endometrial cancer and breast cancer can also be found [34].

Key Message
- Autosomal dominant disorder.
- MPM and early-onset melanoma.
- *POT1* mutation is associated with brain tumor, especially glioma.

Hereditary Melanoma Syndrome Related to MITF *Gene*

Inheritance: Autosomal dominant disorder with intermediate penetrance [32].

Molecular genetics and pathophysiology: The *MITF* gene is responsible for melanocyte homeostasis. It encodes a lineage-specific transcription factor concerning cell differentiation, proliferation and survival [32]. Mutation in variant p.E318K results in a gain of expression [5, 32].

Clinical features: *MITF* mutation carriers present with multiple and atypical nevi, darker hair, non-blue eye color and an increased risk for melanoma and renal carcinoma [5, 31].

Key Message
- Autosomal dominant disorder.
- Mutation in *MITF* gene.
- High nevus count, melanoma and increased risk for renal carcinoma.
- Phenotypic characteristics: Non-blue eye color and dark skin.

Hereditary Melanoma Syndrome Related to MC1R *Gene*

Inheritance: Autosomal dominant disorder with lower penetrance [32]. *MC1R* variants autosomal recessive pattern [34].

Molecular genetics and pathophysiology: *MC1R* gene controls hair and skin pigmentation and after UV exposure this gene regulates melanocytes and stimulates DNA repair mechanisms [5]. *MC1R* variants present a reduced receptor function with a switch from eumelanin to pro-oxidant pheomelanin [32, 36]. There are more than 200 variants associated with *MC1R* gene and these variants are classified as "R" or "RHC" alleles because of its association with red hair color or "r" alleles with no association with this phenotype [36].

Clinical features: *MC1R* variants tend to present melanoma independent of phenotypic characteristics. This risk is increased in variants that present two or more *MC1R* variants, in particular *MC1R* "RHC" variant alleles [32]. Melanoma in *MC1R* "r" variant tends to be more common in children and adolescents under 18 years old [36]. Compared to men, women tend to present a lower incidence of melanoma and a better prognosis when presenting "RHC" alleles [36].

Key Message

- Autosomal dominant and recessive disorder.
- Increased risk of melanoma in young age.

Hereditary Melanoma Syndrome Related to BAP1 *Gene*

Inheritance: Autosomal dominant disorder [37].

Molecular genetics and pathophysiology: *BAP1* gene regulates chromatin modulation, transcriptional regulation and DNA damage repair [5]. Tumors show loss of heterozygosity of *BAP1*.

Clinical features: When a germline mutation in *BAP1* occurs, it predisposes carriers to the *BAP1* tumor predisposition syndrome (BAP1-TPDS) [5]. The main cancer associated to this syndrome is uveal melanoma followed by mesothelioma, cutaneous melanoma and renal cell carcinoma. Less frequently associated cancers include BCC, meningioma, cholangiocarcinoma, breast, pancreatic and thyroid cancer [5].

Patients develop multiple melanocytic lesions that clinically resemble dermal nevi but on histology, they are nevoid melanomas or atypical spitz tumors [30].

Key Message

- Autosomal dominant disorder.
- BAP1 tumor predisposition syndrome: Uveal melanoma, mesothelioma, cutaneous melanoma and renal cell carcinoma.

Li-Fraumeni Syndrome

Inheritance: Autosomal dominant disorder with variable penetrance [38].

Molecular genetics and pathophysiology: Mutations in the suppressor tumor gene *TP53* [38].

Clinical features: Li-Fraumeni syndrome (LFS; OMIM #151623) is a very serious cancer predisposition syndrome with onset at early ages [39]. The variety of tumors present in this syndrome is wide. Patients can exhibit hematologic malignancies, soft tissue sarcomas and bone tumors, brain tumors, adrenocortical carcinoma, breast cancer and other less frequent tumors such as neuroblastoma, lung cancer, skin cancer and tumors that involve the gastrointestinal tract, kidneys and thyroid [39]. The risk of melanoma in these patients is still unclear as there are few reports in the literature about skin cancer in these patients [40].

Key Message
- Autosomal dominant disorder.
- Germline *TP53* mutations.
- High and early-onset cancer risk (more frequently brain tumors, adrenocortical carcinoma, sarcomas, breast cancer).

Hereditary Breast and Ovarian Cancer Syndrome Due to Pathogenic Variants in BRCA1 *and* BRCA2 *Genes*

Inheritance: Autosomal dominant disorder [5].

Molecular genetics and pathophysiology: Mutations in *BRCA1* and *BRCA2* genes. These genes are vital for the process of homologous recombination repair which controls the repair of DNA lesions that stall DNA replication forks and/or cause DNA double-strand breaks [41].

Clinical features: Patients with mutations in *BRCA1* and *BRCA2* have a higher risk of breast and ovarian cancer [41]. Previous reports have shown melanoma cases among *BRCA2* mutation carriers although its correlation has not been confirmed [33, 34].

Key Message
- Autosomal dominant disorder.
- Mutations in *BRCA1* and *BRCA2*.
- Breast and ovarian cancer.

Genetic Counseling and Risk Assessment in Cancer Predisposition Syndromes

Genetic counseling is recommended in patients with early onset skin malignancies and multiple primary cutaneous malignancies. Physicians should suspect DNA repair disorders in such a cases and diagnosis should be based on clinical features and/or history of related malignancies and in high-risk melanoma patients. Defining the molecular pathogenic variant that leads to a hereditary cancer predisposition syndrome may enable families to improve early detection and reduce mortality. Dermatologists are fundamental in identifying patients and families who may have an inherited risk for melanoma. Carriers of a cancer predisposition syndrome and a germline pathogenic variant will benefit from tailored screening recommendations and risk-reducing strategies. Adequate pre- and post-test genetic counseling is a major part of the genetic testing process. Incorporating it in routine clinical practice can be challenging. Thus, partnerships with genetic counselors and geneticists are necessary. Genetic counselors are trained to provide cancer risk assessment, discuss benefits and difficulties that one may face in genetic testing, indicating the appropriate test or panel to each individual, and providing management recommendations. Integrating environmental risk factors and hereditary profile may enable a better risk assessment and provide indications on how to define more accurate management strategies. Cascade testing is the process of providing genetic counseling and testing to family members who may also be at risk. This is a strategy that may save lives in high risk families.

References

1. Jaju PD, Ransohoff KJ, Tang JY, Sarin KY. Familial skin cancer syndromes: increased risk of nonmelanotic skin cancers and extracutaneous tumors. J Am Acad Dermatol. 2016;74(3):437–54. https://doi.org/10.1016/j.jaad.2015.08.073.
2. Nikolaou V, Stratigos AJ, Tsao H. Hereditary nonmelanoma skin cancer. Semin Cutan Med Surg. 2012;31(4):204–10. https://doi.org/10.1016/j.sder.2012.08.005.
3. Schierbeck J, Vestergaard T, Bygum A. Skin cancer associated genodermatoses: a literature review. Acta Derm Venereol. 2019;99(4):360–9. https://doi.org/10.2340/00015555-3123.
4. Ramalingam K, Allamaneni SS. Staging melanoma: what's old and new. Surg Clin North Am. 2020;100(1):29–41. https://doi.org/10.1016/j.suc.2019.09.007.
5. Toussi A, Mans N, Welborn J, Kiuru M. Germline mutations predisposing to melanoma. J Cutan Pathol. 2020;47(7):606–16. https://doi.org/10.1111/cup.13689.
6. D'Orazio J, Jarrett S, Amaro-Ortiz A, Scott T. UV radiation and the skin. Int J Mol Sci. 2013;14(6):12222–48. https://doi.org/10.3390/ijms140612222.
7. Leem JL, Asgari M, Marion DW. Cutaneous squamous cell carcinoma: epidemiology, risk factors, and molecular pathogenesis. In: Post TW, editor. UpToDate. Waltham, MA: UpToDate. Accessed 4 Jul 2018.
8. National Comprehensive Cancer Network. Melanoma: cutaneous (version 2.2021). https://www.nccn.org/professionals/physician_gls/pdf/cutaneous_melanoma.pdf. Accessed 3 Jul 2021.

9. Chen ST, Geller AC, Tsao H. Update on the epidemiology of melanoma. Curr Dermatol Rep. 2013;2(1):24–34. https://doi.org/10.1007/s13671-012-0035-5.
10. Dowd MD. Treatment and prevention of pediatric sunburn. Pediatr Ann. 2019;48(6):e213–4. https://doi.org/10.3928/19382359-20190520-02.
11. Markovic SN, Erickson LA, Rao RD, Weenig RH, Pockaj BA, Bardia A, Vachon CM, Schild SE, McWilliams RR, Hand JL, Laman SD, Kottschade LA, Maples WJ, Pittelkow MR, Pulido JS, Cameron JD, Creagan ET, Melanoma Study Group of the Mayo Clinic Cancer Center. Malignant melanoma in the 21st century, part 1: epidemiology, risk factors, screening, prevention, and diagnosis. Mayo Clin Proc. 2007;82(3):364–80. https://doi.org/10.4065/82.3.364.
12. Qureshi AA, Laden F, Colditz GA, Hunter DJ. Geographic variation and risk of skin cancer in US women. Differences between melanoma, squamous cell carcinoma, and basal cell carcinoma. Arch Intern Med. 2008;168(5):501–7. https://doi.org/10.1001/archinte.168.5.501.
13. Rodriguez-Acevedo AJ, Green AC, Sinclair C, van Deventer E, Gordon LG. Indoor tanning prevalence after the International Agency for Research on Cancer statement on carcinogenicity of artificial tanning devices: systematic review and meta-analysis. Br J Dermatol. 2020;182(4):849–59. https://doi.org/10.1111/bjd.18412.
14. Cust AE, Armstrong BK, Goumas C, Jenkins MA, Schmid H, Hopper JL, Kefford RF, Giles GG, Aitken JF, Mann GJ. Sunbed use during adolescence and early adulthood is associated with increased risk of early-onset melanoma. Int J Cancer. 2011;128(10):2425–35. https://doi.org/10.1002/ijc.25576.
15. Yoshinaga S, Hauptmann M, Sigurdson AJ, Doody MM, Freedman DM, Alexander BH, Linet MS, Ron E, Mabuchi K. Nonmelanoma skin cancer in relation to ionizing radiation exposure among U.S. radiologic technologists. Int J Cancer. 2005;115(5):828–34. https://doi.org/10.1002/ijc.20939.
16. Wheeler BW, Allen J, Depledge MH, Curnow A. Radon and skin cancer in Southwest England: an ecologic study. Epidemiology (Cambridge, Mass.). 2012;23(1):44–52. https://doi.org/10.1097/EDE.0b013e31823b6139.
17. Su F, Viros A, Milagre C, Trunzer K, Bollag G, Spleiss O, Reis-Filho JS, Kong X, Koya RC, Flaherty KT, Chapman PB, Kim MJ, Hayward R, Martin M, Yang H, Wang Q, Hilton H, Hang JS, Noe J, Lambros M, et al. RAS mutations in cutaneous squamous-cell carcinomas in patients treated with BRAF inhibitors. N Engl J Med. 2012;366(3):207–15. https://doi.org/10.1056/NEJMoa1105358.
18. González-Cruz C, Ferrándiz-Pulido C, García-Patos Briones V. Melanoma in solid organ transplant recipients. Melanoma en pacientes receptores de un trasplante de órgano sólido. Actas Derm Sifiliogr. 2021;112(3):216–24. https://doi.org/10.1016/j.ad.2020.11.005.
19. Long MD, Martin CF, Pipkin CA, Herfarth HH, Sandler RS, Kappelman MD. Risk of melanoma and nonmelanoma skin cancer among patients with inflammatory bowel disease. Gastroenterology. 2012;143(2):390–399.e1. https://doi.org/10.1053/j.gastro.2012.05.004.
20. Chen ML, Wang SH, Wei JC, Yip HT, Hung YM, Chang R. The impact of human papillomavirus infection on skin cancer: a population-based cohort study. Oncologist. 2021;26(3):e473–83. https://doi.org/10.1002/onco.13593.
21. Serna-Higuita LM, Harrison SL, Buttner P, Glasby M, Raasch BA, Iftner A, Garbe C, Martus P, Iftner T. Modifiable risk-factors for keratinocyte cancers in Australia: a case-control study. Acta Derm Venereol. 2019;99(4):404–11. https://doi.org/10.2340/00015555-3107.
22. Evans DG, Farndon PA. Nevoid basal cell carcinoma syndrome. In: Adam MP, et al., editors. GeneReviews®. Seattle: University of Washington; 2002.
23. AlSabbagh MM, Baqi MA. Bazex-Dupré-Christol syndrome: review of clinical and molecular aspects. Int J Dermatol. 2018;57(9):1102–6. https://doi.org/10.1111/ijd.14065.
24. Parren LJ, Frank J. Hereditary tumour syndromes featuring basal cell carcinomas. Br J Dermatol. 2011;165(1):30–4. https://doi.org/10.1111/j.1365-2133.2011.10334.x.
25. Santiago KM, Castro LP, Neto J, de Nóbrega AF, Pinto C, Ashton-Prolla P, Pinto E, Vairo F, de Medeiros P, Ribeiro EM, Ribeiro B, do Valle FF, Doriqui M, Leite C, Rocha RM, Moura L, Munford V, Galante P, Menck C, Rogatto SR, Achatz MI. Comprehensive germline mutation

analysis and clinical profile in a large cohort of Brazilian xeroderma pigmentosum patients. J Eur Acad Dermatol Venereol. 2020;34(10):2392–401. https://doi.org/10.1111/jdv.16405.
26. Sharma R, Lewis S, Wlodarski MW. DNA repair syndromes and cancer: insights into genetics and phenotype patterns. Front Pediatr. 2020;8:570084. https://doi.org/10.3389/fped.2020.570084.
27. Simic D, Dummer R, Freiberger SN, Ramelyte E, Barysch MJ. Clinical and molecular features of skin malignancies in Muir-Torre syndrome. Genes. 2021;12(5):781. https://doi.org/10.3390/genes12050781.
28. Soura E, Eliades PJ, Shannon K, Stratigos AJ, Tsao H. Hereditary melanoma: update on syndromes and management: genetics of familial atypical multiple mole melanoma syndrome. J Am Acad Dermatol. 2016;74(3):395–410. https://doi.org/10.1016/j.jaad.2015.08.038.
29. Sá B, Moredo LF, Gomes EE, Araújo E, Duprat JP. Hereditary melanoma: a five-year study of Brazilian patients in a cancer referral center—phenotypic characteristics of probands and pathological features of primary tumors. An Bras Dermatol. 2018;93(3):337–40. https://doi.org/10.1590/abd1806-4841.20186201.
30. Soura E, Eliades PJ, Shannon K, Stratigos AJ, Tsao H. Hereditary melanoma: update on syndromes and management: emerging melanoma cancer complexes and genetic counseling. J Am Acad Dermatol. 2016;74(3):411–22. https://doi.org/10.1016/j.jaad.2015.08.037.
31. Gironi LC, Colombo E, Pasini B, Giorgione R, Farinelli P, Zottarelli F, Esposto E, Zavattaro E, Allara E, Ogliara P, Betti M, Dianzani I, Savoia P. Melanoma-prone families: new evidence of distinctive clinical and histological features of melanomas in CDKN2A mutation carriers. Arch Dermatol Res. 2018;310(10):769–84. https://doi.org/10.1007/s00403-018-1866-0.
32. Rossi M, Pellegrini C, Cardelli L, Ciciarelli V, Di Nardo L, Fargnoli MC. Familial melanoma: diagnostic and management implications. Dermatol Pract Concept. 2019;9(1):10–6. https://doi.org/10.5826/dpc.0901a03.
33. Lee KC, Higgins HW 2nd, Qureshi AA. Familial risk of melanoma and links with other cancers. Melanoma Manag. 2015;2(1):83–9. https://doi.org/10.2217/mmt.14.34.
34. Read J, Wadt KA, Hayward NK. Melanoma genetics. J Med Genet. 2016;53(1):1–14. https://doi.org/10.1136/jmedgenet-2015-103150.
35. Hosler GA, Davoli T, Mender I, Litzner B, Choi J, Kapur P, Shay JW, Wang RC. A primary melanoma and its asynchronous metastasis highlight the role of BRAF, CDKN2A, and TERT. J Cutan Pathol. 2015;42(2):108–17. https://doi.org/10.1111/cup.12444.
36. Manganelli M, Guida S, Ferretta A, Pellacani G, Porcelli L, Azzariti A, Guida G. Behind the scene: exploiting MC1R in skin cancer risk and prevention. Genes. 2021;12(7):1093. https://doi.org/10.3390/genes12071093.
37. Murali R, Wiesner T, Scolyer RA. Tumours associated with BAP1 mutations. Pathology. 2013;45(2):116–26. https://doi.org/10.1097/PAT.0b013e32835d0efb.
38. de Andrade KC, Mirabello L, Stewart DR, Karlins E, Koster R, Wang M, Gapstur SM, Gaudet MM, Freedman ND, Landi MT, Lemonnier N, Hainaut P, Savage SA, Achatz MI. Higher-than-expected population prevalence of potentially pathogenic germline TP53 variants in individuals unselected for cancer history. Hum Mutat. 2017;38(12):1723–30. https://doi.org/10.1002/humu.23320.
39. Kratz CP, Achatz MI, Brugières L, Frebourg T, Garber JE, Greer MC, Hansford JR, Janeway KA, Kohlmann WK, McGee R, Mullighan CG, Onel K, Pajtler KW, Pfister SM, Savage SA, Schiffman JD, Schneider KA, Strong LC, Evans D, Wasserman JD, et al. Cancer screening recommendations for individuals with Li-Fraumeni syndrome. Clin Cancer Res. 2017;23(11):e38–45. https://doi.org/10.1158/1078-0432.CCR-17-0408.
40. Giavedoni P, Ririe M, Carrera C, Puig S, Malvehy J. Familial melanoma associated with Li-Fraumeni syndrome and atypical mole syndrome: total-body digital photography, dermoscopy and confocal microscopy. Acta Derm Venereol. 2017;97(6):720–3. https://doi.org/10.2340/00015555-2639.
41. Johansson PA, Nathan V, Bourke LM, Palmer JM, Zhang T, Symmons J, Howlie M, Patch AM, Read J, Holland EA, Schmid H, Warrier S, Glasson W, Höiom V, Wadt K, Jönsson G, Olsson

H, Ingvar C, Mann G, Brown KM, et al. Evaluation of the contribution of germline variants in BRCA1 and BRCA2 to uveal and cutaneous melanoma. Melanoma Res. 2019;29(5):483–90. https://doi.org/10.1097/CMR.0000000000000613.

Chapter 5
Principles of the Dermatologic Assessment of Cutaneous Lesions

João Paulo Junqueira, Cristina Martinez Zugaib Abdalla, and Fernando Augusto de Almeida

Key Points
- Dermatological skin diseases can often be diagnosed based on physical examination.
- Primary skin lesions are those developed on the onset of a skin disease and secondary lesions are developed secondary to a disease progression.
- Clinical examination represents a gross macroscopy of histopathology.
- The knowledge of dermatological standardized terminology is vital for any physician in oncodermatology care.

Dermatological skin diseases can often be diagnosed based on physical examination. Classifying skin lesions into their specific morphologies is the first step in diagnosing skin diseases [1].

Palpation is essential to assess tenderness, consistency, induration, depth of skin lesions. Additional maneuvers besides palpation like pressing, stretching, rubbing, squeezing, and scratching are important for complementary information.

Some Instrumental tests, such as diascopy with glass spatula, Brocq's methodical curettage (vigorous scratching or picking off the scale produces small bleeding points—Auspitz's sign), and assessment of skin sensibility are part of the physical examination.

The dermatologic lesions can be classified according to some categories as per lesion's morphology. It is divided into primary and secondary lesions [2–4].

J. P. Junqueira · C. M. Z. Abdalla (✉) · F. A. de Almeida
Hospital Sírio-Libanês, São Paulo, Brazil

C. M. Z. Abdalla et al. (eds.), *Oncodermatology*,
https://doi.org/10.1007/978-3-031-29277-4_5

Primary Lesions

Primary skin lesions are those developed on the onset of a skin disease.

Primary Skin Lesions with Liquid-Filled Lesions

Abscess

Collection of purulent material deep in the dermis and/or subcutaneous tissue with or without drainage, usually accompanied by pain, swelling, and erythema. The lesion presents fluid sensation when pressed.

Bullae/Blister

Circumscribed collections of fluid (serous, hematic, or purulent content) secondary to cleavage plane of epidermis or dermal-epidermal junction (blisters are up to 1 cm and bullae upward of 1 cm).

Cyst

Cyst is an encapsulated cavity or sac that contains fluid or semi-fluid material. It may be firm or fluctuant and often distends the overlying skin.

Hematoma

Circumscribed blood collection in the dermis or subcutaneous layer. A possible location is also subungual space and subcorneal layer (palmoplantar lesion).

Pustule

A small, circumscribed raised lesion in the epidermis or infundibulum, measures less than 1 cm, filled with pus. The purulent exudate is made up of leucocytes, may contain cellular debris, bacteria, or fungi.

Vesicle

Vesicle is a fluid-filled cavity smaller than 0.5 cm, tense or flaccid, depending on the cleavage plane of epidermis or dermis (subcorneal, intraepidermal, or subepidermal).

Flat Primary Skin Lesions

Macule

Macules are circumscribed modification of skin color <1 cm, neither elevated nor depressed. It doesn't involve any change in the thickness or texture, could be hyperchromic, hypochromic, and achromic. Vascular macules could be erythematous, purpuric, petechiae, angiomatous, or anemic (Figs. 5.1 and 5.2).

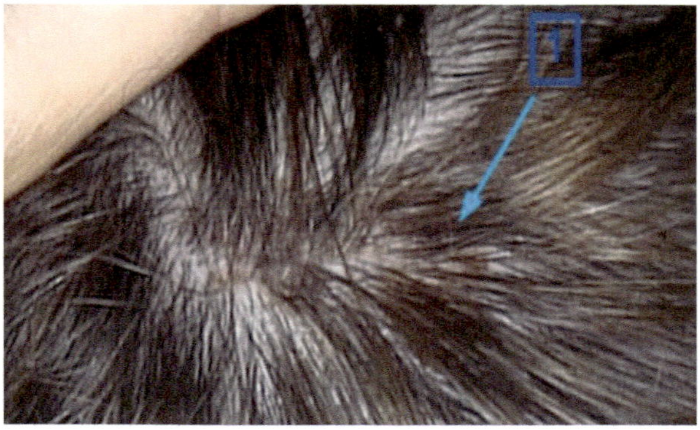

Fig. 5.1 Lentigo maligna—brown irregular macule on the scalp. (Courtesy of Fernando de Almeida, MD)

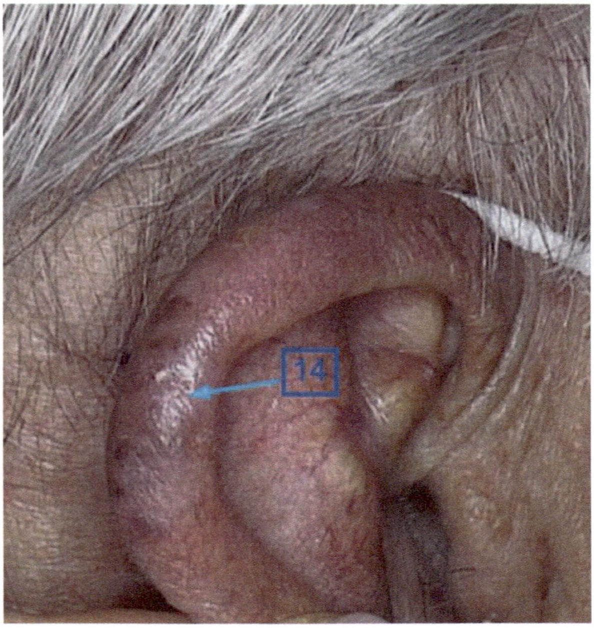

Fig. 5.2 Lentigo maligna—irregular pigmented macule on the helix. (Courtesy of Fernando de Almeida, MD)

Patch

It is similar to a macule, larger, >1 cm and may have surface change such as fine desquamation. These lesions are very important in cutaneous oncology because cutaneous lymphomas, melanomas, and carcinomas could appear as macules and patches.

Telangiectasias

Telangiectasias are small, dilated vessels less than 2 mm on the skin surface. In dermoscopy telangiectasia-like "arborizing vessels" is a characteristic feature of basal cell carcinoma (BCC) with distinct tree-like branching.

Solid Primary Skin Lesions

Most of skin cancers are solid lesions.

Nodule

Solid, circumscribed, and palpable lesions that measure from 1 to 3 cm. Lesions measuring more than 3 cm are called tumor masses. Some skin cancers can be seen as a nodule that enlarges over weeks to months. Some examples are nodular melanoma, cutaneous lymphoma, and even skin metastasis (Fig. 5.3).

Papule

Solid, circumscribed, elevated lesions of less than 1 cm surrounded by plane skin that could be rough or smooth, sessile, flat-topped, or umbilicated. The papules are very common findings in many different skin diseases and skin cancers like BCC, SCC, Merkel carcinoma, nodular melanoma, among others (Figs. 5.4, 5.5, and 5.6).

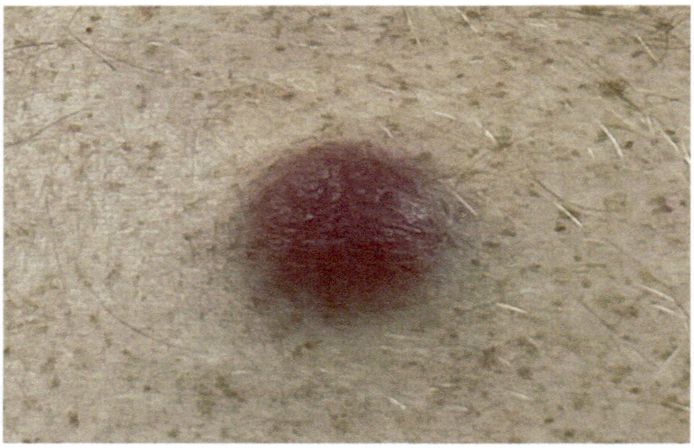

Fig. 5.3 Skin metastasis of small bowel adenocarcinoma—well delimitated nodular lesion. (Courtesy of Cristina Abdalla, MD)

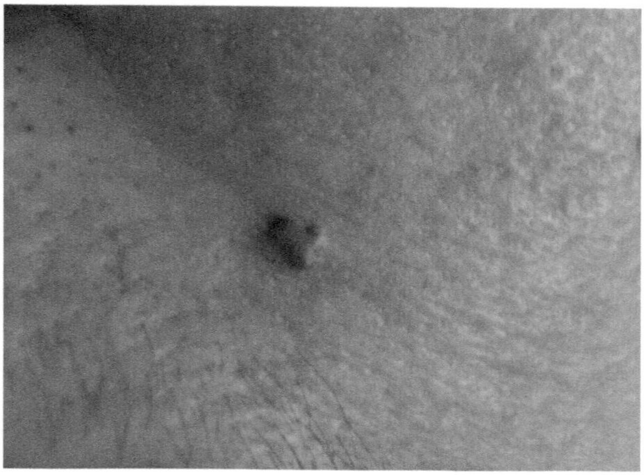

Fig. 5.4 Pigmented BCC—pearly pigmented papule in the nasolabial fold. (Courtesy of Fernando de Almeida, MD)

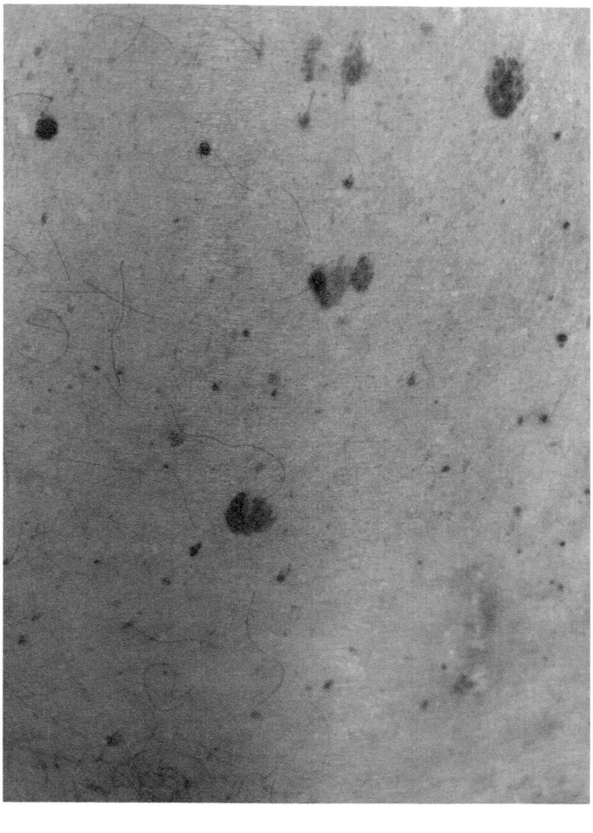

Fig. 5.5 Cherry angiomas and seborrheic keratosis—angiomatous papules and pigmented plaques. (Courtesy of Fernando de Almeida, MD)

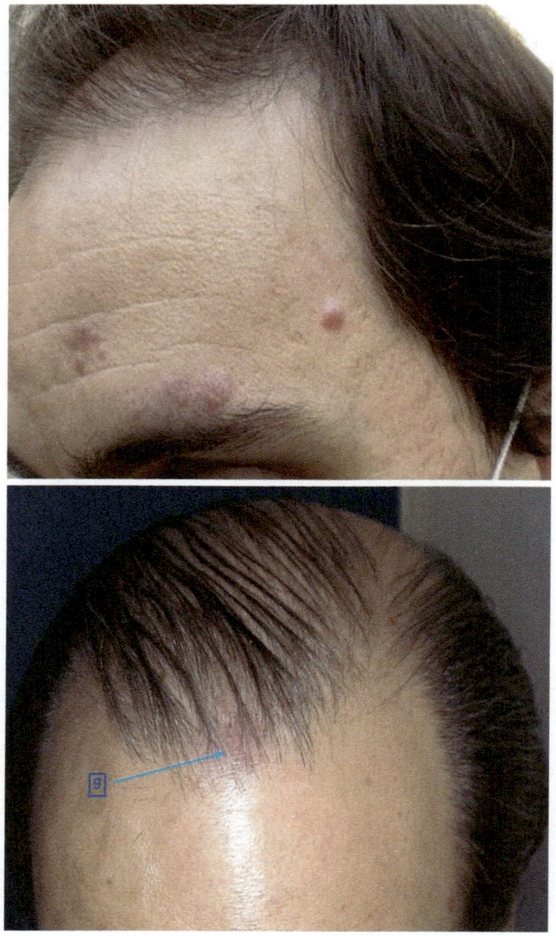

Fig. 5.6 Cutaneous primary B cell follicle center lymphoma—erythematous papules and plaques in the forehead. (Courtesy of Fernando de Almeida, MD)

Plaque

Skin plaques are circumscribed, elevated, plateau-like lesion (>1 cm) with well delimited borders. The lesion could be indurated, scaly, with crusts or maceration. Plaques are commonly described in a variety of skin tumors, like cutaneous lymphomas (Figs. 5.6, 5.7, and 5.8).

Wheals

Wheals are irregularly shaped, elevated, annular, serpiginous, round, or oval tiny papules or giant plaques that are evanescent, disappearing in 24 h. The lesions usually are reddish to pink or could be white-porcelain color. The shape may change, and these lesions are usually pruritic.

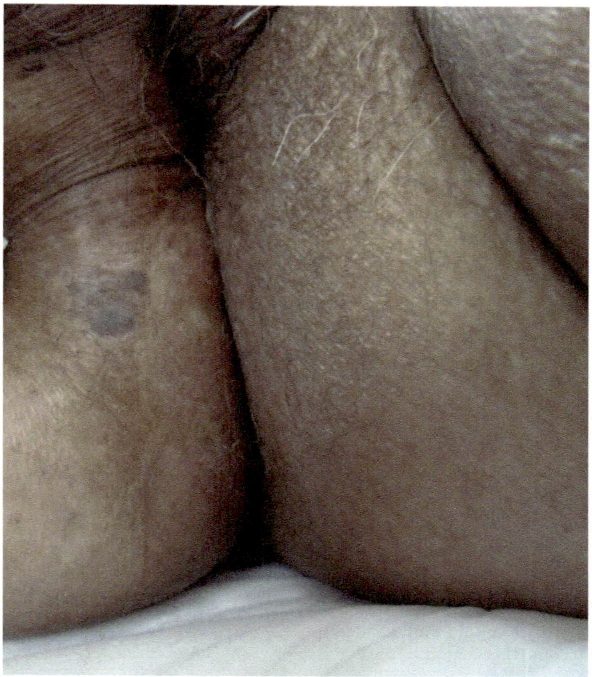

Fig. 5.7 In situ SCC—irregular pigmented plaque mimicking melanocytic lesion. (Courtesy of Fernando de Almeida, MD)

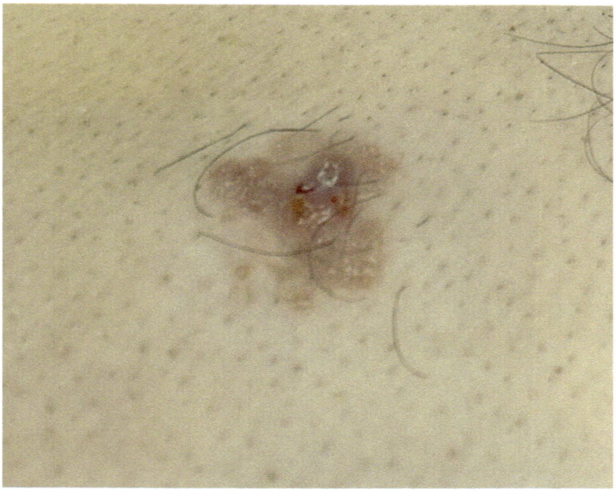

Fig. 5.8 Bowen's disease—erythematous plaque on the thigh. (Courtesy of Cristina Abdalla, MD)

Vegetation

Papillomatous growths of the skin that could be keratotic or friable. It is usually fast-growing skin lesions like in viral warts, but also in skin tumors (Figs. 5.9 and 5.10).

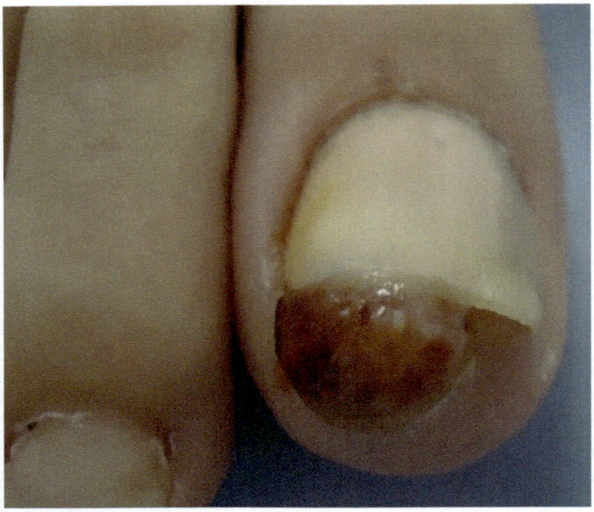

Fig. 5.9 Amelanotic melanoma—subungueal vegetative nodule. (Courtesy of Fernando de Almeida, MD)

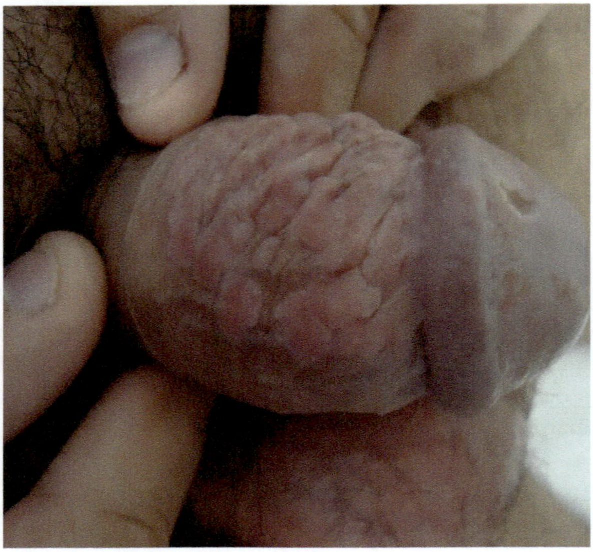

Fig. 5.10 Erythroplasia of Queyrat—penile intraepithelial neoplasia grade III elevated erythematous vegetative plaque on the skin of the penis. (Courtesy of Fernando de Almeida, MD)

Secondary Lesions

Secondary skin lesions are developed from changes secondary to disease progression, even manipulation and/or after treatment.

Atrophy

The atrophy is a thinning of the epidermal and/or dermal tissue. The skin can be thin, roughed/wrinkled, and depressed.

Edema

Edema is an abnormal infiltration and accumulation of serous fluid in the dermis.

Sclerosis

Sclerosis is a circumscribed or diffuse hardening of the skin secondary to dermal fibrosis. This lesion is rather palpable than visible.

Lichenification

Lichenification refers to a thickened, hyperpigmented skin lesion with exaggerated skin lines. It could be secondary to chronic inflammation caused by scratching or other irritation.

Scars

Scar is a permanent fibrotic skin lesion that develops in consequence of an injury in which normal tissue is replaced by fibrous tissue. Scars may be hypertrophic, atrophic, sclerotic, and are secondary to collagen proliferation. Some melanomas can regress producing skin findings described as scar-like appearance which can complicate the determination of Breslow index.

Secondary Elementary Lesions Caused by Substance Loss

Crust

Crust is secondary to dry blood, serum, sebum, or purulent material on skin surface or lesion. It can be present as an evolution of some tumors after ulceration.

Erosion

Erosion is a consequence of the superficial and partial loss of the epidermal layer or mucosal. The lesion is depressed, moist, and raw. Multiple superficial erosions are a dermatoscopic finding described in superficial BCC and larger erosions in nodular BCC.

Ulcer

Ulcers are deeper than erosions with focal loss of epidermis, and that can reach the dermis, subcutaneous, or even muscle and bone depth. Ulceration could be seen in different skin cancers.

Fissure

It's a linear sharp skin cleft of variable depth that is formed when skin is brittle, dry, or thickened.

Fistulae

It's an abnormal connection between the epithelialized surface with or without drainage.

Scale

Scales are the accumulation or excess shedding of the stratum corneum. It is present in actinic keratosis and SCC.

There are other important aspects to consider diagnosing skin diseases like shape, configuration, arrangement, and distribution (Table 5.1).

The first step to diagnose skin tumors depends on the ability to perform skin examination. The knowledge of dermatological standardized terminology is vital for any physician in oncodermatology care.

Table 5.1 Possible clinical findings in skin tumors

Clinical feature	BCC	SCC	Melanoma	Merkel carcinoma	Kaposi sarcoma	Other sarcomas	Cutaneous lymphomas
Macules			✓		✓		✓
Papules	✓	✓	✓	✓	✓	✓	✓
Plaques	✓	✓	✓	✓	✓	✓	✓
Patches							✓
Nodules	✓	✓	✓	✓	✓	✓	✓
Telangiectasia	✓	✓	✓	✓	✓		
Vegetation	✓	✓	✓				✓
Cystic	✓						
Crust	✓	✓	✓	✓	✓		✓
Erosion	✓	✓	✓	✓	✓	✓	✓
Ulcer	✓	✓	✓	✓	✓	✓	✓
Pigmented	✓	Rarely	✓				
Erythematous	✓	✓	Rarely	✓	✓	✓	✓
Violaceus				✓	✓		✓
Angiomatous				✓	✓		✓
Pearly	✓						
Papillomatous/verrucous		✓					
Keratotic		✓					
Infiltrated	✓	✓	✓	✓	✓	✓	✓
Well-delimited	✓	✓	✓		✓	✓	✓
Poor-delimited	✓	✓	✓	✓	✓	✓	✓
Solitary lesion	✓	✓	✓	✓	✓	✓	✓
Multiple lesions	✓	✓			✓	✓	✓

BCC basal cell carcinoma, *SCC* squamous cell carcinoma

References

1. Wilmer EN, Gustafson CJ, Ahn CS, Davis SA, Feldman SR, Huang WW. Most common dermatologic conditions encountered by dermatologists and nondermatologists. Cutis. 2014;94(6):285–92.
2. Cox NH. Palpation of the skin—an important issue. J R Soc Med. 2006;99(12):598–600. https://doi.org/10.1258/jrsm.99.12.598.
3. Rimoin L, Altieri L, Craft N, Krasne S, Kellman PJ. Training pattern recognition of skin lesion morphology, configuration, and distribution. J Am Acad Dermatol. 2015;72(3):489–95. https://doi.org/10.1016/j.jaad.2014.11.016. Epub 2015 Jan 13.
4. Vasconcellos C, Criado PR. Semiologia Dermatológica e Lesões Elementares. In: Belda Junior W, Di Chiacchio N, Criado PR, editors. Tratado de Dermatologia. Rio de Janeiro: Atheneu; 2018. p. 91–112.

Chapter 6
Ancillary Tools for Dermatological Skin Assessment: Dermoscopy, Reflectance Confocal Microscopy and Optical Coherence Tomography

Ana Maria Fagundes Sortino, Cristina Martinez Zugaib Abdalla, Beatrice Martinez Zugaib Abdalla, Juan Manuel Piñeiro-Maceira, Naiara A. Fraga Braghiroli, Juliana Casagrande Tavoloni Braga, Bianca Costa Soares de Sá, Tatiana Cristina Moraes Pinto Blumetti, Elimar Elias Gomes, Ana Carolina Souza Porto Mitsunaga, Lílian Kelly Faria Licarião Rocha, and Maria Fernanda Vianna Hunziker

A. M. F. Sortino (✉) · C. M. Z. Abdalla · B. M. Z. Abdalla · M. F. V. Hunziker
Hospital Sírio-Libanês, São Paulo, Brazil
e-mail: ana.m.sortino@dermatis.com.br

J. M. Piñeiro-Maceira
Universidade do Estado do Rio de Janeiro, Rio de Janeiro, Brazil

N. A. Fraga Braghiroli
Miami Cancer Institute, Miami, FL, USA

J. C. T. Braga · B. C. S. de Sá · T. C. M. P. Blumetti · A. C. S. P. Mitsunaga
AC Camargo Cancer Center, São Paulo, Brazil

E. E. Gomes
BP—A Beneficiência Portuguesa de São Paulo, São Paulo, Brazil

L. K. F. L. Rocha
Hospital das Clínicas de São Paulo, São Paulo, Brazil

C. M. Z. Abdalla et al. (eds.), *Oncodermatology*,
https://doi.org/10.1007/978-3-031-29277-4_6

Key Points

- Dermoscopy, reflectance confocal microscopy (RCM) and optical coherence tomography (OCT) are imaging devices that help to make an early diagnosis with greater accuracy.
- Ancillary tools should be used complementary to a complete skin exam and applied to selected lesions. Decision making to perform an excision should be integrated with medical information, clinical examination, and the patient's context.
- Dermoscopy permits the observation of colors and structures, allowing the clinician to see the correspondence between morphology and histopathology.
- Reflectance confocal microscopy (RCM) is a noninvasive, in vivo, technique that allows the evaluation of the skin with quasi-histological resolution.
- OCT is mostly used to evaluate non-melanoma skin cancers, however there are fewer studies for melanocytic lesions. The black and white images are like conventional histology. The software is also capable of building 3D images.

Dermoscopy

Basic Principles of Dermoscopy, Equipment, and Histopathological Correlations

Dermoscopy, also known as dermatoscopy or epiluminescense microscopy, is a noninvasive method that allows in vivo evaluation of the subsurface of pigmented and non-pigmented skin lesions, using a handheld light examination device, called dermatoscope [1–4]. The principle of dermoscopy is based on the understanding that by assessing a lesion with the naked eye, the stratum corneum reflects light, and structures under the skin are not visible. By applying a dermatoscope, that illuminates and magnifies a skin lesion, the observation of colors and structures of the epidermis, dermo-epidermal junction, and the papillary dermis are possible. This opens a new realm for skin lesions evaluation that, in the hands of experienced users, can improve clinical diagnostic accuracy [5–9].

This technique should be used complementary to a complete skin exam and applied to selected lesions. Decision making to perform an excision should be integrated with medical information, clinical examination, and the patient's context [5, 8]. Over the past years, dermoscopy has evolved and is now widely used for the examination of skin lesions presenting a 60–90% sensitivity in the diagnosis of melanoma [9]. Today dermatoscopes are becoming the dermatologist's stethoscope to aid early skin cancer diagnosis and reduce the number of unnecessarily excised lesions [10].

There is a wide variety of handheld and video dermatoscopes on the market, with different magnification capacities and varied illumination properties. Dermoscopy can be performed with or without contact with skin lesions. First, it's important to understand the devices and dermoscopic modalities described below:

- Nonpolarized dermatoscopes today provide illumination with light-emitting diodes and are equipped with a 10× magnification lens. It's necessary to have direct contact of the device glass plate with the skin. A liquid interface (water, alcohol, gel, or mineral oil) between the dermatoscope glass plate and the skin is required. It decreases light refraction and makes the stratum corneum appear more translucent, allowing for a nonpolarized dermoscopy (NPD). The 70% liquid alcohol is a good choice for skin lesions since it yields fewer air bubbles and provides clearer images, with the added benefit of its cleaning and disinfection properties. However, for nail and convex surfaces' examination ultrasound or antibacterial gels are superior [6, 11].
- Polarized dermatoscopes contain white light-emitting diodes, with 10× optical magnification, and two light polarizers (cross-polarized devices). They capture the backscattered light from deeper layers of the skin, allowing for a polarized dermoscopy (PD). The advantages are elimination of the need for liquid interface, permitting a noncontact examination and a relatively rapid scanning of lesions. Some devices award the option between noncontact and contact polarized dermoscopy; the latter can be used with or without the application of fluid onto the lesion. It's possible to attach this type of dermatoscope to cameras or mobile devices for pictures of the dermoscopic structures, zooming on specific features and storing images for future reference. This is known as digital dermoscopy (DD) [6, 11].
- "Hybrid" dermatoscopes grant the benefit to switch between polarized and nonpolarized dermoscopy using the same device; however, the glass plate must be in direct contact with a liquid interface to allow the observation of the lesion dermoscopic structures in both modes [6].
- Video dermatoscopes are full high-definition (HD) video cameras attached to a dermoscopy microscope that uses white light-emitting diodes, with 20–400× optical magnification. They allow digital dermoscopy, by capturing images of contact NPD and PD, but also noncontact PD images. They are linked to a computer, and they simplify the process of image acquisition, storage, organization, retrieval, image viewing, and comparison over time. Many systems have incorporated computer-based analytical algorithms and artificial intelligence to assist clinicians in managing skin lesions [6, 11]. The importance of digital dermoscopic monitoring (DDM) is the information regarding lesion changes over time and is very useful for diagnosing an early melanoma in high-risk patients [9].

Most lesions can be correctly diagnosed by either NPD or PD; however, there are some important differences that must be known and understood to avoid misdiagnosis (Fig. 6.1). Under NPD the stratum corneum and upper epidermis are well seen; this is the reason why blue-white color (orthokeratosis and/or regression) and milia-like cysts (horn pseudocysts in the epidermis) are better observed on this mode. Under PD the upper skin layers are "blinded" making the blue-white color and milia-like cysts less visible. By toggling between NPD and PD over a lesion one can clearly see the difference, also known as "blink sign," on dermoscopy [6, 11, 12].

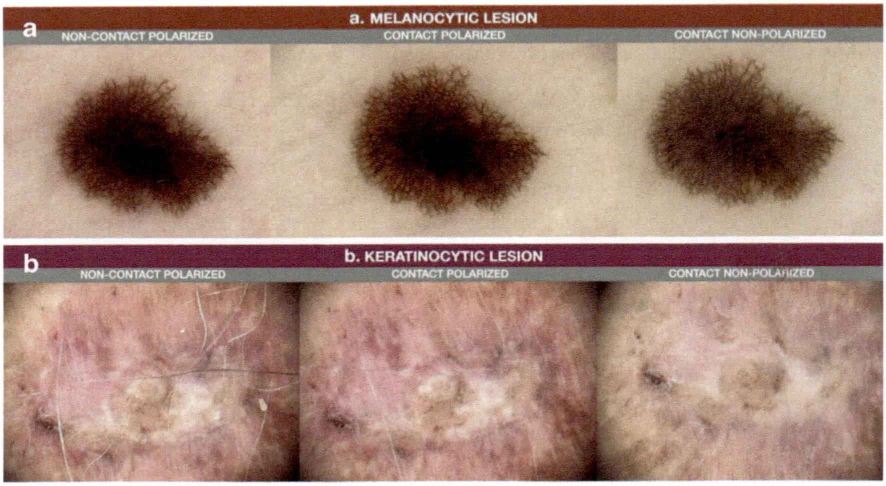

Fig. 6.1 (**a**) Dermoscopy of a MELANOCYTIC LESION under 20× magnification, showing the differences between noncontact polarized, contact polarized, and contact nonpolarized dermoscopy. (**b**) Dermoscopy of a KERATINOCYTIC LESION under 20× magnification, showing the differences between noncontact polarized, contact polarized, and contact nonpolarized dermoscopy. (*Dermoscopy courtesy of Ana Maria Sortino MD, MSc*)

Although PD is not ideal for evaluating the skin superficial layer, it does improve the examination of deeper skin layers, enhancing the melanin pigment that can appear in varying shades of brown and blue (Tyndall effect), allowing better observation of the red and pink colors (vascular structures) and the presence of white shiny areas (chrysalis or white scar). The use of both NPD and PD provides complementary information, and they should be used for the assessment of a suspicious lesion, helping the clinician reach a higher diagnostic accuracy [6].

Colors are fundamental in dermoscopic evaluation, they correlate with different chromophores and skin layers, being useful to evaluate depth (Fig. 6.2). The main chromophore in pigmented lesions is melanin, which can vary from black, different shades of brown to blue. This will depend on its location and concentration. In the stratum corneum, melanin can appear black. In the Malpighian layer, melanin is seen with a light brown color, and when in the dermal epidermal junction it is a darker brown. When melanin reaches the upper dermis, it can be seen as a gray color and more profoundly as a blue color. Other chromophores are hemoglobin, which is perceived as pink to red or blue to purple. Collagen and keratin within cysts appear white. Yellow color can be seen in sebaceous structures and keratin, lipids, pus, serum, and granuloma [6, 13].

Besides colors, dermoscopy allows the observer to identify how these pigments are distributed throughout the lesion. This distribution is called structure and the structures create a pattern. In the very beginning, structures had a metaphoric correspondence. In 2015 a consensus decided to avoid the use of metaphoric terms, affirming that dermoscopic structures should be referred by descriptive terminology. Nowadays both terminologies are used [6, 7, 13–15].

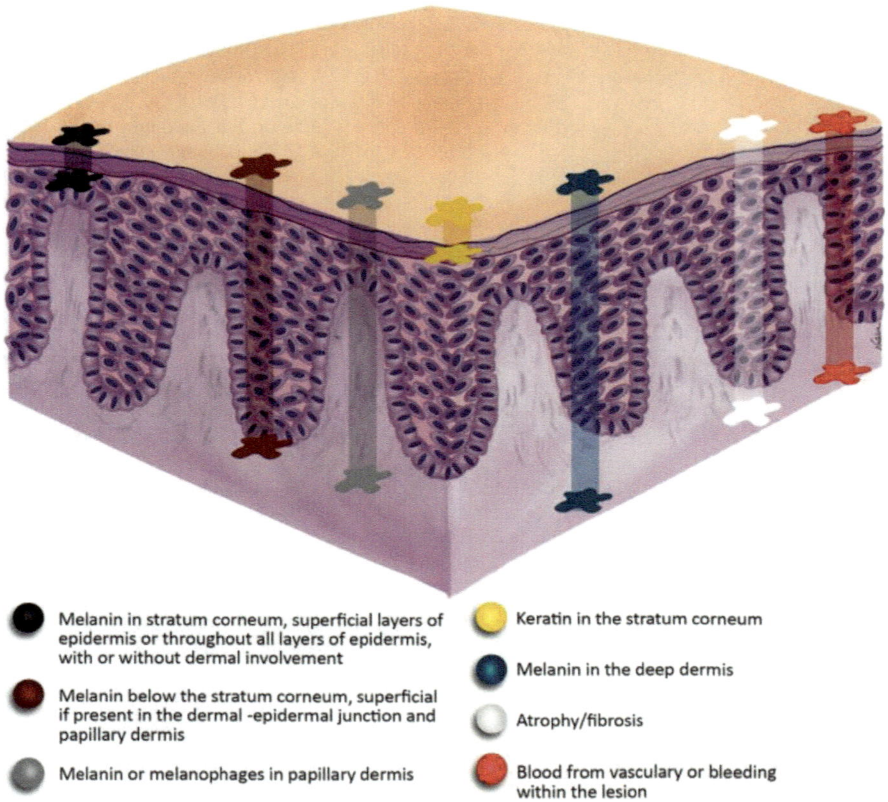

Fig. 6.2 Diagram of colors seen with dermoscopy and histopathologic correlation

Dermoscopy and Histopathological Correlation

Dermoscopy permits the observation of colors and structures, allowing the clinician to see the correspondence between morphology and histopathology (HP). There is correlation of the patterns and features observed on dermoscopy (en-face horizontal view of the entire lesion) and the histopathological structures (in-depth vertical cellular examination) [6, 7].

In benign skin tumors the correlation between dermoscopy and histopathology helps one to understand most of the dermoscopy images (Fig. 6.3). Classical dermatofibroma presents hyperpigmented elongated rete ridges which correspond to the peripheral network on dermoscopy while the effaced non-pigmented epidermis in the central portion correlates with the central white scar-like patch on dermoscopy. These secondary epidermal changes allow the dermoscopic diagnosis; the tumor however is in the reticular dermis. Both dermoscopy and histopathology clearly demonstrate the main diagnostic criteria of seborrheic keratosis: horn pseudocysts

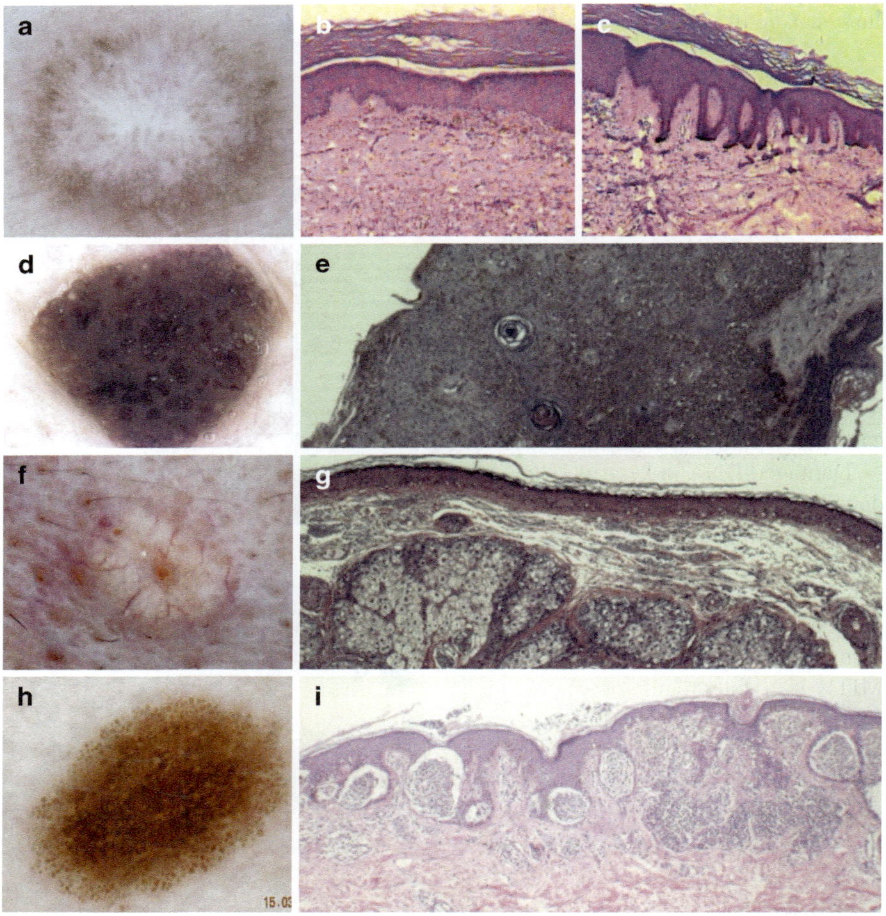

Fig. 6.3 The central white scar-like patch and the peripheral network on dermoscopy (**a**) correlate very well with the histopathology (**b**, **c**) of classic dermatofibroma. Horn pseudocysts inside an amorphous area (**d**) correspond to the pseudocysts encircled by a hyperpigmented acanthotic epidermis (**e**) in seborrheic keratosis. Multilobulated yellowish structures (**f**) correspond to the prominent sebaceous glands in sebaceous hyperplasia (**g**). The combination of reticular, globular, and homogenous patterns (**h**) is reflected in the histopathology of combined nevi by the simultaneous occurrence of elongated rete ridges and junctional nests over sheets of nevus cells in the superficial dermis (**i**). (*Dermoscopy and histopathology images courtesy of Juan Piñeiro-Maceira, MD, MSc, PhD*)

and amorphous areas which indicate an enlarged and hyperpigmented epidermis engulfing cyst-like areas of keratin. The prominent sebaceous glands under an effaced epidermis in sebaceous hyperplasia appear on dermoscopy as multilobulated yellowish structures surrounded by crown vessels that extend toward the center of the lesion without crossing it (the vessels however aren't so exuberant on histopathology). Multiple dilated aggregated vessels in the superficial reticular dermis are responsible for the round to oval reddish-blue areas characteristic of the dermoscopy of hemangiomas. Junctional melanocytic nevi are easily recognized on dermoscopy by the reticular or the globular patterns in different lesions. These are reflected by elongated hyperpigmented rete ridges with an increased number of nevoid melanocytes along the basal layer or the grouping of the proliferating melanocytes into nests along the dermoepidermal junction (DEJ). In compound nevi due to the overlapping of the proliferating nevus cells in the epidermis and in the dermis with an irregular distribution of the melanin pigmentation there is an increased chance of a combination of reticular, globular, and homogenous patterns [6, 7, 13, 14, 16].

In the evaluation of malignant skin tumors or suspicious lesions the differences between dermoscopy and histopathology are striking because in the latter cytopathologic criteria are very important and these are not really depicted on dermoscopy. Therefore, an integrated analysis of both types of microscopies is highly recommended for the correct diagnosis. If a cutaneous lesion cannot be readily classified as benign versus malignant on dermoscopy, usually it will present some degree of difficulty in histopathology as well (Fig. 6.4). Radial streaks and pseudopods on dermoscopy of a pigmented lesion make it highly suspicious for malignancy because they are present in several melanomas; however, they may also occur in atypical nevi and appear on histopathology as intense bridging of proliferating melanocytes

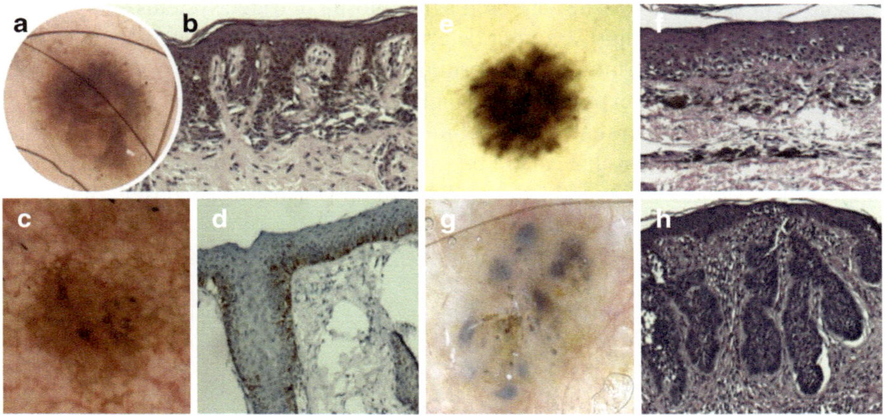

Fig. 6.4 Radial streaks and pseudopods on dermoscopy of a pigmented lesion (**a**) may correspond to the intense bridging of proliferated melanocytes occupying the dermoepidermal junction in atypical nevi (**b**). The characteristic rhomboidal structures of lentigo maligna melanoma (**c**) correspond in histopathology to involvement of the infundibular epithelium by malignant melanocytes (**d**). Heavily pigmented small lesions on dermoscopy (**e**) may represent the early stage of a melanoma showing only a continuous and confluent proliferation of hyperpigmented pleomorphic melanocytes at the DEJ and melanin incontinence into the dermis (**f**). The ovoid nests detected by dermoscopy in basal cell carcinoma (**g**) are reproduced by the islands of basal cells seen in histopathology (**h**). (*Dermoscopy and histopathology images courtesy of Juan Piñeiro-Maceira, MD, MSc, PhD*)

occupying the dermoepidermal junction. Lentigo maligna melanoma of sun damaged skin is characterized by rhomboidal structures that correspond on histopathology to the evident involvement of the infundibular epithelium by proliferation of malignant melanocytes. Intensely pigmented small lesions, which on dermoscopy leave little doubt that they are malignant, may only show a continuous and confluent proliferation of hyperpigmented pleomorphic melanocytes along the dermoepidermal junction accompanied by melanin incontinence, indicating the early development of a malignant melanocytic lesion. Actinic keratosis presents on dermoscopy basically as areas of intense hyperkeratosis and erythema, so the occurrence of whitish cylindrical structures on this background usually indicates its transformation into a squamous cell carcinoma (SCC). The very characteristic ovoid nests of basal cell carcinoma (BCC) are almost exactly reproduced by the islands of basal cells seen in histopathology [6, 7, 13, 14, 16].

Specific Standards and Algorithms in Dermoscopy

The use of dermoscopy in daily practice is high among dermatologists (98% in Brazil and 84% in the US) [17, 18] and has also increased among nondermatologist physicians who actively take part in skin cancer vigilance. Algorithms have been created to interpret the dermoscopic features aiming to make an early and accurate diagnosis of skin tumors. They are used as diagnostic or triage systems and as teaching methodologies to improve tumor detection abilities and management decisions. The main published dermoscopic algorithms are detailed in Table 6.1. As accuracy is dependent upon the experience of examiner [41], the best course of action is to adopt one of them and use it in your clinical practice. It is important to emphasize that all cutaneous lesions that cannot be confidently diagnosed by their macroscopic appearance should be examined by dermoscopy, using the chosen diagnostic algorithm.

Reflectance Confocal Microscopy

Confocal laser scanning microscopy may be used in either reflectance mode for in vivo examination or fluorescence mode for ex vivo analysis. Reflectance confocal microscopy (RCM) is a noninvasive, in vivo, technique that allows the evaluation of the skin with quasi-histological resolution [42, 43]. It's able to capture images at different depths, from the stratum corneum to the superficial dermis, with impaired observation of the deeper dermal layer [43, 44]. RCM improves the clinical diagnosis of malignant lesions while minimizing the number of unnecessary biopsies [43, 44]. We will focus on the use of RCM for real-time diagnosis of skin lesions.

Table 6.1 The main published dermoscopic algorithms over the past three decades

Dermoscopic algorithm	Scores/criteria	Applicability	Sensitivity %	Specificity %
Pattern analysis [19–21]	Irregular or atypical pigment network Pigment network with sharp margins Irregular brown dots and globules Nonuniform radial streaming and pseudopods Nonuniform pigment distribution Structureless light brown areas Dark brown or black homogeneous areas Gray-blue areas Regression pattern Whitish veil Atypical vascular pattern	Melanocytic lesions	83–85	79–83
ABCD rule of dermoscopy [20–26]	A. Asymmetry (points 0–2; weight factor × 1.3; score 0.0–2.6) B. Border (points 0–8; weight factor × 0.1; score 0.0–0.8) C. Color (points 1–6; weight factor × 0.5; score 0.5–3.0) D. Dermatoscopic structures (points 1–5; weight factor × 0.5; score 0.5–2.5) Excision is recommended if the total dermatoscopic score (TDS) ≥4.75	Melanocytic lesions	75–92	45–75
Menzies method [26, 27]	*Positive features (at least one found)* Blue-white veil Multiple brown dots Pseudopods Radial streaming Scar-like depigmentation Peripheral black dots/globules Multiple (5–6) colors Multiple blue/gray dots Broadened network *Negative features (cannot be found)* Point and axial symmetry of pigmentation Presence of a single color	Melanocytic lesions	85–95	25–85

(continued)

Table 6.1 (continued)

Dermoscopic algorithm	Scores/criteria	Applicability	Sensitivity %	Specificity %
Seven-point checklist [20, 23, 24, 26, 28, 29]	Atypical network +2 Blue-white veil +2 Atypical vascular pattern +2 Irregular dots/globules +1 Irregular streaks +1 Irregular blotches +1 Regression structures +1 Excision is recommended if the total dermatoscopic score (TDS) ≥3	Melanocytic lesions	62–95	58–97
Modified ABC-point list of dermoscopy [30]	A. Asymmetry (at least one axis and/or differential structures inside) +1 B. Border (abrupt cutoff of network) +1 C. Color (3 or more colors) +1 D. Dermatoscopic structures (three or more differential structures) +1 E. Evolution (change noticed by patient in the last 3 months +1; no change or uncertain information +0; no change in the last 3 months −1) Excision is recommended if the total dermatoscopic score (TDS) ≥4	Melanocytic lesions	90	87
Three-point checklist [24, 31]	1. Asymmetry (asymmetrical distribution of colors and dermoscopic structures) 2. Atypical network (pigmented network with irregular holes and thick lines) 3. Blue-white structures (any type of blue and/or white color) presence ≥1 criterion suggests a suspicious lesion	Melanocytic lesions	69–96	33–63
CASH (color, architecture, symmetry, homogeneity) [26, 32, 33]	*Color* Light brown +1; dark brown +1; black +1; red +1; white +1; blue +1 *Architectural disorder* None/mild +0; moderate +1; marked +2 *Symmetry* Biaxial symmetry +0; monaxial asymmetry +1; biaxial asymmetry +2 *Dermoscopic structures* Network +1; dots/globules +1; streaks/pseudopods +1; blue-white veil +1; regression structures +1; blotches +1; polymorphous blood vessels +1 Excision is recommended if the total CASH score (TCS) ≥8	Melanocytic lesions	79–98	51–68

Table 6.1 (continued)

Dermoscopic algorithm	Scores/criteria	Applicability	Sensitivity %	Specificity %
Two-step [20, 28]	*First step*: Differentiate melanocytic from non-melanocytic lesions using well-known dermoscopic criterion for the diagnosis of seborrheic keratosis, basal cell carcinoma, vascular lesion, and melanocytic lesion. *Second step*: Differentiate melanoma from benign melanocytic lesions using four different diagnostic algorithms: (1) modified pattern analysis; (2) ABCD rule of dermoscopy; (3) Menzies method; and (4) 7-point checklist	Melanocytic and non-melanocytic lesions	95	90
Modified two-step [6, 20, 34]	*First step*: Make the decision if the lesion is melanocytic or non-melanocytic Level 1. Criteria for melanocytic lesions Level 2. Criteria for basal cell carcinoma Level 3. Criteria for seborrheic keratoses Level 4. Criteria for vascular lesion Level 5. Specific blood vessels in non-melanocytic lesions Level 6. Specific blood vessels in melanocytic lesions Level 7. "Structureless" lesions *Second step*: Make the decision if the lesion is a nevus vs. suspect melanocytic lesion vs. melanoma (need to use any algorithm intended for melanocytic lesions)	Melanocytic and non-melanocytic lesions on glabrous and nonglabrous skin. Not intended for the evaluation of special sites (acral, mucosal, scalp)	85–95	90–94
Chaos and clues pattern recognition [7, 8, 26, 35–37]	*Step 1*: Chaos (asymmetry of structure or color)—if yes move to second step. *Step 2*: Clues (search for the eight clues to malignancy) 1. Eccentric structureless area (of any color, but skin color) 2. Grey or blue structures (including gray or blue structureless) 3. Black dots and clods in the periphery 4. Segmental radial lines or pseudopods at the periphery 5. White lines 6. Thick reticular lines 7. Polymorphous vessels 8. Parallel lines on the ridges (for acral lesions)/chaotic parallel lines (nails) 9. Angulated lines If one or more clues are found a biopsy is indicated	Melanocytic and non-melanocytic lesions	91	63

(continued)

Table 6.1 (continued)

Dermoscopic algorithm	Scores/criteria	Applicability	Sensitivity %	Specificity %
TADA (triage amalgamated dermoscopic algorithm) Three-step [38, 39]	*Step 1*: Is the lesion an unequivocal seborrheic keratosis, cherry hemangioma, or dermatofibroma? Yes—lesion does not enter the algorithm No—lesion is analyzed with polarized light *Step 2*: Does the lesion manifest a disorganized pattern? Yes—consider the distribution of colors and structures within the lesion *Step 3*: Does the organized-appearing lesion manifest 1 of 2 patterns, 2 structures, or 4 colors? Yes—starburst pattern; blue-black or gray color; shiny white structures; negative network; ulcer/erosion; and vessels If the answer for steps 2 or 3 is yes, a skin biopsy is recommended to rule out skin cancer	Melanocytic and non-melanocytic lesions	94	75
Top-down two-step pattern analysis approach (revised two-step) [40]	*Step 1*: To establish a specific diagnosis (if possible) – Not necessary to differentiate melanocytic from non-melanocytic lesions – Requires a specific diagnosis by recognizing the classic patterns/structures associated with nevi, dermatofibromas (DF), intradermal nevi (IDN), basal cell carcinomas (BCC), squamous cell carcinomas (SCC), lentigines and seborrheic keratoses (SK), angiomas, angiokeratomas, sebaceous hyperplasias, and clear cell acanthoma (CCA) *Step 2*: To rule out melanoma – Requires the observer to acknowledge the nevus patterns that require context for their interpretation and the patterns and structures associated with melanoma	Melanocytic and non-melanocytic lesions	–	–

Basic Principles of In Vivo RCM, Equipment, and Image Acquisition

The light source used in RCM is a near-infrared, low-power laser beam (830 nm diode laser with a power less than 35 mW) that emits monochromatic coherent light [44], that doesn't cause tissue damage [43] (Fig. 6.5). RCM uses backscattered light from cell structures which is based on refractive index of cell structures and organelles, with keratin, melanin, and collagen ("endogenous chromophores") showing higher refractive indices compared to water [43]. RCM images obtained in the dermatologic setting are black, gray, and white [42, 44]. The high-resolution horizontal images of cells and nuclear structures at epidermal level, collagen, and circulating blood cells at dermal layer allow the identification of clues for diagnosis of different skin conditions [43].

There are two types of RCM devices available for bedside use: the wide probe and handheld, both requiring skin contact, with lateral resolution of 0.5–1 μm for single RCM images, an axial resolution of 3–5 μm (section thickness), and a depth up to 200 μm, depending on the anatomical site [42–45]. The basic RCM optical section image is comparable to histopathology at about 30× magnification [45].

The wide probe RCM must be fixed to the skin, requires an immersion oil between the skin and the ring or window, and is limited to flat surfaces. It allows stitching together 0.5 × 0.5 mm adjacent optical sections at the same image depth or plane, into a two-dimensional block, or mosaic, with a field of view up to 8 × 8 mm, simulating a shave biopsy procedure [42–45]. Mosaic images can be acquired at different skin layers and can overlap with the dermoscopic image through a device built-in dermatoscope [43, 44]. When necessary to evaluate non-flat surfaces or lesions by RCM, it's important to remember it will result in oblique mosaic images, showing more than one depth (i.e., epidermis and DEJ at the same image block).

The handheld RCM has a smaller probe that requires contact, but not fixation to the skin. After applying mineral oil to the surface, it is moved manually on the lesion, enabling imaging of curved anatomic sites, such as nose, ears, scalp, eyelids,

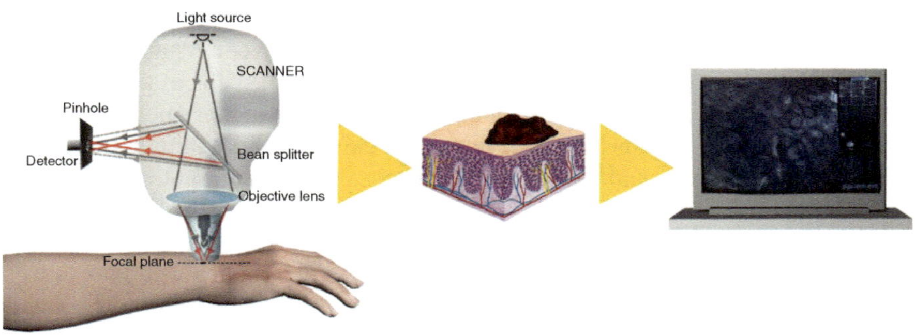

Fig. 6.5 Schematic image of optical basis of the RCM laser device. The laser light passes through a system of optical lenses and mirrors, finds a focal tissue point, and reflects from the tissue through the pinhole, creating gray-scale horizontal images of cells [44]

palmoplantar, and mucosae [43, 44, 46]. The automated 0.75 × 0.75 mm optical sections are stacked vertically, from the skin surface to superficial dermis, at the same point in the tissue [47]. RCM stacks have a limited view [43, 44], simulating a less-than 1 mm punch procedure.

RCM revealed a sensitivity of 94–95% and a specificity of 85–95% for the diagnosis of basal cell carcinoma (BCC) diagnosis, and a sensitivity of 92% and a specificity of 70% for melanoma diagnosis [43]. One should be aware of the limitations and pitfalls of RCM, especially with nodular lesions (limited RCM depth penetration), hyperkeratotic, crusting, or ulcerated lesions (highly reflective surface may reduce imaging quality), and lesions with discrepancy between the clinical-dermoscopic and RCM findings [44]. Even today, histopathology is still considered an important accessory examination for the diagnosis of skin cancers [43].

RCM and Histopathological Correlation

There is a very good correlation between the histopathological characteristics of normal skin from different anatomical sites and what is seen on RCM.

The main differences observed on histopathology (HP) when looking at facial, palmoplantar, or trunk skin are reflected very clearly on RCM. These are: the thick compact horny layer on palmoplantar skin which makes it difficult on RCM to see the basal cell layer of the epidermis in these areas, the numerous sweat ducts on these anatomical sites and follicular openings on facial skin, and the effaced dermoepidermal junction (DEJ) on facial skin which hampers the detection of the limit between epidermis and dermis, the so-called edged papillae. Changes in superficial dermis elastic tissue due to cumulative solar damage are also highlighted on RCM as well as on HP. In trunk skin it's easy to identify the four layers of the epidermis: the cells in the horny layer are large, polygonal, refractive, and non-nucleated. Skin markings are noted at this level. In the thinner granular layer, the cells present a central dark nucleus and granules in the cytoplasm just as in HP. The thicker spinous layer is recognized by the "honeycomb" pattern of well-organized polygonal cells with an oval central nucleus. The cells of the basal layer are smaller and may contain large amounts of melanin in higher phototypes creating a melanin cap over the nucleus. In normal skin it's impossible to distinguish between keratinocytes and melanocytes because the latter are not dendritic. The basal layer of the epidermis borders on the papillary dermis, which is recognized by delicate collagen fibers, a few resident inflammatory cells, and small vessels. RCM highlights the main characteristics of basal cell carcinoma well known from dermoscopy and HP: hyporeflective tumor islands surrounded by bright collagen bundles (tumor stroma) and dilated vessels coursing in the en face plane of imaging [16, 46] (Fig. 6.6).

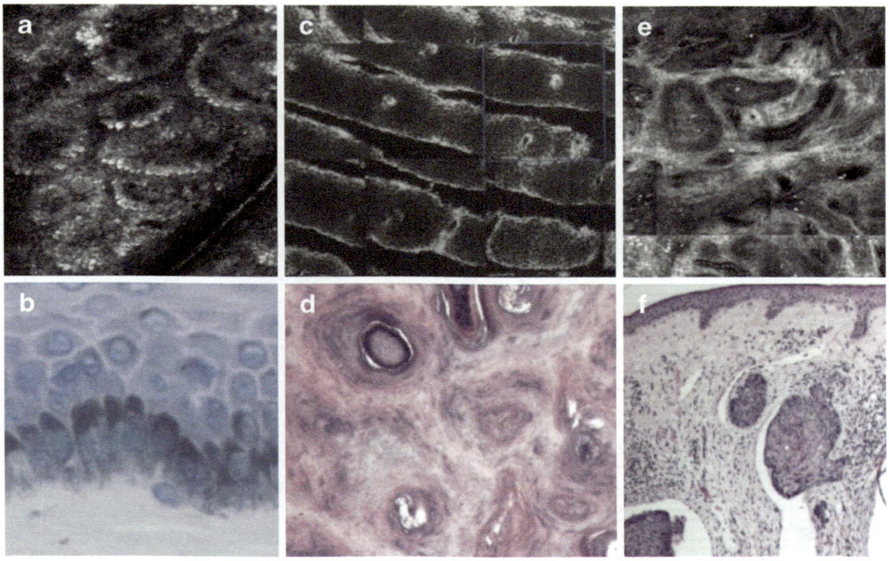

Fig. 6.6 In normal skin it's impossible to distinguish between keratinocytes and melanocytes because the latter are not dendritic. Under RCM the cells of the basal layer are small and may contain large amounts of melanin (**a**) in higher phototypes creating a melanin cap over the nucleus as also seen in HP (**b**). Numerous acrosyringia cross palmoplantar epidermis and are easily identified in both RCM (**c**) and HP (**d**). Hyporeflective tumor islands surrounded by bright collagen bundles (tumor stroma) and dilated vessels coursing in the "en-face" plane of imaging characterize basal cell carcinoma in RCM (**e**) and correspond to the classic HP of this neoplasia (**f**). (*RCM and histopathology images courtesy of Juan Piñeiro-Maceira, MD, MSc, PhD*)

An irregular meshwork pattern correlates with the ill-defined grouping of pleomorphic melanocytes in the DEJ junction seen both in horizontal and vertical histopathological sections in dysplastic nevi. Aggregates of bright cells in dense nonhomogeneous nests close to the epidermis may be seen both in melanomas and in atypical nevi and correlate very well with the HP of these lesions. Pleomorphic atypical bright cells in the so-called pagetoid spread pattern in the epidermis are one of the main diagnostic features of melanoma both in RCM and HP [16, 46] (Fig. 6.7).

Specific Standards and Algorithms in RCM

RCM imaging can be time consuming compared to dermoscopy and therefore should be used as a highly selective complementary exam for equivocal lesions of concern, based on dermoscopic findings. The association of these techniques

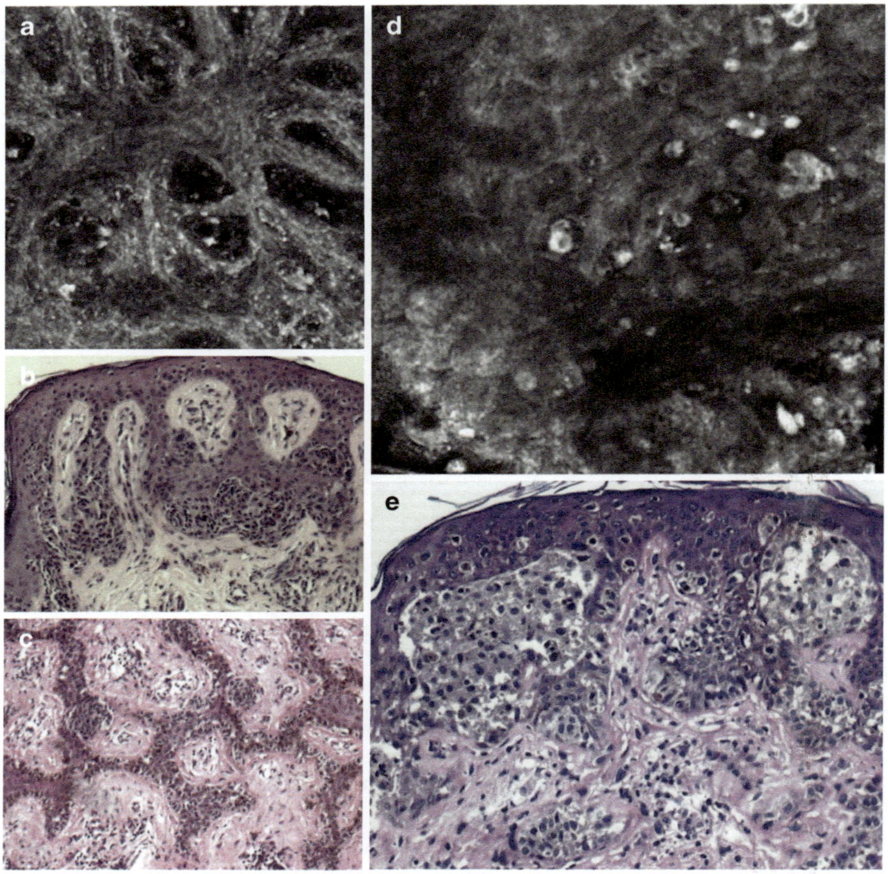

Fig. 6.7 An irregular meshwork pattern (**a**) correlates clearly with the ill-defined grouping of pleomorphic melanocytes in the DEJ seen both in vertical (**b**) and horizontal (**c**) histopathological sections in dysplastic nevi. Pleomorphic atypical bright cells in the so-called pagetoid spread pattern (**d**) in the epidermis is one of the main diagnostic features of melanoma both in RCM and HP (**e**). (*RCM and histopathology images courtesy of Juan Piñeiro-Maceira, MD, MSc, PhD*)

significantly improves the early diagnosis of melanocytic and non-melanocytic skin tumors [44, 46, 48]. The use of RCM by Brazilian dermatologists is limited to university hospitals (public), or specialized hospitals/skin cancer clinics (private). Conversely, in the US reimbursement codes have been stablished and a consequent rise in the integration of RCM into clinical practice is expected [49]. Training is required for optimal proficiency and to reach an acceptable level of diagnostic skill and expertise. The accuracy of diagnosis has been related to the experience of RCM readers [43]. RCM algorithms have been created and validated to interpret the images and aid the novice user (Table 6.2) [48, 50–53].

Table 6.2 The main four microscopic scores/algorithms over the past two decades

Algorithm	Scores/criteria	Applicability	Sensitivity %	Specificity %
Pellacani 2005 (RCM only) [50]	Cytologic atypia (mild or marked) +2 Non-edged papillae at basal layer +2 Roundish cells in superficial layers spreading upward in a pagetoid fashion +1 Pagetoid cells widespread throughout the lesion +1 Cerebriform clusters in the papillary dermis +1 Nucleated cells within dermal papillae +1 Biopsy is recommended if the total score ≥3	Melanoma diagnosis	97	72
Segura 2009 (RCM only) [51]	Typical basal cells −1 Edged papillae −1 Roundish pagetoid cells +1 Atypical nucleated dermal cells +1 Biopsy is recommended if the total score ≥0	Melanoma diagnosis	86	95
Borsari 2018 (Dermoscopy and RCM) [52]	Atypical network (dermoscopy) +1 Regression (dermoscopy) +1 Pagetoid cells +1 Cytologic atypia focal +1 Cytologic atypia widespread +2 Dense nests −1 Melanophages −1 Biopsy is recommended if the total score ≥2	In situ melanoma diagnosis	93	61
Pellacani 2019 (RCM only) [53]	Four key features *Two melanoma features* – Atypical cells (roundish and/or dendritic cells in the suprabasal epidermis and/or DEJ and/or dermis, either presenting as single isolated cells or forming clusters) – DEJ disarray (architectural disorder at the DEJ includes non-edged papillae, disorganized/chaotic pattern of ringed, meshwork, and/or clod, with asymmetrical distribution) *One basal cell carcinoma feature* – Basaloid cords/islands (roundish, elongated, or polycyclic refractive structures with cellular palisading at the periphery, frequently outlined by a "dark cleft" that separates the refractive structure from the surrounding stroma or dark homogeneous areas with lobulated contours embedded in bright fibrotic stroma "dark silhouettes") *One squamous cell carcinoma feature* – Keratinocyte disarray (irregular honeycomb pattern of the epidermis or lack of a recognizable epidermal pattern) – Biopsy is recommended if ≥1 feature	Skin cancer diagnosis	91	57

Clinical Examination, Total Body Photography (TBP), and Serial Digital Dermoscopy (SDD)

Clinical Examination

Total-body skin examination (TBSE) is the *hallmark* for skin cancer clinical detection [54–56]. Although there have been controversies in the past, whether it should be performed for all patients, it's clear that TBSE is a safe procedure that can be easily performed by dermatologists who are specifically trained and skilled in diagnosing skin disorders [56–59]. Adopting a standardized TBSE can increase time efficiency and minimize the chance of missing a body area [57]. It's important to acknowledge that TBSE includes the genitalia, mucous membranes, conjunctiva, inframammary folds, intergluteal cleft, scalp, and examination between digits and nails [56, 58, 59]. Patients over 40 years old, with history of NMSC, and fair skin type should be prioritized [55, 56].

Patients with multiple nevi can be challenging for the naked eye examination. Nevi count and size matter. The number of histologically confirmed dysplastic nevi is a tenfold risk factor for melanoma. It is known that nevus remnants (of any type) are associated with more than 50% of diagnosed melanomas [16]. These patients are often subjected to unnecessary biopsies by TBSE alone, so adding the comparative approach (ugly duckling sign), with dermoscopic examination and comparison, digital monitoring with total body photography (TBP), and digital dermoscopy (DD), is a necessary strategy for a cost-efficient early melanoma detection [60].

Total Body Photography (TBP)

Patients have a significantly increased risk for melanoma when they have a personal or family history of the tumor, a known high penetrance gene mutation, a high nevi count, and atypical mole syndrome (AMS) [60]. TBP is recommended for AMS patients, as well as for adults with more than 50 nevi that have one or more of the following: personal history of multiple cutaneous melanomas; personal history of melanoma or amelanotic melanoma; multiple pink nevi, multiple clinically atypical nevi, family history, and/or a genetic syndrome that predisposes to the development of cutaneous melanoma. Other considerations that support using TBP include presence of significant photodamage, patient history of many biopsies, and patient anxiety [61].

Digital Dermoscopy (DD)

Even for the eyes of experienced dermatologists, early melanomas may be difficult to diagnose because they can exhibit few malignancy criteria and be clinically symmetrical [60, 62]. Dermoscopy can increase the index of suggestion to perform biopsy in difficult-to-diagnose melanomas [62]. DD is more reassuring for the clinician, due to the possibility to store dermoscopic images, asses them for detailed examination, and compare with other lesions on the patient (nevi pattern) prior to the decision for biopsy [60, 62]. Pigmented lesions with obviously malignant dermoscopic features should be biopsied in totum [61].

Serial Digital Dermoscopy (SDD)

Lesions with equivocal dermoscopic features can be followed up. SDD is used alone or in conjunction with TBP for monitoring suspicious macular melanocytic lesions over predetermined intervals, and then must be re-assessed (Fig. 6.8). Palpable lesions showing suspect dermoscopic criteria should be immediately removed, not followed by SDD [60, 61].

Two-Dimensional (2D) Mapping System

TBP associated with SDD is a form of 2D mole monitoring. TBP is a baseline set of digital photographs of every part of the skin surface. Comparing the regional photographs with the TBSE on subsequent visits allows the detection of new lesions and macroscopic changes in preexisting moles, by providing a comparative reference point of areas of the skin [63]. SDD allows the precise detection of changes in structures and colors of the melanocytic lesions that are not visible to the naked eye. Recognition of featureless melanomas can be enhanced by SDD since it allows observation of changes over time. Dermoscopic changes in a melanocytic lesion may represent an early sign of malignant transformation and stability of a lesion speaks against a diagnosis of melanoma [60, 63–66]. It is recommended that new TBP images should be obtained once previous images are not easily comparable to the patient's current appearance [61] (Fig. 6.9).

SDD can be performed in short or long-term follow-up. In short-term SDD, monitoring period is up to 3 months and is used to evaluate suspicious melanocytic lesions that lack dermoscopy features of melanoma. Long term follow-up (6–12 months) is indicated for high-risk patients with multiple nevi, including AMS individuals [67]. A combination of short and long-term SDD is considered a major surveillance strategy and follow-up must be maintained throughout life in patients at high risk for developing melanoma [68].

Early diagnosis is key for melanoma management. Patients at high risk for melanoma, mainly AMS individuals and patients with multiple nevi associated with personal and/or family history of melanoma, should have TBP combined with SDD—the so-called two-step method—which is one of the most efficient strategies to detect early melanomas while minimizing unnecessary biopsies [65, 68]. The accuracy of the two-step method is directly related to the examiner's experience.

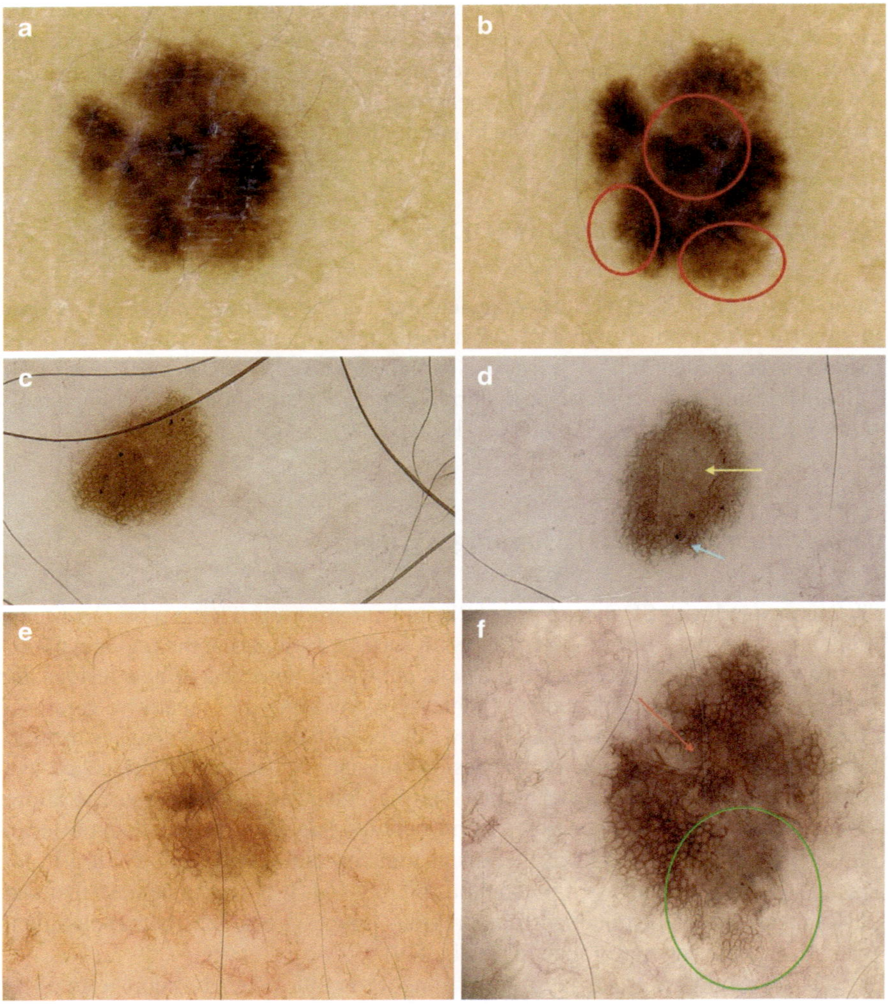

Fig. 6.8 Three examples of dermoscopic change during follow-up of melanocytic lesions. (**a**) Dermoscopy at first visit. (**b**) Dermoscopy with immersion fluid on the 3-month follow-up showing new streaks at the periphery, growth of the lesion, and increased dark structures area at the center (red circles). Final diagnosis was a MELANOMA IN SITU. (**c**) Baseline dermoscopy of a small trunk lesion with regular network and diffuse black globules. (**d**) Dermoscopy after 1-year follow-up showing a slight growth, peripheral atypical network (teal arrow), and structureless tan color in the center of the lesion (yellow arrow). Final diagnosis was a COMPOUND DYSPLASTIC NEVUS, with moderate atypia. (**e**) Baseline dermoscopy of a lentigo-like small shoulder lesion with regular network and focal area of structureless brown. (**f**) Patient skipped regular follow-up time and a new dermoscopy image was taken after 3 years showing an impressive growth, atypical network in 2/3 of the lesion (orange arrow) and a peripheral regression area with gray-blue hue and gray dots and granules (green circle). Final diagnosis was an ATYPICAL LENTIGINOUS COMPOUND NEVUS associated with focal lichenoid infiltrate (mild atypia). All images show PD (20×). (*Dermoscopy images courtesy of Naiara Fraga-Braghiroli, MD, PhD, and Ana Maria Sortino, MD, MSc*)

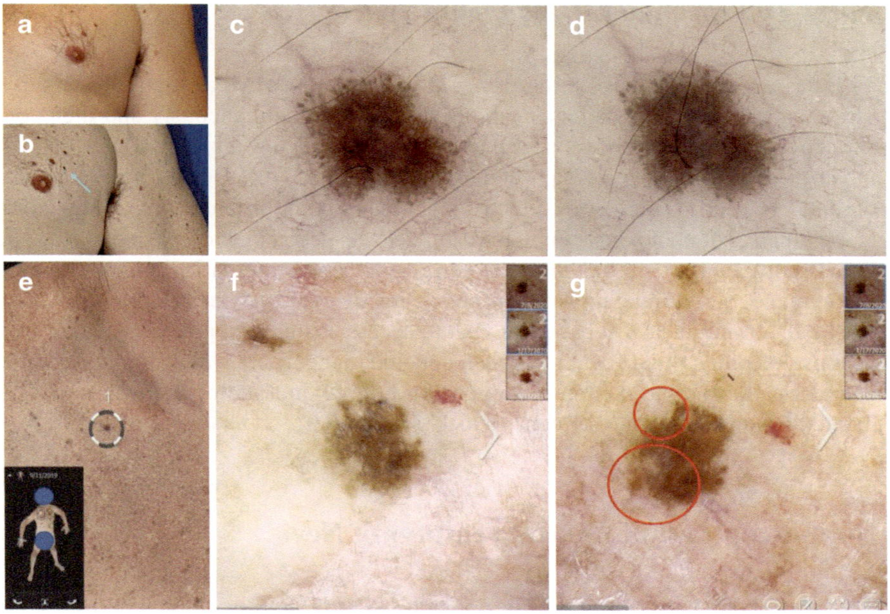

Fig. 6.9 Example of a 2D mapping system (**a**) first visit clinical image. (**b**) Follow-up clinical image showing a new melanocytic lesion (teal arrow). (**c**) PD (20×) with evident peripheral teared globules, structureless center, and hyperpigmented irregular areas. (**d**) NPD enhancing the central regression with gray-brown color, it was considered a very suspicious lesion and referred for full excision. Final diagnosis was a severely COMPOUND DYSPLASTIC NEVUS (mild atypia). Example of a 3D mapping system (**e**) lower left square: 3D total body image; upper left: lesion marked on the 3D image. (**f**) Dermoscopic image of the marked lesion at the first visit. (**g**) 6-month follow-up dermoscopic image showing new structures (red circles). Final diagnosis was a severely DYSPLASTIC NEVUS. (*Clinical and dermoscopy images courtesy of Ana Maria Sortino, MD, MSc, and Naiara Fraga-Braghiroli, MD, PhD*)

Although it is of great relevance for the diagnosis of macular slow-growing melanomas, it is not adequate for suspicious papular or nodular melanocytic lesions which may represent fast-growing tumors [69].

The optimal body mapping system for melanocytic lesions follow-up and melanoma screening should improve diagnostic accuracy, be time and cost efficient, and accessible to patients. Instruments and systems for performing TBP and SDD are based on a digital camera and a dermoscopic device coupled to a computer for capturing images from the patients and their melanocytic lesions. Specifically designed software permits the management of the image database, including image acquisition, storage, organization, analysis, and retrieval. Different systems are available on the market and some of these can calculate mathematical parameters allowing the so-called computer-assisted diagnosis; more recently artificial intelligence has been incorporated to these devices [70].

Three-Dimensional (3D) Mapping System

TBP has undergone an evolution from 2D imaging to a 3D realistic representation of the patient. Multiple cameras capture the images simultaneously and then construct a digital 3D full-body avatar that rotates 360° to view all body angles, including curved surfaces which are particularly compromised on 2D imaging. Additional digital dermoscopic images of selected melanocytic lesions that showed some atypical features, but do not have enough features to suspect a melanoma, are taken. The dermoscopy images are linked to the corresponding lesion marked on the 3D total body image. Serial imaging sessions consisting of total body and dermoscopy data can be reviewed in each subsequent visit to access changes on previous nevi or new lesions. Recently, the software has been updated to incorporate an automatic change detector and artificial intelligence algorithm to track morphologic changes on pigmented lesions during subsequent visits [71] (Fig. 6.9).

Dermoscopic and Confocal Features of Nevi

Melanocytic nevi are benign skin lesions due to proliferation of cells derived from melanocytes. The subtypes of nevi are categorized based on the level of the nevus cells in the skin. Dermoscopy and RCM have been valuable noninvasive diagnostic tools for assessment of benign and malignant melanocytic neoplasms of the skin. Use of both modalities combined led to fewer biopsies of benign lesions (Fig. 6.10). The use of RCM with the wide probe is preferred due the possibility of evaluating the entire architecture of the lesion, and correlating it to the dermoscopic image, which is essential when analyzing melanocytic lesions [72, 73].

Junctional Melanocytic Nevi

A junctional melanocytic nevus (JMN) is formed by proliferation of nevus cells at the DEJ. The main dermoscopic features of JMN are a regular network and regular edges. The pigmentation is distributed homogenously throughout the lesion and gradually fades at the periphery [74, 75]. On RCM, JMN displays a regular honeycomb pattern at the epidermal level. At the DEJ, it can show two main patterns: ringed, characterized by a rim of bright cells forming the edged papillae; and meshwork, characterized by elongated cords and junctional thickening. Histopathologically, the ringed pattern represents elongated rete-ridges with an increased number of single melanocytes at the basal layer. In contrast, the meshwork pattern corresponds on histopathology to the enlargement of the interpapillary space formed by aggregated melanocytes, with predominantly small, non-confluent nests at the tips of the rete ridges [73, 75, 76] (Fig. 6.11).

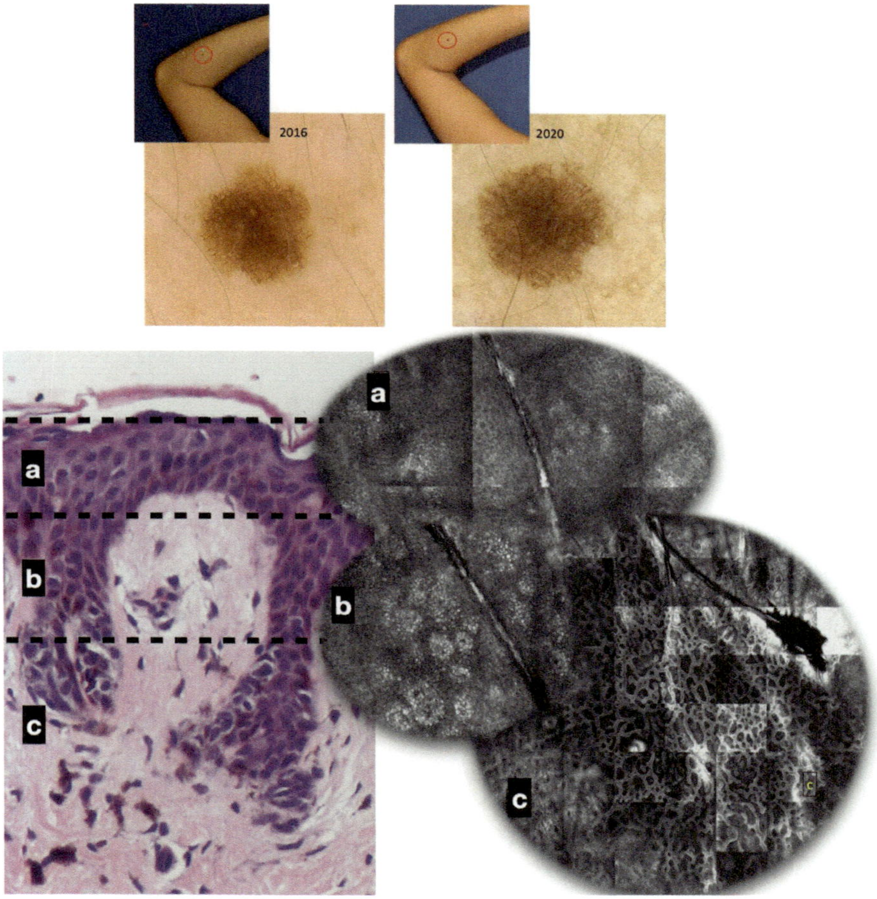

Fig. 6.10 Female patient in her thirties with family history of multiple melanomas, intense photodamage, and a growing lesion on the left forearm, noticed by the patient. Baseline PD (20×) in 2016 shows a symmetric lesion with a regular pigment network. In 2020, follow-up PD (20×) shows an enlarging lesion that maintained the symmetric and regular network pattern. (**a**) RCM of the upper epidermis showing a regular honeycomb pattern. (**b**) RCM of the basal epidermal layer showing a regular cobblestone pattern. (**c**) RCM of the DEJ shows a regular ringed pattern. The clinical diagnosis of a benign acquired nevus was made, and an excision was spared. The lesion is under clinical follow-up. RCM images are close-ups of wide probe 8 × 8 mm mosaics. (*Clinical, dermoscopy and RCM images courtesy of Ana Maria Sortino, MD, MSc*)

Compound and Dermal Melanocytic Nevi

Compound nevus represents acquired and/or congenital type nevus with a junctional and a dermal component. Dermoscopically, it is represented by at least two of the following patterns: reticular, globular, homogeneous, and multicomponent pattern, usually distributed symmetrically throughout the lesion [75]. On RCM, it

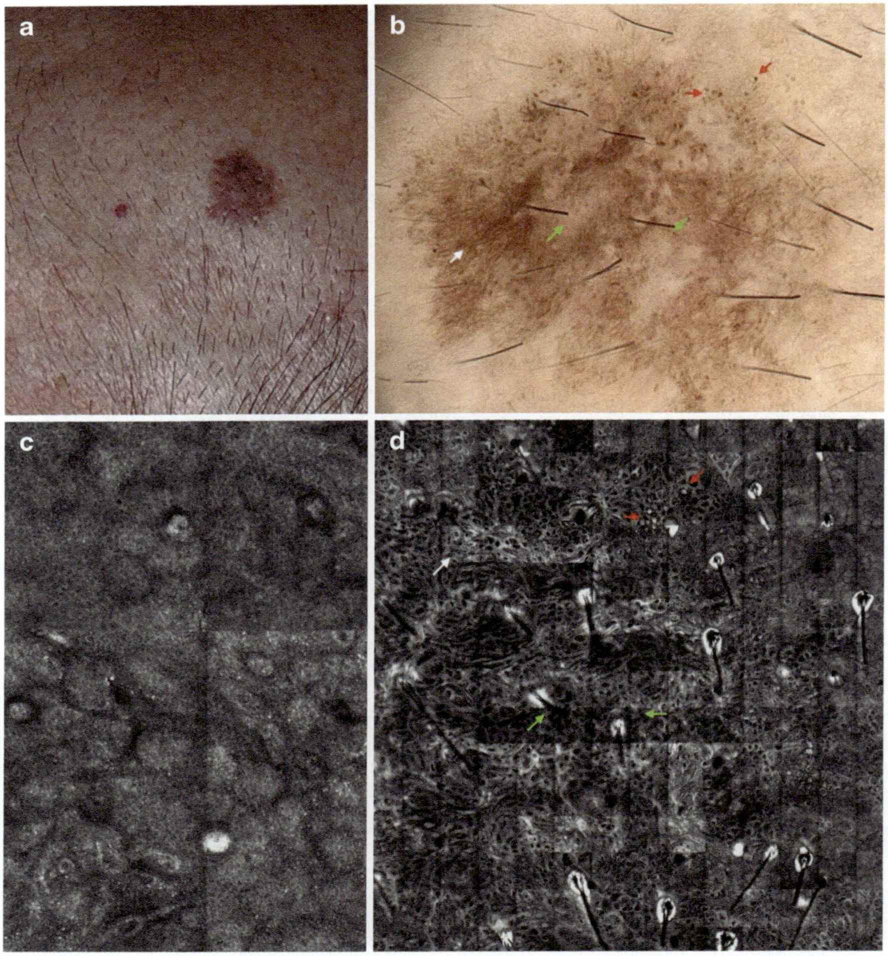

Fig. 6.11 Male patient in his forties with intense photodamage and a stand-out isolated forehead lesion. (**a**) Clinical image of the pigmented lesion. (**b**) PD (30×) shows an asymmetric multicomponent pattern with an atypical network (white arrow), peripheral diffuse brown globules (red arrow), a few structureless hypopigmented areas around the follicles (green arrows) not reassuring of the lesion benignity. (**c**) RCM image shows a regular honeycomb pattern at the epidermal level. (**d**) RCM image at the DEJ shows a regular meshwork characterized by elongated cords and junctional thickening (white arrow hyperreflective and green arrows hyporeflective meshwork) and, small non-confluent nests at the tip of the rete ridges (red arrows). RCM images are wide probe 8 × 8 mm mosaics. Patient was asked for old pictures and showed a few (from over 5 years ago) with no clinical change of the lesion. The diagnosis favoring a stable lesion was made, and an excision at first visit was spared. The lesion is probably an acquired junctional or compound nevus and is under strict clinical follow-up. (*Clinical, dermoscopy and RCM images courtesy of Ana Maria Sortino, MD, MSc*)

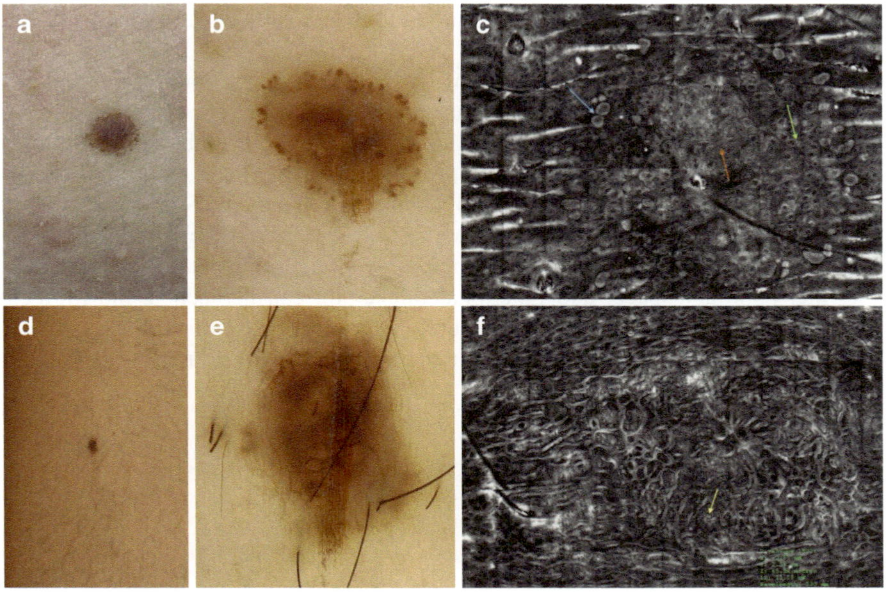

Fig. 6.12 (**a**) Clinical aspect of a COMPOUND NEVUS. (**b**) PD (20×) showing regular peripheral globules and a structureless brown center. (**c**) RCM at the DEJ shows a central regular meshwork pattern (orange arrow), areas of ringed pattern (green arrow), and dense nests at the periphery (blue arrow). (**d**) Clinical aspect of a pigmented and flat DERMAL NEVUS. (**e**) PD (20×) showing an enlarged central pigment network and structureless tan peripheral areas. (**f**) RCM at the DEJ shows a regular meshwork and grouped dense nests (yellow arrow). RCM images are wide probe 8 × 8 mm mosaics. (*Clinical, dermoscopy and RCM images courtesy of Ana Maria Sortino, MD, MSc*)

presents features of the junctional component (ringed and/or meshwork pattern at the DEJ) and of the dermal component, with dense compact nests visible within the dermal papillae with little or no cytologic atypia. Aggregates of numerous dense nests at the DEJ/upper dermis form the clod pattern [77] (Fig. 6.12).

The classical model of nevus evolution implies that benign melanocytic proliferations start to develop at the DEJ, then become compound, and finally dermal over time [76]. Confocal microscopy of dermal nevus is characterized by the presence of dermal dense nests (clod pattern), which correlate dermoscopically with the globular pattern [77].

Congenital Melanocytic Nevi

A congenital melanocytic nevus (CMN) is characterized by a dome-shaped papule with homogeneous color. CMN under dermoscopy can show a globular/cobblestone pattern, focal broadened network, target globules, milia-like cysts, hypopigmentation in skin furrows and around the hair follicles, terminal hairs, and comma-like vessels [75, 78].

The most common RCM features of CMN are a typical honeycomb and/or a typical cobblestone pattern at the spinous granular level. The cobblestone pattern is formed by monomorphic bright cells due to transfer of melanin to the keratinocytes. It is common to see dark linear structures (fissures) and small dark circles due to the invagination of the epidermis with a non-flat surface. Small, bright white structures are present; they represent the milia-like cysts. At the DEJ level a combination of a meshwork and clod pattern, meshwork, and ring pattern, thickening of the inter-papillary space, and junctional thickening can be seen. Dendritic cells may be occasionally seen in CMN, usually in a focal distribution. At the dermal level there are large oval bright structures representing the dermal nests [73, 76] (Fig. 6.13).

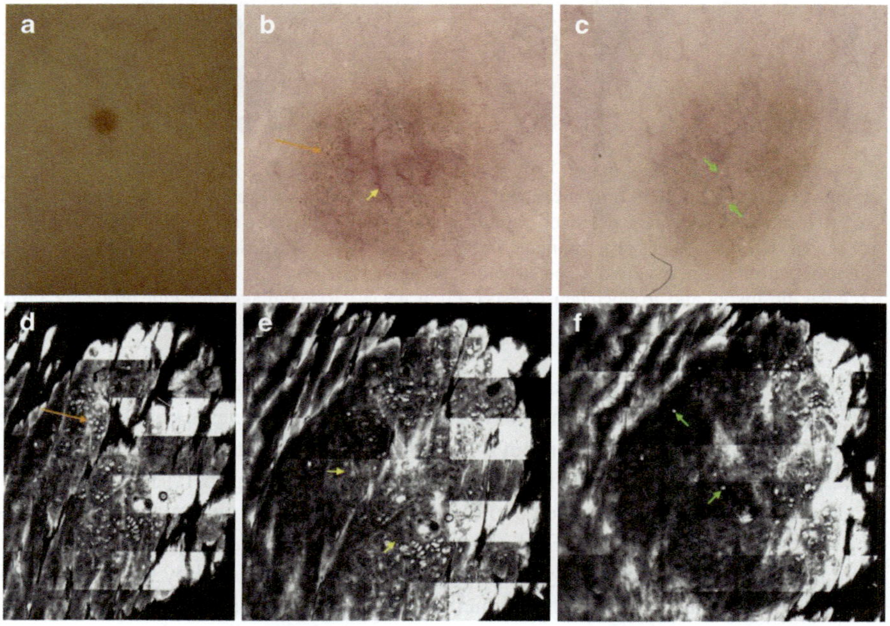

Fig. 6.13 (**a**) Clinical image of a CONGENITAL COMPOUND MELANOCYTIC NEVUS. (**b**) PD (20×) showing regular brown dots and globules (orange arrow) with a diffuse distribution, and central linear vessels (yellow arrow). (**c**) NPD (20×) allowing the observation of milia-like cysts (green arrows). (**d**) RCM image at the suprabasal epidermal level shows multiple small hyperreflective nests (orange arrow) diffusely distributed within the lesion. (**e**) RCM image at the DEJ shows a combination of meshwork and clod pattern with a higher number of linear vessels (yellow arrows). (**f**) RCM image at dermal level shows small bright white structures that represent the milia-like cysts (green arrows). RCM images are wide probe 8 × 8 mm mosaics. (*Clinical, dermoscopy and RCM images courtesy of Ana Maria Sortino, MD, MSc*)

Dysplastic Melanocytic Nevi

Dysplastic Melanocytic nevi (DMN) are nevi with some degree of cytologic atypia. The significance of DMN is that they are biomarkers of increased risk for melanoma, are potential precursors of melanoma, and they may coexist with melanoma. DMN are classified histopathologically as mildly, moderate, or severely dysplastic based on the degree of epidermal melanocytic atypia and architecture asymmetry. A new WHO classification has been proposed in 2018, classifying DMN into low-grade and high-grade dysplasia [16]. Because of the variability in atypia, DMN can present diverse clinical and dermoscopic features. They can range from a slightly asymmetric pigmented macule to a chaotic lesion with irregularly distributed brown globules, with either discrete or prominent irregular network, abrupt or gradual edges, irregular depigmentation, and focal gray-dots and granules. The main confocal features of DMN at the epidermal level are a typical or slightly atypical honeycomb or cobblestone pattern with a granular appearance. When atypical dendritic cells are present, they are few in numbers and usually located at the center of the lesion. At the DEJ level, there are typical or atypical rings, meshwork, or a mixed pattern. An atypical clod pattern, with ovoid bright large structures at the DEJ and dermal level, comprised of cells with different degrees of reflectivity represent the junctional and dermal nests, respectively. They can form bridges interconnecting the atypical nests. Atypical dendritic shaped cells or round nucleated cells, representing the atypical melanocytes, are present at areas with a dermal-epidermal disarrangement [79, 80]. DMN are a lot more common than melanomas, and the risk of progression is low. Yet, DMN with severe or high-grade dysplasia should be considered for complete excision [16] (Fig. 6.14).

Spitz Nevi

Spitzoid melanocytic lesions may represent a challenging situation in clinical practice, due to a distinctive histological architecture [16]. They can demonstrate a wide variety of clinical and dermoscopic patterns. The most relevant dermoscopic feature is the starburst pattern, characterized by multiple streaks of pigmentation or large globules arranged symmetrically at the periphery of the lesion, in a radiating pattern. Some spitzoid lesions may show a negative network, a superficial black network, or be a non-pigmented lesion [81, 82].

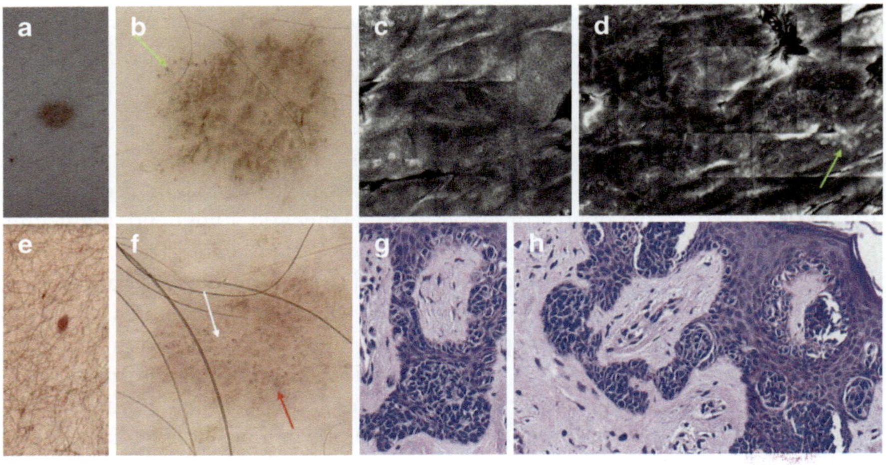

Fig. 6.14 (**a**) Clinical image of macular suspect melanocytic lesion. (**b**) PD (20×) shows irregular hyperpigmentation, multiple orthogonal white lines, and peripheral teared globules (green arrow). (**c**) RCM image shows an atypical honeycomb pattern at the epidermal level. (**d**) RCM image at the DEJ shows an irregular meshwork, with focal areas of non-edged papillae and dense-sparse nests with a linear arrangement at the periphery (green arrow). RCM images are close-up of wide probe 8 × 8 mm mosaics. The lesion was excised with a final diagnosis of COMPOUND NEVUS, with moderate cytologic atypia. (**e**) Clinical image of a palpable melanocytic pink lesion. (**f**) PD (20×) revealing irregular hyperpigmentation, multiple orthogonal bright-white central lines (white arrow), and dotted vessels (red arrow). (**g**, **h**) Histological sections (400×) of a skin fragment that presents, at the dermoepidermal junction and superficial dermis, an accumulation of nevus cells, arranged in nests. There is moderate continuous melanocytic proliferation, containing numerous atypical cells, with an epithelioid appearance, moderately hyperchromatic nuclei, and small nucleoli. Nests cause fusion of epithelial cones. On the periphery of the main lesion, there is a continuous proliferation of melanocytic cells at the dermoepidermal junction that exceeds the dermal component. In the dermis, there is concentric lamellar fibrosis around the epithelial cones and a mild perivascular lymphocytic inflammatory infiltrate. The final diagnosis was COMPOUND NEVUS, with severe junctional cytologic atypia. The lesion was treated with 0.5 cm margins. (*Clinical, dermoscopy and RCM images courtesy of Ana Maria Sortino, MD, MSc. Histopathology images courtesy of Melissa Lissae Fugimori, MD*)

Classical Spitz nevi are compounded by large spindle and/or epithelioid cells that are mainly arranged in nests on histology [16]. Therefore, RCM is characterized by the presence of spindled cells at the DEJ and numerous homogeneous dense nests at the DEJ and upper dermis. Spitz nevi can often present a pagetoid distribution of melanocytes (roundish and dendritic shape) mainly centrally located. A broadened honeycombed pattern, non-edged papillae, and atypical cells at the DEJ can also be present. The atypical cells may be distributed widespread throughout the lesion, making their differentiation from melanoma very challenging [83]. A less common variety of Spitz nevus is the pigmented spindle cell nevus, also called Reed nevus. They usually have a dark color (black, blue, and brown) and a history of recent onset or change, being frequently clinically mistaken for melanoma [16] (Fig. 6.15).

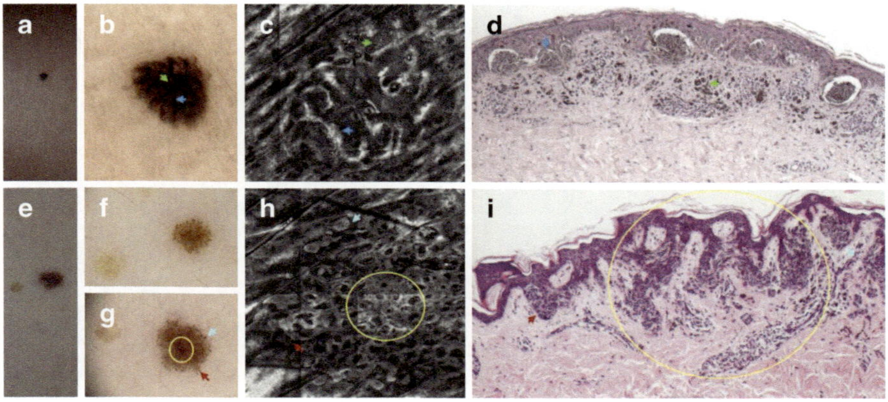

Fig. 6.15 Phototype III, female, in her forties, with severe sun damage, presenting a clinically brown-black 2-mm papule of unknown duration and regarded as new. (**a**) Clinical image of a dark palpable small melanocytic lesion. (**b**) PD (30×) showing a structureless grayish-black background (green arrow) and dark-brown polygonal lines (blue arrow). (**c**) RCM wide probe 2.5 × 2.5 mm mosaic at the DEJ shows juncional nests forming lines (blue arrow) and abundance of melanophages in the dermis (green arrow). (**d**) Histological examination (100×) reveals at the dermoepidermal junction a proliferation of fusiform melanocytic elements, richly pigmented by melanin, whose nuclei show a slight degree of variation of size and shape. They are arranged in nests parallel to the epidermis, and sometimes these penetrate the epidermis (blue arrow). At dermis there is dense proliferation of melanophages (green arrow) and vascular ectasia, with a diagnosis of REED NEVUS. Phototype I, male, in his thirties, with moderate sun damage, presenting a clinically small brown macular lesion that almost doubled its size after 1-year follow-up. (**e**) Clinical image of a macular melanocytic lesion. (**f**) Baseline PD (20×) revealing a central atypical network and large globules arranged symmetrically at the periphery of the lesion in a radiating pattern. (**g**) Follow-up PD (20×) showing the lesion enlargement and change to a structureless brown center (yellow circle), with areas of hyperpigmentation and peripheral isolated globules (turquoise arrow) and teared globules (red arrow). (**h**) Close-up of RCM wide probe 8 × 8 mm mosaic at the DEJ shows a central atypical meshwork (yellow circle), multiple juncional nests (red arrow), and peripheral dense isolated dermal nests (turquoise arrow). (**i**) Histology at 100× magnification shows a proliferation of typical epithelioid cells, distributed singly or forming nests of varying sizes, which in the epidermis are at the ends of the slightly elongated interpapillary ridges. Some spindle cells are present. The cells exhibit varying amounts of melanin pigment in the cytoplasm, with an uneven increase in melanin pigmentation in the keratinocytes. In the papillary dermis, these cells form small nests surrounded by lymphocytes and melanophages. A final diagnosis of COMPOUND PIGMENTED SPITZ NEVUS was made. (*Clinical, dermoscopy and RCM images courtesy of Dra. Ana Maria Sortino. Histopathology images courtesy of Dr. Gilles Landman, Dr. Alexandre Michalany and Dr. Nílceo Michalany*)

Dermoscopic and Confocal Feature of Cutaneous Melanoma

When a melanoma is clinically suspicious (e.g., asymmetry, irregular borders, varied colors, diameter greater than 6 mm, evolution, or ulceration) the tumor is likely in an invasive phase. Nodular melanoma is known to have a poorer prognosis, because it may stay unnoticed, both by patients and by physicians, due to its

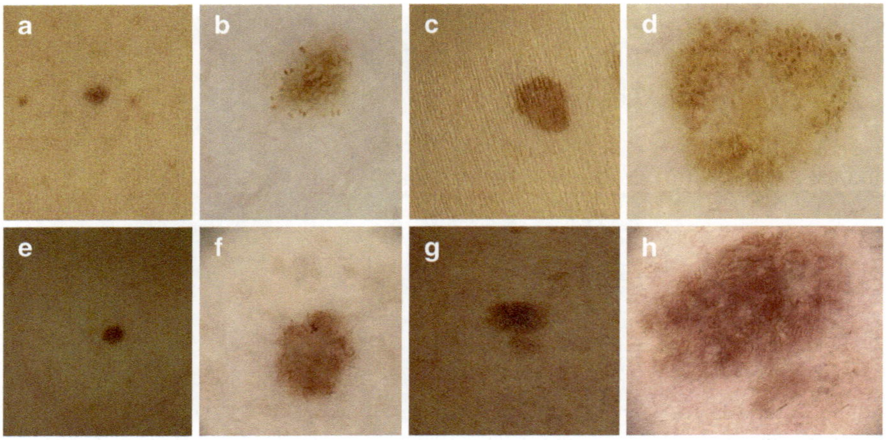

Fig. 6.16 Four examples of nevus-like in situ melanomas. All dermoscopy images are PD (20×). (**a**) Clinical image of a LENTIGINOUS MELANOMA IN SITU, not associated with nevus (de novo). (**b**) Dermoscopy: atypical network and peripheral irregular globules and pseudopods. (**c**) Clinical image of a SUPERFICIAL SPREADING MELANOMA IN SITU, ASSOCIATED WITH A JUNCIONAL NEVUS. (**d**) Dermoscopy: atypical network, peripheral irregular aggregated globules, structureless central area with orthogonal bright-white lines. (**e**) Clinical image of a SUPERFICIAL SPREADING MELANOMA IN SITU, ASSOCIATED WITH A COMPOUND NEVUS. (**f**) Dermoscopy: atypical network, peripheral brown circles, structureless central area, and irregular hyperpigmentation. (**g**) Clinical image of a SUPERFICIAL SPREADING MELANOMA IN SITU, ASSOCIATED WITH A DERMAL NEVUS. (**h**) Dermoscopy: atypical network, irregular globules, structureless peripheral areas with irregular gray dots. (*Clinical and dermoscopy images courtesy of Dra. Ana Maria Sortino*)

symmetry, a diameter less than 6 mm, and uniform red to blue color [9, 84]. Five common melanoma morphologic groups were identified: typical, nevus-like, amelanotic/non-melanoma skin cancer-like, seborrheic keratosis-like, and lentigo maligna-like. The awareness of the variety of melanoma appearances helps to improve clinical diagnosis [85]. Historically, the addition of dermoscopy in the daily practice of dermatologists was an important step toward early diagnosis of melanoma, due to improvement on the recognition of both early and peculiar melanomas, leading to patient's better outcomes [9] (Fig. 6.16).

Conversely, very early and featureless melanomas may escape detection by dermoscopy-specific melanoma patterns [86]. Reflectance confocal microscopy was introduced as a third step for the evaluation of equivocal or difficult-to-diagnose lesions [50]. The correlation between dermoscopic structures and confocal features increased the diagnostic accuracy for melanoma, except for rare variants of melanoma with a predominance of dermal tumor [87, 88] (Fig. 6.17).

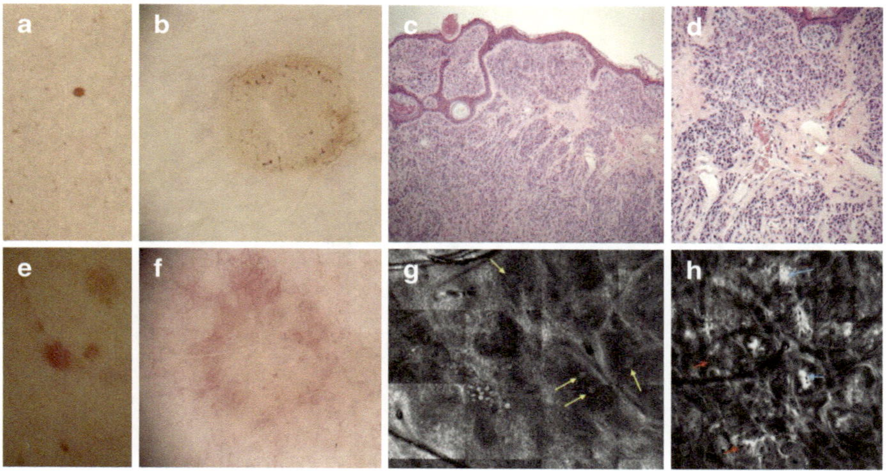

Fig. 6.17 Two palpable nodular pink melanocytic lesions. (**a**) Clinical image of a COMPOUND NEVUS. (**b**) PD (20×) allows the observation of comma-like vessels around the lesion, bright-white central lines, and comedo-like openings. (**c**) Histopathology (40×) showing intraepidermal and dermal nests of melanocytes. (**d**) Histopathology (200×) ectatic capillaries in between the nests. (**e**) Clinical image of an AMELANOTIC MELANOMA IN SITU, SUPERFICIAL SPREADING TYPE, ASSOCIATED WITH COMPOUND NEVUS. (**f**) PD (20×) shows polymorphous vessels irregularly distributed, multiple orthogonal bright-white central lines. (**g**) RCM image at the DEJ showing hyporeflective dense and sparse dermal nests (yellow arrows). (**h**) RCM image at the upper dermis with hyperreflective collagen bundles (blue arrows) and an increased number of linear/perpendicular vessels (red arrows). RCM images are close-ups of wide probe 8 × 8 mm mosaics. (*Clinical, dermoscopy and RCM images courtesy of Dra. Ana Maria Sortino. Histopathology images courtesy of Dra. Rafaela Brito de Paula*)

Dermoscopy of Melanoma

Melanoma diagnostic accuracy and sensitivity is increased by dermoscopy. The technic also improves the detection of thinner tumors [9, 18, 89]. Dermoscopy must be analyzed in context with the clinical findings of a lesion (flat, elevated, degree of firmness), comparative reasoning, patient history (age, gender, skin type, location, extent of sun damage) and "gut feeling," because melanomas, as well as other skin cancers, may lack specific dermoscopic features [9, 89] (Fig. 6.18). A melanoma may become recognizable only with time, and information if it's a new or changing lesion may be very helpful [9, 90] (Fig. 6.19).

The main dermoscopic melanoma-specific structures are atypical pigment network, negative pigment network, irregular dots and globules, peripheral irregular streaks (pseudopods and radial streaming), regression structures as gray dots and granules and scar-like depigmented areas, blue-white veil, shiny white streaks, dark

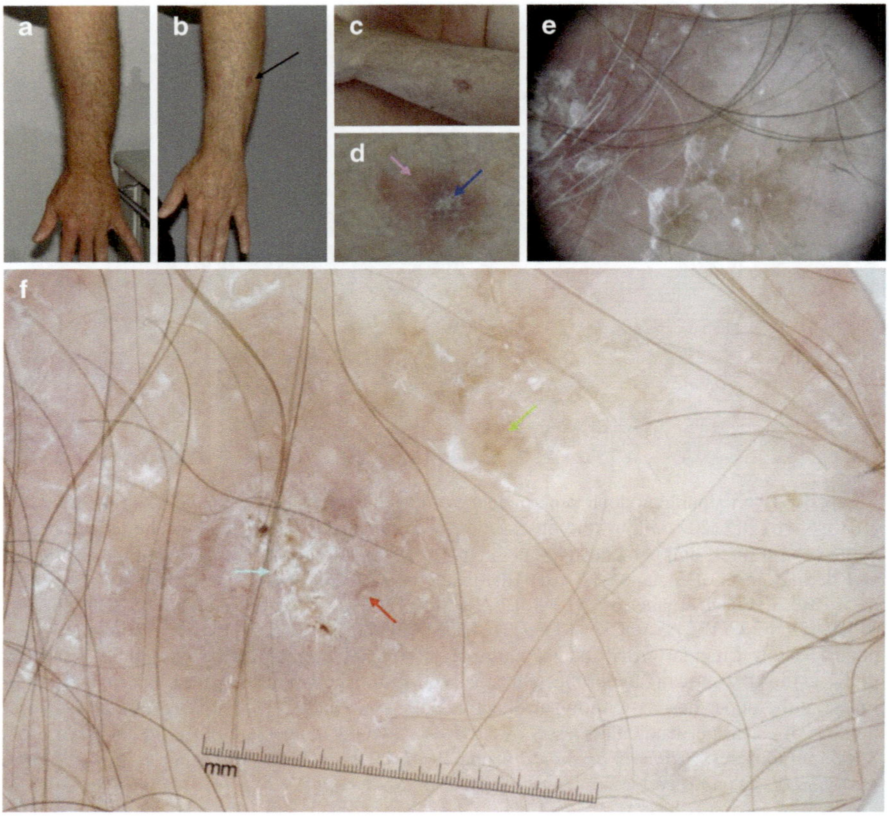

Fig. 6.18 Male patient in his fifties, phototype I, and family history of melanoma. (**a**) Clinical baseline image (**b**) 4-year follow-up clinical image with the presence of a new hypertrophic and erythematous lesion. (**c**) An image with a better clinical view. (**d**) Close-up image of the lesion with scales (blue arrow) and eczema-like erythema (pink arrow), also known as Meyerson phenomenon. (**e**) Contact PD (10×) showing central structureless pink area and scales. (**f**) Close-up of PD (10×) image showing linear atypical vessels (red arrow), peripheral structureless tan area (green arrow), and central scales (teal arrow). The lesion was fully excised with 2 mm margins. The final diagnosis was SUPERFICIAL SPREADING INVASIVE MELANOMA, NOT ASSOCIATED WITH NEVUS, Breslow 1.3 mm. (*Clinical and dermoscopy images courtesy of Ana Maria Sortino MD, MSc*)

structureless areas (off-centered or multiple blotches), and polymorphous vessels [89, 91]. Nonfacial melanoma on chronic sun damaged skin mostly shows one of the three main patterns: patchy peripheral pigmented islands, angulated lines, and tan structureless areas with granularity [92]. Nodular melanomas are known to show an overall homogeneous or featureless pattern; however, when melanoma specific structures are present, they show a disorganized and asymmetric arrangement [84]. Amelanotic and uncommon histologic variants of melanomas may be more difficult to recognize [93]. Amelanotic and hypomelanotic melanomas commonly show linear irregular vessels as the predominant type, or the combination of dotted

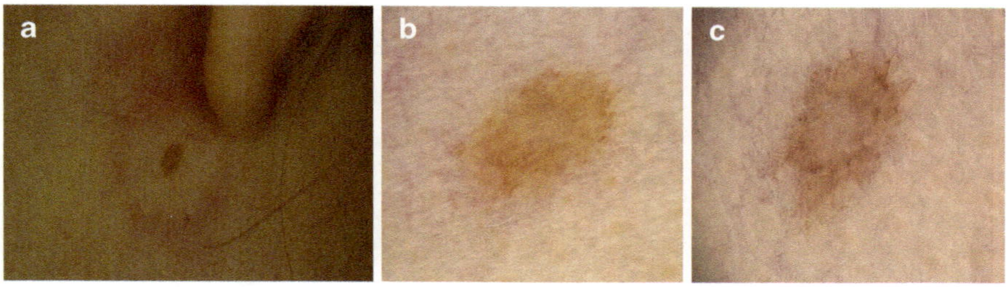

Fig. 6.19 Third decade female patient with personal history of multiple melanomas. (**a**) New clinical symmetric light brown flat lesion on the posterior aspect of the neck. (**b**) Baseline dermoscopic image showing a structureless tan lesion. (**c**) After 16 months, follow-up dermoscopic image demonstrates gain of peripheral irregular brown hyperpigmentation. Both images are PD (20×). The lesion was excised with a final diagnosis of SUPERFICIAL SPREADING INVASIVE MELANOMA, NOT ASSOCIATED WITH NEVUS, Clark II, Breslow 0.2 mm. (*Clinical and dermoscopy images courtesy of Ana Maria Sortino MD*)

and linear irregular vessels, more than one shade of pink, milky-red globules, and irregularly shaped depigmentation [94] (Fig. 6.17). Nevoid melanomas have a nevus-like pattern, but with irregular globules/dots and atypical vascular structures [93, 95, 96]. Desmoplastic melanoma usually presents at least one melanoma-specific clue under dermoscopy, with a high prevalence of atypical vessels, regression structures, and more than three colors [93, 97, 98]. Spitzoid, nested, and balloon cell melanomas may display an asymmetric multicomponent pattern, and verrucous melanoma a homogeneous color with crusts and a rough surface [93] (Fig. 6.20).

Dermoscopy can be used to estimate tumor thickness. Dermoscopic indicative patterns of melanoma in situ are atypical network, regression, irregular hyperpigmented areas, and angulated lines [99–101]. Common patterns of thick melanomas are blue-white veil, scar-like depigmentation, shiny white structures, and milky-red areas [100, 101] (Fig. 6.21).

RCM of Melanoma

When a lesion looks clinically benign, dermoscopic melanoma-specific criteria may fail to be present or may not be clearly identified, and yet the physician feels it's suspicious, considering its solitary nature ("only son of a widowed mother" sign), or the dermoscopic pattern differs from the patient's nevus signature ("ugly duckling" sign), or it's a pinky lesion in an individual with fair skin and light-colored hair ("little red riding hood" sign), or on digital dermoscopy follow-up, it shows enlargement and/or gain/loss of pattern. In those situations, RCM can be used to provide additional information, and may facilitate the correct clinical diagnosis [9, 102–104]. RCM criteria for the diagnosis of melanoma are shown on Table 6.2.

Dark lesions are usual suspects. They can be a challenge to confidently rule out a melanocytic tumor, despite clinical and dermoscopic information. A recent study

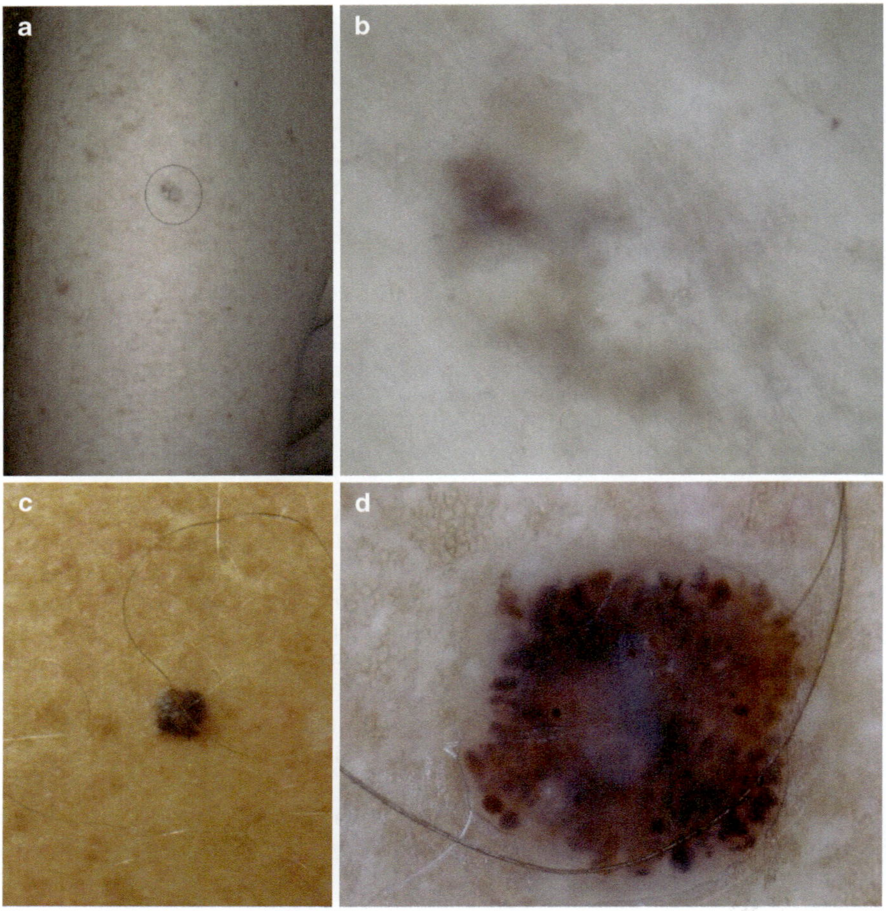

Fig. 6.20 Two uncommon histologic variants of melanomas. (**a**) Female in her eighties, skin type I, intense photodamage. A skin-colored depressed and indurated lesion on the right arm, found on palpation during the clinical exam. The lesion was unknown to the patient. (**b**) Dermoscopy shows an asymmetric pattern with more than three colors (white, brown, and gray). Pathology diagnosis was DESMOPLASTIC MELANOMA. (**c**) Male in his seventies, skin type I, intense photodamage. A dark stand-out nodular lesion on the left arm, found on total body skin exam. The lesion was unknown to the patient. (**d**) Dermoscopy reveals a central blue-white veil and irregular globules (different shapes and colors) in a starburst pattern. Histological diagnosis was SPITIZOID AND SUPERFICIAL SPREADING INVASIVE MELANOMA, Clark II, Breslow 0.6 mm. Dermoscopic images are close-up of PD (10×). (*Clinical and dermoscopy images courtesy of Ana Maria Sortino MD, MSc*)

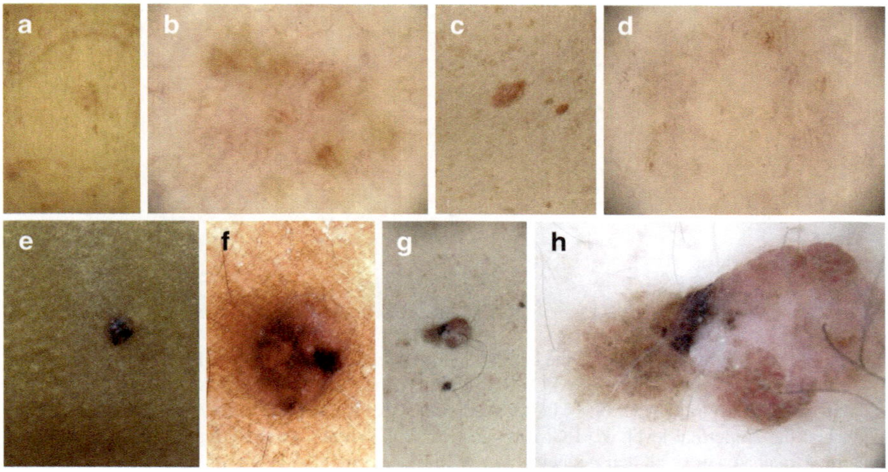

Fig. 6.21 Four invasive melanomas. (**a**) Male in his seventies, skin type III, brown hair when young, intense photodamage and personal history of multiple melanomas. A skin-colored flat lesion was followed for 3 years until it became mildly pinkish. (**b**) PD (20×) showing central polymorphous atypical vessels, irregular peripheral brown hyperpigmentation, and focal grayish granularity. Pathology diagnosis was SUPERFICIAL SPREADING INVASIVE MELANOMA, NOT ASSOCIATED WITH NEVUS, Clark III, Breslow 0.3 mm. (**c**) Female in her thirties, skin type I, red hair, personal and family history of multiple melanomas. A pinky stand-out slightly palpable lesion on the posterior aspect of the left shoulder. (**d**) PD (20×) showing central shiny orthogonal white lines, diffuse polymorphous atypical vessels, and focal irregular peripheral globules. Pathology disclosed a SUPERFICIAL SPREADING INVASIVE MELANOMA, ASSOCIATED WITH DERMAL NEVUS, Clark III, Breslow 0.4 mm. (**e**) Female in her fifties, skin type IV, noticed a growing lesion on the left arm for 9 months. (**f**) PD (10×) allows the observation of peripheral shiny orthogonal white lines, central pigmented atypical network, eccentric black blotch (island), and focal irregular globules. Histological diagnosis was SUPERFICIAL SPREADING INVASIVE MELANOMA, NOT ASSOCIATED WITH NEVUS, Clark III, Breslow 0.8 mm. (**g**) Male in his thirties, skin type II. An upper posterior trunk multicolored nodular lesion. (**h**) Close-up image of PD (10×) shows on the palpable aspect of the lesion, a milky-red structureless center, within grouped red clods and a focal area of dark brown/black irregular globules. The flat peripheral area of the lesion discloses an island of irregular brown hyperpigmentation. Histological diagnosis was SUPERFICIAL SPREADING INVASIVE MELANOMA, ASSOCIATED WITH CONGENITAL DERMAL NEVUS, Clark IV, Breslow 1.3 mm. (*Clinical and dermoscopy images courtesy of Ana Maria Sortino MD, MSc; Monica Freitas, MD; Marcos Martins, MD, MSc, PhD*)

integrated RCM for the analysis of 370 dark pigmented lesions and found 89 melanomas (93.3% "de novo"/6.7% nevus associated), with a median Breslow thickness of 0.9 mm. The clinical/dermoscopy/RCM approach avoided 60.6% of unnecessary excisions. Almost all melanomas (96.6%) were diagnosed; there were three false negative cases at baseline, but after digital follow-up they were recognized [105].

Our personal experience shows that incipient, nevus-like, and other benign-looking melanomas may be diagnosed by the integrated approach (clinical/dermoscopic/RCM) (Figs. 6.22, 6.23, 6.24, 6.25, and 6.26).

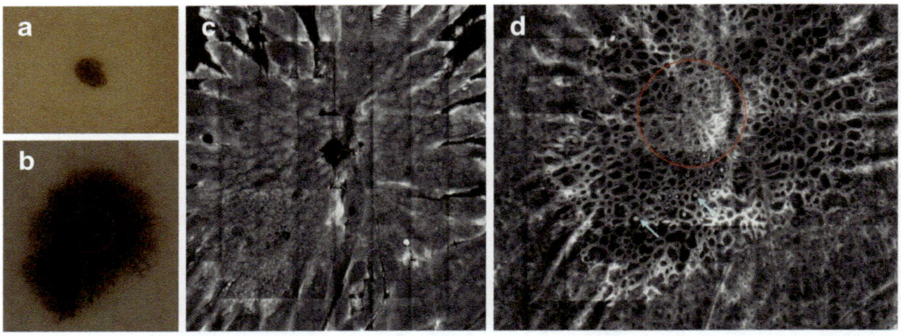

Fig. 6.22 Dark pigmented lesion on the lumbar region of female patient in her fifties. (**a**) Clinical image of a macular brown-black mole. (**b**) NPD (10×) built into the RCM machine, showing peripheral atypical network and central brown-black blotch (red circle). (**c**) RCM image shows a typical honeycomb pattern at the epidermal level. (**d**) RCM image at the DEJ shows a mostly regular peripheral ringed pattern, a focal area of small dense juncional nests (turquoise arrows), and a central irregular meshwork with cytologic atypia. RCM images are wide probe 8 × 8 mm mosaics. Final histologic diagnosis was ATYPICAL LENTIGINOUS JUNCTIONAL MELANOCYTIC PROLIFERATION. Despite the intense cytoarchitectural atypia, the suspected area was not represented in the serial sections and the lesion didn't fully meet the criteria for in situ melanoma. The lesion was treated with 0.5 cm margins. (*Clinical, dermoscopy and RCM images courtesy of Ana Maria Sortino MD, MSc*)

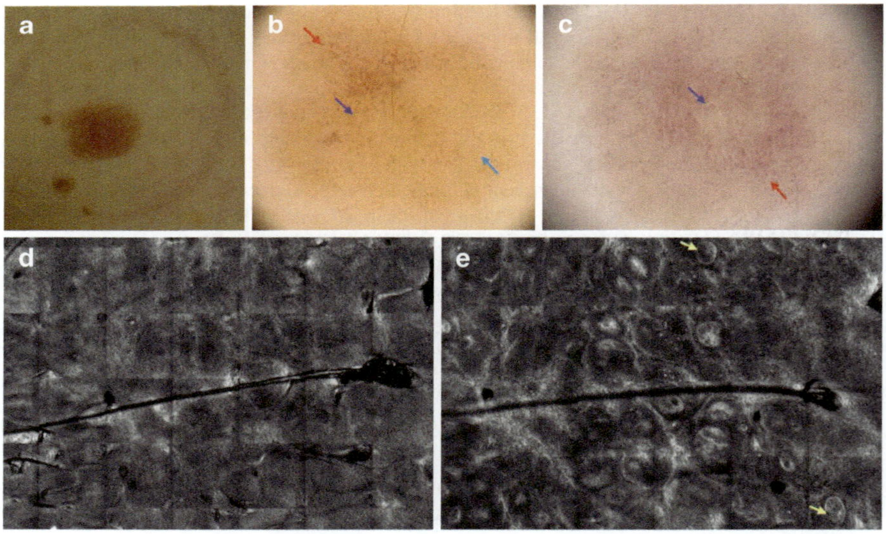

Fig. 6.23 Female patient in her thirties that wanted to avoid excision of a suspicious pink lesion on a flexural area (medial knee). (**a**) Clinical image of a slightly palpable, large, atypical mole. (**b**) Baseline PD (20×) reveals a structureless tan background (blue arrow), central negative network (purple arrow), and polymorphous vessels (red arrow). (**c**) 3-year follow-up PD (20×) image showing increase of both central negative network (purple arrow) and polymorphous vessels (red arrow). (**d**) RCM image shows an atypical honeycomb pattern at the epidermal level. (**e**) RCM image at the DEJ shows multiple irregular dense-sparse nests with hyporeflective cells (yellow arrow) and areas of cytologic atypia. RCM images are close-ups of wide probe 8 × 8 mm mosaics. The patient finally agreed to have the lesion excised and the histologic diagnosis was SUPERFICIAL SPREADING MELANOMA IN SITU, ASSOCIATED WITH COMPOUND NEVUS. (*Clinical, dermoscopy, and RCM images courtesy of Ana Maria Sortino MD, MSc*)

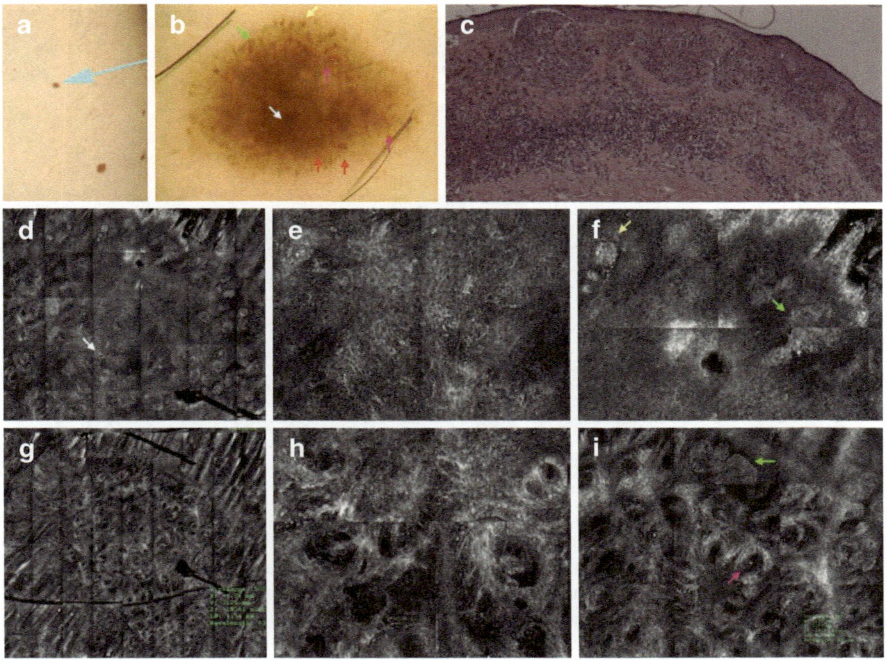

Fig. 6.24 New nevus-like pigmented lesion on the right hypochondrium of a male AMS patient in his forties, with family history of melanoma. (**a**) Clinical image of a new slightly palpable brown melanocytic lesion (turquoise arrow). (**b**) PD (30×) showing peripheral pseudopods (green arrow) and atypical globules (yellow arrow), irregular hyperpigmented areas (white arrow), linear vessels (red arrows), and dotted vessels within brown rim circles (pink arrows). (**c**) Histological examination reveals a neoplasm characterized by proliferation of cells with abundant cytoplasm, sometimes containing melanin pigment. The nuclei are hyperchromatic, polymorphic, with evident nucleoli. They spread side by side or form nests along the dermo-epidermal junction and above it. Neoplastic cells infiltrate the papillary dermis in the form of nests or isolated cells. In the dermis there are melanophages and lymphocytic inflammatory infiltrate. (**d**) RCM at the epidermal level shows an irregular honeycomb pattern with epidermal infiltration of polymorphous atypical cells (white arrow). (**e**) RCM image of the pagetoid cell infiltrate. (**f**) RCM image of the periphery shows presence of epidermal dense-sparse isolated nests (yellow arrow) and confluent nests (green arrow). (**g**) RCM at the DEJ shows an atypical meshwork. (**h**) RCM image of the lesion center discloses non-edged papillae and enlarged juncional spaces with infiltration of atypical cells. (**i**) RCM image of the lesion periphery showing dense-sparse nests (green arrow), and perpendicular vessels within the papillae (pink arrow). RCM images are close-ups of wide probe 8 × 8 mm mosaics. Final histologic diagnosis was SUPERFICIAL SPREADING INVASIVE MELANOMA, NOT ASSOCIATED WITH NEVUS, Clark III, Breslow 0.4 mm. (*Clinical, dermoscopy and RCM images courtesy of Ana Maria Sortino MD, MSc. Histopathology images courtesy of Gilles Landman MD, PhD*)

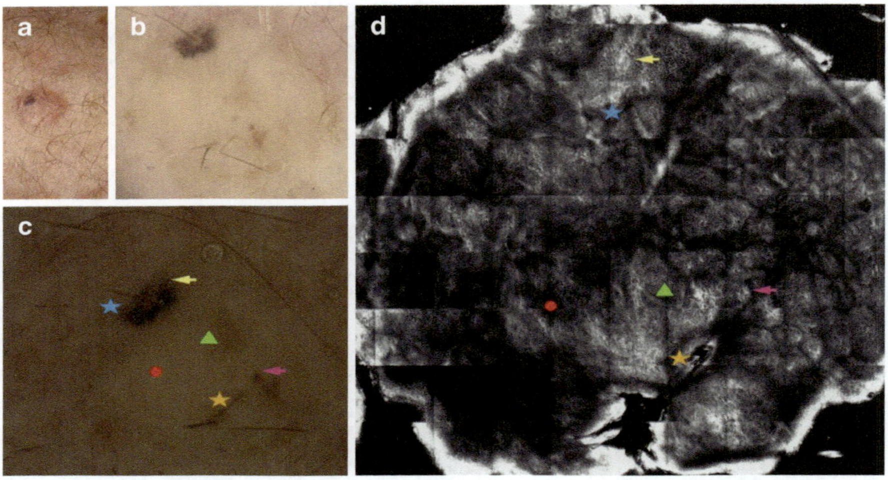

Fig. 6.25 New dermal nevus-like hypopigmented lesion on the left arm of a male patient in his sixties with personal history of multiple melanomas. (**a**) Clinical image of a new palpable firm pink lesion. (**b**) PD (20×) showing peripheral hair follicle surrounded by bluish-gray granules, structureless tan color, brown irregular pigmentation, and a focal area of atypical brown globules. (**c**) NPD (10x) built into the RCM machine. Blue/orange star: hair follicle, yellow arrow: bluish-gray granules, red dot: structureless area, green triangle: brown irregular pigmentation, and pink arrow: atypical brown globules. (**d**) RCM wide probe 8 × 8 mm mosaic at the DEJ level and respective structures highlighted by blue/orange star: hair follicle, yellow arrow/green triangle: bright irregular cells in sheet-like manner, red dot: non-edged papillae, and pink arrow: aggregated irregular cells forming nests. Final histologic diagnosis was SUPERFICIAL SPREADING INVASIVE MELANOMA, NOT ASSOCIATED WITH NEVUS, Clark IV, Breslow 1.5 mm. (*Clinical, dermoscopy and RCM images courtesy of Ana Maria Sortino MD, MSc*)

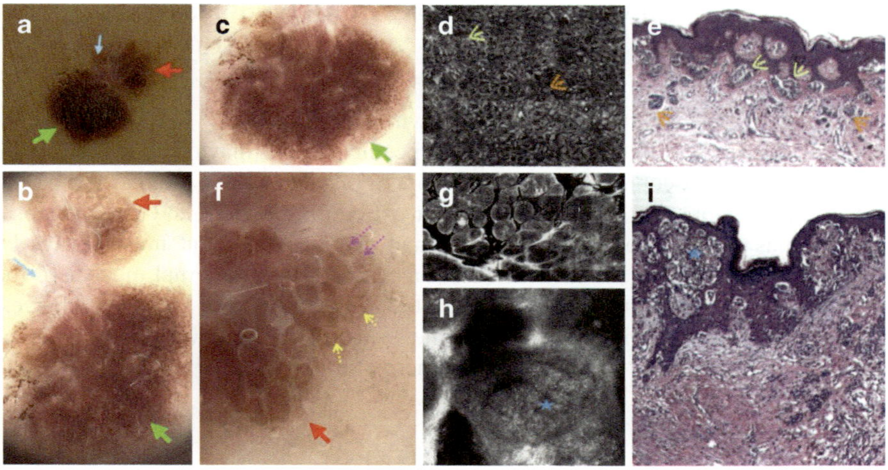

Fig. 6.26 Female in her fifties noticed a peripheral palpable enlargement of a long-standing nevus. She has intense sun-damaged skin and more than 50 moles. No personal history of skin cancer. A 3 mm punch biopsy was performed by the first dermatologist that saw the patient, with a diagnosis of invasive melanoma. The patient was then referred to a skin cancer clinic. (**a**) Clinical image of the lesion. Green arrow showing the flat nevus, red arrow the palpable area, and blue arrow the biopsy scar. (**b**) PD (20×) of the nevus flat component (green arrow), the palpable component (red arrow), and the milky-red scar area with shiny white lines (blue arrow). (**c**) PD (20×) showing central structureless brown, areas of irregular hyperpigmentation, and peripheral teared globules (green arrow). (**d**) RCM at the DEJ level reveals an irregular meshwork with juncional (lime arrowhead) and dermal (orange arrowhead) atypical nests**.** (**e**) Histopathology of a DYSPLASTIC COMPOUND NEVUS that shows juncional (lime arrowhead) and dermal (orange arrowhead) atypical nests**.** (**f**) PD (40×) showing irregular aggregated dark and light globules (red arrow), some globules with a brown rim forming circles (yellow dotted arrow), and very thin polymorphous vessels are seen within the globules (pink dotted arrows). (**g**) RCM oblique image reveals at the epidermal level an atypical honeycomb pattern, and dark oval areas at the DEJ. (**h**) RCM at the dermal level shows cerebriform nests (blue star)**.** RCM images are close-ups of wide probe 8 × 8 mm mosaics. (**i**) The lesion was fully excised, and histology shows confluent epidermal atypical nests (blue star) and involvement of the superficial dermis. The final histologic diagnosis was a SUPERFICIAL SPREADING INVASIVE MELANOMA, ASSOCIATED WITH DYSPLASTIC COMPOUND NEVUS, Clark II, Breslow 0.3 mm. This case had a good outcome; however, we want to address the need for full excision of suspicious melanocytic nevi. If the punch biopsy had been performed in the nevus component of the lesion, it could have had a disastrous outcome for both patient and the first attending physician. (*Clinical, dermoscopy and RCM images courtesy of Ana Maria Sortino MD, MSc., Maria Fernanda Hunziker, MD, Carlos Barcaui, MD, PhD. Histopathology images courtesy of Juan Piñeiro-Maceira, MD, MSc, PhD*)

Dermoscopic and Confocal Features of Melanomas at "Special Sites"

Melanoma in some parts of the body, known as "special sites," may show specific criteria, due to the different anatomy. The specific patterns may occur in addition to the classic dermoscopic features [6, 7, 13]. Acral melanomas include lesions on volar skin of palms and soles, non-volar skin extremities, fingers, and nails. Mucosal melanomas can develop on visible oral and genital areas, that must always be included in the TBSE. However, melanoma can happen on internal mucosa of the nasopharynx, larynx, respiratory/gastrointestinal/genitourinary tracts, and eyes. These areas must be remembered on the exam of patients with melanoma of unknown primary (MUP) and on management of high-risk patients [106].

Acral

Acral lentiginous melanoma (ALM) can be very challenging to diagnose at an early stage. It's frequently invasive when diagnosed, with poor patient outcome. Integrating dermoscopy and, when possible, RCM to exam acral lesions may help early detection of ALM [107, 108].

On dermoscopy ALM usually shows a parallel ridge pattern (PRP), characterized by a band-like pigmentation on the ridges of skin markings, and obscuring the acrosyringia. Irregular diffuse pigmentation with different shades of color is also an important diagnostic feature [107–109] (Fig. 6.27). PRP is the primary dermoscopic pattern in early lesions of ALM, conversely more advanced tumors may present more colors (red, blue, white), atypical vascular patterns, white scar-like depigmentation, and/or blue pepper-like granules, blue-white veil, and ulcers [107, 108] (Fig. 6.28). The BRAAFF checklist is a specific algorithm for acral melanocytic lesions, with 93.1% sensitivity and 86.7% specificity for melanoma diagnosis, that helps with biopsy decision [108]. Amelanotic melanoma on volar skin is rare and may display a "vascularized parallel ridge pattern," defined as erythema and dotted vessels filling the ridges and sparing the furrows [110, 111].

Subungual melanoma occurs secondary to proliferation of atypical melanocytes on the nail matrix. A complete history of the nail lesion may provide clues for the correct diagnosis. A previous trauma, recent irregular pigmentation, rapid growth, and nail plate dystrophy are alert signs for suspecting subungual melanoma [6]. Dermoscopy of early nail apparatus melanoma presents as pigmented lines of the nail plate with a progressive enlarging width, forming a triangular shape at the base. The dermoscopic features of more advanced subungual melanoma include irregular brown to black bands with different shades of color, 7 mm or larger width, irregular spacing and parallelism of the bands, pigmentation of the proximal nailfold cuticle

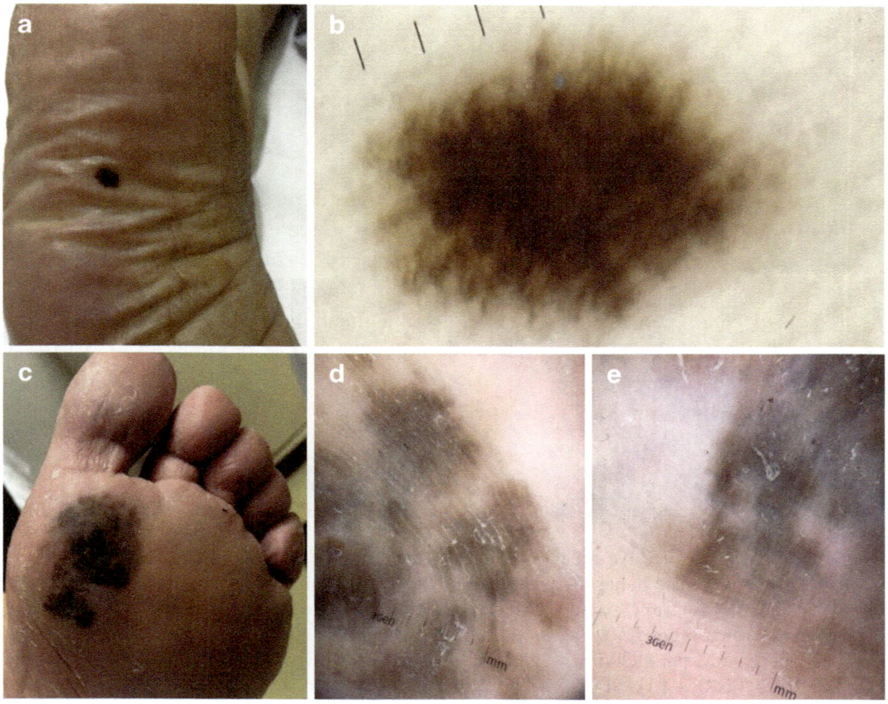

Fig. 6.27 Volar skin early melanomas. (**a**) Clinical image of a new hyperpigmented flat lesion on the left plantar arch of a female in her fifties. (**b**) Dermoscopic image showing irregular diffuse pigmentation with different shades of brown and peripheral parallel ridge pattern. Final histologic diagnosis was a LENTIGINOUS ACRAL MELANOMA IN SITU. (**c**) Clinical image of a large hyperpigmented flat lesion, with a 10-year history of growth, on the left plantar forefoot of a male patient in his eighties. (**d**) Dermoscopic image reveals parallel ridge pattern. (**e**) Dermoscopic image showing irregular diffuse pigmentation with different shades of brown, black, gray, and white. Final histologic diagnosis was a LENTIGINOUS ACRAL MELANOMA IN SITU. Images are PD (10×). (*Clinical and dermoscopy images courtesy of Adriana Mendes, MD, MSc, Gisele Barros, MD, MSc, and Anna Rita Ferrante Mitidieri de Oliveira, MD*)

(micro-Hutchison's sign), pigmentation of the surrounding skin (Hutchison's sign), and nail dystrophy [6, 109, 112] (Fig. 6.29).

RCM is less frequently used on volar skin due to stratum corneum thickness. Skin scraping prior to RCM examination allows for better imaging of the lesion. At the epidermal level, in situ ALM frequently presents an irregular honeycomb pattern, whereas invasive ALM shows a disarranged pattern. Another epidermal finding is granular dust-like hyper-reflective particles. At the DEJ a proliferation of atypical melanocytes may be seen. When the dermis is visible, sheets and/or nests of large, atypical cells are present [113] (Fig. 6.30).

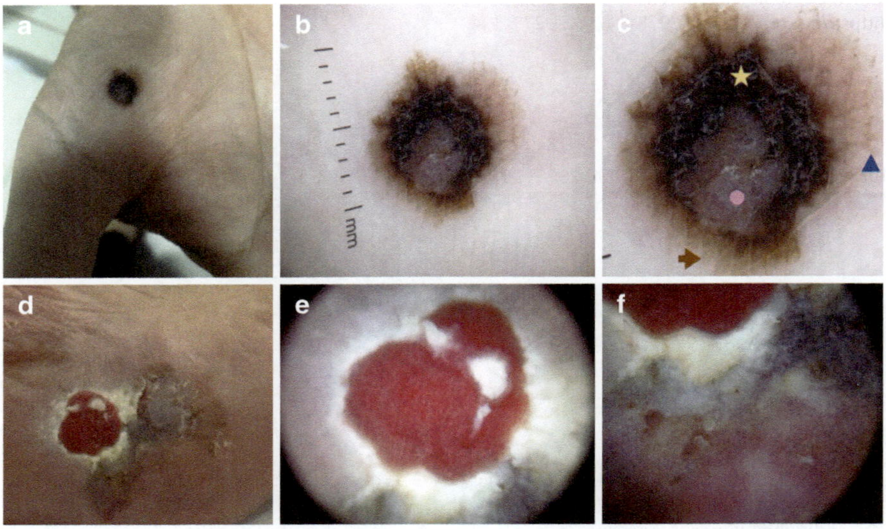

Fig. 6.28 Volar skin invasive melanomas. (**a**) Clinical image of a palpable multicolored right palmar lesion of a female in her fifties. (**b**) Dermoscopy highlights the lesion multiple colors (tan, dark brown, and gray). (**c**) Close-up of dermoscopic image showing parallel ridge pattern (brown arrow), dark brown pigment obliterating the acrosyringial (yellow star), central red clods (pink dot), and peripheral parallel furrow pattern (blue triangle). Final histologic diagnosis was an INVASIVE SUPERFICIAL SPREADING MELANOMA, Clark IV, Breslow 1.2 mm, with perineural infiltration. (**d**) Clinical image of a very large lesion with nodule and plaque on the right plantar forefoot of a male patient in his eighties. (**e**) Dermoscopy of the nodular component showing homogeneous red and white areas. (**f**) Dermoscopic image of the flat area showing multicolored pigmentation with shades of blue, purple, gray, pink, and light brown. Final histologic diagnosis was an ULCERATED INVASIVE LENTIGINOUS ACRAL MELANOMA, Clark IV, Breslow 4.1 mm, not associated with nevus. Images are PD (10×). (*Clinical and dermoscopy images courtesy of Flávia Brandão, MD and Marcos Martins, MD, PhD*)

Face

Lentigo maligna (LM) is a subtype of melanoma that mostly occurs on the face and chronic sun-damaged skin, in elderly patients [114]. Initial lesions may appear as clinically inconspicuous uniform pigmented macules [115]. The earliest dermoscopic signs of LM are related to pigmentation involving the follicular openings, such as asymmetric pigmented follicular openings, slate-gray dots, and globules. With further progression, rhomboidal structures appear and finally the follicular invasion is characterized by the development of obliterated hair follicles [116]. Although each dermatoscopic LM criterion may be also seen in solar lentigo, flat seborrheic keratosis and pigmented actinic keratosis (PAK), the presence of all four features is strongly suggestive of LM, reaching 89% of sensitivity and 93% of specificity for LM diagnosis [116, 117]. Additional notable features include a follicular

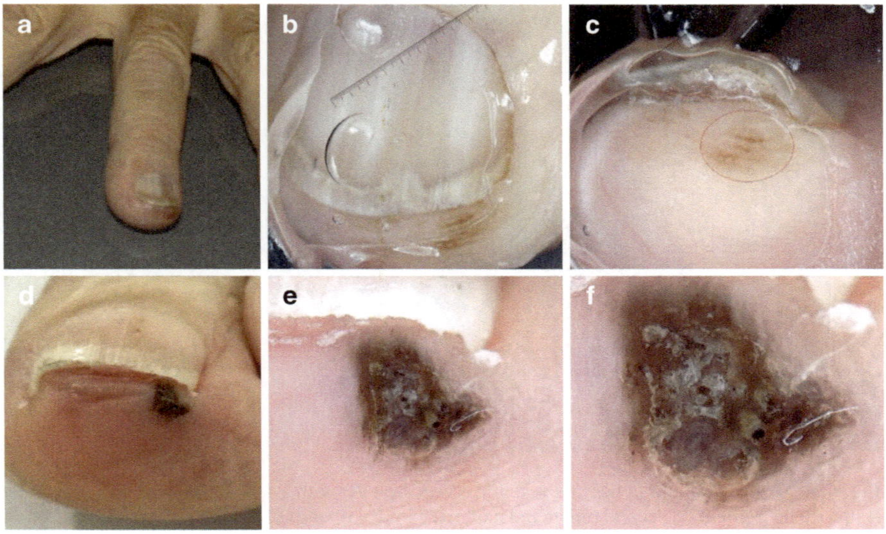

Fig. 6.29 Subungual melanomas. (**a**) Clinical image of a hypopigmented lesion of the nail and hyponychium, present for 1 year, on the left hand third finger. The patient is a male in his eighties. He complains of local pain and difficulty to play the piano. (**b**) Dermoscopic image shows pale gray-brown irregular nail bands, hyponychial brown pigmentation, and nail dystrophy. (**c**) Dermoscopic image reveals a parallel ridge pattern on the hyponychial skin (red circle). Final histologic diagnosis was a LENTIGINOUS ACRAL MELANOMA IN SITU. (**d**) Clinical image of a new hyperpigmented lesion on the left hallux hyponychium. The patient is a female in her eighties. (**e**) Dermoscopic image shows a diffuse brownish base and a hyperkeratotic center. (**f**) Dermoscopy close-up reveals red clods, and brown-black irregular globules within the keratin. Final histologic diagnosis was an INVASIVE LENTIGINOUS ACRAL MELANOMA, Clark IV, Breslow 1.2 mm. Images are close-ups of PD (10×). (*Clinical and dermoscopy images courtesy of Ana Maria Sortino MD, MSc, and Marcos Martins, MD, PhD*)

circle within a circle pattern, indicative of atypical melanocytes extending down adnexa [115]. Gray pigmentation might be the most common finding in early LM and it was found in 88.6% of LM cases in one study [118–120]. Lallas et al. observed that the most potent predictors of LM are gray rhomboids, non-evident follicles, and intense pigmentation [121].

The dermoscopic diagnosis of initial LM can be challenging because it presents overlapping characteristics with other pigmented macules on chronic sun-damaged skin [122]. RCM improves diagnostic accuracy of facial melanoma and can aid in diagnosis [123–125]. Presence of dendritic and/or roundish cells has been established as a highly specific RCM pattern for LM diagnosis [126]. The presence of few dendritic cells in the epidermal layer around the hair follicle is described in PAK, but the infiltration of the hair follicle by many of these cells, corresponding to folliculotropism (called "medusa head" feature), is a specific feature of LM [127] (Fig. 6.31).

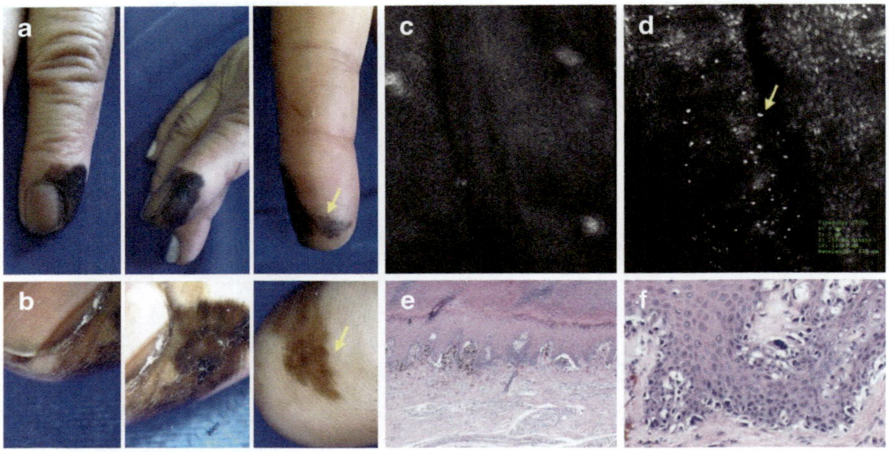

Fig. 6.30 Female patient in her late seventies, skin type IV, with a 10-year history of a pigmented lesion on the right hand second finger and nail. (**a**) Clinical images of the lesion with three different views: nail, lateral finger, and palmar region (yellow arrow). (**b**) PD (10×) showing brown to black irregular nail bands, hyponychial pigmentation, irregular diffuse pigmentation of the lateral finger, and parallel ridge pattern of the palmar aspect (yellow arrow). (**c**) RCM at the epidermal level of normal volar skin, typical honeycomb pattern, and eccrine ducts are seen on patient's second finger of the left hand. (**d**) RCM at the epidermal level of the pigmented lesion on volar skin, irregular honeycomb pattern with multiple dust-like bright particles (yellow arrow) and diffuse small roundish bright pagetoid cells around acrosyringia on patient's second finger of the right hand. (**e**) Histology (40×) shows a thick compact horny layer, intraepithelial atypical melanocytic neoplasm with lentiginous pattern, and nest formation. (**f**) Histology (200×) shows lentiginous proliferation of anaplastic melanocytes. Final histologic diagnosis was a LENTIGINOUS ACRAL MELANOMA IN SITU. RCM 0.75 × 0.75 mm individual images from handheld probe. (*Clinical and dermoscopy images courtesy of Carolina Malavassi Murari MD, RCM images courtesy of Ana Maria Sortino MD, MSc, and Histopathology images courtesy of Alexandre O. Michalany, MD*)

Scalp

Scalp melanoma is responsible for 5% of all melanomas and it has worse prognosis than melanoma located elsewhere. Late diagnosis due to disguising by the hair coverage and difficulties in interpreting dermoscopy findings are possible explanations for that [128–130]. Until 2012, only two case reports described dermoscopic patterns of scalp melanomas—the first one referred similar patterns as melanomas on the trunk and limbs [131] while the second one referred similar pattern of melanoma on the face [132]. In 2012 Stanganelli et al. described dermoscopic patterns of 71 scalp melanomas: regression and atypical network/pseudo-network were more common in thin melanomas (in situ and Breslow thickness <1 mm), and irregular

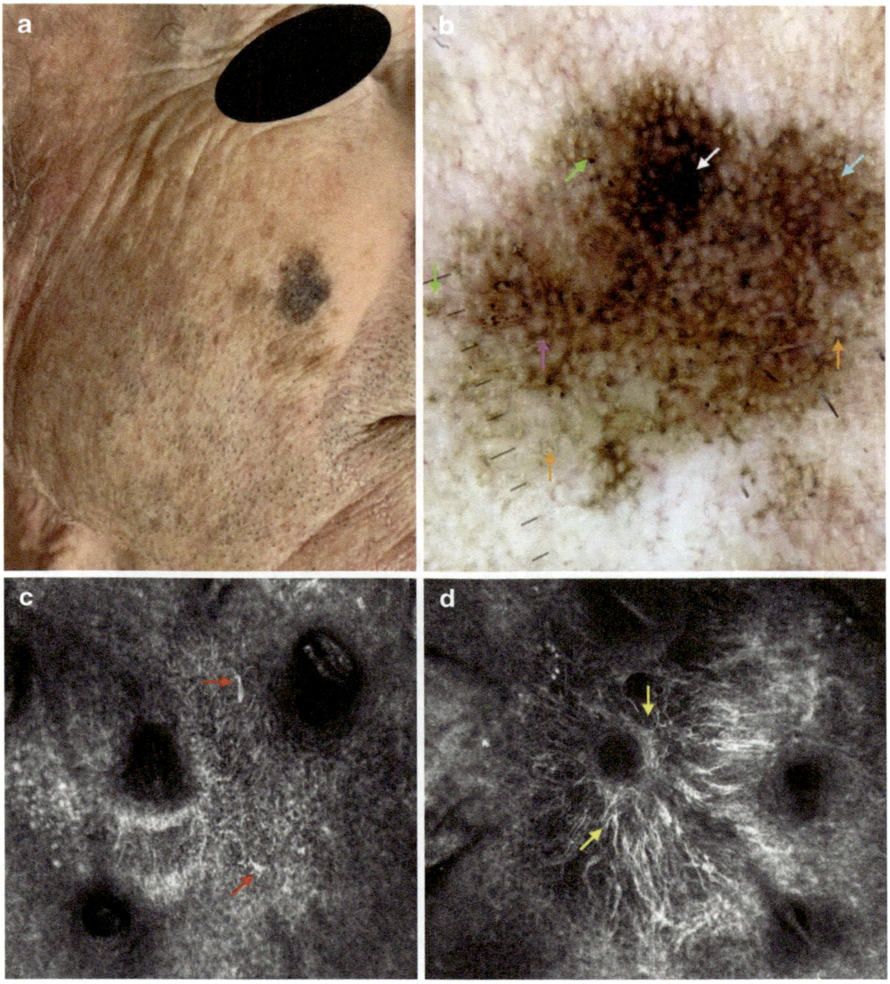

Fig. 6.31 (**a**) An isolated blackish-brown macula was observed on the right cheek. (**b**) Close-up of PD (10×) shows intense pigmentation, asymmetric pigmented follicular opening (pink arrow), slate-gray dots and globules (green arrows), rhomboidal structures (teal arrow), non-evident follicles (white arrow), and circles within circles (orange arrows). (**c**) RCM at the level of the epidermis: presence of dendritic pagetoid cells (red arrows). (**d**) RCM at the level of the dermoepidermal junction: presence of dendritic cells arranged radially from the hair follicle, forming the "medusa head" (yellow arrows). Histopathologic analysis confirmed a MELANOMA IN SITU, LENTIGO MALIGNA TYPE. RCM 0.75 × 0.75 mm individual images from handheld probe. (*Clinical, dermoscopy, and RCM images courtesy of Ana Carolina S. Porto Mitsunaga MD, and Juliana Casagrande T. Braga, MD, PhD*)

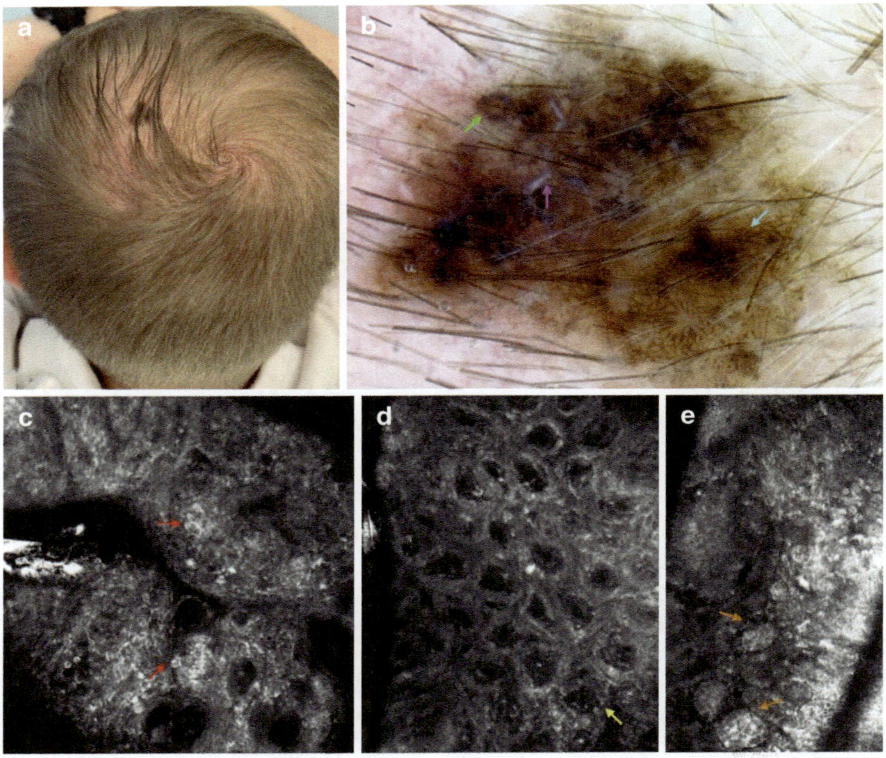

Fig. 6.32 (**a**) A brownish macula was observed on the vertex. (**b**) Dermoscopic evaluation shows regression (green arrow), atypical network (teal arrow), and white shiny lines (pink arrow). (**c**) RCM at the level of the epidermis: presence of atypical cobblestone with scattered nucleated pleomorphic cells (red arrows). (**d**) RCM at the level of the DEJ: presence of nucleated cells and non-edged papillae (yellow arrow). (**e**) RCM at the dermal level: presence of heterogeneous melanocytic nests (orange arrows). Histopathologic analysis confirmed a SUPERFICIAL SPREADING INVASIVE MELANOMA, Breslow 0.3 mm. Dermoscopic image is a close-up of PD (10×) and RCM 0.75 × 0.75 mm individual images from handheld probe. (*Clinical, dermoscopy and RCM images courtesy of Ana Carolina S. Porto Mitsunaga MD, and Juliana Casagrande T. Braga, MD, PhD*)

pigmented blotches, blue-white veil, and unspecific pattern were more common in thick lesions [133]. In 2017, Benati et al. observed that the most frequent dermoscopic features in scalp melanoma were regression, atypical pseudo-network, and irregular pigmented blotches [134].

One study evaluated RCM features of scalp melanomas and the authors concluded that RCM features of scalp melanomas seem not to differ from RCM features of melanomas on the trunk. Pagetoid infiltration of round and dendritic atypical cells in the epidermis, and irregular meshwork at the DEJ were the most common features [134] (Fig. 6.32).

Mucosal Melanoma

Mucosal melanoma is responsible for 1% of all melanomas and can affect the glabrous portion of the lips, oral, anorectal, conjunctival, and other mucosal locations. Due to lack of early visible signs and symptoms, it is usually diagnosed at an advanced stage. Clinically, it's usually a solitary brown to black macule. In several studies, the dermoscopic features most observed are blue-white veil, followed by the presence of two or more colors and irregular vessels [135–138]. The International Dermoscopy Society affirmed that the presence of blue, gray, or white color is the most effective dermoscopic clue to distinguish between melanoma and benign mucosal lesions. Additionally, the association of at least one of the three colors and the existence of structureless zones had a higher diagnostic precision for mucosal melanoma [139]. A multicenter retrospective study focusing in thin (Breslow thickness <0.5 mm) and in situ mucosal melanomas found that the most frequent features were structureless areas, gray areas, irregular black-brown dots, and blue-white structures [140].

Under RCM examination, mucosal melanoma is characterized by the presence of pagetoid hyperreflective large and polymorphous cells in the epithelium (roundish or dendritic), high density of basal hyperreflective large dendritic and round cells, and loss of normal papillae architecture [141, 142]. The main differential diagnosis of mucosal melanoma is a melanotic macule, where dendritic bright cells can also be observed in basal layer of the epithelium, but usually are less numerous and smaller in size, with thinner dendrites [143, 144] (Fig. 6.33).

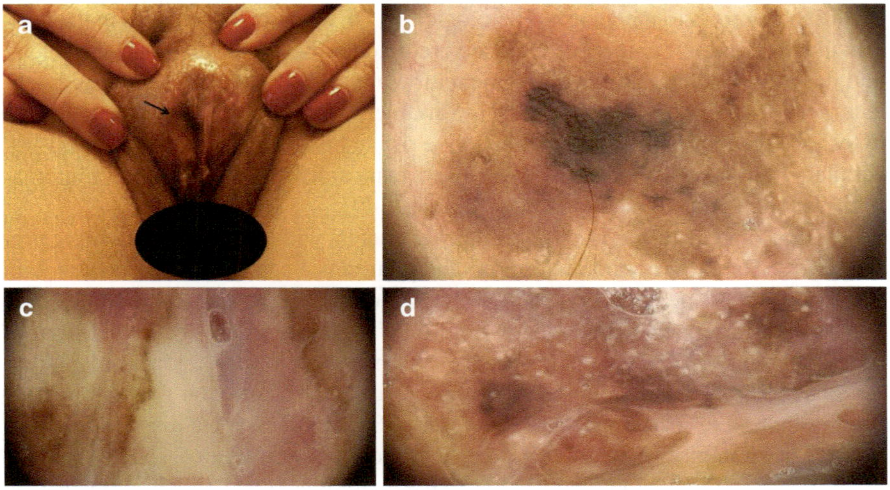

Fig. 6.33 (**a**) A solitary brown to black macule on the vulva (black arrow). (**b**–**d**) PD (20×) images show presence of three colors (black, gray, and white), and presence of structureless areas. Histopathologic analysis confirmed a SUPERFICIAL SPREADING MELANOMA. (*Clinical, dermoscopy and RCM images courtesy of Ana Carolina S. Porto Mitsunaga MD, and Juliana Casagrande T. Braga, MD, PhD*)

Dermoscopic and Reflectance Confocal Microscopy Features of Melanoma Mimickers: Dermatofibroma, Seborrheic Keratosis/Melanoacanthoma, Lichen Planus-Like Keratosis

There isn't a noninvasive skin imagining technique that's 100% accurate. A better comprehension of the benign skin tumors' universe may enhance the dermoscopic diagnosis accuracy. False positive diagnosis usually leads to unnecessary excisions and its unpleasant consequences. On the other hand, a false negative diagnosis is a worrisome scenario, because the diagnosis of a cancer may be overlooked [13]. This section will explore the main great mimickers of melanoma: dermatofibroma (DF), seborrheic keratosis (SK), and lichen planus-like keratosis (LPLK). There are other benign lesions that may be misdiagnosed as skin cancer; however, they won't be discussed in this chapter.

Dermatofibroma

DF is a common benign papular or nodular skin lesion comprising fibroblasts, histiocytes, coarse collagen, and blood vessels [145]. DFs are found predominantly on the limbs of middle-aged adults [146]. Clinically, they may be pink, red, or brown, small (<2 cm), firm, and well circumscribed. Most have a characteristic dimple when laterally compressed (dimple sign). Pigmented variants may represent a differential diagnosis to melanoma. Histologically, DF is typically centered in the mid-reticular dermis. The epidermal elongated rete ridges that are often broad, confluent, and flat at the bottom, with hyperpigmentation of basal keratinocytes, seen as a delicate network with dermoscopy [147]. Variable proportions of fibroblasts, histiocytes, collagenous and vascular stroma give rise to histopathological variants [148]: cellular, lipidized, angiomatous (vascular), hemosiderotic, aneurismal (angiomatoid), keloidal, and atypical dermatofibromas [149].

DF may display different morphological variants, with diverse dermoscopic presentations. The most common dermoscopic pattern is a central scar-like patch with a peripheric delicate network. Under polarized dermoscopy, shiny white lines may be present in the center, surrounded by a light pigmented network. Other dermoscopic findings of DF are negative network, homogeneous areas, and vascular structures (dotted, linear, irregular, and hairpin vessels). Less common features include dots, globule-like structures, scale-crust [150]. Some DF can be a diagnostic pitfall [144]. For example, when a central negative network is present in DF, ruling out Spitz nevus and melanoma is necessary [151]. Homogeneous bluish pigmentation may be an indicator for hemosiderotic variant of DF, but blue nevus and melanoma can be a differential diagnosis. Moreover, globules-like structures can be seen in pigmented DF, and it may lead to a misdiagnosis of a melanocytic lesion [148, 152].

RCM images of DF show a normal honeycomb or cobblestone pattern in the epidermis. In the DEJ, dermal papillae are seen as rings of bright monomorphic round cells that correspond to the pigmented keratinocytes in the basal layer. The central white scar-like area or negative network observed with dermoscopy is seen on RCM as bright thick fibrillar structures that correspond to the thick collagen bundles in the dermis [153]. Also, the dermoscopy-RCM correlation shows that globule-like structures seen in DF are wider bright rings, that correspond to pigmented rete ridges separated by a broadened dermal papilla [148] (Fig. 6.34). One limitation of RCM is imaging depth. Important histologic clues to DF diagnosis are in the dermis and may be out of the deep penetration power of RCM. Moreover, when the DF is nodular, the extensive acanthosis may not allow visualization of the deeper layers of the epidermis [154]. Doubtful lesions should be biopsied [102].

Seborrheic Keratosis

Seborrheic keratosis (SK) is a very common benign intraepidermal neoplasm that arises from epidermal keratinocytes and most commonly occurs in the aging skin [16]. Clinically, SK presents as a solitary or multiple stuck-on waxy patches, papules, or plaques. A brown or black appearance is typical, but some lesions can be

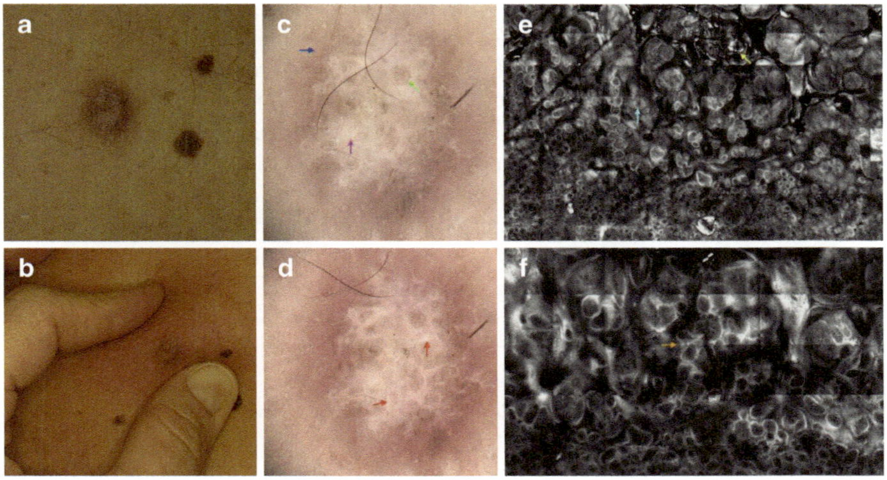

Fig. 6.34 (**a**) Clinical image of a nodular lesion on the back of a male patient in his thirties. (**b**) Lateral compression of the lesion showing the dimple sign. (**c**) NPD (20×) showing central scar-like patch (pink arrow), brown circles (green arrow), and a peripheric delicate network (blue arrow). (**d**) PD (20×) reveals orthogonal shiny white lines between brown circles (red arrows). (**e**) RCM at the epidermal level shows a central keratin mass (yellow arrow) surrounded by globule-like structures with typical honeycomb pattern (teal arrow), and rings. (**f**) RCM at the DEJ shows wider bright rings corresponding to broadened dermal papilla (orange arrow) and bright homogeneous areas (dense collagen). A clinical diagnosis of DERMATOFIBROMA was made, and the lesion is under follow-up due to size and unusual location. RCM images are close-ups of wide probe 8 × 8 mm mosaics. (*Clinical, dermoscopy and RCM images courtesy of Ana Maria Sortino MD, MSc*)

pale or gray. Usually, the SK diagnosis is straightforward after the clinical and dermoscopic examination. However, due to its multiple presentations, the differential diagnosis with melanoma can sometimes be challenging. Some melanomas present a verrucous surface and can be misdiagnosed as an SK [6, 16, 155].

Seborrheic keratoses are well-demarcated epidermal neoplasms comprised of a proliferation of basaloid keratinocytes. Hyperkeratosis, acanthosis, papillomatosis, pseudo-horn cyst formation, and increased basal layer pigmentation are common histopathologic features. Several histopathological variants are recognized. The most common is the *acanthotic type*, that is characterized by a regular architecture with broad adjoining columns of acanthotic epidermis, a flat base, and pseudo-horn cysts. Other histological variants: *keratotic*, with prominent hyperkeratosis; *adenoid*, with thin and elongated rete ridges; *clonal*, with the proliferation of sharply demarcated intraepidermal nests of basaloid or pale cells; *irritated*, with hyperkeratotic stratum corneum, scale crust, apoptosis, and lichenoid inflammation in the DEJ; *pigmented*, with increased pigmented keratinocytes; and *macular*, with mild acanthosis [16, 153, 156].

From the dermoscopic point of view, the most significant features for SK identification are milia-like cysts and comedo-like openings, that represent intraepidermal pseudo-horn cysts and keratin filled invaginations of the epidermis, respectively; ridges and fissures (brain-like appearance); light brown fingerprint-like structures; looped or hairpin vessels within a white halo; sharp demarcation; and moth-eaten border [157]. Some SK may display network-like structures, blue-black hue, and pink color with atypical vessels. In this scenario, the differentiation with melanoma and other skin cancers can be difficult. Using contact dermoscopy the "wobble test/sign" may help differentiate SK from nevi. SK will be fixed (negative wobble) and nevi will roll under the glass plate (positive wobble) [6, 14].

Melanoacanthoma, a highly pigmented variant of SK, and the clonal variant of SK can be clinically and dermoscopically equivocal [156, 158, 159]. Also, irritation and regression can cause alterations within an SK, like pink and gray pigmentation, mimicking melanoma, and other skin cancers [158]. None of the above-mentioned dermoscopic features are specific to SK and they can be seen in other skin tumors, including melanoma [160]. Therefore, the absence of melanocytic criteria associated with clinical and dermoscopic features of SK are the combination for the correct diagnosis. Nevertheless, in some cases, further evaluation with RCM or histopathology is necessary (Fig. 6.35).

The most common confocal features of SK are epidermal projections and keratin-filled invaginations; epidermal regular honeycomb pattern (non-pigmented SK) or cobblestone pattern (pigmented SK); corneal plugs, that are well-circumscribed, round, bright reflecting structures at various epidermal levels and correspond to the milia-like cysts seen on dermoscopy; densely packed round to polycyclic edged dermal papillae (non-pigmented SK can present non-edged papillae); cord-like rete ridges and bulbous projections; mixed vascular pattern; and bright, round to triangular ill-defined cells that correspond to melanophages [158, 161]. On RCM, clonal SK presents a clod pattern, compatible with the clustered globules seen on dermoscopy. The clods appear as compact nests of keratinocytes that have a polygonal

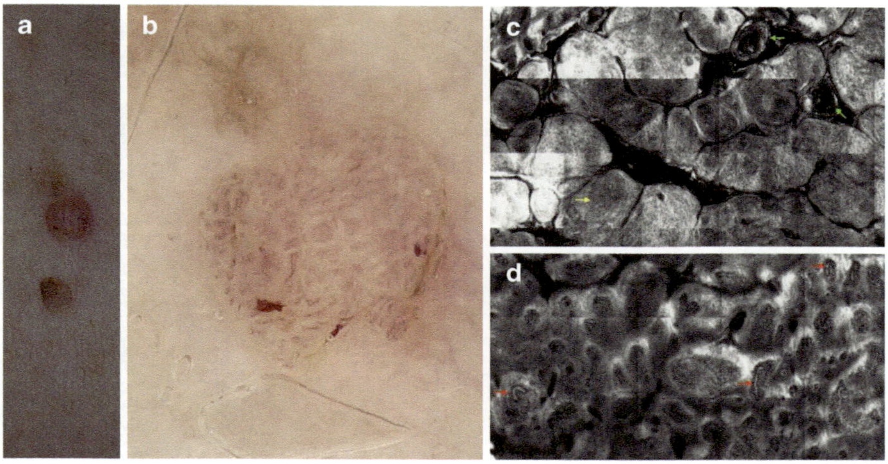

Fig. 6.35 (**a**) Clinical baseline image of a new nodular lesion, above an old SK, on the clavicular region of a female patient in her forties. She is a patient with AMS, but no personal/family history of melanoma. (**b**) PD (20×) showing orthogonal shiny white lines between polymorphous vessels (linear, hairpin, and looped). (**c**) RCM at the epidermal level shows horn plugs (green arrows) and an irregular honeycomb pattern (yellow arrow). (**d**) RCM at the DEJ shows polymorphous and polycyclic dermal papillae with an increased number of vessels (red arrows). A biopsy was done with the final diagnosis of IRRITATED SK. RCM images are close-ups of wide probe 8 × 8 mm mosaics. (*Clinical, dermoscopy and RCM images courtesy of Ana Maria Sortino MD, MSc*)

shape. Differently, melanocytes are larger and with round or dendritic morphology [156]. Irritated SK presents on RCM with small bright inflammatory cells on the DEJ [152]. RCM has a high agreement with histopathology for SK and may obviate the need for biopsy of equivocal lesions [162] (Fig. 6.36).

Lichen Planus-Like Keratosis

Lichen planus-like keratosis (LPLK) or lichenoid keratosis is a benign squamous-proliferative lesion showing chronic interface inflammation [59]. The precise nature of LPLK is uncertain, but it has been proposed that it represents an SK or solar lentigo undergoing regression [163]. It usually presents as solitary macules or papules, with varying presentations, depending on its stage of evolution. It is sharply demarcated, often scaly, and colors vary between pink, pink-brownish, pinkish-orange, dusky-violaceous, or bluish-gray to black [164].

The lesions are well demarcated and present acanthosis, hyperkeratosis, parakeratosis, and band-like lymphocytic inflammation in the superficial dermis. Interface changes with necrotic keratinocytes and basal layer vacuolar degeneration in the basal epidermal layer is seen. Prominent keratinocytic degeneration can result

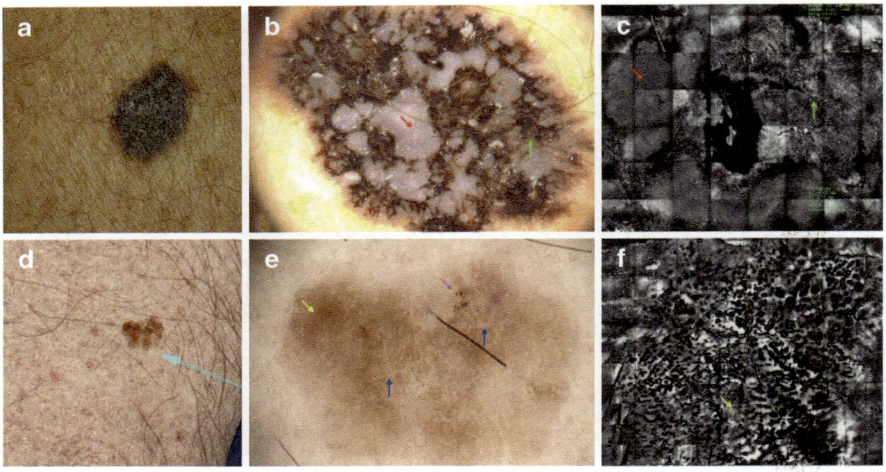

Fig. 6.36 Mimickers. (**a**) Clinical image of a false negative verrucous brown-black plaque, present for over a year, on the right calf of a male patient in his forties. (**b**) PD (20×) showing dusky-violaceous structureless areas (red arrow) intermingled with gray-black granules and polygonal lines (green arrow). (**c**) RCM shows a poorly circumscribed lesion with epidermal alternation of disarranged (green arrow) and atypical honeycomb (red arrow) patterns. RCM was reassuring for the need of a full thickness excision of a large lesion in a difficult closure area. Final diagnosis was SUPERFICIAL SPREADING INVASIVE MELANOMA, not associated with nevus, Clark II, Breslow 0.3 mm. (**d**) Clinical image of a false positive brown plaque of unknown duration, on the left calf of a male patient in his sixties. (**e**) PD (30×) exhibiting a negative network (blue arrow), structureless brown/tan areas (yellow arrow), and focal dark brown irregular globules (pink arrow). (**f**) RCM shows epidermal projections, keratin-filled invaginations (pink arrow), and regular honeycomb pattern (yellow arrow). RCM was reassuring for the clinical diagnosis of SK and the lesion remains under follow-up. RCM images are close-ups of wide probe 8 × 8 mm mosaics. (*Clinical, dermoscopy and RCM images courtesy of Ana Maria Sortino MD, MSc*)

in cleft and blister formation. Late-stage lesions present with an atrophic epidermis and superficial dermal fibrosis [16].

Regression features are the hallmark of LPLK and the clinical-dermoscopic presentation can vary depending on the lesion stage. The characteristic dermoscopic findings are blue-gray dots and granules with or without white areas. The granules are typically coarse, and the distribution can be either diffuse or localized. Dermoscopic elements of pre-existing lesion, e.g., SK or SL, may be identified (Fig. 6.37). On the other hand, regression in melanoma is seen on dermoscopy as blue-gray dots and fine granules (peppering), with a multifocal distribution. Also, other dermoscopic features of melanocytic lesion can be identified [164, 165]. Shiny white structures can be observed under polarized light in a percentage of cases of LPLK [166].

LPLK can be clinically and dermoscopically equivocal and simulate melanoma or other skin cancers. RCM can be a useful adjunct to diagnosis in doubtful cases.

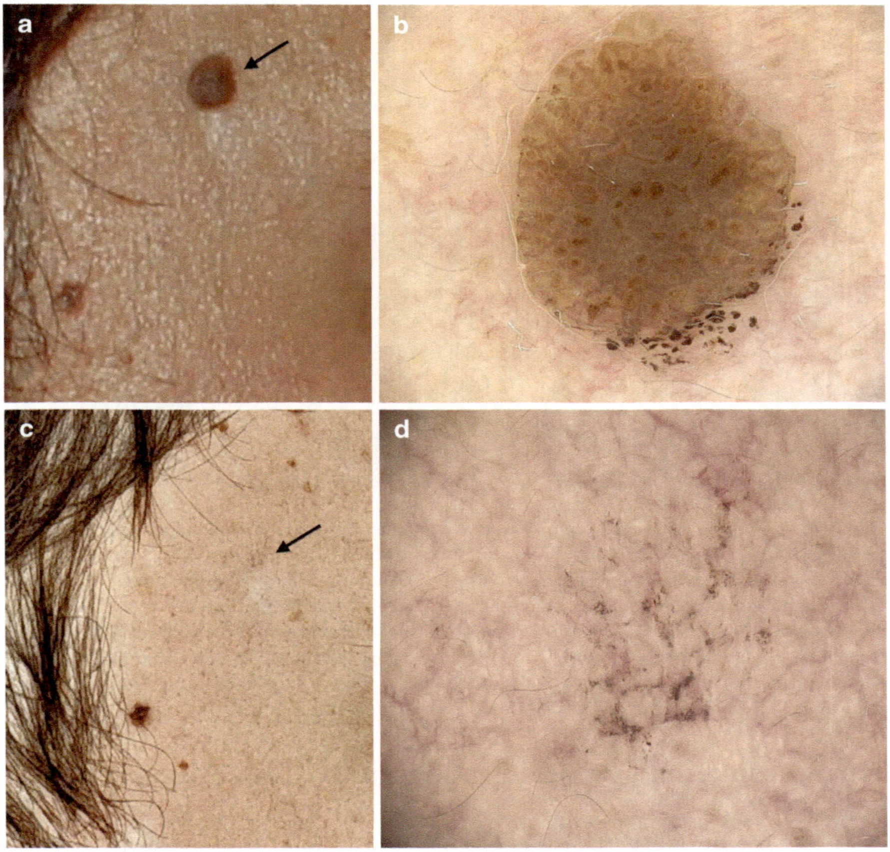

Fig. 6.37 Regressing SK. (**a**) Clinical baseline image of a palpable, dome-shaped, brown lesion. (**b**) PD (20×) showing ridges, fissures, and focal coarse gray granules. (**c**) Clinical 1-year follow-up image of a completely regressed lesion with remains of gray pigmentation (the scar underneath the lesion is an old one and not associated with the lesion). (**d**) PD (20×) exhibiting gray granules with diffuse distribution. (*Clinical, dermoscopy and RCM images courtesy of Elisabeth Callegaro, MD, and Ana Maria Sortino MD, MSc*)

Bassoli et al. described RCM criteria for LPLK diagnosis and its correlations with histopathology. The diagnosis of LPLK should be considered when a solitary lesion shows the following criteria: typical honeycomb pattern of the spinous layer; elongated cords and/or bulbous projections at the dermal epidermal junction; numerous plump-bright cells and/or bright stellate spots in the superficial dermis; absence of bright nucleated round or dendritic cells in a pagetoid pattern in the epidermis; absence of atypical honeycomb pattern; no tumor islands in the epidermis [153, 167] (Fig. 6.38).

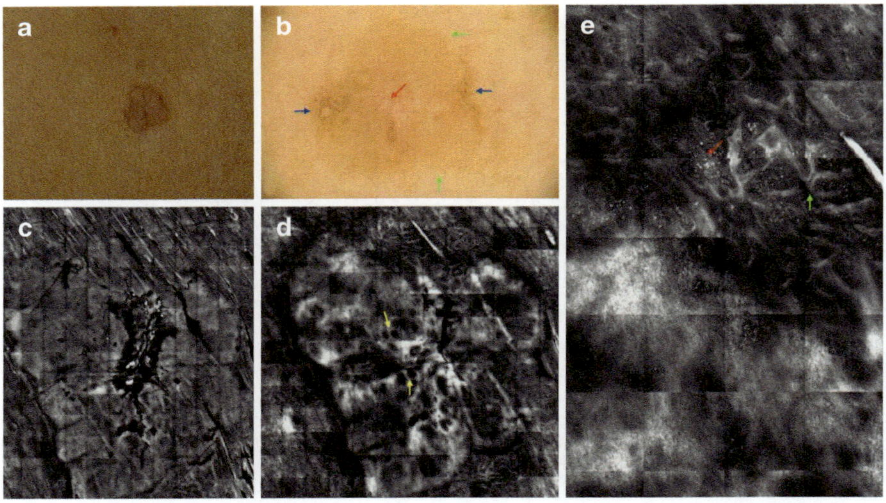

Fig. 6.38 LPLK. (**a**) Clinical image of a new palpable, solitary, hypopigmented lesion. (**b**) PD (20×) showing central shiny white bright lines (red arrow), focal peripheral gray granules (blue arrows), and sharp demarcation (green arrows). (**c**) RCM shows a well circumscribed lesion with typical honeycomb pattern at the epidermal level. (**d**) RCM at the DEJ shows central oval dark silhouettes (yellow arrows), without clefting or linear dilated vessels. (**e**) Close-up RCM reveals peripheral elongated cords (green arrow) and numerous plump-bright cells (red arrow) in the superficial dermis. RCM images are close-ups of wide probe 8 × 8 mm mosaics. (*Clinical, dermoscopy and RCM images courtesy of Ana Maria Sortino MD, MSc*)

Dermoscopic and Confocal Features of BCC and Mimickers

Basal cell carcinoma (BCC) derives from epidermal and/or hair follicle keratinocytes of the basal layer and it's the most frequent type of skin cancer [59]. Dermoscopy has improved the diagnosis with 91.2% sensitivity and 95% specificity, enabling its detection in early stages [168]. There are many lesions that dermoscopy can help discriminate such as actinic keratosis, squamous cell carcinoma (SCC), melanoma, and other inflammatory skin diseases, such as psoriasis or dermatitis. In contrast, dermoscopy seems insufficient to differentiate it from adnexal tumors characterized as dermoscopic "mimickers" of BCC, such as, trichoblastoma, trichoepithelioma, pilomatrichoma, and cylindroma [169]. New criteria for eccrine poroma have been recently described [13].

BCCs have a variety of clinical presentations ranging from pigmented to non-pigmented, patches to ulcerated nodules, depending on their histopathological subtypes. Low risk of recurrence BCCs are the subtypes: nodular, superficial, infundibulocystic, and fibroepithelial (Pinkus tumor). High risk of recurrence BCCs are the subtypes: basosquamous, sclerosing/morphoeic (morpheaform tumor), infiltrating, sarcomatoid, and micronodular. Mixed histological types may occur and up to 30% of BCCs present pigment on dermoscopy [6, 16, 170] (Fig. 6.39).

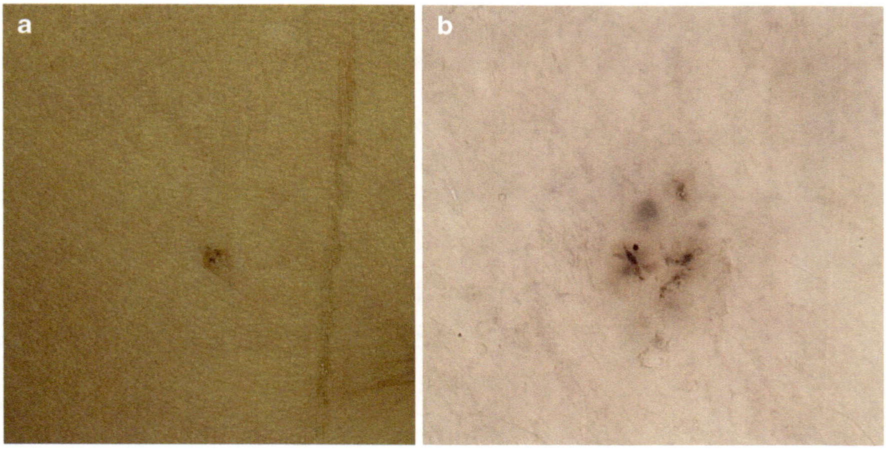

Fig. 6.39 Superficial and nodular pigmented BCC. (**a**) Clinical image of a small palpable, solitary, hypopigmented lesion, unknown to the patient, and immediately treated by full excision with adequate margins. (**b**) PD (20×) showing blue-gray ovoid nests and gray-black dots and globules. (*Clinical and dermoscopy images courtesy of Ana Maria Sortino MD, MSc*)

Dermoscopy

The diagnosis of BCC is based on the detection of one or more of the dermoscopic criteria described in Table 6.3. BCC does not present network, pseudopods, nor aggregated globules. When globules are present in BCCs they are multiple and not aggregated, usually blue-gray and less frequently brown (Fig. 6.40). Non-pigmented BCCs may present only short, fine telangiectasia, multiple small erosions, and shiny white blotches and strands [6, 13].

Dermoscopy is a valuable tool for the diagnosis and management of BCCs. The correspondence of dermoscopic structures and histological subtypes, such as, superficial fine telangiectasia, shiny white-red structureless areas, multiple small erosions, and leaf-like structures in superficial BCC; blue-gray ovoid nests and arborizing vessels in nodular BCC; shiny white-red structureless areas and arborizing vessels for infiltrative subtypes, allows the best treatment approach. Therefore, dermoscopic knowledge can avoid topical treatments for nodular or more aggressive subtypes of BCC [171].

Microscopically controlled surgery is the gold standard for BCC treatment. Nonetheless, initial assessment of margins using dermoscopy helps to discriminate tumoral arborizing vessels from normal vessels, and peripheral white-red structureless areas that should be included in the initial surgical margins. Moreover, dermoscopy is a tool that helps in clinical follow-up, by evaluating if there are features suggestive of residual and/or recurrent BCC in the treated area [169, 170].

Table 6.3 Dermatoscopic criteria for BCC [6, 7, 13, 14]

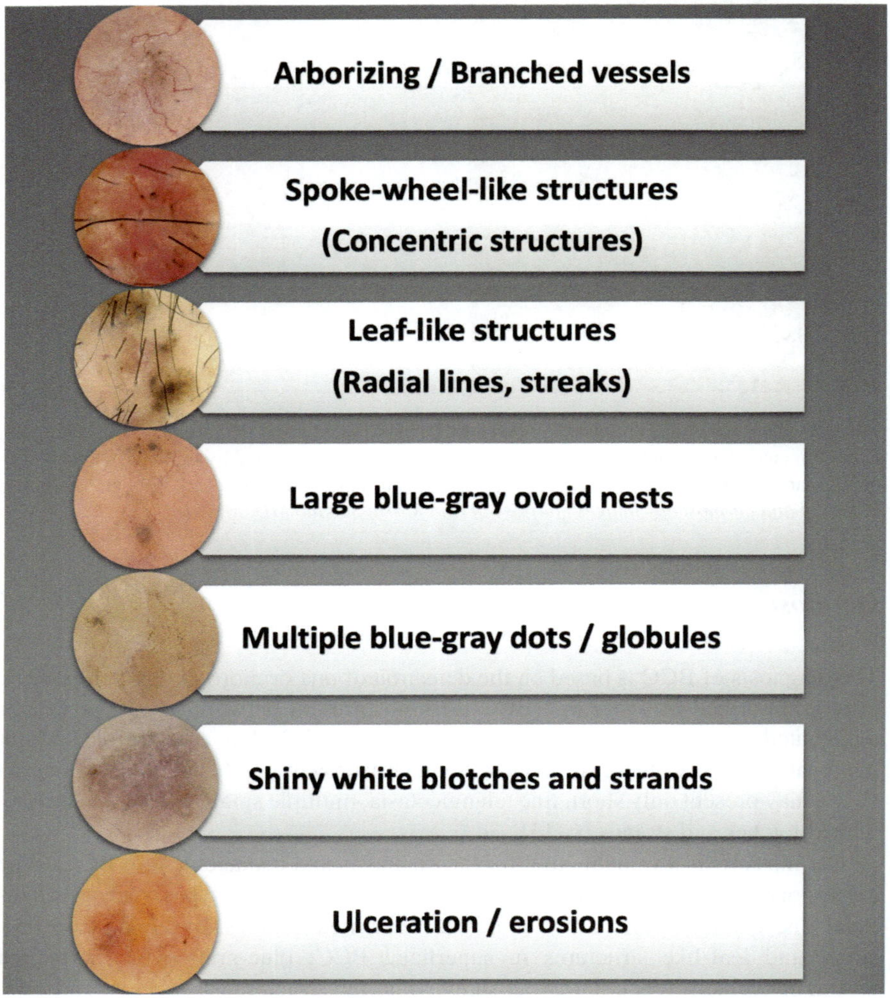

Reflectance Confocal Microscopy (RCM)

The first RCM feature for BCC was described in 2002 by Gonzales et al. as "tumor islands." These structures correspond to compact aggregates of tightly packed basaloid cells with peripheral palisading of nuclei [172]. On RCM, BCC features are perceived from the epidermis down to the dermis (Table 6.4). The epidermis presents variable degrees of irregular honeycomb patterns due to the keratinocytic atypia linked to the degree of actinic damage. The most sensitive and specific feature for BCC is the presence of elongated monomorphic keratinocytes above the tumor

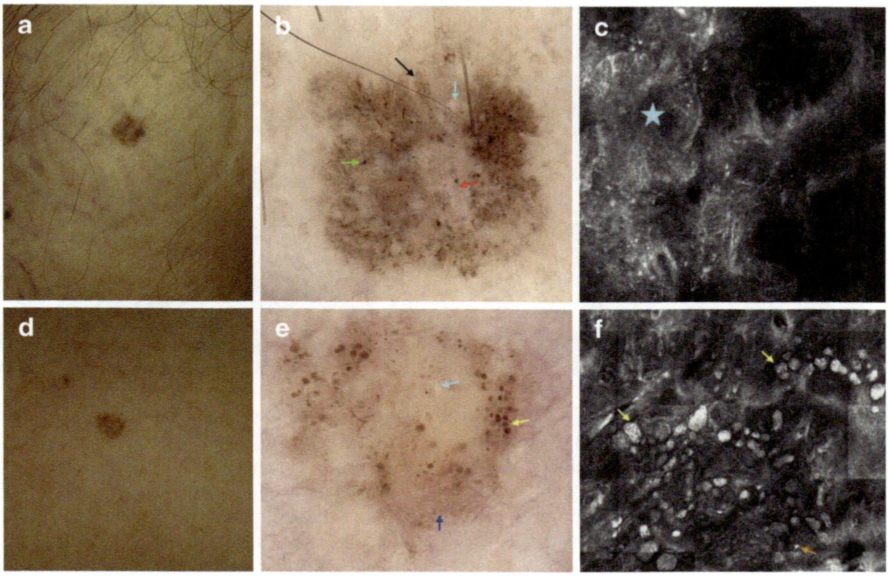

Fig. 6.40 Male patient in his sixties with a solitary macule on the lower right leg, unknown to the patient. (**a**) Clinical image of the flat pigmented lesion. (**b**) PD (30×) showing opaque central structureless area with bright white strands (teal arrow), multiple blue gray/brown non-aggregated dots/globules (green arrow), peripheral leaf-like structures (black arrow), and very thin telangiectatic vessels (red arrow). (**c**) RCM individual image (0.75 × 0.75 mm) at the DEJ shows tumor islands (teal star) surrounded by dark cleft-like spaces, and refractive dendritic cells within the neoplastic aggregate. Histopathology revealed a SUPERFICIAL PIGMENTED BCC. Female patient in her thirties with AMS. (**d**) Clinical image of a palpable sub clavicular pigmented lesion. (**e**) PD (30×) a central structureless area with shiny white lines (teal arrow), multiple aggregated irregular globules, with different shapes, colors, and sizes (yellow arrow), peripheral atypical pigment network (blue arrow). (**f**) RCM (close-up of 8 × 8 mm mosaic) shows multiple irregular dense-sparse (heterogeneous) nests (yellow arrows) and single enlarged atypical cells (orange arrow). Histopathology revealed a SUPERFICIAL SPREADING MELANOMA IN SITU. (*Clinical, dermoscopy and RCM images courtesy of Ana Maria Sortino MD, MSc*)

Table 6.4 RCM features and histology correspondence of BCC [46]

RCM feature	Histology
Dark silhouettes	Hyporeflective aggregates of basaloid cells with peripheral palisading of nuclei in non-pigmented BCC
Bright tumor islands	Hyperreflective aggregates of basaloid cells with peripheral palisading of nuclei in pigmented BCC
Cleft-like dark spaces	Mucin or cleft around tumor aggregates
Dendritic cells	Dendritic melanocytes inside the tumor in pigmented BCC or epidermal Langerhans cells
Plump-bright cells	Melanophages
Canalicular vessels	Telangiectatic blood vessels

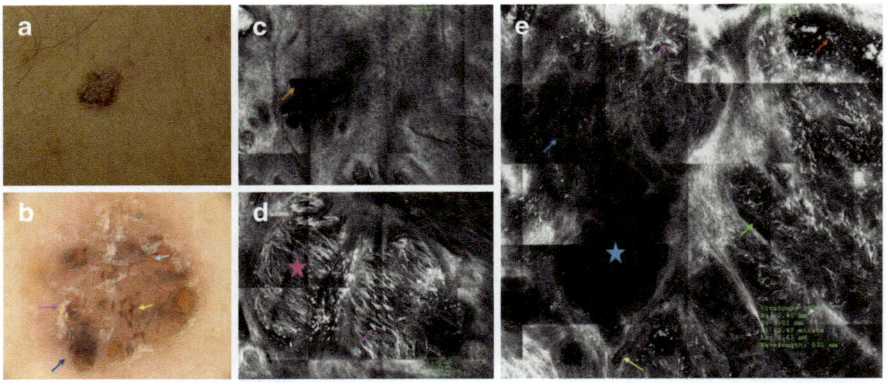

Fig. 6.41 Nodular pigmented BCC. (**a**) Clinical image of a palpable, solitary, pigmented lumbar lesion, unknown to the patient in his eighties. (**b**) PD (20×) showing large blue-gray ovoid nests (blue arrow), multiple gray dots and globules (yellow arrow), arborizing vessels (teal arrow), and scales (pink arrow). (**c**) RCM at the epidermal level shows an irregular honeycomb pattern with shadows and dark silhouettes (orange arrow). (**d**) RCM at the DEJ shows hyperreflective tumor islands (pink star) with dendritic cells (pink arrow). (**e**) RCM at the superficial dermis shows multiple dark silhouettes (blue star), hyporeflective tumor islands (blue arrow), cleft-like dark spaces (green arrow), canalicular vessels (yellow arrow), dendritic cells (pink arrow), and plump-bright cells (red arrow). RCM images are close-ups of wide probe 8 × 8 mm mosaics. (*Clinical, dermoscopy and RCM images courtesy of Ana Maria Sortino MD, MSc*)

islands (streaming). At the DEJ, one of the most characteristic features of pigmented BCCs is the identification of bright tumor islands, which are well-demarcated by surrounding dark cleft-like spaces, corresponding to mucin surrounding neoplastic aggregates, bright round large plump cells and/or small bright particles (melanophages), and dendritic cells (Langerhans cells or dendritic melanocytes) [171] (Fig. 6.41).

Non-pigmented BCC shows dark silhouettes of cell islands as hyporeflective areas, surrounded by dense and bright collagen bands. Canalicular vessels are present as abundant, elongated, and/or twisted blood vessels, visible immediately beneath the epidermis, sometimes presenting the rolling of leukocytes along the lumen [171, 173].

Regarding the differences between BCC subtypes, nodular variants also present aggregated tumor cell islands in the upper dermis that are often adjacent to large and dilated blood vessels. Superficial BCCs present aggregates of polarized cells with elongated nuclei oriented along the same axis in the epidermal basal cell layer and in the superficial dermis. Pigmented BCC shows greater brightness of the tumoral islands, which also show highly refractive dendritic cells (Fig. 6.41). RCM features for infiltrating BCCs are multiple dark silhouettes outlined by bright collagen [171, 173–175] (Fig. 6.42).

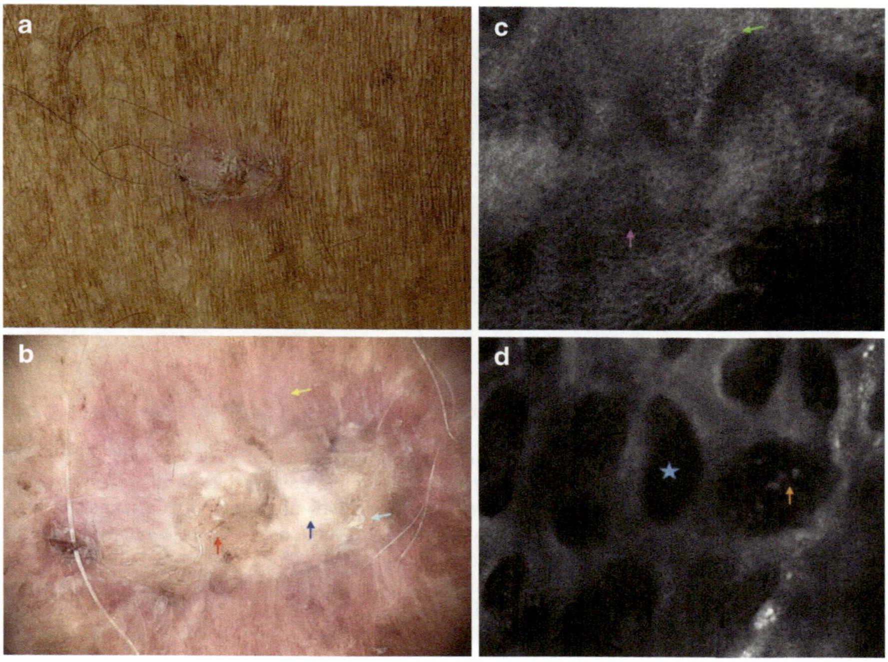

Fig. 6.42 Ulcerated and infiltrating BCC. (**a**) Clinical image of a scar-like lesion on the right shoulder, unknown to the patient in his seventies, with a personal history of multiple keratinocytic tumors. (**b**) PD (20×) showing a central shiny white blotch (blue arrow) with ulceration—"sticky fiber sign" (red arrow), rim of scales (teal arrow), and reddish-white peripheral area (yellow arrow). (**c**) RCM at the epidermal level shows an irregular honeycomb pattern with focal streaming (green arrow) and shadows (pink arrow). (**d**) RCM at the DEJ shows dark papillae (blue star), and plump-bright cells (orange arrow). RCM individual images of 0.75 × 0.75 mm handheld probe. In this case specific BCC structures on RCM were very subtle epidermal clues, probably due to ulceration, but also because of a mainly dermal histological subtype. A combination of clinical and dermoscopy knowledge were enough for the indication of a full excision with margin control. (*Clinical, dermoscopy and RCM images courtesy of Ana Maria Sortino MD, MSc*)

Dermoscopic and Confocal Features of Actinic Keratosis and Squamous Cell Carcinoma

Skin cancer of keratinocytic origin includes actinic keratosis (AK), intraepidermal carcinoma (in situ carcinoma, also named Bowen's disease), and invasive squamous cell carcinoma (SCC) [176]. There is an important correlation between the clinical and dermoscopic aspects and the degree of atypia observed in reflectance confocal microscopy (RCM) [177].

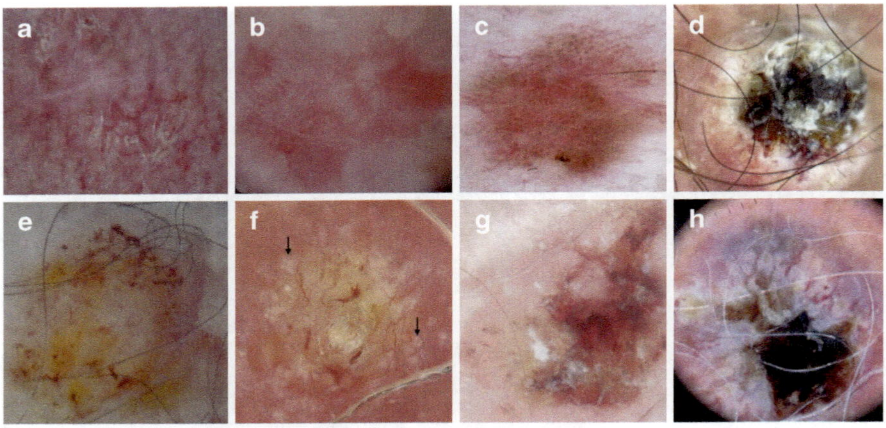

Fig. 6.43 Dermatoscopic images under polarized light of actinic keratosis showing red pseudo network and scales (**a**), intraepidermal squamous cell carcinoma showing glomerular vessels in clusters and white scales (**b**), pigmented Bowen's disease showing brown dots arranged in lines (**c**), keratoacanthoma showing central mass of keratin surrounded by linear-irregular and dotted peripheral vessels (**d**), moderately differentiated squamous cell carcinoma showing diffuse yellow to white amorphous areas (keratin) associated with ulceration and linear vessels; rosettes are also seen (black arrow) (**e**, **f**), and poorly differentiated squamous cell carcinoma showing bleeding and dense vascularity (**g**, **h**). (*Dermoscopy images courtesy of Ana Carolina S. Porto Mitsunaga MD, and Juliana Casagrande T. Braga, MD, PhD*)

Dermoscopy

This method plays an important role in the early detection of SCC and in its differentiation from precursor lesions (AKs) (Fig. 6.43).

Dermoscopy is helpful in recognizing the three different grades of classical non-pigmented facial AK: grade 1—red pseudo network and mild white scales; grade 2—"strawberry pattern" of whitish-yellow, keratotic, and enlarged follicular openings on an erythematous background; grade 3—yellow background intermingled with enlarged follicular openings filled with keratotic plugs or white to yellow structureless areas [176, 178–181]. In AK and related conditions, the rosette sign can be seen under contact PD. It's characterized by four white points localized inside the hair follicle opening [180, 182]. The typical dermoscopic pattern of facial pigmented actinic keratosis (pAK) is a superficial brown network surrounding keratotic and variable follicular openings [183]. AKs may occur simultaneously in facial and nonfacial skin. The most frequent NPD structures found in non-pigmented nonfacial AKs are white scales and erythema, while yellow scales and homogeneous pigmentation are found on pigmented nonfacial AKs. Under PD monomorphous vessels, rosettes and scales are seen [184, 185].

In most cases of intraepidermal SCC, dermoscopy shows glomerular vessels arranged in groups with a scaly white surface on an erythematous to yellow background [176, 180, 183]. Pigmented Bowen's disease is characterized by brown dots arranged in lines and structureless gray-brown pigmentation [180, 183].

The main dermatoscopic patterns of invasive SCC are radial linear irregular and hairpin vessels, white circles around hair follicles, central keratin with hemorrhagic spots, white structureless areas, and ulceration [180, 186, 187]. The well-differentiated SCC (keratoacanthoma-type) frequently shows exophytic growth and a central mass of keratin surrounded by elongated telangiectasias [176, 180, 186, 188]. Compared to keratoacanthoma, moderately differentiated SCC reveals peripheral hairpin/linear vessels and diffuse yellow to white amorphous areas (keratin) associated with ulceration, whereas poorly differentiated SCC reveals bleeding and/or dense vascularity (red color) in the absence of keratin or other white-colored criteria [180, 186].

Reflectance Confocal Microscopy (RCM)

RCM helps differentiate the various grades of AK, intraepidermal carcinoma, and invasive SCC [189, 190]. RCM is also a useful tool to select the better place for biopsy in the field of cancerization and to monitor treatment response over time [191, 192]. The three grades of AK may be differentiated by RCM based on the keratinocyte atypia reflecting the architectural disarray of the epidermis [192, 193]. AK and SCC have some overlapping features in RCM and histopathology, but the architectural disarrangement at the epidermis is more pronounced and prevalent in SCC [192].

The main RCM features of actinic keratosis are disruption of the stratum corneum by overlying hyperkeratotic scale; detached keratinocytes and bright cells corresponding to parakeratosis; atypical honeycomb pattern (pleomorphism of atypical keratinocytes defined as variations in their size and shape with architectural disruption of the epidermis) corresponding to atypical proliferation of keratinocytes in histopathology; collagen in bundles, corresponding to solar elastosis and elongated vessels; small, highly refractive cells at the epidermal layer and/or superficial dermis, corresponding to inflammatory cells [192, 193] (Fig. 6.44).

The examination of SCC in situ/Bowen's disease by RCM reveals hyperkeratosis and parakeratosis; atypical honeycomb and/or disarranged pattern involving all of the epidermis, with marked atypia in the stratum granulosum; targetoid cells in the epidermis (apoptotic keratinocytes) shown as bright round cells; buttonhole and round to S-shaped vessels in the center of dermal papillae and solar elastosis [192, 194, 195] (Fig. 6.45).

Pigmented SCC in situ is a known melanoma mimicker. RCM can be useful in establishing its specific diagnosis by displaying, at the epidermal level, an atypical and/or disarranged honeycomb pattern; numerous suprabasal bright dendritic cells (Langerhans cells); small rings of bright polygonal keratinocytes around the dermal papillae with widened interpapillary spaces at the DEJ [196–198].

RCM features of invasive SCC are severe hyperkeratosis, architectural disarray of the stratum granulosum (loss of the honeycomb pattern), nest-like structures (bright tumor nests) that represent the most important feature for invasive SCC, and elongated vessels (dilated hairpin vessels) [191, 192, 195] (Fig. 6.46).

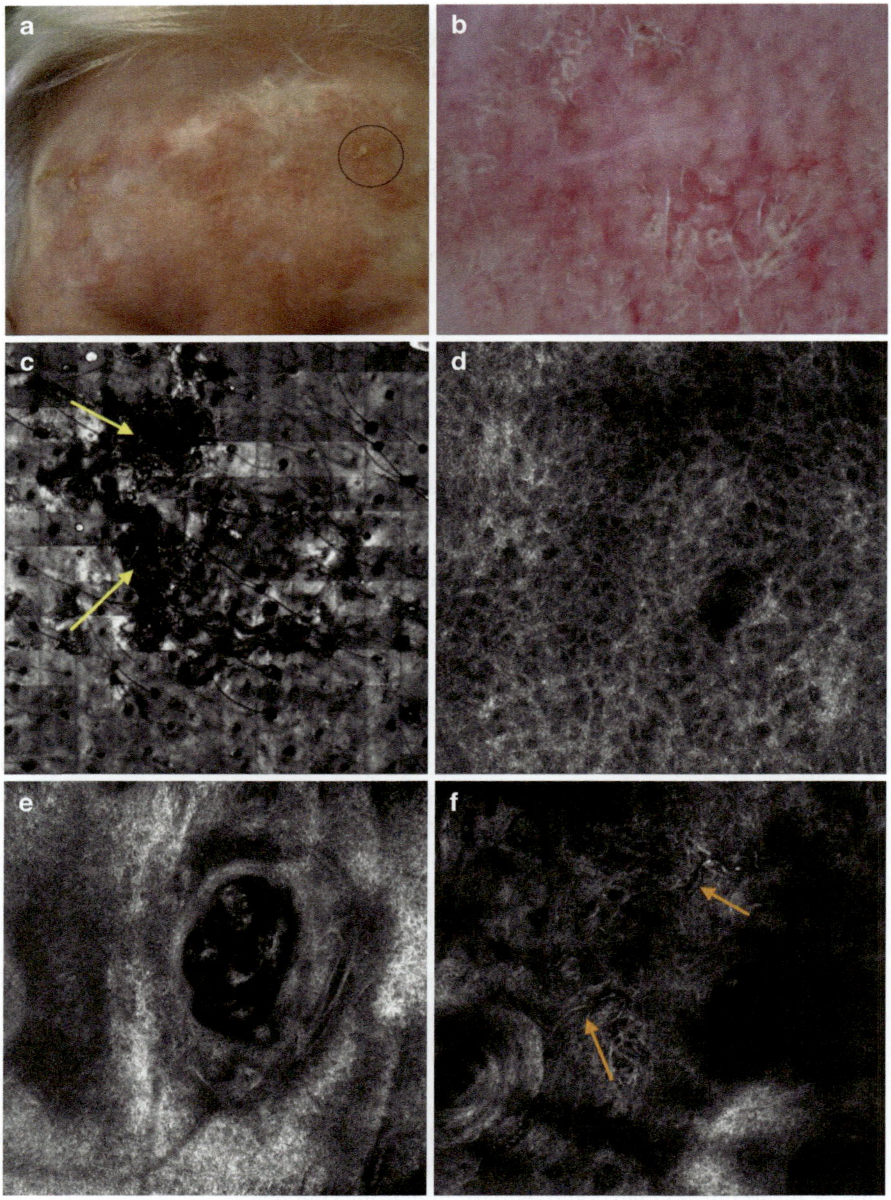

Fig. 6.44 Clinical (**a**) and dermoscopic (**b**) images of actinic keratosis. RCM mosaic image (6 × 6 mm) at the level of epidermis showing several areas of overlying scale (yellow arrows) at the stratum corneum (**c**). RCM individual image at the stratum spinosum showing atypical honeycomb pattern (**d**). RCM individual image at the stratum granulosum/spinosum showing disarray of the epidermal architecture (**e**). RCM individual image of the dermis showing solar elastosis and small dilated vessels (orange arrows) (**f**). (*Dermoscopy images courtesy of Ana Carolina S. Porto Mitsunaga MD, and Juliana Casagrande T. Braga, MD, PhD*)

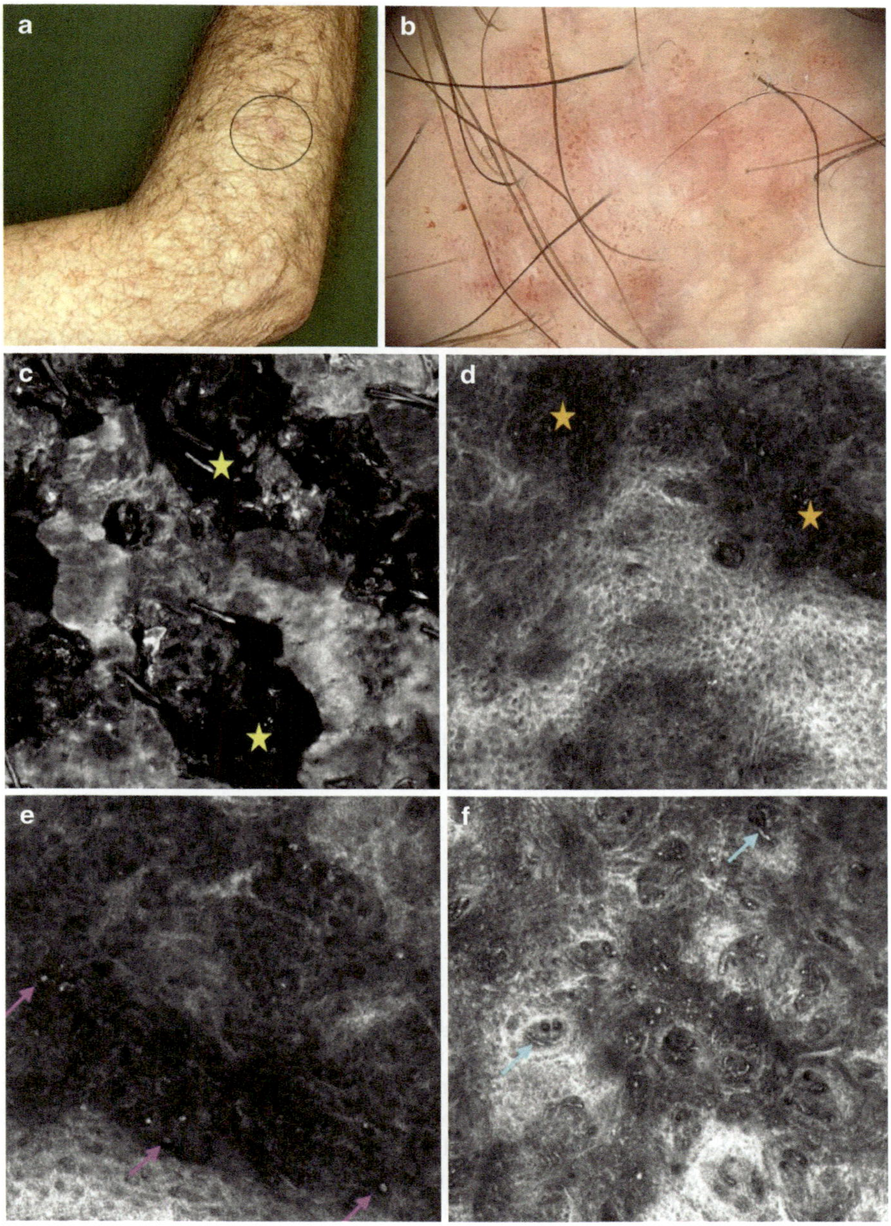

Fig. 6.45 Clinical (**a**) and dermoscopic (**b**) images of SCC in situ. RCM mosaic image (8 × 8 mm) at the level of epidermis showing disruption of the stratum corneum with areas of scale (yellow stars) (**c**). RCM individual image at the stratum granulosum/spinosum showing pleomorphism of the keratinocytes (atypical honeycomb pattern) and areas of complete disarray of the epidermal architecture (orange stars) (**d**). RCM single image of the stratum spinosum showing architecture disarray and the presence of targetoid cells (pink arrows) (**e**). RCM individual image at the level of upper dermis showing buttonhole and dilated vessels in the center of dermal papillae (teal arrows) and solar elastosis (**f**). (*Dermoscopy images courtesy of Ana Carolina S. Porto Mitsunaga MD, and Juliana Casagrande T. Braga, MD, PhD*)

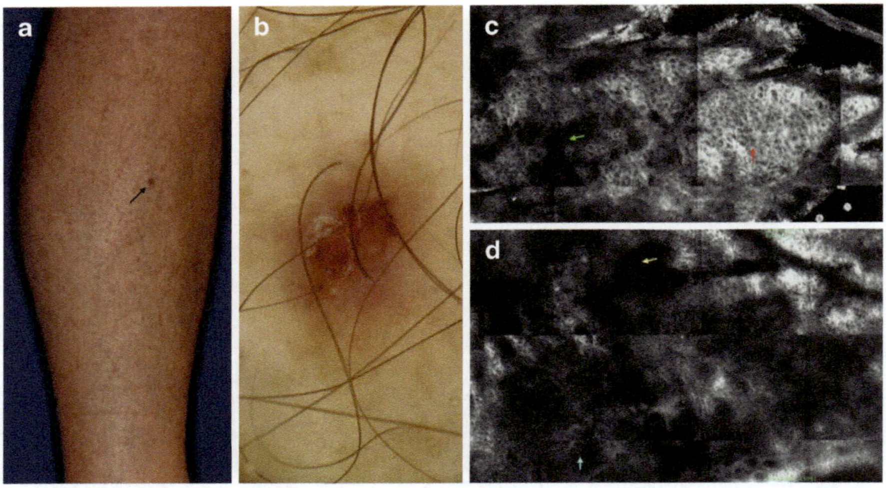

Fig. 6.46 Invasive SCC. (**a**) Clinical image of a small solitary pink lesion (black arrow), unknown to the patient in his sixties. (**b**) PD (20×) showing central red clods with scales and a structureless pink area. (**c**) RCM at the epidermal level shows areas of architectural disarray (green arrow) and areas of atypical honeycomb pattern (red arrow). (**d**) RCM at the DEJ shows buttonhole vessels (teal arrow) and multiple dark silhouettes (yellow arrow). RCM images are close-ups of wide probe 8 × 8 mm mosaics. (*Clinical, dermoscopy and RCM images courtesy of Ana Maria Sortino MD, MSc*)

The main limitations of RCM in the spectrum of keratinocytic tumors are hyperkeratosis which can impair the assessment of the deeper layers and the fact that the en face evaluation of this technique can limit the detection of early invasion [192].

RCM in Practice

RCM Indications

RCM is a complementary in vivo imaging technique that has proven useful in avoiding unnecessary excisions of benign lesions that can be dermoscopically suspicious of malignancy. It is currently a validated instrument for noninvasive diagnosis of skin tumors, already counting over 1000 indexed articles. The main application of RCM is for the diagnosis of skin lesions that display equivocal clinical and dermoscopic features of malignancy, especially in cosmetically sensitive areas, regions with poor wound healing characteristics, or difficult anatomic sites for biopsy [45].

An optimal indication of RCM is for suspicious macules and non-pigmented papules located on sun-damaged areas, especially head and neck. The technique allows the observer to suspect the diagnosis of basal cell carcinoma, squamous cell carcinoma, actinic keratosis, nevi, melanoma, and lentigo maligna with extra confidence. The association of RCM, to a previous dermoscopic examination, is ideal for

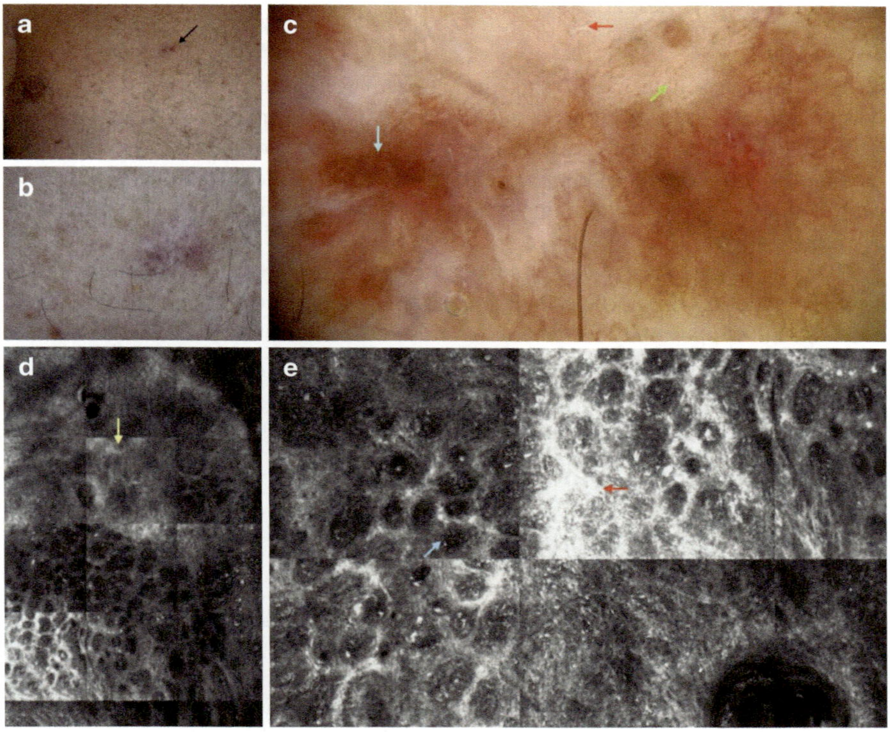

Fig. 6.47 Male patient in his seventies with personal history of multiple skin cancers. (**a**) Clinical image of chest lesion that was previously electrocoagulated without pathology examination. (**b**) Close-up of the clinical image showing pigmentation around the scar. (**c**) PD (20×) reveals central whitish scar-like area with shiny white lines (red arrow), atypical linear vessels (green arrow), and irregular hyperpigmented areas at the periphery (teal arrow). (**d**) RCM shows an epidermal disarray and both edged and non-edged papillae at the DEJ. (**e**) RCM at the DEJ reveals focal areas of non-edged papillae (blue arrow) and infiltration of juncional spaces by polymorphic atypical cells, forming "sheets of cells" (red arrow). RCM images are close-ups of wide probe 8 × 8 mm mosaics. The lesion was excised with 2 mm margins and pathology diagnosis was a LENTIGINOUS INVASIVE MELANOMA, NOT ASSOCIATED WITH NEVUS, Clark IV, Breslow 0.6 mm. A second surgery was done for ideal surgical margins. This is a good example of how RCM helps in management of high-risk patients. He was reluctant to have the scar excised after dermoscopy, but after RCM he understood the need for excisional biopsy without further delay. This is also a good case for understanding that destructive methods shouldn't be used without a sample in totum for histological examination. (*Clinical, dermoscopy and RCM images courtesy of Ana Maria Sortino MD, MSc*)

surgical referral or follow-up decision. Lateral and superficial surgical margins, of a suspicious or previously biopsied malignant lesion, can be planned with RCM for ill-defined BCCs and melanomas. Other important applications for RCM are monitoring of ablative and noninvasive therapies, surveillance for tumor recurrence or residual neoplasia (Fig. 6.47), and applications in inflammatory disorders. Nowadays, an ex vivo device is available to be used in microscopically controlled surgery [44, 45].

RCM Limitations

Skin-depth assessment is the main limitation of RCM impairing the detection of dermal tumors. Hyperkeratotic skin and verrucous lesions may be difficult to access and debulking the top of the lesion may be necessary prior to RCM exam. This technique should not be used on the nail plate. For ulcerated lesions, the skin adjacent to the ulcer may be examined; however it's very challenging for an accurate diagnosis [44, 45] (Fig. 6.42).

RCM is still an expensive imaging technique that requires a considerable immersion for reader training. The establishment of reimbursement codes in the US may soon open the opportunity for other countries to follow the trend and integrate RCM into clinical practice [44, 45].

Optical Coherence Tomography (OCT)

Basic Principles and Equipment

Optical coherence tomography (OCT) is a noninvasive diagnostic tool which allows the analysis of the morphology of biologic tissues in vivo with micro-resolution. It was first used in ophthalmology and first applied to image the skin by Welzel et al. [199]. This technology allows imaging of the human skin with different ranges of resolution depending on the device in use (3–15 μm). OCT works through a laser light that scans across the skin. The backscattered light from the surface of the skin returns with coherence to the receptor beam and is processed producing a black and white image that reaches up to 2 mm in depth [200, 201]. The devices produce 2D or 3D black and white images and more recently it is also able to recognize movement from blood and produce linear red drawings that correspond to blood vessels [202]. A line-field OCT that offers higher resolution has been recently released, but there aren't enough clinical studies [203] (Fig. 6.48).

OCT Terminology and Specific Standards

Different models of OCT devices have been used for clinical and research purposes, with image quality improvement over time. With better image definition, it became possible to observe skin appendages as hair follicles, sebaceous glands, and the transition from epidermis to dermis [204]. It was possible to notice different reflective properties in a variety of skin structures. Since the phenomenon that produces the image is basically the light reflection from the skin, the terminology to describe structures is based on it. Collagen, melanin, keratinocytes are hyperreflective (brighter), whereas blood vessels, water/other fluids, and air have shown to be hyporeflective (darker, with color close to black) [205]. Newly described structures (as

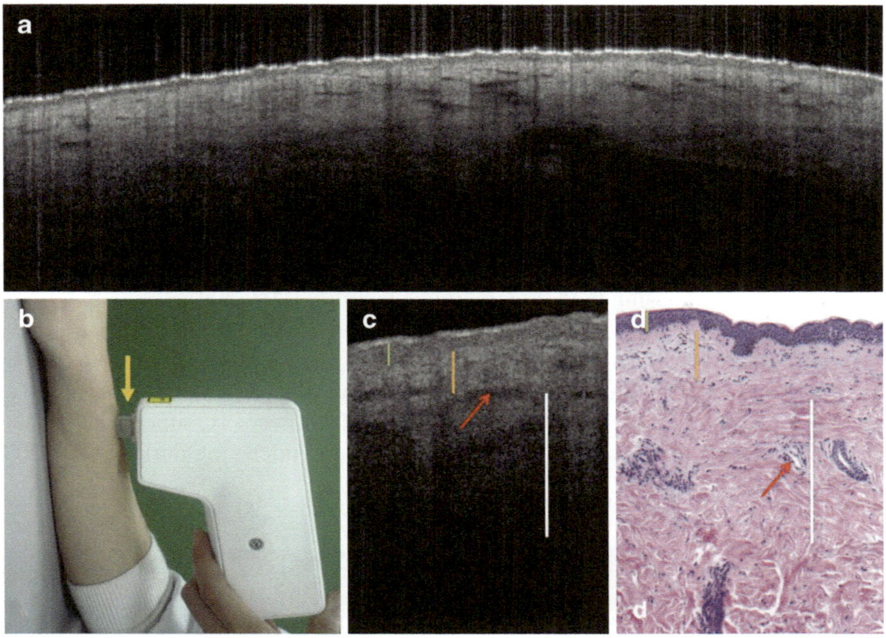

Fig. 6.48 (**a**) Example of an OCT image from Vivosight OCT scanner (Michelson diagnostics, Orpington, England). The produced image is 6 × 2 mm in diameter. (**b**) OCT probe; the image is obtained by touching the skin with an adaptor chosen according to the lesion height. (**c**, **d**) OCT and Histopathology image (H&E—40×) showing the skin structures seen by OCT; epidermis characterized by a hyporeflective layer bellow the hyperreflective transition line (green line), papillary dermis shown as a hyperreflective area bellow epidermis (orange line), vessels seen as hyporeflective linear structures in the dermis (red arrow) and reticular dermis (white line). (*Clinical, histological and OCT images courtesy of Tatiana Cristina Moraes Pinto Blumetti, MD, PhD*)

tumor cells in a non-pigmented basal cell carcinoma) are recognized mainly based on their differences of reflectivity from the normal surrounding skin [206] (Fig. 6.48).

Regarding the terminology of skin tumors, there is no standardization in nomenclature for the structures detected in skin tumors and there is a variety of different researchers using different names for the same structures. In this chapter, the terms used will be based on the papers with high level of citation and published in high-impact journals.

OTC in Practice

For conventional OCT, the image is obtained through a probe in contact with the skin that emits the laser light over the target area and produces 60–120 "axial cuts" within seconds. The black and white images are like conventional histology. Images are seen on a computer screen, and it is possible to analyze each of the sections individually. The software is also capable of building 3D images where "transversal cuts" can also be obtained.

OCT has been used to evaluate especially non-melanoma skin cancers, but it was also studied to analyze melanocytic lesions, inflammatory and bullous diseases, as well as research of topical cream absorptions and effectivity. Basal cell carcinoma (BCC) is the skin cancer where OCT has shown to be effective in the diagnosis as well as in the follow-up after treatment [206, 207]. Squamous cell carcinoma (SCC) and melanoma were also extensively studied on OCT; however, the need of cellular resolution for diagnosing both tumors limits its utility [208, 209].

Nodular BCC tumor is seen as a well circumscribed round hyperreflective (when pigmented) or hyporeflective (when non-pigmented) area surrounded by the hyperreflective collagen of the dermis. When present, inner cystic areas or mucin deposition are seen as hyporeflective [208]. Conversely, superficial BCC is detected as a focal thickening of epidermis with an underlying dark border [209, 210] (Fig. 6.49).

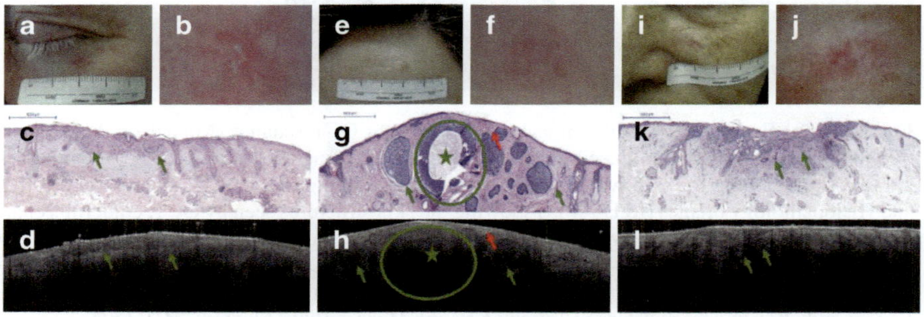

Fig. 6.49 Clinical, dermoscopy, histopathologic, and OCT images from three different BCC subtypes. (**a**) Superficial basal cell carcinoma located in the lower eyelid presenting as an erythematous scaling plaque. (**b**) Thin short telangiectasia on dermoscopy. (**c**) Histopathology image (H&E 40×) showing islands of basaloid cells connected to the epidermis (green arrows). (**d**) The corresponding OCT image showing epidermal hyporeflective islands with dark borders (green arrows). (**e**) Nodular basal cell carcinoma on the forehead. (**f**) Seen as an erythematous papule with telangiectasia on dermoscopy. (**g**) Histopathology image (H&E 40×) showing basaloid islands in the dermis. (**h**) The corresponding OCT image showing dermal basaloid islands seen as dermal hyporeflective areas (green line) or as dermal ovoid structures (green arrows), an inner cyst is seen as a black area (green star) and papillary dermis is shown as a hyperreflective stroma (red arrow). (**i**) Infiltrating basal cell carcinoma located in the cheek. (**j**) Presenting as an erythematous plaque with white lines, erythema, and ill-defined borders on dermoscopy. (**k**) Histopathology image (H&E 40×) showing epidermal and dermal basaloid islands (green arrows). (**l**) The corresponding OCT image showing dermal basaloid islands with an infiltrated pattern described as "fish shoal" area (green arrows) [210]. (*Clinical, histological and OCT images courtesy of Tatiana Cristina Moraes Pinto Blumetti, MD, PhD. and Elimar Gomes, MD, PhD*)

SCC often shows loss of the common morphology of the epidermis due to scaling and ulceration. When the horny layer is preserved and the tumor is in situ, it is possible to observe an irregular thickening of epidermis. When SCC is invasive, there is loss of the transition from epidermis to dermis [211].

Nevus and melanoma have different patterns on OCT. While nevi show well circumscribed areas with preserved architecture, melanomas change the normal reflectivity of collagen and the transition seen at the derma-epidermal junction [212]. As mentioned before, the lack of cellular resolution is a limitation to rely on OTC as a single technique for the diagnosis of melanoma [213] (Fig. 6.50).

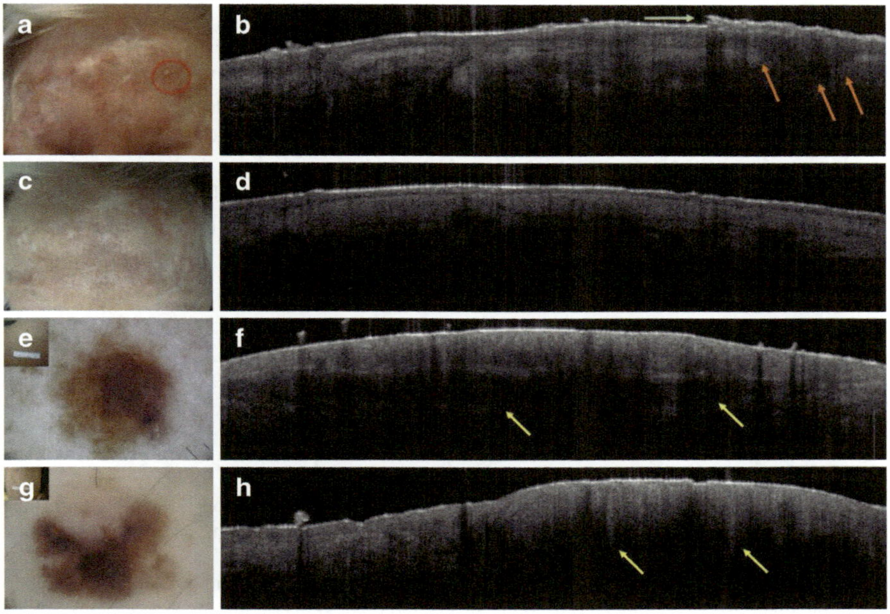

Fig. 6.50 Example of OCT use for follow-up of patient's with field cancerization under topical treatment. (**a**) Clinical picture of a forehead lesion before treatment (red circle is the analyzed area). (**b**) OCT image showing the disruption of epidermal layer (green arrow) and irregular thickening of epidermis (orange arrows). (**c**) Clinical picture after treatment with a cycle of topical ingenol mebutate showing clinical clearance of actinic keratosis. (**d**) Improvement shown on OCT image. Example of melanocytic compound nevus and melanoma on OCT. (**e**) Dermoscopic image of a compound nevus (inset showing the clinical image). (**f**) OCT showing a hyporeflective well demarcated area in yellow arrows nominated as a hyporeflective band representing a symmetrical and homogeneous dermal nest of melanocytes. (**g**) Dermoscopy image of a cutaneous melanoma, Breslow 0.95 mm (inset showing the clinical image). (**h**) OCT showing a disarranged pattern with non-visualized collagen in dermis and "spiculated" hyperreflective structures nominated as "icicle shaped structures." (*Clinical, histological and OCT images courtesy of Tatiana Cristina Moraes Pinto Blumetti, MD, PhD*)

Final Notes

Early detection of skin cancers is associated with better survival, less morbidity from treatment, and lower health system costs. Like patients with keratinocytic tumors, those who develop an in situ or invasive primary melanoma are at much greater risk of developing subsequent melanomas compared with the general population, especially for individuals with additional risk factors, such as multiple primary melanomas, dysplastic nevi, family history, or a melanoma-predisposing gene variant. A recent study showed that new melanomas were most likely to be detected by a clinician with the aid of TBP followed by digital dermoscopy monitoring [214, 215].

The authors aimed to show a brief and practical overview of the everyday use of skin cancer imaging techniques. A small sample of the skin cancer early detection universe is represented in this chapter. It's important to remember that there are many more benign and malignant skin tumors that can be studied with these technologies. As enthusiasts in the field, we hope to have aided the novice to understand how the clinical examination, dermoscopy, RCM, OCT, and future technologies may complement each other, collaborating to a deeper understanding of cutaneous tumors dynamics.

References

1. Schneider SL, Kohli I, Hamzavi IH, Council ML, Rossi AM, Ozog DM. Emerging imaging technologies in dermatology: part I: basic principles. J Am Acad Dermatol. 2019;80(4):1114–20. https://doi.org/10.1016/j.jaad.2018.11.042.
2. Schneider SL, Kohli I, Hamzavi IH, Council ML, Rossi AM, Ozog DM. Emerging imaging technologies in dermatology: part II: applications and limitations. J Am Acad Dermatol. 2019;80(4):1121–31. https://doi.org/10.1016/j.jaad.2018.11.043.
3. Malvehy J, Pellacani G. Dermoscopy, confocal microscopy and other non-invasive tools for the diagnosis of non-melanoma skin cancers and other skin conditions. Acta Derm Venereol. 2017;218(Suppl):22–30. https://doi.org/10.2340/00015555-2720.
4. Tkaczyk E. Innovations and developments in dermatologic non-invasive optical imaging and potential clinical applications. Acta Derm Venereol. 2017;218(Suppl):5–13. https://doi.org/10.2340/00015555-2717.
5. Sonthalia S, Yumeen S, Kaliyadan F. Dermoscopy overview and extradiagnostic applications. In: StatPearls. Treasure Island, FL: StatPearls Publishing; 2020. Available from: https://www.ncbi.nlm.nih.gov/books/NBK537131/.
6. Marghoob A, Braun R, editors. An atlas of dermoscopy. 2nd ed. CRC Press; 2013. https://doi.org/10.3109/9781841847627.
7. Kittler H, Rosendahl C, Cameron A, Tschandl P. Dermatoscopy. An algorithmic method based on pattern analysis. Wien: Facultas Universitatsverlag; 2011. ISBN: 978-3-7089-0717-8.
8. Weber P, Tschandl P, Sinz C, Kittler H. Dermatoscopy of neoplastic skin lesions: recent advances, updates, and revisions. Curr Treat Options Oncol. 2018;19(11):56. https://doi.org/10.1007/s11864-018-0573-6.
9. Conforti C, Giuffrida R, Vezzoni R, Resende F, di Meo N, Zalaudek I. Dermoscopy and the experienced clinicians. Int J Dermatol. 2019; https://doi.org/10.1111/ijd.14512. Advance online publication.

10. Zalaudek I, Lallas A, Moscarella E, Longo C, Soyer HP, Argenziano G. The dermatologist's stethoscope-traditional and new applications of dermoscopy. Dermatol Pract Concept. 2013;3(2):67–71. https://doi.org/10.5826/dpc.0302a11.
11. Wilkinson D, Argenziano G, Lallas A. The definitive guide [to] dermoscopy & diagnosis of benign and malignant skin lesions. Singapore: HealthCert; 2018. ISBN: 978-981-11-7124-6.
12. Braun RP, Scope A, Marghoob AA. The "blink sign" in dermoscopy. Arch Dermatol. 2011;147(4):520. https://doi.org/10.1001/archdermatol.2011.82.
13. https://www.dermoscopedia.org.
14. Rosendal C, Marozava A. Dermoscopy and skin cancer. 1st ed. Scion Publishing Ltd.; 2019.
15. Kittler H, Marghoob AA, Argenziano G, Carrera C, Curiel-Lewandrowski C, Hofmann-Wellenhof R, Malvehy J, Menzies S, Puig S, Rabinovitz H, Stolz W, Saida T, Soyer HP, Siegel E, Stoecker WV, Scope A, Tanaka M, Thomas L, Tschandl P, Zalaudek I, et al. Standardization of terminology in dermoscopy/dermatoscopy: results of the third consensus conference of the International Society of Dermoscopy. J Am Acad Dermatol. 2016;74(6):1093–106. https://doi.org/10.1016/j.jaad.2015.12.038.
16. Elder DE, Massi D, Scolyer RA, Willemze R. WHO classification of skin tumours. 4th ed. WHO; 2018. ISBN-13: 978-92-832-2440-2 (Print Book).
17. Barcaui CB, Miot HA. Profile of the use of dermoscopy among dermatologists in Brazil (2018). An Bras Dermatol. 2020;95(5):602–8. https://doi.org/10.1016/j.abd.2020.04.007.
18. Wolner ZJ, Yélamos O, Liopyris K, Rogers T, Marchetti MA, Marghoob AA. Enhancing skin cancer diagnosis with dermoscopy. Dermatol Clin. 2017;35(4):417–37. https://doi.org/10.1016/j.det.2017.06.003.
19. Pehamberger H, Steiner A, Wolff K. In vivo epiluminescence microscopy of pigmented skin lesions. I. Pattern analysis of pigmented skin lesions. J Am Acad Dermatol. 1987;17(4):571–83. https://doi.org/10.1016/s0190-9622(87)70239-4.
20. Argenziano G, Soyer HP, Chimenti S, Talamini R, Corona R, Sera F, Binder M, Cerroni L, De Rosa G, Ferrara G, Hofmann-Wellenhof R, Landthaler M, Menzies SW, Pehamberger H, Piccolo D, Rabinovitz HS, Schiffner R, Staibano S, Stolz W, Bartenjev I, et al. Dermoscopy of pigmented skin lesions: results of a consensus meeting via the internet. J Am Acad Dermatol. 2003;48(5):679–93. https://doi.org/10.1067/mjd.2003.281.
21. Annessi G, Bono R, Sampogna F, Faraggiana T, Abeni D. Sensitivity, specificity, and diagnostic accuracy of three dermoscopic algorithmic methods in the diagnosis of doubtful melanocytic lesions: the importance of light brown structureless areas in differentiating atypical melanocytic nevi from thin melanomas. J Am Acad Dermatol. 2007;56(5):759–67. https://doi.org/10.1016/j.jaad.2007.01.014.
22. Nachbar F, Stolz W, Merkle T, Cognetta AB, Vogt T, Landthaler M, Bilek P, Braun-Falco O, Plewig G. The ABCD rule of dermatoscopy. High prospective value in the diagnosis of doubtful melanocytic skin lesions. J Am Acad Dermatol. 1994;30(4):551–9. https://doi.org/10.1016/s0190-9622(94)70061-3.
23. Argenziano G, Fabbrocini G, Carli P, De Giorgi V, Sammarco E, Delfino M. Epiluminescence microscopy for the diagnosis of doubtful melanocytic skin lesions. Comparison of the ABCD rule of dermatoscopy and a new 7-point checklist based on pattern analysis. Arch Dermatol. 1998;134(12):1563–70. https://doi.org/10.1001/archderm.134.12.1563.
24. Unlu E, Akay BN, Erdem C. Comparison of dermatoscopic diagnostic algorithms based on calculation: the ABCD rule of dermatoscopy, the seven-point checklist, the three-point checklist and the CASH algorithm in dermatoscopic evaluation of melanocytic lesions. J Dermatol. 2014;41(7):598–603. https://doi.org/10.1111/1346-8138.12491.
25. Ahnlide I, Bjellerup M, Nilsson F, Nielsen K. Validity of ABCD rule of dermoscopy in clinical practice. Acta Derm Venereol. 2016;96(3):367–72. https://doi.org/10.2340/00015555-2239.
26. Carrera C, Marchetti MA, Dusza SW, Argenziano G, Braun RP, Halpern AC, Jaimes N, Kittler HJ, Malvehy J, Menzies SW, Pellacani G, Puig S, Rabinovitz HS, Scope A, Soyer HP, Stolz W, Hofmann-Wellenhof R, Zalaudek I, Marghoob AA. Validity and reliability of dermoscopic criteria used to differentiate nevi from melanoma: a web-based International

Dermoscopy Society Study. JAMA Dermatol. 2016;152(7):798–806. https://doi.org/10.1001/jamadermatol.2016.0624.
27. Menzies SW, Ingvar C, Crotty KA, McCarthy WH. Frequency and morphologic characteristics of invasive melanomas lacking specific surface microscopic features. Arch Dermatol. 1996;132(10):1178–82.
28. Argenziano G, Catricalà C, Ardigo M, Buccini P, De Simone P, Eibenschutz L, Ferrari A, Mariani G, Silipo V, Sperduti I, Zalaudek I. Seven-point checklist of dermoscopy revisited. Br J Dermatol. 2011;164(4):785–90. https://doi.org/10.1111/j.1365-2133.2010.10194.x.
29. Haenssle HA, Korpas B, Hansen-Hagge C, Buhl T, Kaune KM, Rosenberger A, Krueger U, Schön MP, Emmert S. Seven-point checklist for dermatoscopy: performance during 10 years of prospective surveillance of patients at increased melanoma risk. J Am Acad Dermatol. 2010;62(5):785–93. https://doi.org/10.1016/j.jaad.2009.08.049.
30. Blum A, Rassner G, Garbe C. Modified ABC-point list of dermoscopy: a simplified and highly accurate dermoscopic algorithm for the diagnosis of cutaneous melanocytic lesions. J Am Acad Dermatol. 2003;48(5):672–8. https://doi.org/10.1067/mjd.2003.282.
31. Soyer HP, Argenziano G, Zalaudek I, Corona R, Sera F, Talamini R, Barbato F, Baroni A, Cicale L, Di Stefani A, Farro P, Rossiello L, Ruocco E, Chimenti S. Three-point checklist of dermoscopy. A new screening method for early detection of melanoma. Dermatology (Basel, Switzerland). 2004;208(1):27–31. https://doi.org/10.1159/000075042.
32. Henning JS, Dusza SW, Wang SQ, Marghoob AA, Rabinovitz HS, Polsky D, Kopf AW. The CASH (color, architecture, symmetry, and homogeneity) algorithm for dermoscopy. J Am Acad Dermatol. 2007;56(1):45–52. https://doi.org/10.1016/j.jaad.2006.09.003.
33. Henning JS, Stein JA, Yeung J, Dusza SW, Marghoob AA, Rabinovitz HS, Polsky D, Kopf AW. CASH algorithm for dermoscopy revisited. Arch Dermatol. 2008;144(4):554–5.
34. Chen LL, Dusza SW, Jaimes N, Marghoob AA. Performance of the first step of the 2-step dermoscopy algorithm. JAMA Dermatol. 2015;151(7):715–21.
35. Rosendahl C, Tschandl P, Cameron A, Kittler H. Diagnostic accuracy of dermatoscopy for melanocytic and nonmelanocytic pigmented lesions. J Am Acad Dermatol. 2011;64(6):1068–73. https://doi.org/10.1016/j.jaad.2010.03.039.
36. Rosendahl C, Cameron A, McColl I, Wilkinson D. Dermatoscopy in routine practice—'chaos and clues'. Aust Fam Physician. 2012;41(7):482–7.
37. Ramji R, Valdes-Gonzalez G, Oakley A, Rademaker M. Dermoscopic 'Chaos and Clues' in the diagnosis of melanoma in situ. Australas J Dermatol. 2018;59(3):201–5. https://doi.org/10.1111/ajd.12740.
38. Rogers T, Marino M, Dusza SW, Bajaj S, Marchetti MA, Marghoob A. Triage amalgamated dermoscopic algorithm (TADA) for skin cancer screening. Dermatol Pract Concept. 2017;7(2):39–46. https://doi.org/10.5826/dpc.0702a09.
39. Jaimes N, Marghoob AA. Triage amalgamated dermoscopic algorithm. J Am Acad Dermatol. 2020;82(6):1551–2. https://doi.org/10.1016/j.jaad.2020.01.079.
40. Revised two-step algorithm. Dermoscopedia. 6 Jun 2019. https://dermoscopedia.org/w/index.php?title=Revised_two-step_algorithm&oldid=16401. Retrieved 7 Jun 2021.
41. Vestergaard ME, Macaskill P, Holt PE, Menzies SW. Dermoscopy compared with naked eye examination for the diagnosis of primary melanoma: a meta-analysis of studies performed in a clinical setting. Br J Dermatol. 2008;159(3):669–76. https://doi.org/10.1111/j.1365-2133.2008.08713.x.
42. Calzavara-Pinton P, Longo C, Venturini M, Sala R, Pellacani G. Reflectance confocal microscopy for in vivo skin imaging. Photochem Photobiol. 2008;84(6):1421–30. https://doi.org/10.1111/j.1751-1097.2008.00443.x.
43. Guida S, Arginelli F, Farnetani F, Ciardo S, Bertoni L, Manfredini M, Zerbinati N, Longo C, Pellacani G. Clinical applications of in vivo and ex vivo confocal microscopy. Appl Sci. 2021;11:179. https://doi.org/10.3390/app11051979.
44. Shahriari N, Grant-Kels JM, Rabinovitz H, Oliviero M, Scope A. Reflectance confocal microscopy: principles, basic terminology, clinical indications, limitations, and practical considerations. J Am Acad Dermatol. 2021;84(1):1–14. https://doi.org/10.1016/j.jaad.2020.05.153.

45. Que SK, Fraga-Braghiroli N, Grant-Kels JM, Rabinovitz HS, Oliviero M, Scope A. Through the looking glass: basics and principles of reflectance confocal microscopy. J Am Acad Dermatol. 2015;73(2):276–84. https://doi.org/10.1016/j.jaad.2015.04.047.
46. Hoffmann-Wellenhof R, Pellacani G, Malvehy J, Soyer HP, editors. Reflectance confocal microscopy for skin disase. 1st ed. Berlin: Springer-Verlag; 2012. https://doi.org/10.1007/978-3-642-21997-9.
47. Ahlgrimm-Siess V, Laimer M, Rabinovitz HS, Oliviero M, Hofmann-Wellenhof R, Marghoob AA, Scope A. Confocal microscopy in skin cancer. Curr Dermatol Rep. 2018;7(2):105–18. https://doi.org/10.1007/s13671-018-0218-9.
48. Pampena R, Borsari S, Lai M, Benati E, Longhitano S, Mirra M, Kyrgidis A, Pellacani G, Longo C. External validation and comparison of four confocal microscopic scores for melanoma diagnosis on a retrospective series of highly suspicious melanocytic lesions. J Eur Acad Dermatol Venereol. 2019;33(8):1541–6. https://doi.org/10.1111/jdv.15617.
49. Navarrete-Dechent C, Liopyris K, Monnier J, Aleissa S, Boyce LM, Longo C, Oliviero M, Rabinovitz H, Marghoob AA, Halpern AC, Pellacani G, Scope A, Jain M. Reflectance confocal microscopy terminology glossary for melanocytic skin lesions: a systematic review. J Am Acad Dermatol. 2021;84(1):102–19. https://doi.org/10.1016/j.jaad.2020.05.097.
50. Pellacani G, Cesinaro AM, Seidenari S. Reflectance-mode confocal microscopy of pigmented skin lesions—improvement in melanoma diagnostic specificity. J Am Acad Dermatol. 2005;53(6):979–85. https://doi.org/10.1016/j.jaad.2005.08.022.
51. Segura S, Puig S, Carrera C, Palou J, Malvehy J. Development of a two-step method for the diagnosis of melanoma by reflectance confocal microscopy. J Am Acad Dermatol. 2009;61(2):216–29. https://doi.org/10.1016/j.jaad.2009.02.014.
52. Borsari S, Pampena R, Benati E, Bombonato C, Kyrgidis A, Moscarella E, Lallas A, Argenziano G, Pellacani G, Longo C. In vivo dermoscopic and confocal microscopy multistep algorithm to detect in situ melanomas. Br J Dermatol. 2018;179(1):163–72. https://doi.org/10.1111/bjd.16364.
53. Pellacani G, Scope A, Gonzalez S, Guitera P, Farnetani F, Malvehy J, Witkowski A, De Carvalho N, Lupi O, Longo C. Reflectance confocal microscopy made easy: the 4 must-know key features for the diagnosis of melanoma and nonmelanoma skin cancers. J Am Acad Dermatol. 2019;81(2):520–6. https://doi.org/10.1016/j.jaad.2019.03.085.
54. Ali Z, Todd PM. Total body skin examination increases squamous cell carcinoma detection: a retrospective cohort study. Clin Exp Dermatol. 2020;45(1):86–8. https://doi.org/10.1111/ced.14013.
55. Omara S, Wen D, Ng B, Anand R, Matin RN, Taghipour K, Esdaile B. Identification of incidental skin cancers among adults referred to dermatologists for suspicious skin lesions. JAMA Netw Open. 2020;3(12):e2030107. https://doi.org/10.1001/jamanetworkopen.2020.30107.
56. Argenziano G, Zalaudek I, Hofmann-Wellenhof R, Bakos RM, Bergman W, Blum A, Broganelli P, Cabo H, Caltagirone F, Catricalà C, Coppini M, Dewes L, Francia MG, Garrone A, Turk BG, Ghigliotti G, Giacomel J, Gourhant JY, Hlavin G, Kukutsch N, et al. Total body skin examination for skin cancer screening in patients with focused symptoms. J Am Acad Dermatol. 2012;66(2):212–9. https://doi.org/10.1016/j.jaad.2010.12.039.
57. Helm MF, Hallock KK, Bisbee E, Miller JJ. Optimizing the total-body skin exam: an observational cohort study. J Am Acad Dermatol. 2019;81(5):1115–9. https://doi.org/10.1016/j.jaad.2019.02.028.
58. Nielson CB, Grant-Kels JM. Commentary on "Optimizing the total-body skin exam: an observational cohort study". J Am Acad Dermatol. 2019;81(5):e131. https://doi.org/10.1016/j.jaad.2019.04.065.
59. Helm MF, Hallock KK, Bisbee E, Miller JJ. Reply to: "Commentary on 'Optimizing the total-body skin exam: an observational cohort study'". J Am Acad Dermatol. 2019;81(5):e133. https://doi.org/10.1016/j.jaad.2019.05.010.
60. Puig S, Malvehy J. Monitoring patients with multiple nevi. Dermatol Clin. 2013;31(4):565–577, viii. https://doi.org/10.1016/j.det.2013.06.004.

61. Waldman RA, Grant-Kels JM, Curiel CN, Curtis J, Rodríguez SG, Hu S, Kerr P, Marghoob A, Markowitz O, Pellacani G, Rabinovitz H, Rao B, Scope A, Stein JA, Swetter SM. Consensus recommendations for the use of non-invasive melanoma detection techniques based on results of an international DELPHI process. J Am Acad Dermatol. 2019; https://doi.org/10.1016/j.jaad.2019.09.046. pii: S0190-9622(19)32794-X. Advance online publication.
62. Argenziano G, Zalaudek I, Ferrara G, Johr R, Langford D, Puig S, Soyer HP, Malvehy J. Dermoscopy features of melanoma incognito: indications for biopsy. J Am Acad Dermatol. 2007;56(3):508–13. https://doi.org/10.1016/j.jaad.2006.10.029.
63. Salerni G, Carrera C, Lovatto L, Martí-Laborda RM, Isern G, Palou J, Alós L, Puig S, Malvehy J. Characterization of 1152 lesions excised over 10 years using total-body photography and digital dermatoscopy in the surveillance of patients at high risk for melanoma. J Am Acad Dermatol. 2012;67(5):836–45. https://doi.org/10.1016/j.jaad.2012.01.028.
64. Nathansohn N, Orenstein A, Trau H, Liran A, Schachter J. Pigmented lesions clinic for early detection of melanoma: preliminary results. Israel Med Assoc J. 2007;9(10):708–12.
65. Salerni G, Carrera C, Lovatto L, Puig-Butille JA, Badenas C, Plana E, Puig S, Malvehy J. Benefits of total body photography and digital dermatoscopy ("two-step method of digital follow-up") in the early diagnosis of melanoma in patients at high risk for melanoma. J Am Acad Dermatol. 2012;67(1):e17–27. https://doi.org/10.1016/j.jaad.2011.04.008.
66. Moscarella E, Tion I, Zalaudek I, Lallas A, Kyrgidis A, Longo C, Lombardi M, Raucci M, Satta R, Alfano R, Argenziano G. Both short-term and long-term dermoscopy monitoring is useful in detecting melanoma in patients with multiple atypical nevi. J Eur Acad Dermatol Venereol. 2017;31(2):247–51. https://doi.org/10.1111/jdv.13840.
67. Adler NR, Kelly JW, Guitera P, Menzies SW, Chamberlain AJ, Fishburn P, Button-Sloan AE, Heal C, Soyer HP, Thompson JF. Methods of melanoma detection and of skin monitoring for individuals at high risk of melanoma: new Australian clinical practice. Med J Aust. 2019;210(1):41–7. https://doi.org/10.5694/mja2.12033.
68. Thomas L, Puig S. Dermoscopy, digital dermoscopy and other diagnostic tools in the early detection of melanoma and follow-up of high-risk skin cancer patients. Acta Derm Venereol. 2017;218(Suppl):14–21. https://doi.org/10.2340/00015555-2719.
69. Barcaui C, Bakos RM, Paschoal FM, Bittencourt FV, Sá B, Miot HA. Total body mapping in the follow-up of melanocytic lesions: recommendations of the Brazilian Society of Dermatology. An Bras Dermatol. 2021; https://doi.org/10.1016/j.abd.2020.10.005. pii: S0365-0596(21)00105-7. Advance online publication.
70. Malvehy J, Puig S. Follow-up of melanocytic skin lesions with digital total-body photography and digital dermoscopy: a two-step method. Clin Dermatol. 2002;20(3):297–304. https://doi.org/10.1016/s0738-081x(02)00220-1.
71. Rayner JE, Laino AM, Nufer KL, Adams L, Raphael AP, Menzies SW, Soyer HP. Clinical perspective of 3D total body photography for early detection and screening of melanoma. Front Med. 2018;5:152. https://doi.org/10.3389/fmed.2018.00152.
72. Lovatto L, Carrera C, Salerni G, Alós L, Malvehy J, Puig S. In vivo reflectance confocal microscopy of equivocal melanocytic lesions detected by digital dermoscopy follow-up. J Eur Acad Dermatol Venereol. 2015;29(10):1918–25. https://doi.org/10.1111/jdv.13067.
73. Serban ED, Farnetani F, Pellacani G, Constantin MM. Role of in vivo reflectance confocal microscopy in the analysis of melanocytic lesions. Acta Derm Venerol Croat. 2018;26(1):64–7.
74. Marghoob AA, Korzenko AJ, Changchien L, Scope A, Braun RP, Rabinovitz H. The beauty and the beast sign in dermoscopy. Dermatol Surg. 2007;33(11):1388–91. https://doi.org/10.1111/j.1524-4725.2007.33298.x.
75. Scope A, Burroni M, Agero AL, Benvenuto-Andrade C, Dusza SW, Rubegni P, Bono R, Dell'Eva G, Salaro C, Marghoob AA. Predominant dermoscopic patterns observed among nevi. J Cutan Med Surg. 2006;10(4):170–4.
76. Pellacani G, Scope A, Ferrari B, Pupelli G, Bassoli S, Longo C, Cesinaro AM, Argenziano G, Hofmann-Wellenhof R, Malvehy J, Marghoob AA, Puig S, Seidenari S, Soyer HP, Zalaudek I. New insights into nevogenesis: in vivo characterization and follow-up of mela-

nocytic nevi by reflectance confocal microscopy. J Am Acad Dermatol. 2009;61(6):1001–13. https://doi.org/10.1016/j.jaad.2009.04.018.
77. Pellacani G, Scope A, Farnetani F, Casaretta G, Zalaudek I, Moscarella E, Casari A, Cesinaro AM, Argenziano G, Longo C. Towards an in vivo morphologic classification of melanocytic nevi. J Eur Acad Dermatol Venereol. 2014;28(7):864–72. https://doi.org/10.1111/jdv.12181.
78. Ingordo V, Iannazzone SS, Cusano F, Naldi L. Dermoscopic features of congenital melanocytic nevus and Becker nevus in an adult male population: an analysis with a 10-fold magnification. Dermatology (Basel, Switzerland). 2006;212(4):354–60. https://doi.org/10.1159/000092286.
79. Fraga-Braghiroli N, Grant-Kels JM, Oliviero M, Rabinovitz H, Ferenczi K, Scope A. The role of reflectance confocal microscopy in differentiating melanoma in situ from dysplastic nevi with severe atypia: a cross-sectional study. J Am Acad Dermatol. 2020;83(4):1035–43. https://doi.org/10.1016/j.jaad.2020.05.071.
80. Pellacani G, Farnetani F, Gonzalez S, Longo C, Cesinaro AM, Casari A, Beretti F, Seidenari S, Gill M. In vivo confocal microscopy for detection and grading of dysplastic nevi: a pilot study. J Am Acad Dermatol. 2012;66(3):e109–21. https://doi.org/10.1016/j.jaad.2011.05.017.
81. Steiner A, Pehamberger H, Binder M, Wolff K. Pigmented Spitz nevi: improvement of the diagnostic accuracy by epiluminescence microscopy. J Am Acad Dermatol. 1992;27(5 Pt 1):697–701. https://doi.org/10.1016/0190-9622(92)70240-g.
82. Ferrara G, Argenziano G, Soyer HP, Chimenti S, Di Blasi A, Pellacani G, Peris K, Piccolo D, Rubegni P, Seidenari S, Staibano S, Zalaudek I, De Rosa G. The spectrum of Spitz nevi: a clinicopathologic study of 83 cases. Arch Dermatol. 2005;141(11):1381–7. https://doi.org/10.1001/archderm.141.11.1381.
83. Pellacani G, Cesinaro AM, Grana C, Seidenari S. In vivo confocal scanning laser microscopy of pigmented Spitz nevi: comparison of in vivo confocal images with dermoscopy and routine histopathology. J Am Acad Dermatol. 2004;51(3):371–6. https://doi.org/10.1016/j.jaad.2003.12.041.
84. Kalkhoran S, Milne O, Zalaudek I, Puig S, Malvehy J, Kelly JW, Marghoob AA. Historical, clinical, and dermoscopic characteristics of thin nodular melanoma. Arch Dermatol. 2010;146(3):311–8. https://doi.org/10.1001/archdermatol.2009.369.
85. Klebanov N, Gunasekera NS, Lin WM, Hawryluk EB, Miller DM, Reddy BY, Christman MP, Beaulieu D, Rajadurai S, Duncan LM, Sober AJ, Tsao H. Clinical spectrum of cutaneous melanoma morphology. J Am Acad Dermatol. 2019;80(1):178–188.e3. https://doi.org/10.1016/j.jaad.2018.08.028.
86. Skvara H, Teban L, Fiebiger M, Binder M, Kittler H. Limitations of dermoscopy in the recognition of melanoma. Arch Dermatol. 2005;141(2):155–60. https://doi.org/10.1001/archderm.141.2.155.
87. Pellacani G, Longo C, Malvehy J, Puig S, Carrera C, Segura S, Bassoli S, Seidenari S. In vivo confocal microscopic and histopathologic correlations of dermoscopic features in 202 melanocytic lesions. Arch Dermatol. 2008;144(12):1597–608. https://doi.org/10.1001/archderm.144.12.1597.
88. Guitera P, Menzies SW, Longo C, Cesinaro AM, Scolyer RA, Pellacani G. In vivo confocal microscopy for diagnosis of melanoma and basal cell carcinoma using a two-step method: analysis of 710 consecutive clinically equivocal cases. J Invest Dermatol. 2012;132(10):2386–94. https://doi.org/10.1038/jid.2012.172.
89. Yélamos O, Braun RP, Liopyris K, Wolner ZJ, Kerl K, Gerami P, Marghoob AA. Usefulness of dermoscopy to improve the clinical and histopathologic diagnosis of skin cancers. J Am Acad Dermatol. 2019;80(2):365–77. https://doi.org/10.1016/j.jaad.2018.07.072.
90. Babino G, Lallas A, Agozzino M, Alfano R, Apalla Z, Brancaccio G, Giorgio CM, Fulgione E, Kittler H, Kyrgidis A, Papageorgiou C, Argenziano G. Melanoma diagnosed on digital dermoscopy monitoring: a side-by-side image comparison is needed to improve early detection. J Am Acad Dermatol. 2020; https://doi.org/10.1016/j.jaad.2020.07.013. pii: S0190-9622(20)32177-0. Advance online publication.

91. Braun RP, Rabinovitz HS, Oliviero M, Kopf AW, Saurat JH. Dermoscopy of pigmented skin lesions. J Am Acad Dermatol. 2005;52(1):109–21. https://doi.org/10.1016/j.jaad.2001.11.001.
92. Jaimes N, Marghoob AA, Rabinovitz H, Braun RP, Cameron A, Rosendahl C, Canning G, Keir J. Clinical and dermoscopic characteristics of melanomas on nonfacial chronically sun-damaged skin. J Am Acad Dermatol. 2015;72(6):1027–35. https://doi.org/10.1016/j.jaad.2015.02.1117.
93. Pampena R, Lai M, Lombardi M, Mirra M, Raucci M, Lallas A, Apalla Z, Argenziano G, Pellacani G, Longo C. Clinical and dermoscopic features associated with difficult-to-recognize variants of cutaneous melanoma: a systematic review. JAMA Dermatol. 2020;156(4):430–9. https://doi.org/10.1001/jamadermatol.2019.4912.
94. Menzies SW, Kreusch J, Byth K, Pizzichetta MA, Marghoob A, Braun R, Malvehy J, Puig S, Argenziano G, Zalaudek I, Rabinovitz HS, Oliviero M, Cabo H, Ahlgrimm-Siess V, Avramidis M, Guitera P, Soyer HP, Ghigliotti G, Tanaka M, Perusquia AM, et al. Dermoscopic evaluation of amelanotic and hypomelanotic melanoma. Arch Dermatol. 2008;144(9):1120–7. https://doi.org/10.1001/archderm.144.9.1120.
95. Martín-Alcalde J, Gamo-Villegas R, Floristán-Muruzábal MU, Pampín-Franco A, Pinedo-Moraleda F, López-Estebaranz JL. Nevoid melanoma: Dermoscopic and in vivo reflectance confocal microscopic aspects in 4 cases. JAAD Case Rep. 2021;11:132–6. https://doi.org/10.1016/j.jdcr.2021.03.044.
96. Jain M, Marghoob AA. Integrating clinical, dermoscopy, and reflectance confocal microscopy findings into correctly identifying a nevoid melanoma. JAAD Case Rep. 2017;3(6):505–8. https://doi.org/10.1016/j.jdcr.2017.08.006.
97. Maher NG, Solinas A, Scolyer RA, Puig S, Pellacani G, Guitera P. Detection of desmoplastic melanoma with dermoscopy and reflectance confocal microscopy. J Eur Acad Dermatol Venereol. 2017;31(12):2016–24. https://doi.org/10.1111/jdv.14381.
98. Debarbieux S, Ronger-Salve S, Dalle S, Balme B, Thomas L. Dermoscopy of desmoplastic melanoma: report of six cases. Br J Dermatol. 2008;159(2):360–3. https://doi.org/10.1111/j.1365-2133.2008.08687.x.
99. Lallas A, Longo C, Manfredini M, Benati E, Babino G, Chinazzo C, Apalla Z, Papageorgiou C, Moscarella E, Kyrgidis A, Argenziano G. Accuracy of dermoscopic criteria for the diagnosis of melanoma in situ. JAMA Dermatol. 2018;154(4):414–9.
100. Martínez-Piva MM, Vacas AS, Rodríguez Kowalczuk MV, Gallo F, Rodrígues Vasconcelos M, Mazzuoccolo LD. Dermoscopy as a tool for estimating Breslow thickness in melanoma. La dermatoscopia como herramienta para inferir el Breslow del melanoma. Acta Derm Sifiliogr. 2021;112(5):434–40. https://doi.org/10.1016/j.ad.2020.11.015.
101. Reiter O, Kurtansky N, Nanda JK, Busam KJ, Scope A, Musthaq S, Marghoob AA. The differences in clinical and dermoscopic features between in situ and invasive nevus-associated melanomas and de novo melanomas. J Eur Acad Dermatol Venereol. 2021;35(5):1111–8. https://doi.org/10.1111/jdv.17133.
102. Zalaudek I, Ferrara G, Di Stefani A, Argenziano G. Dermoscopy for challenging melanoma; how to raise the 'red flag' when melanoma clinically looks benign. Br J Dermatol. 2005;153(1):200–2. https://doi.org/10.1111/j.1365-2133.2005.06617.x.
103. Kamińska-Winciorek G, Placek W. The most common mistakes on dermatoscopy of melanocytic lesions. Postepy Dermatol Alergol. 2015;32(1):33–9. https://doi.org/10.5114/pdia.2014.44029.
104. Sanchez MI, Rabinovitz HS, Oliverio MC, Elgart GW, Grichnik JM. Confocal microscopy of challenging dermoscopic diagnoses. Arch Dermatol. 2012;148(10):1224. https://doi.org/10.1001/archdermatol.2012.2538.
105. Longo C, Mazzeo M, Raucci M, Cornacchia L, Lai M, Bianchi L, Peris K, Pampena R, Pellacani G. Dark pigmented lesions: diagnostic accuracy of dermoscopy and reflectance confocal microscopy in a tertiary referral center for skin cancer diagnosis. J Am Acad Dermatol. 2021;84(6):1568–74. https://doi.org/10.1016/j.jaad.2020.07.084.

106. Rigel DS, Robinson JK, Ross M, Friedman RJ, Cockerell CJ, Lim HW, Stockfleth E, Kirkwood JM, editors. Cancer of the skin. 2nd ed. Elsevier Inc.; 2011. ISBN: 978-1-4377-1788-4.
107. Darmawan CC, Jo G, Montenegro SE, Kwak Y, Cheol L, Cho KH, Mun JH. Early detection of acral melanoma: a review of clinical, dermoscopic, histopathologic, and molecular characteristics. J Am Acad Dermatol. 2019;81(3):805–12. https://doi.org/10.1016/j.jaad.2019.01.081.
108. Lallas A, Kyrgidis A, Koga H, Moscarella E, Tschandl P, Apalla Z, Di Stefani A, Ioannides D, Kittler H, Kobayashi K, Lazaridou E, Longo C, Phan A, Saida T, Tanaka M, Thomas L, Zalaudek I, Argenziano G. The BRAAFF checklist: a new dermoscopic algorithm for diagnosing acral melanoma. Br J Dermatol. 2015;173(4):1041–9. https://doi.org/10.1111/bjd.14045.
109. Thomas L, Phan A, Pralong P, Poulalhon N, Debarbieux S, Dalle S. Special locations dermoscopy: facial, acral, and nail. Dermatol Clin. 2013;31(4):615–24. https://doi.org/10.1016/j.det.2013.06.006.
110. Liopyris K, Navarrete-Dechent C, Mancebo SE, Busam KJ, Pulitzer MP, Marghoob AA, Marchetti MA. Dermoscopic appearance of amelanotic volar melanoma compared with volar angioma. JAMA Dermatol. 2019;155(4):500–1. https://doi.org/10.1001/jamadermatol.2018.5487.
111. Marghoob N, Navarrete-Dechent C, Liopyris K, Apalla Z, Lallas A, Marghoob AA. Dermoscopic features of benign vascular lesions presenting on volar skin: a case series and literature review. J Eur Acad Dermatol Venereol. 2019;33(12):e444–5. https://doi.org/10.1111/jdv.15758.
112. Jaimes N, Marghoob AA. The morphologic universe of melanoma. Dermatol Clin. 2013;31(4):599–613. https://doi.org/10.1016/j.det.2013.06.010.
113. Cinotti E, Debarbieux S, Perrot JL, Labeille B, Long-Mira E, Habougit C, Douchet C, Depaepe L, Hammami-Ghorbel H, Lacour JP, Thomas L, Cambazard F, Bahadoran P, Groupe Imagerie Cutanée Non Invasive de la Société Française de Dermatologie. Reflectance confocal microscopy features of acral lentiginous melanoma: a comparative study with acral nevi. J Eur Acad Dermatol Venereol. 2016;30(7):1125–8. https://doi.org/10.1111/jdv.13399.
114. Zalaudek I, Cota C, Ferrara G, Moscarella E, Guitera P, Longo C, Piana S, Argenziano G. Flat pigmented macules on sun-damaged skin of the head/neck: junctional nevus, atypical lentiginous nevus, or melanoma in situ? Clin Dermatol. 2014;32(1):88–93. https://doi.org/10.1016/j.clindermatol.2013.05.029.
115. Pralong P, Bathelier E, Dalle S, Poulalhon N, Debarbieux S, Thomas L. Dermoscopy of lentigo maligna melanoma: report of 125 cases. Br J Dermatol. 2012;167(2):280–7. https://doi.org/10.1111/j.1365-2133.2012.10932.x.
116. Schiffner R, Schiffner-Rohe J, Vogt T, Landthaler M, Wlotzke U, Cognetta AB, Stolz W. Improvement of early recognition of lentigo maligna using dermatoscopy. J Am Acad Dermatol. 2000;42(1 I):25–32. https://doi.org/10.1016/S0190-9622(00)90005-7.
117. Lallas A, Argenziano G, Moscarella E, Longo C, Simonetti V, Zalaudek I. Diagnosis and management of facial pigmented macules. Clin Dermatol. 2014;32(1):94–100. https://doi.org/10.1016/j.clindermatol.2013.05.030.
118. Tiodorovic-Zivkovic D, Zalaudek I, Lallas A, Stratigos A, Piana S, Argenziano G. The importance of gray color as a dermoscopic clue in facial pigmented lesion evaluation: a case report. Dermatol Pract Concept. 2013;3(4):37–9. https://doi.org/10.5826/dpc.0304a09.
119. Tiodorovic-Zivkovic D, Argenziano G, Lallas A, Thomas L, Ignjatovic A, Rabinovitz H, Moscarella E, Longo C, Hofmann-Wellenhof R, Zalaudek I. Age, gender, and topography influence the clinical and dermoscopic appearance of lentigo maligna. J Am Acad Dermatol. 2015;72(5):801–8. https://doi.org/10.1016/j.jaad.2015.01.030.
120. Tschandl P, Rosendahl C, Kittler H. Dermatoscopy of flat pigmented facial lesions. J Eur Acad Dermatol Venereol. 2015;29(1):120–7. https://doi.org/10.1111/jdv.12483.
121. Lallas A, Tschandl P, Kyrgidis A, Stolz W, Rabinovitz H, Cameron A, Gourhant JY, Giacomel J, Kittler H, Muir J, Argenziano G, Hofmann-Wellenhof R, Zalaudek I. Dermoscopic clues

to differentiate facial lentigo maligna from pigmented actinic keratosis. Br J Dermatol. 2016;174(5):1079–85. https://doi.org/10.1111/bjd.14355.
122. Costa-silva M, Calistru A, Barros AM. Dermatoscopy of flat pigmented facial lesions—evolution of lentigo maligna diagnostic criteria. Dermatol Pract Concept. 2018;8(3):198–203.
123. Pellacani G, Guitera P, Longo C, Avramidis M, Seidenari S, Menzies S. The impact of in vivo reflectance confocal microscopy for the diagnostic accuracy of melanoma and equivocal melanocytic lesions. J Invest Dermatol. 2007;127(12):2759–65. https://doi.org/10.1038/sj.jid.5700993.
124. de Carvalho N, Farnetani F, Ciardo S, Ruini C, Witkowski AM, Longo C, Argenziano G, Pellacani G. Reflectance confocal microscopy correlates of dermoscopic patterns of facial lesions help to discriminate lentigo maligna from pigmented nonmelanocytic macules. Br J Dermatol. 2015;173(1):128–33. https://doi.org/10.1111/bjd.13546.
125. De Carvalho N, Fagundes Sortino AM, Martinez Zugaib Abdalla B, Martinez Zugaib Abdalla C. How can reflectance confocal microscopy help in the diagnosis of pigmented facial macules: a series of 3 cases. Australas J Dermatol. 2021;62(2):e244–8. https://doi.org/10.1111/ajd.13542.
126. Guitera P, Pellacani G, Crotty KA, Scolyer RA, Li LX, Bassoli S, Vinceti M, Rabinovitz H, Longo C, Menzies SW. The impact of in vivo reflectance confocal microscopy on the diagnostic accuracy of lentigo maligna and equivocal pigmented and nonpigmented macules of the face. J Invest Dermatol. 2010;130(8):2080–91. https://doi.org/10.1038/jid.2010.84.
127. Persechino F, De Carvalho N, Ciardo S, De Pace B, Casari A, Chester J, Kaleci S, Stanganelli I, Longo C, Farnetani F, Pellacani G. Folliculotropism in pigmented facial macules: differential diagnosis with reflectance confocal microscopy. Exp Dermatol. 2018;27(3):227–32. https://doi.org/10.1111/exd.13487.
128. Dabouz F, Barbe C, Lesage C, Le Clainche A, Arnoult G, Hibon E, Bernard P, Grange F. Clinical and histological features of head and neck melanoma: a population-based study in France. Br J Dermatol. 2015;172(3):707–15. https://doi.org/10.1111/bjd.13489.
129. Lachiewicz AM, Berwick M, Wiggins CL, Thomas NE. Survival differences between patients with scalp or neck melanoma and those with melanoma of other sites in the Surveillance, Epidemiology, and End Results (SEER) program. Arch Dermatol. 2008;144(4):515–21. https://doi.org/10.1001/archderm.144.4.515.
130. Xie C, Pan Y, McLean C, Mar V, Wolfe R, Kelly JW. Scalp melanoma: distinctive high risk clinical and histological features. Australas J Dermatol. 2017;58(3):181–8. https://doi.org/10.1111/ajd.12437.
131. Zalaudek I, Leinweber B, Soyer HP, Petrillo G, Brongo S, Argenziano G. Dermoscopic features of melanoma on the scalp. J Am Acad Dermatol. 2004;51(2 Suppl):S88–90. https://doi.org/10.1016/j.jaad.2003.12.024.
132. Torres F, Fabbrocini G, Hirata SH, Yamada S, De Vita V, Annunziata MC, Tosti A. Dermoscopy of scalp melanoma: report of three cases. Cancers. 2010;2(3):1597–601. https://doi.org/10.3390/cancers2031597.
133. Stanganelli I, Argenziano G, Sera F, Blum A, Ozdemir F, Karaarslan IK, Piccolo D, Peris K, Kirchesch H, Bono R, Pizzichetta MA, Gasparini S, Braun RP, Correia O, Thomas L, Zaballos P, Puig S, Malvehy J, Scalvenzi M, Rabinovitz H, et al. Dermoscopy of scalp tumours: a multi-centre study conducted by the international dermoscopy society. J Eur Acad Dermatol Venereol. 2012;26(8):953–63. https://doi.org/10.1111/j.1468-3083.2011.04188.x.
134. Benati E, Longo C, Piana S, Moscarella E. Preliminary evaluation of reflectance confocal microscopyfeatures of scalp melanoma. Austral J Dermatol. 2017; https://doi.org/10.1111/ajd.12690.
135. Hajar-Serviansky T, Gutierrez-Mendoza D, Galvan IL, Lammoglia-Ordiales L, Mosqueda-Taylor A, de Hernandez-Cázares ML, Toussaint-Caire S. A case of oral mucosal melanoma. Clinical and dermoscopic correlation. J Dermatol Case Rep. 2012;6(1):1–4. https://doi.org/10.3315/jdcr.2012.1085.

136. Matsushita S, Kageshita T, Ishihara T. Comparison of dermoscopic and histopathological findings in a mucous melanoma of the lip. Br J Dermatol. 2005;152(6):1324–6. https://doi.org/10.1111/j.1365-2133.2005.06463.x.
137. Simionescu O, Dumitrescu D, Costache M, Blum A. Dermatoscopy of an invasive melanoma on the upper lip shows possible association with Laugier-Hunziker syndrome. J Am Acad Dermatol. 2008;59(5 Suppl):S105–8. https://doi.org/10.1016/j.jaad.2008.07.023.
138. Virgili A, Zampino MR, Corazza M. Primary vulvar melanoma with satellite metastasis: dermoscopic findings. Dermatology. 2004;208(2):145–8. https://doi.org/10.1159/000076490.
139. Blum A, Simionescu O, Argenziano G, Braun R, Cabo H, Eichhorn A, et al. Dermoscopy of pigmented lesions of the mucosa and the mucocutaneous junction: results of a multicenter study by the International Dermoscopy Society (IDS). Arch Dermatol. 2011;147(10):1181–7. https://doi.org/10.1001/archdermatol.2011.155.
140. Vaccari S, Barisani A, Salvini C, Pirola S, Preti EP, Pennacchioli E, et al. Thin vulvar melanoma: a challenging diagnosis. Dermoscopic features of a case series. Clin Exp Dermatol. 2020;45(2):187–93. https://doi.org/10.1111/ced.14068.
141. Cinotti E, Perrot JL, Labeille B, Adegbidi H, Cambazard F. Reflectance confocal microscopy for the diagnosis of vulvar melanoma and melanosis: preliminary results. Dermatol Surg. 2012;38(12):1962–7. https://doi.org/10.1111/dsu.12009.
142. Debarbieux S, Perrot JL, Erfan N, Ronger-Savlé S, Labeille B, Cinotti E, et al. Reflectance confocal microscopy of mucosal pigmented macules: a review of 56 cases including 10 macular melanomas. Br J Dermatol. 2014;170(6):1276–84. https://doi.org/10.1111/bjd.12803.
143. De Pascalis A, Perrot JL, Tognetti L, Rubegni P, Cinotti E. Review of dermoscopy and reflectance confocal microscopy features of the mucosal melanoma. Diagnostics. 2021;11(1):91. https://doi.org/10.3390/diagnostics11010091.
144. Porto AC, Fraga-braghiroli N, Blumetti P. Reflectance confocal microscopy features of labial melanotic macule: report of three cases. JAAD Case Rep. 2018;4:1000–3.
145. Zaballos P, Puig S, Llambrich A, Malvehy J. Dermoscopy of dermatofibromas: a prospective morphological study of 412 cases. Arch Dermatol. 2008;144(1):75–83. https://doi.org/10.1001/archdermatol.2007.8.
146. Mentzel T. Cutaneous mesenchymal tumours: an update. Pathology. 2014;46(2):149–59. https://doi.org/10.1097/PAT.0000000000000046.
147. Luzar B, Calonje E. Cutaneous fibrohistiocytic tumours—an update. Histopathology. 2010;56(1):148–65. https://doi.org/10.1111/j.1365-2559.2009.03447.x.
148. Scope A, Ardigo M, Marghoob AA. Correlation of dermoscopic globule-like structures of dermatofibroma using reflectance confocal microscopy. Dermatology (Basel, Switzerland). 2008;216(1):81–2. https://doi.org/10.1159/000109364.
149. Weedon DE. Skin pathology. London: Churchill-Livingstone; 2002.
150. Ferrari A, Argenziano G, Buccini P, Cota C, Sperduti I, De Simone P, Eibenschutz L, Silipo V, Zalaudek I, Catricalà C. Typical and atypical dermoscopic presentations of dermatofibroma. J Eur Acad Dermatol Venereol. 2013;27(11):1375–80. https://doi.org/10.1111/jdv.12019.
151. Zaballos P, Puig S, Malvehy J. Dermoscopy of atypical dermatofibroma: central white network. Arch Dermatol. 2006;142(1):126. https://doi.org/10.1001/archderm.142.1.126.
152. Kilinc Karaarslan I, Gencoglan G, Akalin T, Ozdemir F. Different dermoscopic faces of dermatofibromas. J Am Acad Dermatol. 2007;57(3):401–6. https://doi.org/10.1016/j.jaad.2006.10.984.
153. Gonzalés S. Reflectance confocal microscopy of cutaneous tumors. 2nd ed. CRC Press Taylor & Francis Group; 2018.
154. Moscarella E, Zalaudek I, Agozzino M, Vega H, Cota C, Catricalà C, Argenziano G, Ardigò M. Reflectance confocal microscopy for the evaluation of solitary red nodules. Dermatology (Basel, Switzerland). 2012;224(4):295–300. https://doi.org/10.1159/000339339.
155. Carrera C, Segura S, Aguilera P, Scalvenzi M, Longo C, Barreiro A, Broganelli P, Cavicchini S, Llambrich A, Zaballos P, Thomas L, Malvehy J, Puig S, Zalaudek I. Dermoscopic clues for diagnosing melanomas that resemble seborrheic keratosis. JAMA Dermatol. 2017;153(6):544–51. https://doi.org/10.1001/jamadermatol.2017.0129.

156. Longo C, Zalaudek I, Moscarella E, Lallas A, Piana S, Pellacani G, Argenziano G. Clonal seborrheic keratosis: dermoscopic and confocal microscopy characterization. J Eur Acad Dermatol Venereol. 2014;28(10):1397–400. https://doi.org/10.1111/jdv.12261.
157. Braun RP, Rabinovitz HS, Krischer J, Kreusch J, Oliviero M, Naldi L, Kopf AW, Saurat JH. Dermoscopy of pigmented seborrheic keratosis: a morphological study. Arch Dermatol. 2002;138(12):1556–60. https://doi.org/10.1001/archderm.138.12.1556.
158. Ahlgrimm-Siess V, Cao T, Oliviero M, Laimer M, Hofmann-Wellenhof R, Rabinovitz HS, Scope A. Seborrheic keratosis: reflectance confocal microscopy features and correlation with dermoscopy. J Am Acad Dermatol. 2013;69(1):120–6. https://doi.org/10.1016/j.jaad.2012.12.969.
159. Hunziker MF, Guaraldo GR, Michalany NS, Michalany A, de Andrade A, Fagundes Sortino AM. Melanoacanthoma on the nipple of a middle-aged woman: a diagnostic challenge. JAAD Case Rep. 2021;9:93–6. https://doi.org/10.1016/j.jdcr.2021.01.026.
160. Lin J, Han S, Cui L, Song Z, Gao M, Yang G, Fu Y, Liu X. Evaluation of dermoscopic algorithm for seborrhoeic keratosis: a prospective study in 412 patients. J Eur Acad Dermatol Venereol. 2014;28(7):957–62. https://doi.org/10.1111/jdv.12241.
161. Shahriari N, Grant-Kels JM, Rabinovitz H, Oliviero M, Scope A. Reflectance confocal microscopy: Diagnostic criteria of common benign and malignant neoplasms, dermoscopic and histopathologic correlates of key confocal criteria, and diagnostic algorithms. J Am Acad Dermatol. 2021;84(1):17–31. https://doi.org/10.1016/j.jaad.2020.05.154.
162. Pezzini C, Mandel VD, Persechino F, Ciardo S, Kaleci S, Chester J, De Carvalho N, Persechino S, Pellacani G, Farnetani F. Seborrheic keratoses mimicking melanoma unveiled by in vivo reflectance confocal microscopy. Skin Res Technol. 2018;24(2):285–93. https://doi.org/10.1111/srt.12427.
163. Ackerman AB, Shapiro L. Lichen-planus-like keratosis. Arch Dermatol. 1970;101(6):705.
164. Zaballos P, Blazquez S, Puig S, Salsench E, Rodero J, Vives JM, Malvehy J. Dermoscopic pattern of intermediate stage in seborrhoeic keratosis regressing to lichenoid keratosis: report of 24 cases. Br J Dermatol. 2007;157(2):266–72. https://doi.org/10.1111/j.1365-2133.2007.07963.x.
165. Bugatti L, Filosa G. Dermoscopy of lichen planus-like keratosis: a model of inflammatory regression. J Eur Acad Dermatol Venereol. 2007;21(10):1392–7. https://doi.org/10.1111/j.1468-3083.2007.02296.x.
166. Liebman TN, Rabinovitz HS, Dusza SW, Marghoob AA. White shiny structures: dermoscopic features revealed under polarized light. J Eur Acad Dermatol Venereol. 2012;26(12):1493–7. https://doi.org/10.1111/j.1468-3083.2011.04317.x.
167. Bassoli S, Rabinovitz HS, Pellacani G, Porges L, Oliviero MC, Braun RP, Marghoob AA, Seidenari S, Scope A. Reflectance confocal microscopy criteria of lichen planus-like keratosis. J Eur Acad Dermatol Venereol. 2012;26(5):578–90. https://doi.org/10.1111/j.1468-3083.2011.04121.x.
168. Peris K, Fargnoli MC, Garbe C, Kaufmann R, Bastholt L, Seguin NB, Bataille V, Marmol VD, Dummer R, Harwood CA, Hauschild A, Höller C, Haedersdal M, Malvehy J, Middleton MR, Morton CA, Nagore E, Stratigos AJ, Szeimies RM, Tagliaferri L, et al. Diagnosis and treatment of basal cell carcinoma: European consensus-based interdisciplinary guidelines. Eur J Cancer (Oxford, England: 1990). 2019;118:10–34. https://doi.org/10.1016/j.ejca.2019.06.003.
169. Lallas A, Apalla Z, Argenziano G, Longo C, Moscarella E, Specchio F, Raucci M, Zalaudek I. The dermatoscopic universe of basal cell carcinoma. Dermatol Pract Concept. 2014;4(3):11–24. https://doi.org/10.5826/dpc.0403a02.
170. Wozniak-Rito A, Zalaudek I, Rudnicka L. Dermoscopy of basal cell carcinoma. Clin Exp Dermatol. 2018;43(3):241–7. https://doi.org/10.1111/ced.13387.
171. Longo C, Lallas A, Kyrgidis A, Rabinovitz H, Moscarella E, Ciardo S, Zalaudek I, Oliviero M, Losi A, Gonzalez S, Guitera P, Piana S, Argenziano G, Pellacani G. Classifying distinct basal cell carcinoma subtype by means of dermatoscopy and reflectance confocal microscopy. J Am Acad Dermatol. 2014;71(4):716–724.e1. https://doi.org/10.1016/j.jaad.2014.04.067.

172. González S, Tannous Z. Real-time, in vivo confocal reflectance microscopy of basal cell carcinoma. J Am Acad Dermatol. 2002;47(6):869–74. https://doi.org/10.1067/mjd.2002.124690.
173. Navarrete-Dechent C, DeRosa AP, Longo C, Liopyris K, Oliviero M, Rabinovitz H, Marghoob AA, Halpern AC, Pellacani G, Scope A, Jain M. Reflectance confocal microscopy terminology glossary for nonmelanocytic skin lesions: a systematic review. J Am Acad Dermatol. 2019;80(5):1414–1427.e3. https://doi.org/10.1016/j.jaad.2018.12.007.
174. Nori S, Rius-Díaz F, Cuevas J, Goldgeier M, Jaen P, Torres A, González S. Sensitivity and specificity of reflectance-mode confocal microscopy for in vivo diagnosis of basal cell carcinoma: a multicenter study. J Am Acad Dermatol. 2004;51(6):923–30. https://doi.org/10.1016/j.jaad.2004.06.028.
175. Hofmann-Wellenhof R, Pellacani G, Malvehy J, Soyer P, editors. Reflectance confocal microscopy for skin diseases. Berlin: Springer-Verlag; 2012. https://doi.org/10.1007/978-3-642-21997-9.
176. Deinlein T, Richtig G, Schwab C, Scarfi F, Arzberger E, Wolf I, Hofmann-Wellenhof R, Zalaudek I. The use of dermatoscopy in diagnosis and therapy of nonmelanocytic skin cancer. J German Soc Dermatol. 2016;14(2):144–51. https://doi.org/10.1111/ddg.12903.
177. Tavoloni Braga JC, de Paula Ramos Castro R, Moraes Pinto Blumetti TC, Rocha Mendes FB, Arêas de Souza Lima Beltrame Ferreira J, Rezze GG. Opening a window into living tissue: histopathologic features of confocal microscopic findings in skin tumors. Dermatol Clin. 2016;34(4):377–94. https://doi.org/10.1016/j.det.2016.05.002.
178. Röwert-Huber J, Patel MJ, Forschner T, Ulrich C, Eberle J, Kerl H, Sterry W, Stockfleth E. Actinic keratosis is an early in situ squamous cell carcinoma: a proposal for reclassification. Br J Dermatol. 2007;156(Suppl 3):8–12. https://doi.org/10.1111/j.1365-2133.2007.07860.x.
179. Zalaudek I, Giacomel J, Argenziano G, Hofmann-Wellenhof R, Micantonio T, Di Stefani A, Oliviero M, Rabinovitz H, Soyer HP, Peris K. Dermoscopy of facial nonpigmented actinic keratosis. Br J Dermatol. 2006;155(5):951–6. https://doi.org/10.1111/j.1365-2133.2006.07426.x.
180. Zalaudek I, Giacomel J, Schmid K, Bondino S, Rosendahl C, Cavicchini S, Tourlaki A, Gasparini S, Bourne P, Keir J, Kittler H, Eibenschutz L, Catricalà C, Argenziano G. Dermatoscopy of facial actinic keratosis, intraepidermal carcinoma, and invasive squamous cell carcinoma: a progression model. J Am Acad Dermatol. 2012;66(4):589–97. https://doi.org/10.1016/j.jaad.2011.02.011.
181. Zalaudek I, Piana S, Moscarella E, Longo C, Zendri E, Castagnetti F, Pellacani G, Lallas A, Argenziano G. Morphologic grading and treatment of facial actinic keratosis. Clin Dermatol. 2014;32(1):80–7. https://doi.org/10.1016/j.clindermatol.2013.05.028.
182. Cuellar F, Vilalta A, Puig S, Palou J, Salerni G, Malvehy J. New dermoscopic pattern in actinic keratosis and related conditions. Arch Dermatol. 2009;145(6):732. https://doi.org/10.1001/archdermatol.2009.86.
183. Zalaudek I, Argenziano G. Dermoscopy of actinic keratosis, intraepidermal carcinoma and squamous cell carcinoma. Curr Probl Dermatol. 2015;46:70–6. https://doi.org/10.1159/000366539.
184. Reinehr C, Garbin GC, Bakos RM. Dermatoscopic patterns of nonfacial actinic keratosis: characterization of pigmented and nonpigmented lesions. Dermatol Surg. 2017;43(11):1385–91. https://doi.org/10.1097/DSS.0000000000001210.
185. Papageorgiou C, Lallas A, Manoli SM, Longo C, Lai M, Liopyris K, Lallas K, Lazaridou E, Apalla Z. Evaluation of dermatoscopic criteria for early detection of squamous cell carcinoma arising on an actinic keratosis. J Am Acad Dermatol. 2021; https://doi.org/10.1016/j.jaad.2021.03.111. pii: S0190-9622(21)00760-X. Advance online publication.
186. Lallas A, Pyne J, Kyrgidis A, Andreani S, Argenziano G, Cavaller A, Giacomel J, Longo C, Malvestiti A, Moscarella E, Piana S, Specchio F, Hofmann-Wellenhof R, Zalaudek I. The clinical and dermoscopic features of invasive cutaneous squamous cell carcinoma depend on the histopathological grade of differentiation. Br J Dermatol. 2015;172(5):1308–15. https://doi.org/10.1111/bjd.13510.

187. Kupsa R, Deinlein T, Woltsche N, Hofmann-Wellenhof R, Zalaudek I. Dermoscopy of keratinocyte skin cancer. G Ital Dermatol Venereol. 2016;151(6):649–62.
188. Conforti C, Giuffrida R, Pizzichetta MA, Di Meo N, Magaton-Rizzi G, Zalaudek I. Integrating the concept of field cancerization in the classification and risk assessment of cutaneous squamous cell carcinoma: proposal for a new classification and terminology of keratinocyte skin cancer. J Eur Acad Dermatol Venereol. 2019;33(9):e327–30. https://doi.org/10.1111/jdv.15624.
189. Rishpon A, Kim N, Scope A, Porges L, Oliviero MC, Braun RP, Marghoob AA, Fox CA, Rabinovitz HS. Reflectance confocal microscopy criteria for squamous cell carcinomas and actinic keratoses. Arch Dermatol. 2009;145(7):766–72. https://doi.org/10.1001/archdermatol.2009.134.
190. Nguyen KP, Peppelman M, Hoogedoorn L, Van Erp PE, Gerritsen MP. The current role of in vivo reflectance confocal microscopy within the continuum of actinic keratosis and squamous cell carcinoma: a systematic review. Eur J Dermatol. 2016;26(6):549–65. https://doi.org/10.1684/ejd.2016.2872.
191. Peppelman M, Nguyen KP, Hoogedoorn L, van Erp PE, Gerritsen MJ. Reflectance confocal microscopy: non-invasive distinction between actinic keratosis and squamous cell carcinoma. J Eur Acad Dermatol Venereol. 2015;29(7):1302–9. https://doi.org/10.1111/jdv.12806.
192. Ulrich M, Zalaudek I, Welzel J. Shining into the white: the spectrum of epithelial tumors from actinic keratosis to squamous cell carcinoma. Dermatol Clin. 2016;34(4):459–67. https://doi.org/10.1016/j.det.2016.05.008.
193. Ulrich M, Maltusch A, Rius-Diaz F, Röwert-Huber J, González S, Sterry W, Stockfleth E, Astner S. Clinical applicability of in vivo reflectance confocal microscopy for the diagnosis of actinic keratoses. Dermatol Surg. 2008;34(5):610–9. https://doi.org/10.1111/j.1524-4725.2007.34117.x.
194. Ulrich M, Kanitakis J, González S, Lange-Asschenfeldt S, Stockfleth E, Roewert-Huber J. Evaluation of Bowen disease by in vivo reflectance confocal microscopy. Br J Dermatol. 2012;166(2):451–3. https://doi.org/10.1111/j.1365-2133.2011.10563.x.
195. Manfredini M, Longo C, Ferrari B, Piana S, Benati E, Casari A, Pellacani G, Moscarella E. Dermoscopic and reflectance confocal microscopy features of cutaneous squamous cell carcinoma. J Eur Acad Dermatol Venereol. 2017;31(11):1828–33. https://doi.org/10.1111/jdv.14463.
196. Fraga-Braghiroli N, Stephens A, Oliviero M, Rabinovitz H, Scope A. Small brown circles: an important diagnostic clue for pigmented squamous cell carcinoma. J Am Acad Dermatol. 2013;69(4):e161–3. https://doi.org/10.1016/j.jaad.2013.04.024.
197. Shahriari N, Grant-Kels JM, Rabinovitz HS, Oliviero M, Scope A. Reflectance confocal microscopy criteria of pigmented squamous cell carcinoma in situ. Am J Dermatopathol. 2018;40(3):173–9. https://doi.org/10.1097/DAD.0000000000000938.
198. Blumetti TP, Scope A, de Macedo MP, Ferreira JB, Gomes EE, Enokihara MY, Pinto CA, Nascimento MM, Rezze GG, Braga JC. Dermoscopic and reflectance confocal microscopy findings in extra-genital HPV16-associated pigmented squamous cell carcinoma in situ. Acta Derm Venereol. 2016;96(6):836–7. https://doi.org/10.2340/00015555-2399.
199. Welzel J, Lankenau E, Birngruber R, Engelhardt R. Optical coherence tomography of the human skin. J Am Acad Dermatol. 1997;37(6):958–63. https://doi.org/10.1016/s0190-9622(97)70072-0.
200. Schmitz L, Reinhold U, Bierhoff E, Dirschka T. Optical coherence tomography: its role in daily dermatological practice. J German Soc Dermatol. 2013;11(6):499–507. https://doi.org/10.1111/ddg.12073.
201. Schuh S, Kaestle R, Sattler E, Welzel J. Comparison of different optical coherence tomography devices for diagnosis of non-melanoma skin cancer. Skin Res Technol. 2016;22(4):395–405. https://doi.org/10.1111/srt.12277.
202. Wang RK. Optical microangiography: a label free 3D imaging technology to visualize and quantify blood circulations within tissue beds in vivo. IEEE J Sel Top Quant Electron. 2010;16(3):545–54. https://doi.org/10.1109/JSTQE.2009.2033609.
203. Dubois A, Levecq O, Azimani H, Siret D, Barut A, Suppa M, Del Marmol V, Malvehy J, Cinotti E, Rubegni P, Perrot JL. Line-field confocal optical coherence tomography for high-

resolution noninvasive imaging of skin tumors. J Biomed Opt. 2018;23(10):1–9. https://doi.org/10.1117/1.JBO.23.10.106007.
204. Mogensen M, Morsy HA, Thrane L, Jemec GB. Morphology and epidermal thickness of normal skin imaged by optical coherence tomography. Dermatology (Basel, Switzerland). 2008;217(1):14–20. https://doi.org/10.1159/000118508.
205. Welzel J. Optical coherence tomography in dermatology: a review. Skin Res Technol. 2001;7(1):1–9. https://doi.org/10.1034/j.1600-0846.2001.007001001.x.
206. Ferrante di Ruffano L, Dinnes J, Deeks JJ, Chuchu N, Bayliss SE, Davenport C, Takwoingi Y, Godfrey K, O'Sullivan C, Matin RN, Tehrani H, Williams HC, Cochrane Skin Cancer Diagnostic Test Accuracy Group. Optical coherence tomography for diagnosing skin cancer in adults. Cochrane Database Syst Rev. 2018;12(12):CD013189. https://doi.org/10.1002/14651858.CD013189.
207. Pomerantz R, Zell D, McKenzie G, Siegel DM. Optical coherence tomography used as a modality to delineate basal cell carcinoma prior to mohs micrographic surgery. Case Rep Dermatol. 2011;3(3):212–8. https://doi.org/10.1159/000333000.
208. Gambichler T, Orlikov A, Vasa R, Moussa G, Hoffmann K, Stücker M, Altmeyer P, Bechara FG. In vivo optical coherence tomography of basal cell carcinoma. J Dermatol Sci. 2007;45(3):167–73. https://doi.org/10.1016/j.jdermsci.2006.11.012.
209. Cheng HM, Lo S, Scolyer R, Meekings A, Carlos G, Guitera P. Accuracy of optical coherence tomography for the diagnosis of superficial basal cell carcinoma: a prospective, consecutive, cohort study of 168 cases. Br J Dermatol. 2016;175(6):1290–300. https://doi.org/10.1111/bjd.14714.
210. Gomes EE, Moraes Pinto Blumetti TC, de Macedo MP, Cohen MP, Bergami MD, Rezze GG. Optical coherence tomography in the diagnosis of basal cell carcinoma. Surg Cosm Dermatol. 2013;5(3):241–3.
211. Batz S, Wahrlich C, Alawi A, Ulrich M, Lademann J. Differentiation of different nonmelanoma skin cancer types using OCT. Skin Pharmacol Physiol. 2018;31(5):238–45. https://doi.org/10.1159/000489269.
212. Moraes Pinto Blumetti TC, Cohen MP, Gomes EE, Petaccia de Macedo M, Ferreira de Souza Begnami MD, Tavares Guerreiro Fregnani JH, Duprat JP, Pellacani G, Rezze GG. Optical coherence tomography (OCT) features of nevi and melanomas and their association with intraepidermal or dermal involvement: a pilot study. J Am Acad Dermatol. 2015;73(2):315–7. https://doi.org/10.1016/j.jaad.2015.05.009.
213. Maher NG, Blumetti TP, Gomes EE, Cheng HM, Satgunaseelan L, Lo S, Rezze GG, Scolyer RA, Guitera P. Melanoma diagnosis may be a pitfall for optical coherence tomography assessment of equivocal amelanotic or hypomelanotic skin lesions. Br J Dermatol. 2017;177(2):574–7. https://doi.org/10.1111/bjd.15187.
214. Ferrone CR, Ben Porat L, Panageas KS, Berwick M, Halpern AC, Patel A, Coit DG. Clinicopathological features of and risk factors for multiple primary melanomas. JAMA. 2005;294(13):1647–54. https://doi.org/10.1001/jama.294.13.1647.
215. Guitera P, Menzies SW, Coates E, Azzi A, Fernandez-Penas P, Lilleyman A, Badcock C, Schmid H, Watts CG, Collgros H, Liu R, van Kemenade C, Mann GJ, Cust AE. Efficiency of detecting new primary melanoma among individuals treated in a high-risk clinic for skin surveillance. JAMA Dermatol. 2021;157(5):521–30. https://doi.org/10.1001/jamadermatol.2020.5651.

Chapter 7
Topical Treatments for Skin Cancer

Vera Maria Bacelar de Barros, Carolina Atallah Pontes da Silva, and Marcelo Neira Ave

Key Points

- The gold standard treatment for skin cancers is surgery.
- Topical therapies should be reserved when surgery or radiotherapy are contraindicated or inappropriate.
- Topical treatment requires knowledge and deep understanding of the drug, pathophysiology and evolution of skin cancer.
- Complications such as skin irritation, erythema, blistering, scaling, necrosis, erosions, burning and pruritus may arise but usually offer good cosmetic results.
- Adherence to topical treatment varies between patients and is associated with treatment outcome.

Introduction

Skin cancer, mostly basal cell carcinoma (BCC) and squamous cell carcinoma (SCC), as known as non-melanoma skin cancer (NMSC), are the most common of all types of cancer in the world, with constantly rising incidence [1]. According to the National Comprehensive Cancer Network (NCCN), the incidence of BCC is two times more common than SCC [2]. These ratios are in dependence of population, sample size, and inclusion and exclusion criteria.

V. M. B. de Barros (✉)
NOCS, Sírio-Libanês Hospital, São Paulo, Brazil
e-mail: vera@verabarros.com.br

C. A. P. da Silva · M. N. Ave
Sírio-Libanês Hospital, São Paulo, Brazil

C. M. Z. Abdalla et al. (eds.), *Oncodermatology*,
https://doi.org/10.1007/978-3-031-29277-4_7

Table 7.1 Risk stratification of BCC according to NCCN version 2.2021 [2]

Risk group	Low risk	High risk
Localization/size	Trunk, extremities <2 cm	– Trunk, extremities ≥2 cm – Cheeks, forehead, scalp, neck and pretibial any size – Mask areas of face (central face, eyelids, eyebrows, periorbital, nose, lips (cutaneous and vermilion), chin, mandible, preauricular and postauricular skin/sulci, temple and ear), genitalia, hands and feet
Borders	Well-defined	Poorly defined
Primary vs recurrent	Primary	Recurrent
Immunosuppression	(−)	(+)
Site of prior radiotherapy	(−)	(+)
Subtype	Nodular, superficial	Aggressive growth pattern
Perineural involvement	(−)	(+)

The risk stratification of BCC and SCC depends on the location and size of the tumor, pathologic risk factors and immunosuppression (Tables 7.1 and 7.2).

It is well known that BCC and SCC on H zone or mask area of the face, such as central face, eyelids, eyebrows, periorbital, nose, lips, chin, mandible, preauricular and postauricular, temple, and ear (Fig. 7.1), is considered high-risk tumor, as well as scalp, genitalia, hands and feet [2, 3].

Actinic keratosis (AK), also known as solar keratosis, is one of the most common diseases diagnosed and treated by dermatologists. They are precancerous lesions that could progress to SCC, if left untreated [2, 4, 5].

The therapeutic approach of AK includes field direct treatment, such as photodynamic therapy (PDT) and topical medications, for example 5-fluorouracil and imiquimod, and lesion direct treatment, as cryosurgery, curettage and electrocauterization, and laser ablation [4, 6].

According to NCCN, the gold standard treatment for BCC and SCC is surgery; topical therapies should be reserved when surgery or radiotherapy are contraindicated or inappropriate [2, 7].

Nonsurgical treatment for skin cancer includes topical medications, photodynamic therapy, cryosurgery, radiation therapy, target therapies, such as Hedgehog pathway inhibitors, immune checkpoint inhibitors like programmed cell death protein 1 (PD-1) inhibitors.

In this chapter, we will discuss the nonsurgical topical treatments for actinic keratosis and non-melanoma skin cancer.

Table 7.2 Risk stratification of SCC according to NCCN version 2.2021 [2]

Risk group	Low risk	High risk	Very high risk
Localization/size	Trunk, extremities <2 cm	– Trunk, extremities >2 to <4 cm – Head, neck, hands, feet, pretibia and anogenital (any size)	≥4 cm (any location)
Borders	Well-defined	Poorly defined	
Primary vs recurrent	Primary	Recurrent	
Immunosuppression	(−)	(+)	
Site of prior radiotherapy or chronic inflammatory process	(−)	(+)	
Rapidly growing tumor	(−)	(+)	
Neurologic symptoms	(−)	(+)	
Degree of differentiation	Well or moderately differentiated		Poor differentiation
Histologic features: acantholytic (adenoid), adenosquamous (showing mucin production) or metaplastic (Carcinosarcomas) subtypes	(−)	(+)	Dermoplastic SCC
Depth: thickness or level of invasions	≤6 mm and no invasion beyond subcutaneous fat		>6 mm or invasion beyond subcutaneous fat
Perineural involvement	(−)	(+)	Tumor cells within the nerve sheath of a nerve lying deeper than the dermis or measuring ≥0.1 mm
Lymphatic or vascular involvement	(−)	(−)	(+)

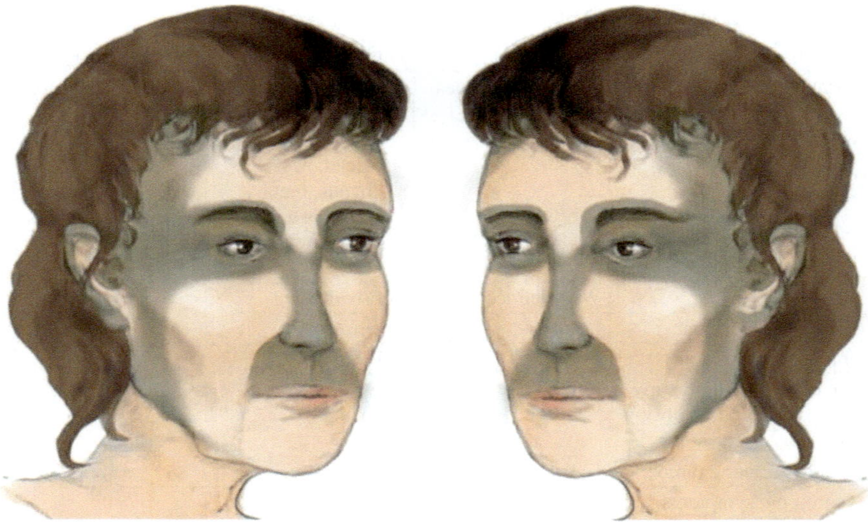

Fig. 7.1 H zone or mask area of the face

Topical Treatments

5-Fluorouracil (5-FU)

Mechanism of Action

Topical 5-FU is a pyrimidine analogue that inhibits thymidylate synthase by inducing cell cycle arrest and apoptosis (Fig. 7.2) [5, 6, 8].

Indications and Formulations

Topical 5-FU is approved for the treatment of premalignant actinic keratosis (AK), superficial basal cell carcinoma (sBCC) and could be used off-label to treat in situ squamous cells carcinoma (SCC) [5, 6, 9] (see Table 7.3).

Topical 5-FU is available as a 2% or 5% solution; or a 0.5%, 1%, 2%, 4% or 5% cream [5, 6, 10].

For the treatment of AK of any location, topical 5-FU (1%, 2% or 5%) can be used two times a day for 2–4 weeks. The 0.5% cream is approved only for the treatment of face and scalp AK and it is recommended as a daily application for 2–4 weeks. It also can be used for field cancerization treatment. In Europe, the maximum area that topical 5-FU 5% cream could be used is 500 cm^2 [4–6, 11]. 5-FU 4% cream is approved for the treatment of AK on the face, scalp or ears and it is recommended as a daily treatment for 4 weeks [10].

For sBCC, when conventional treatments are contraindicated, topical 5-FU 5% cream should be applied twice a day for 2–4 weeks. It is important to avoid treating

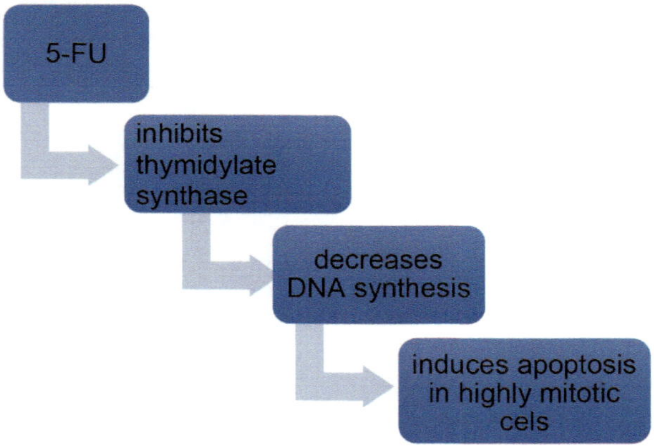

Fig. 7.2 5-FU: mechanism of action in neoplastic cells

Table 7.3 5-FU: indications, dosage and side effects

Drug	Available formulation (%)	Indications	Dosage	Off-label indication	Side effects
5-FU	0.5%, 1%, 2%, 4% or 5%	AK and superficial BCC	AK: – 5-FU (1%, 2% or 5%) Twice a day (BID) for 2–4 weeks – 5 -FU 0.5% (face and scalp) daily for 2–4 weeks – 5-FU 4% (face, scalp and ears) daily for 4 weeks sBCC: – 5-FU 5% BID for 2–4 weeks	Bowen's disease, actinic cheilitis	Skin irritation, erythema, blistering, scaling, necrosis and erosions

BCC located in mask zone and terminal hair-bearing areas (scalp, pubic and axillary regions, and beard area in men) [5, 12].

The treatment of Bowen's disease with topical 5-FU is off-label [5].

Side Effects and Contraindications

The most common skin side effects are skin irritation, erythema, blistering, scaling, necrosis and erosions that can be accompanied by pruritus and burning (see Figs. 7.3 and 7.4) [5, 6, 9].

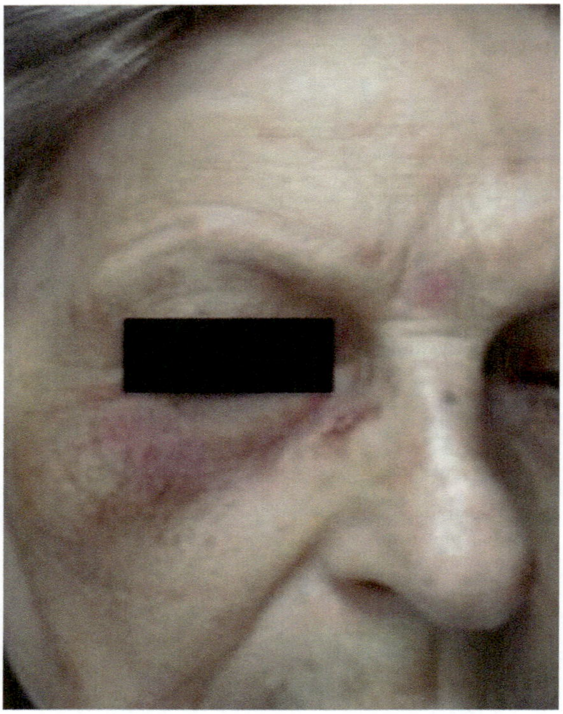

Fig. 7.3 5-FU side effects: erythema. (Courtesy of Carolina AP da Silva MD)

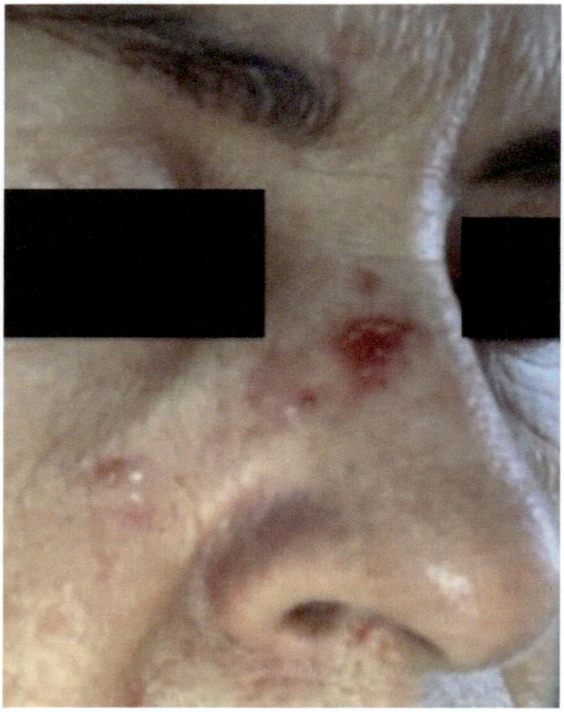

Fig. 7.4 5-FU side effects: erosions. (Courtesy of Carolina AP da Silva MD)

Topical 5-FU is formally contraindicated for fertile and pregnant women because of its teratogenicity [5].

New Formulations Combined with 5-Fluorouracil

5-Fluorouracil Combined with Calcipotriol

The combination of 5-FU and calcipotriol has a synergistic effect in the treatment of actinic keratosis [4, 11, 13] (see Table 7.4).

The studies recommend the use of the combination (5% 5-FU + 0.005% calcipotriol ointment) twice a day for 4 days for the treatment of AK on the face, scalp and upper extremities with 87.8% versus 26.3% (control group) mean reduction in the number of AK ($P < 0.0001$) [4, 11, 13].

The use of the association of 5% 5-FU cream + 0.005% calcipotriol ointment for the treatment of AK is off-label, but is a promising mode of chemoprevention because of the short treatment duration [4, 11, 13].

Chemowraps with 5-FU

The use of 5-FU over large areas can be challenging, especially if the patient uses it at home. It is a good option for the treatment of extensive areas of actinic keratoses or as an option for palliative management of lower or upper limbs SCC in patients who are not good candidates for surgery or refuse surgery, or as neoadjuvant to surgery to help define the tumor borders [6, 14, 15] (see Table 7.5).

The treatment regimen consists of weekly wraps with 5% 5-FU occluded with a gauze impregnated by zinc oxide (Unna wrap) covered by a compression wrap and gauze bandages. The chemowrap is changed once a week and the treatment should last for 4–8 weeks [6, 14, 15].

Table 7.4 5-FU + calcipotriol: indications, dosage and side effects

Drug	Available formulation	Indication (off-label)	Dosage	Side effects
5-FU combined with calcipotriol	5% 5-FU + 0.005% calcipotriol ointment	AK on scalp, face and limbs	BID for 4 days	Skin irritation, erythema, blistering, scaling, necrosis and erosions

Table 7.5 Chemowraps with 5-FU: indications, dosage and side effects

Drug	Available formulation	Indication (off-label)	Side effects
Chemowraps with 5-FU	5% 5-FU occluded with a gauze impregnated by zinc oxide	AK's extensive areas, palliative management of lower or upper limbs SCC	Skin irritation, erythema, blistering, scaling, necrosis and erosions

The use of chemowraps with 5-FU is off-label, but is a promising treatment for AK, especially in the upper and lower limbs [6, 14, 15].

Imiquimod

Mechanism of Action

Imiquimod (IQ) is an immune response modulator that works by stimulating toll-like receptors 7 and 8, present on immune cells, causing a release of proinflammatory cytokines that contribute to tumor destruction (Fig. 7.5) [5, 6, 9, 16–18].

Indications and Formulations

IQ is approved for the treatment of AK on the face and scalp in immunocompetent patients and for the treatment of sBCC lesser than 2 cm in diameter in any location, except on zone mask of the face or located in terminal hair-bearing areas, such as scalp, pubic and axillary regions, and beard area in men. It could be used off-label in other types of skin cancer, such as nodular BCC, in situ SCC, erythroplasia of Queyrat, lentigo maligna (LM), melanoma metastases, extramammary Paget disease and cutaneous T-cell lymphomas [4, 6] (see Table 7.6).

Topical formulations available are 5%, 3.75% and 2.5% IQ cream. The IQ 5% cream may be used to treat a surface area of 25 cm^2, and the other formulations may be used to treat larger areas, up to 200 cm^2. All formulation should be applied at bedtime, and left for 8 h, and washed in the morning with water and soap.

For AK's treatment, in the USA the standard regimen of IQ 5% cream consists of two applications per week for 16 weeks, the regimen for European countries consists of one or two courses of treatment three times per week for 4 weeks. The IQ 3.75% and 2.5% cream are used on a daily application for 2-week treatment cycles, followed for 2-week interval [5, 6, 9, 16–18].

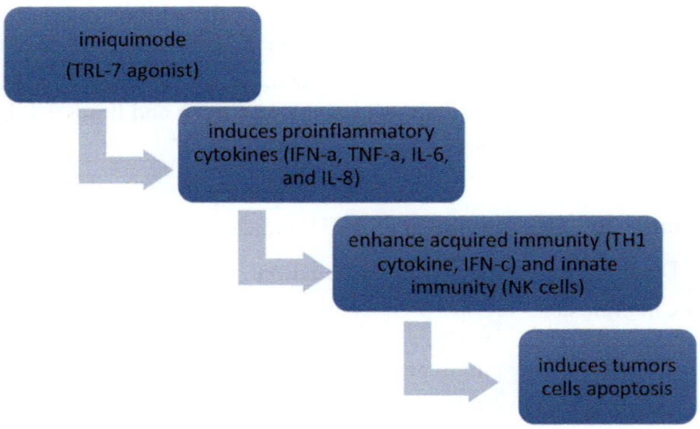

Fig. 7.5 Imiquimod: mechanism of action in neoplastic cells

Table 7.6 Imiquimod: indications, dosage and side effects

Drug	Available formulation	Indications	Dosage	Off-label indication	Side effects
Imiquimod	5%, 3.75% and 2.5% IQ cream	AK Superficial BCC	AK: – USA: IQ 5% two applications per week for 16 weeks – Europe: One or two courses of treatment three times per week for 4 weeks sBCC: – Once a day for five times a week for 6–16 weeks	Nodular BCC, Bowen's disease, lentigo maligna, erythroplasia of Queyrat, extramammary Paget disease, melanoma metastases, cutaneous T-cell lymphomas	Skin irritation, erythema, blistering, scaling, necrosis, erosions, burning and pruritus

IQ 5% cream is approved for the treatment of sBCC and the treatment regimen consists of daily applications five times a week for 6–16 weeks. IQ represents a useful alternative to surgery in the treatment of low-risk sBCC [5, 6, 9, 16–18].

Side Effects and Contraindications

The most common skin side effects are skin irritation, erythema, blistering, scaling, necrosis, erosions, burning and pruritus. Occasionally, the skin reactions could be extending beyond the application site (Fig. 7.6). IQ could lead to systemic side effects such as flu-like or gastrointestinal symptoms (fatigue, fever, chills, arthralgias, myalgias, nausea and diarrhea) especially when larger areas are treated [5, 6, 9, 17, 18].

It should be avoided during pregnancy (category C).

Photodynamic Therapy (PDT)

Mechanism of Action

PDT combines the use of a photosensitizing agent, such as 5-aminolevulinic acid (ALA) or methyl (MAL), and a light source to selectively destroy premalignant and malignant cells. Both ALA and MAL are precursors of protoporphyrin IX (PpIX) an

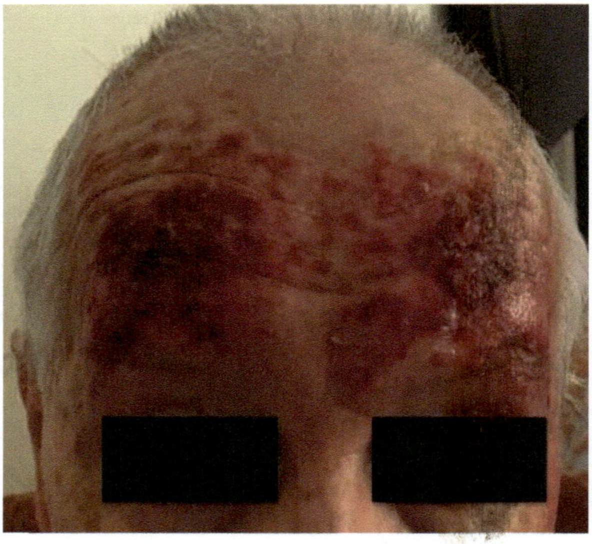

Fig. 7.6 Imiquimod side effects: erythema, blistering and erosions. (Courtesy of Carolina AP da Silva MD)

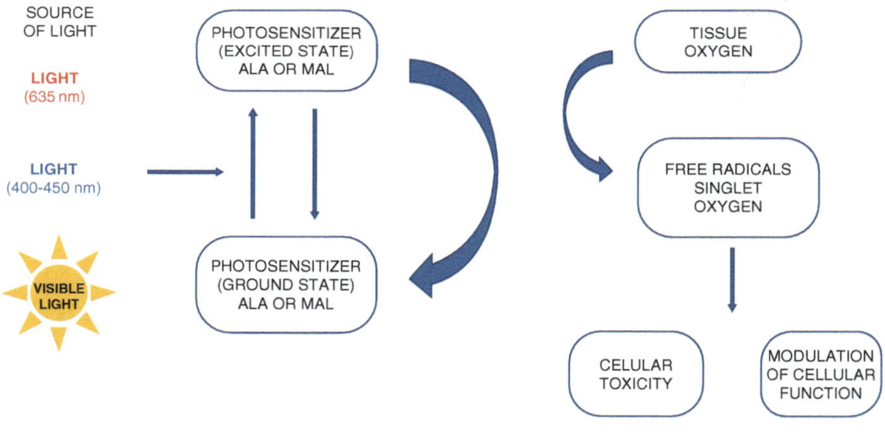

Fig. 7.7 PDT: mechanism of action in dysplastic cells

endogenous photosensitizer, that accumulates in dysplastic cells. PpIX is synthesized in mitochondria and there is evidence that mitochondrial toxicity is the primary cause of cell death (Fig. 7.7) [4, 7, 17].

Topical application of ALA or MAL, after a light exposure, such as red light (635 nm), blue light (405–420 nm) or visible light, leads to a chemical reaction that selectively produces reactive oxygen species and death of premalignant and malignant cells [4, 7].

The difference between ALA and MAL is that the first one is hydro soluble and the second is lipophilic increasing its penetration into deeper tissues.

Indications and Formulations

Topical ALA 20% combined to a blue light (400–450 nm, 10 J/cm^2) and topical ALA 10% in a nano emulsion gel combined to red light (635 nm, 37 J/cm^2) are approved for lesion-directed, or field-directed treatment of mild to moderate AK on the face and scalp. Both ALA 20% and ALA 10% are applied on skin under occlusion for 3–4 h and then illuminated with an appropriate light source [4, 6, 7] (see Table 7.7).

Topical MAL 16.8% cream combined with a red light (635 nm) is approved for the treatment of AK, superficial BCC, nodular BCC and in situ SCC. The period of MAL incubation under occlusion is 3 h, followed by cleaning the area with saline and irradiation with a red LED (635 nm, 37 J/cm^2). For the treatment of superficial and nodular BCC and in situ SCC, it is recommended two treatments 1 week apart [4, 6, 7] (see Table 7.7, Fig. 7.8).

Daylight PDT (DL-PDT) with ALA or MAL is a new treatment for mild and moderate AK on scalp and face. Recent studies have shown similar short-term efficacy compared to conventional PDT. Treatment consists in applying the photosensitizer agent (ALA or MAL) without occlusion, for 30 min, exposing the affected area to ambient daylight for 2 h. Application of chemical sunscreen during the exposure is recommended to prevent sunburn [4, 6, 7, 19].

Side Effects and Contraindications

The most common skin side effects with conventional PDT are pain, burning, pruritus, followed by skin irritation, erythema, blistering, scaling, erosions, phototoxicity, sterile pustular eruption in the treated area, and rarely superinfection [4, 6, 7, 20].

Table 7.7 PDT: indications and side effects

Drug	Available formulation	Indications	Off-label indication	Side effects
ALA-PDT	ALA 20% ALA 10%	Mild and moderate AK on scalp and face	Superficial BCC, <2 mm nodular BCC	Pain, burning, pruritus, followed by skin irritation, erythema, blistering, scaling, erosions, phototoxicity, sterile pustular eruption in the treated area; and rarely superinfection
MAL-PDT	MAL 16.8%	Mild and moderate AK on scalp and face, superficial BCC, <2 mm nodular BCC, in situ SCC	Actinic cheilitis, mycosis fungoides	Pain, burning, pruritus, followed by skin irritation, erythema, blistering, scaling, erosions, phototoxicity, sterile pustular eruption in the treated area; and rarely superinfection
DL-PDT	ALA 20% ALA 10% MAL 16.8%	Mild and moderate AK on scalp and face		Mild discomfort, erythema, scaling, less often blistering and crusting

Common adverse reactions of DL-PDT are mild discomfort, erythema, scaling, less often blistering and crusting. Phototoxicity and pustular eruptions have been described [19, 21, 22].

Tirbanibulin

Mechanism of Action

Topical tirbanibulin is a novel microtubule inhibitor, with a possible mechanism of inhibition of Src protein tyrosine kinase and tubulin polymerization (see Fig. 7.9) [23–25].

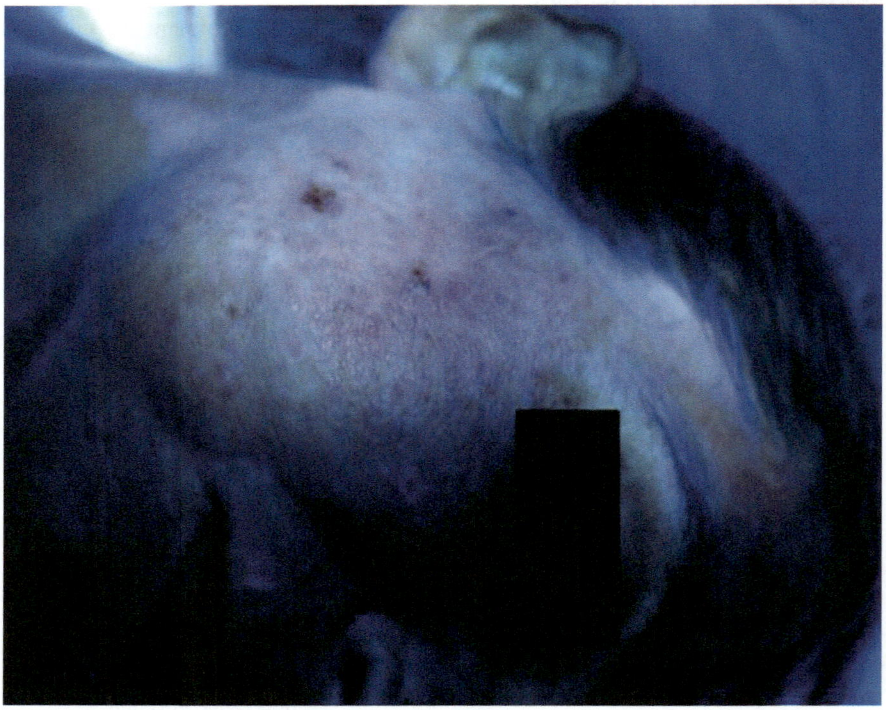

Fig. 7.8 Mal-PDT: lesions fluorescence after 3 h of MAL occlusion. (Courtesy of Carolina AP da Silva MD)

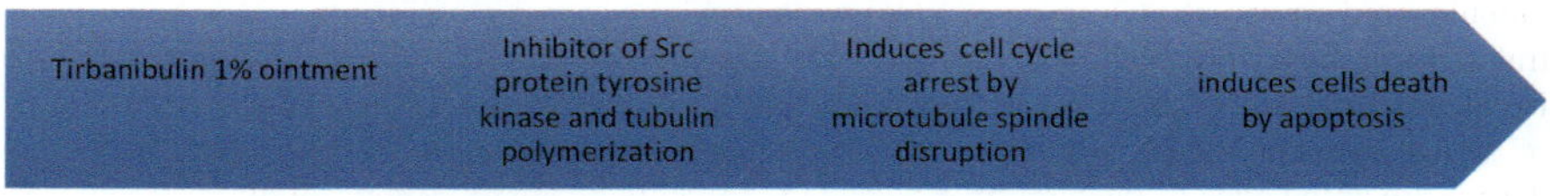

Fig. 7.9 Tirbanibulin: mechanism of action

Indications and Formulations

Topical tirbanibulin is approved to treat facial and scalp AK; therefore increased Src activity has been detected [4, 23, 24] (see Table 7.8).

Topical tirbanibulin is available as 1% ointment in packets [23–25].

For the treatment of AK of face or scalp turbanibulin, 1% ointment should be used once a day for 5 days up to 25 cm^2 [23–25].

Side Effects and Contraindications

The most common skin side effects are edema, erythema, pruritus, erosion, irritation and ulceration of de skin treated area. Pruritus, pain and burning sensation might result after application [23–25].

It is contraindicated in pregnancy, breast feeding, occlusive dressing and ocular exposure [23–25].

Diclofenac Gel

Diclofenac is a nonsteroidal anti-inflammatory (NSAID) drug that induces apoptosis, inhibits angiogenesis and alters cellular proliferation by downregulating cyclooxygenase enzymes, mostly cyclooxygenase 2 (COX-2), leading to death of cells typical (see Fig. 7.10) [5, 6, 16, 20].

Indications and Formulations

Topical diclofenac 3% in 2.5% acid hyaluronic gel is approved for the treatment of AK in immunocompetent and immunosuppressed patients. The regimen consists of twice-daily application for 12 weeks [5, 6, 16, 20] (see Table 7.9).

Table 7.8 Tirbanibulin: indications, dosage and side effects

Drug	Available formulation	Indications	Side effects
Tirbanibulin	1% ointment	AK of face and scalp	Skin irritation Erythema Edema Pruritus Pain Burning

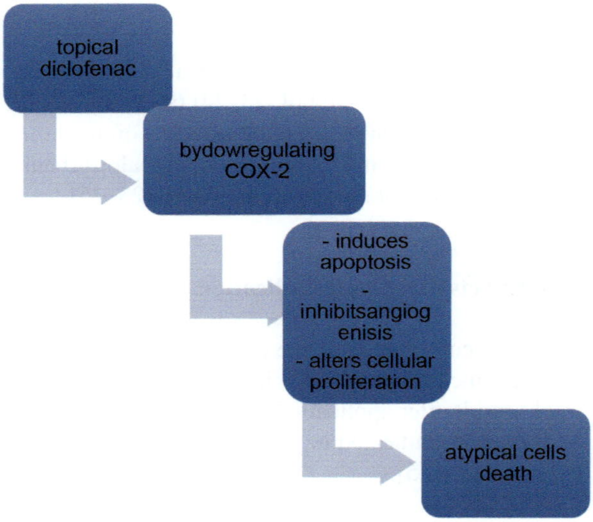

Fig. 7.10 Diclofenac: mechanism of action

Table 7.9 Topical diclofenac: indications, dosage and side effects

Drug	Available formulation	Indications	Side effects
Topical diclofenac	Diclofenac 3% + 2.5% hyaluronic acid	AK	Mild irritation Erythema Scaling Dry skin Erosions Pruritus

Side Effects and Contraindications

The most common skin side effects are mild irritation, such as erythema, scaling, dry skin, erosions and pruritus [5, 6, 16, 20].

It should be avoided in pregnant women, patients with history of cardiovascular thrombotic events, gastrointestinal complications and patients with NSAID hypersensitivity. Patients should avoid sun exposure during the treatment with topical diclofenac due the risk of photosensitivity [4–6, 16, 20].

Ingenol Mebutate

Mechanism of Action

Ingenol mebutate (IM) is a natural extract from *Euphorbia peplus.* IM induces a rapid cellular death in the treated area, by mitochondrial disruptions leading to necrosis, followed by an inflammatory response via activation of protein kinase C pathway and apoptosis [4, 5, 11].

Indications and Formulations

IM 0.015% was approved for treatment of AK on face and scalp once a day for 3 days and IM 0.05% was approved for treatment of AK on trunk and extremities once a day for 2 days [4, 5, 11].

The use of IM was discontinued in the European Union, after a safety data reviewed by the European Medicines Agency's Pharmacovigilance Risk Committee reported an incidence of skin cancer in the treatment area with IM three times more than observed with imiquimod. IM was discontinued in the USA and Canada, as well [4].

Conclusion

The approach of melanoma and non-melanoma skin cancer patients must follow some basic principles:

- Complete excision of the lesion
- Preservation of the normal tissue
- Maintenance of function
- Best cosmetic result

Following the guidelines of treatment of skin cancer, the first choice is surgical excision with safe margins considering the tumor localization and histological type.

The peripheral and deep surgical margins of the excised tissue examined histologically intraoperative using frozen sections or Mohs micrographic surgery are mandatory for recurrences or primary tumors with poorly defined edges and high and very high-risk tumor stratification according to NCCN version 2.2021 [2].

The radiotherapy is a choice when surgery is not feasible.

For the superficial BCC or in situ SCC that surgery is not suitable there are topical treatments, each one with some pros and cons.

Dermatologists must select the method that is more suitable for each case and always consider the NMSC subtype (aggressive or nonaggressive BCC or SCC), location, immunosuppression, time of onset and previous treatment. Follow-up patient's lesions treated with topical therapy are imperative because, in addition to the treated tumor, these patients are susceptible to develop new tumors [26, 27].

References

1. Ciążyńska M, Kamińska-Winciorek G, Lange D, Lewandowski B, Reich A, Sławińska M, Pabianek M, Szczepaniak K, Hankiewicz A, Ułańska M, et al. The incidence and clinical analysis of non-melanoma skin cancer. Sci Rep. 2021;11:1–10.
2. NCCN guidelines for squamous cell skin cancer (version 2.2021). https://www.nccn.org/professionals/physician_{g}{l}{s}/pdf/squamous.pdf. Accessed 2021.

3. Swanson NA. Mohs surgery: technique, indications, applications, and the future. Arch Dermatol. 1983;119:761–73.
4. Eisen DB, Asgari MM, Bennett DD, Connolly SM, Dellavalle RP, Freeman EE, Goldenberg G, Leffell DJ, Peschin S, Sligh JE, et al. Guidelines of care for the management of actinic keratosis. J Am Acad Dermatol. 2021;85:e209.
5. Micali G, Lacarrubba F, Nasca MR, Ferraro S, Schwartz RA. Topical pharmacotherapy for skin cancer: part II. Clinical applications. J Am Acad Dermatol. 2014;70:979–e1.
6. Nemer KM, Council ML. Topical and systemic modalities for chemoprevention of nonmelanoma skin cancer. Dermatol Clin. 2019;37:287–95.
7. Braathen LR, Szeimies R-M, Basset-Seguin N, Bissonnette R, Foley P, Pariser D, Roelandts R, Wennberg A-M, Morton CA. Guidelines on the use of photodynamic therapy for nonmelanoma skin cancer: an international consensus. J Am Acad Dermatol. 2007;56:125–43.
8. Thomson J, Hogan S, Leonardi-Bee J, Williams HC, Bath-Hextall FJ. Interventions for basal cell carcinoma of the skin. Cochrane Database Syst Rev. 2020;11:CD003412.
9. Dianzani C, Conforti C, Giuffrida R, Corneli P, di Meo N, Farinazzo E, Moret A, Magaton Rizzi G, Zalaudek I. Current therapies for actinic keratosis. Int J Dermatol. 2020;59:677–84.
10. Dohil MA. Efficacy, safety, and tolerability of 4% 5-fluorouracil cream in a novel patented aqueous cream containing peanut oil once daily compared with 5% 5-fluorouracil cream twice daily: meeting the challenge in the treatment of actinic keratosis. J Drugs Dermatol. 2016;15:1218–24.
11. Cornejo CM, Jambusaria-Pahlajani A, Willenbrink TJ, Schmults CD, Arron ST, Ruiz ES. Field cancerization: treatment. J Am Acad Dermatol. 2020;83:719–30.
12. Peris K, Fargnoli MC, Garbe C, Kaufmann R, Bastholt L, Seguin NB, Bataille V, Del Marmol V, Dummer R, Harwood CA, et al. Diagnosis and treatment of basal cell carcinoma: European consensus-based interdisciplinary guidelines. Eur J Cancer. 2019;118:10–34.
13. Cunningham TJ, Tabacchi M, Eliane J-P, Tuchayi SM, Manivasagam S, Mirzaalian H, Turkoz A, Kopan R, Schaffer A, Saavedra AP, et al. Randomized trial of calcipotriol combined with 5-fluorouracil for skin cancer precursor immunotherapy. J Clin Investig. 2017;127:106–16.
14. Goon PKC, Clegg R, Yong ASW, Lee ASW, Lee KYC, Levell NJ, Tan EKH, Shah SN. 5-Fluorouracil chemowraps in the treatment of multiple actinic keratoses: a Norwich experience. Dermatol Ther. 2015;5:201–5.
15. Tallon B, Turnbull N. 5% fluorouracil chemowraps in the management of widespread lower leg solar keratoses and squamous cell carcinoma. Austral J Dermatol. 2013;54:313–6.
16. Collins A, Savas J, Doerfler L. Nonsurgical treatments for nonmelanoma skin cancer. Dermatol Clin. 2019;37:435–41.
17. Tanese K. Diagnosis and management of basal cell carcinoma. Curr Treat Options Oncol. 2019;20:1–13.
18. Hanna E, Abadi R, Abbas O. Imiquimod in dermatology: an overview. Int J Dermatol. 2016;55:831–44.
19. Wiegell SR, Wulf HC, Szeimies R-M, Basset-Seguin N, Bissonnette R, Gerritsen M-JP, Gilaberte Y, Calzavara-Pinton P, Morton CA, Sidoroff A, et al. Daylight photodynamic therapy for actinic keratosis: an international consensus: International Society for Photodynamic Therapy in Dermatology. J Eur Acad Dermatol Venereol. 2012;26:673–9.
20. Jetter N, Chandan N, Wang S, Tsoukas M. Field cancerization therapies for management of actinic keratosis: a narrative review. Am J Clin Dermatol. 2018;19:543–57.
21. Rubel DM, Spelman L, Murrell DF, See J-A, Hewitt D, Foley P, Bosc C, Kerob D, Kerrouche N, Wulf HC, et al. Daylight photodynamic therapy with methyl aminolevulinate cream as a convenient, similarly effective, nearly painless alternative to conventional photodynamic therapy in actinic keratosis treatment: a randomized controlled trial. Br J Dermatol. 2014;171:1164–71.
22. Wiegell SR, Haedersdal M, Eriksen P, Wulf HC. Photodynamic therapy of actinic keratoses with 8% and 16% methyl aminolaevulinate and home-based daylight exposure: a double-blinded randomized clinical trial. Br J Dermatol. 2009;160:1308–14.

23. Blauvelt A, Kempers S, Lain E, Schlesinger T, Tyring S, Forman S, Ablon G, Martin G, Wang H, Cutler DL, et al. Phase 3 trials of tirbanibulin ointment for actinic keratosis. N Engl J Med. 2021;384:512–20.
24. Kempers S, DuBois J, Forman S, Poon A, Cutler E, Wang H, Cutler D, Fang J, Kwan R. Tirbanibulin ointment 1% as a novel treatment for actinic keratosis: phase 1 and 2 results. J Drugs Dermatol. 2020;19:1093–100.
25. Smolinski MP, Bu Y, Clements J, Gelman IH, Hegab T, Cutler DL, Fang JWS, Fetterly G, Kwan R, Barnett A, et al. Discovery of novel dual mechanism of action Src signaling and tubulin polymerization inhibitors (KX2-391 and KX2-361). ACS Publications; 2018.
26. Nasca M, Lacarrubba F. Topical pharmacotherapy for skin cancer. J Am Acad Dermatol. 2014;70:965.
27. Knackstedt TJ, Knackstedt RW, Djohan M, Djohan R, Gastman BR, Crowe DR. New developments in the management of cutaneous squamous cell carcinoma. Plast Reconstr Surg. 2021;147:492–504.

Chapter 8
Biopsy Techniques

Beatrice Martinez Zugaib Abdalla and Reinaldo Tovo Filho

Key Points
- Biopsy is important for diagnosis and management of skin cancers.
- Knowledge of different biopsy techniques provides better diagnosis.
- Melanocytic lesions that are suspicious of melanoma should undergo excisional biopsy, with rare exceptions.

Skin Biopsy

Introduction

A biopsy is an important step to diagnose skin cancer. It is indicated when clinical diagnosis of a cutaneous disorder is unclear or must be defined before a therapeutic decision is made. This is also true for lesions that are suspicious for malignancy, where the biopsy can sustain the appropriate surgical plan for the patient [1, 2].

The procedure allows the histologic examination of the lesion in question. Although experts can diagnose a suspicious lesion clinically and with complementary imaging, pathology remains the gold standard [1, 2]. Now-a-days there are various techniques which allow efficient cutaneous biopsies to be performed with less tissue damage. The modalities include curettage, shave, saucerization, punch, and

Observation: Figures provided for this chapter are from Hospital Sírio-Libanês Institute of Knowledge and Research Center. The images were performed in the facility's laboratory using pig's skin to demonstrate the different types of biopsies.

B. M. Z. Abdalla (✉) · R. T. Filho
Hospital Sírio-Libanês, São Paulo, Brazil

C. M. Z. Abdalla et al. (eds.), *Oncodermatology*,
https://doi.org/10.1007/978-3-031-29277-4_8

incisional and excisional biopsy. These types of biopsies must be well known technically to provide a correct and complete diagnosis [1–4].

When analyzing a lesion for biopsy, depending on size and technique used, there are some modalities which may even be curative. Also, the experience of the physician influences the choice and result of this biopsy [3, 4].

Methods

Curettage

This can be used to remove clinically benign epidermal lesions such as seborrheic keratosis, actinic keratosis (AKs), and may even be used to remove superficial basal cell carcinomas (BCCs). Histologic interpretation of this material may be difficult due to the fragmented tissue provided and lack of orientation of the specimen [1, 3, 4].

Shave Biopsy

Shave biopsies can be performed with a scalpel (Fig. 8.1), scissors, Dermablade®, consisting of a representative sample of the lesion [1]. It may include epidermis, papillary, and at times the reticular dermis [1–3]. When performing the shave

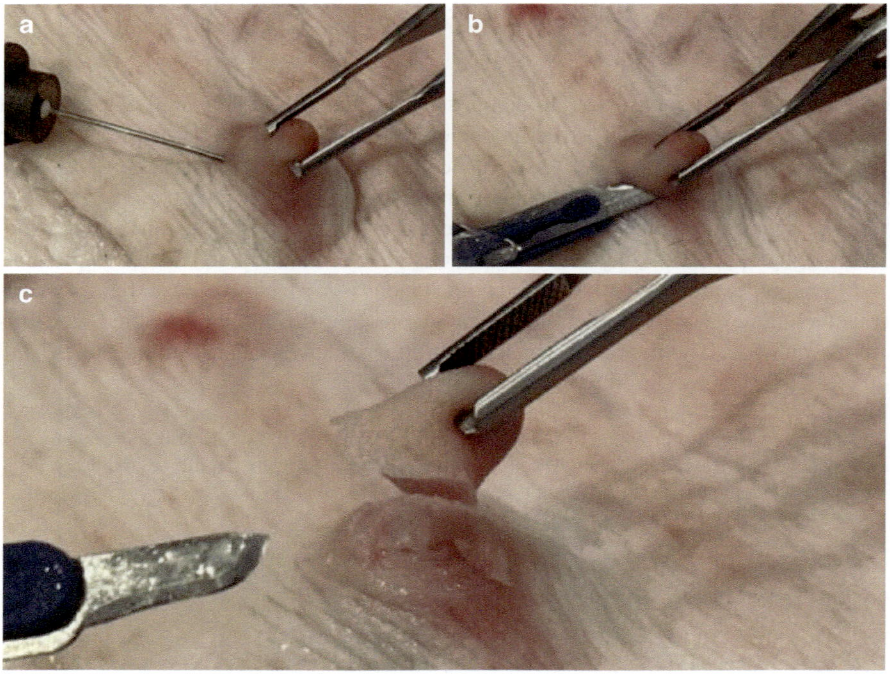

Fig. 8.1 Example of shave biopsy being performed on pig's skin: (**a**) local anesthesia performed on the base of the lesion; (**b**) shave biopsy being performed; (**c**) specimen of shave biopsy

biopsy, after anesthesia infiltration, the edematous wheel can raise the lesion and allow an easier access to perform the biopsy [1, 4]. The shave technique is a quick, low-cost technique, with less instrumentation, does not require suture closure, and the resulting bleeding can be stopped with chemical cautery or electrocoagulation [1, 4, 5]. It may be performed to diagnose clinically benign lesions, such as melanocytic nevi, fibrous papules, as well as malignant lesions like BCCs, squamous cell carcinoma (SCC), and lentigo maligna [1, 2].

Saucerization Biopsy

Saucerization biopsy is a deeper biopsy than shave biopsy due to angulation of the blade [3, 4]. This type of biopsy can be used for melanocytic nevi with atypical features when the differential diagnosis includes a thin melanoma, as well as non-melanoma carcinomas [1–5]. It allows histologic examination of the entire lesion, which increases diagnostic accuracy, especially in the case of larger lesions [4, 5].

Punch Biopsy

For the punch biopsy we use a cylindrical instrument that can vary from 2 to 6 mm, to obtain a conically shaped specimen that may reach past the dermis to subcutaneous tissue (Fig. 8.2) [3, 5]. The volume of tissue sampled correlates with the size of the punch biopsy instrument. This biopsy modality can be used for inflammatory lesions or large-sized tumors with sample biopsies [3, 5].

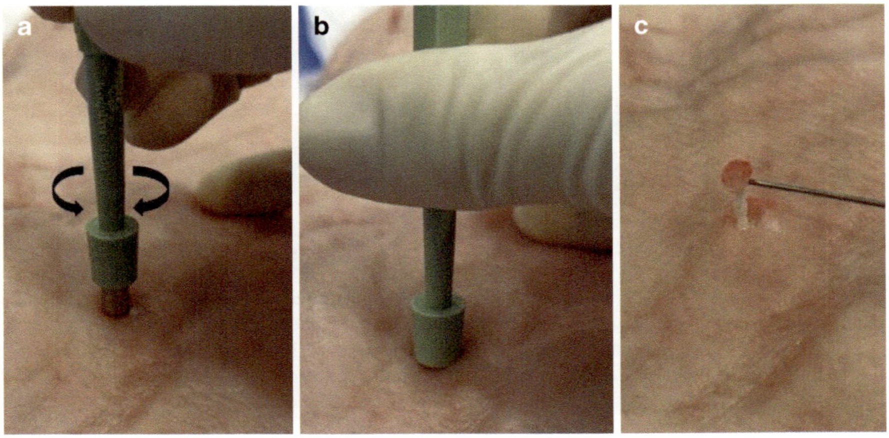

Fig. 8.2 Example of punch biopsy: (**a**) movement of punch biopsy (twisting); (**b**) demonstrating the end point of the punch biopsy; (**c**) specimen of the biopsy, carefully removed not to harm the tissue

Incisional Biopsy

Incisional biopsy removes a sample of the tissue and usually contains epidermis, dermis, and subcutaneous fat or even fascia and muscle (Fig. 8.3). It can be used to remove a part of large-sized tumors [1–5].

Excisional Biopsy

This modality removes the entire lesion and reaches subcutaneous fat (Fig. 8.4). This can be used when there is a suspicion of cutaneous melanoma and in some cases excisional biopsies can be curative for other tumors [1–5].

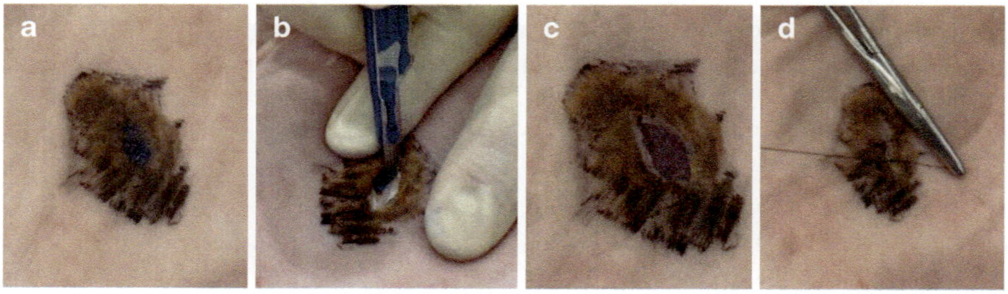

Fig. 8.3 Example of incisional biopsy: (**a**) lesion demonstrated with ink markings, central part with darker pigment to demonstrate where incisional biopsy should be performed; (**b**) using a scalpel, the incisional biopsy should be performed with the blade at 90° on skin surface; (**c**) final view of specimen removal, showing muscle tissue, therefore specimen removed should contain epidermis, dermis, and subcutaneous fat; (**d**) closing wound with primary sutures. Suture knot should be left adjacent to the wound closure

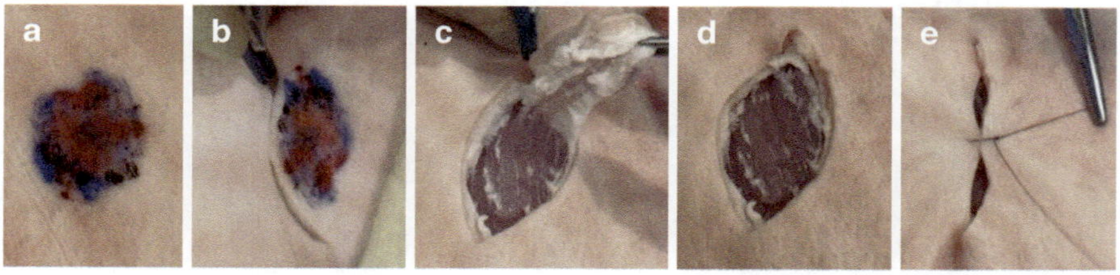

Fig. 8.4 Example of excisional biopsy: (**a**) lesion demonstrated with ink markings; (**b**) using a scalpel, the excisional biopsy should be performed with the blade at 90° on skin surface, removing the lesion with a 2–3 mm margin; (**c**) removing specimen containing epidermis, dermis, and subcutaneous fat; (**d**) final view of specimen removal, showing muscle tissue; (**e**) closing wound with primary sutures. Suture knot should be left adjacent to the wound closure

Procedure Steps

1. When deciding to biopsy, patient must first be advised about the procedure and sign informed consent. This must include the risk of bleeding, discomfort, infection, and scarring [1, 2, 5].
2. The chosen site of biopsy should be photographed. In some cases, other imaging techniques may be added to the lesion documentation, such as dermoscopy [1, 2, 5]. The use of confocal microscopy, high-frequency ultrasound using 24–33 MHz and optimal computerized tomography can be helpful and in a near future more accessible to physicians.
3. The lesion can be delineated with a surgical marking dye prior to injection, if needed [1, 2, 5].
4. The lesion must then be cleaned with antiseptic with chlorhexidine solution. For sensitive areas, such as, around the eyes, aqueous chlorhexidine solution is best to avoid irritation [5].
5. The area is then draped for the instillation of local anesthesia. Usually, lidocaine at 1% with or without epinephrine (1:100,000) is used for local anesthesia [1]. This is instilled into a deeper layer (subcutaneous layer) and takes up to 10 min to act on the biopsy site, so epinephrine can cause vasoconstriction [1, 5]. If instilled superficially, creating an edematous wheal, action is almost immediate, however the patient may feel more pain. The anesthesia may last locally up to 2 h [1, 5].
6. The excision can be done by stabilizing the biopsy site with the non-dominant hand, while using a #15 blade or a punch instrument to cut the epidermis with the dominant hand [5]. It is very important to handle the specimen with care, not to macerate the skin [5]. Therefore, the use of delicate forceps, such as Adson's forceps or skin hooks, such as Joseph's or Gillies' skin hooks.
7. Hemostasis is usually obtained with suturing when biopsies, such as a punch biopsy, are done [1, 5]. When incisional or excisional biopsies are performed, electrocoagulation may be required for hemostasis. Other forms of hemostasis include wound pressure, gel foam, or aluminum chloride solution [1, 5].
8. Wound closure may occur by either primary or second-intention healing. Sutures can be removed around 7–15 days depending on the biopsy site [1, 5].

Wound Healing

Primary intention healing occurs when the lesion is closed with suturing. Sutures can be done in the dermis, usually with synthetic absorbable materials and epidermal sutures with monofilament nylon or polypropylene [2, 3, 5]. Second intension healing repairs wounds without sutures. In both healing processes, there is the formation of granulation tissue, epidermal cell migration, and contraction [2, 3, 5]. The difference is that primary healing happens at a faster rate. After complete re-epithelization the scar still undergoes maturation and with time, a better cosmetic aspect [2, 3, 5].

Indications/Contraindications

In most cases, patients can safely undergo a skin biopsy, since there are no absolute contraindications to performing a skin biopsy [1–5]. Anyways, a clinician must be aware of the patient's medical history in order to make an adequate surgical plan and to predict any complications that can be managed [2, 4, 5]. For patients with primary coagulation or platelet disorders, it may be preferable to biopsy a site that can be compressed to produce hemostasis [2, 4, 5]. Patients on warfarin, heparin, clopidogrel, apixaban, rivaroxaban, or aspirin can be biopsied if there is planning for hemostasis [2, 4, 5]. When patients are on anticoagulants, it may be possible to pause medication to perform the biopsy.

If the lesion is on an anatomical site that could injure a vital structure, multidisciplinary decision should be made to provide the best option for the patient [5].

Specimen Fixation

Biopsy fixation consists of placing the biopsy specimen in a specific liquid for preservation [3–5]. Any skin fragment removed from the body should be handled with care, since this keeps the material in a state similar to live tissue [3, 4]. A fixator must have rapid action, high penetration and not induce artifacts or provoke lesion retraction [3, 4]. Formaldehyde at 10% or buffered formaldehyde are considered good fixators [3, 4]. For nail preservation, 10% formaldehyde or trichloroacetic acid can be used. The specimen must be placed in the fixating liquid as soon as it is removed from the skin [3, 4]. The recommended liquid volume is 10–20 times greater than the size or volume of the tissue fragment. This vile with the biopsy can be left 24 h for fixation [3–5].

Recommendations for Biopsying a Suspicious Lesion: Non-Melanoma and Melanoma

Basal Cell Carcinoma (BCC) and Squamous Cell Carcinoma (SCC)

A biopsy specimen can be obtained before planning a definitive treatment [1–6].

Shave biopsy is usually a preferred technique for superficial or nodular BCC or Bowen's disease (SCC in situ). However, a small (2–3 mm) punch biopsy specimen obtained from the center of the lesion may have advantages over a shave biopsy specimen [2, 6]. When performing a punch biopsy, superficial tumor margins can remain visible and can provide greater information on tumor growth pattern [2, 6]. When a broad shave is done, surrounding erythema can leave tumor margin as indistinct and deeper growth patterns may not be visible [2, 6]. Both modalities are superior to biopsy via curettage, which rarely allows accurate assessment of tumor growth [2, 6].

Melanoma

When analyzing pigmented lesions and there is suspicion of malignancy, a biopsy is key to provide an early diagnosis and intervention plan to improve prognosis [1, 2, 6]. A complete excision of a suspicious pigmented lesions is the method of choice. This form of biopsy gives the pathologist the possibility to view the lesion in its entirety, evaluating symmetry, architecture, depth, and invasion of other structures [1, 2, 6]. Therefore, it is important to include up to the subcutaneous tissue. This allows the possibility to measure Breslow and Clark's depth [1, 2, 6].

A partial/incisional biopsy is usually not recommended for pigmented lesions, however there is the exception if the lesion is very large in size and an excisional biopsy is not possible [1, 2, 6]. It must be known that with an incisional biopsy, sampling error may occur. The greatest limitation of partial biopsy is the possibility of compromising both diagnostic accuracy and staging. If chosen, the areas with darker pigment or elevated areas are chosen for incisional biopsy [1, 2, 6].

When performing an excisional biopsy, dermatologists should respect lymphatic drainage and perform the biopsy on a longitudinal axis [5, 6]. If a biopsy is performed on the limbs, the cut will go against the skin tension lines to respect lymphatic drainage and not compromise a sentinel lymph node investigation, if necessary [5]. The margin of the biopsy should be 1–3 mm wide and with deep margins [5].

When discussing difficult locations such as lentigo maligna on the face, the large size of the lesion often excludes the possibility of a complete excision. In some cases, a punch biopsy is performed and may provide a false-negative result [6]. Also, in photodamaged areas, there may be collision non-melanocytic pigmented lesions, such as benign lentigines and pigmented actinic keratosis, which can cause a misdiagnosis [6]. A broad thin shave biopsy can provide a broad view of the lesion without creating a large wound. Another possibility is to perform various small shave biopsies that sample the different structures seen clinically and in dermoscopy [6].

Pigmented volar lesions sometimes can be completely removed via saucerization [2].

References

1. Sobanko JF, Leitenberger JJ, Neil AS, Lee KK. Biopsy techniques. In: Rigel DS, editor. Cancer of the skin. Saunders, Elsevier Inc.; 2011. p. 434–42.
2. Elston DM, Stratman EJ, Miller SJ. Skin biopsy: biopsy issues in specific diseases. J Am Acad Dermatol. 2016;74(1):1–18. https://doi.org/10.1016/j.jaad.2015.06.033.
3. Olbricht S. Biopsy techniques and basic excisions. In: Bolognia JL, Schaffer J, Cerroni L, editors. Dermatology. New York: Elsevier Science; 2018. p. 2478–94.
4. Werner B. Biópsia de pele e seu estudo histológico: por quê? para quê? como? parte II. An Bras Dermatol. 2009;84(5):507–13. https://doi.org/10.1590/S0365-05962009000500010.
5. Galdelha AR. Biópsia de Pele. In: Gadelha AR, Costa IMC, editors. Cirurgia Dermatológica em consultório. São Paulo: Ed. Atheneu; 2016. p. 209–16.

6. Swetter SM, Tsao H, Bichakjian CK, Curiel-Lewandrowski C, Elder DE, Gershenwald JE, Guild V, Grant-Kels JM, Halpern AC, Johnson TM, Sober AJ, Thompson JA, Wisco OJ, Wyatt S, Hu S, Lamina T. Guidelines of care for the management of primary cutaneous melanoma. J Am Acad Dermatol. 2019;80(1):208–50. https://doi.org/10.1016/j.jaad.2018.08.055.

Chapter 9
Principles of Surgical Oncology

Fabio de Oliveira Ferreira, Eduardo Hiroshi Akaishi, and Flavio Cavarsan

F. de Oliveira Ferreira (✉)
General Surgery, Faculdade de Medicina da Universidade de São Paulo, São Paulo, SP, Brazil

Sarcoma and Melanoma Group, Instituto do Câncer do Estado de São Paulo—ICESP, São Paulo, SP, Brazil

Cutaneous Oncology and Sarcomas Center, Hospital Sírio-Libanês de São Paulo—HSL/SP, São Paulo, SP, Brazil

High-Risk Clinic of the Oncogenetics Service, Hospital Beneficência Portuguesa de São Paulo, São Paulo, SP, Brazil

E. H. Akaishi
Sarcoma and Melanoma Group, Instituto do Câncer do Estado de São Paulo—ICESP, São Paulo, SP, Brazil

Cutaneous Oncology and Sarcomas Center, Hospital Sírio-Libanês, São Paulo, SP, Brazil

F. Cavarsan
Brazilian Melanoma Group, São Paulo, SP, Brazil

Intensive Training in Mohs Surgery (TIMOS), São Paulo, SP, Brazil

Cutaneous Oncology of Honcord Clinic, Goiânia, GO, Brazil

C. M. Z. Abdalla et al. (eds.), *Oncodermatology*,
https://doi.org/10.1007/978-3-031-29277-4_9

Key Points

- The importance of the multidisciplinary approach is pointed out by the authors, with emphasis on cutaneous oncological surgery.
- Concepts and technical principles about oncological surgery are discussed in the second part of the chapter, considering that is essential to know the disease's natural history.
- The correct and necessary aspects of staging the patients before any kind of treatment are analyzed.
- Different forms of biopsy, surgical margins, and lymphadenectomies are exposed.
- The relationship between minimally invasive surgery and cancer is analyzed, discussing the pros and cons about this procedure.

Principles of Surgical Oncology

Oncology evolves from the interaction of the work of physicians, scientists, and professionals from related fields involved in the care of cancer patients. The principles of current oncological treatment are focused on the concept of a multidisciplinary approach in the different phases of the disease's evolution and in the patient's physical and psychological care. In recent years, translational research has definitively been incorporated into the daily life of oncologists, increasing the interaction between the basic and clinical science, and contributing to an accelerated transformation in the bases of cancer treatment. Thus, the multidisciplinary approach is the result of the application of knowledge that comes from a multi-professional interaction, where cancer surgery has an important contribution.

In the first part of this chapter, we present a brief history about cancer surgery, highlighting in chronological order remarkable facts that contributed to the development of the specialty and cancer treatment, in a few moments with greater emphasis on historical aspects related to cutaneous tumors. In the second part, we will discuss important concepts for the correct exercise of surgical oncology.

Brief History of Surgical Oncology

3000 BC—The first signs of cancer were found in fossilized bones of mummies in ancient Egypt and Peru and date back to 3000 BC. Imhotep, the founder of Egyptian medicine, is credited with recording the earliest accounts of cancer. The document known as the Edwin Smith Papyrus, acquired in 1862 by Edwin Smith in Luxor, Egypt, possibly originally written by Imhotep, has the earliest written description of the existence of cancer. This document reports eight cases of breast tumors ("ulcers") treated with cauterization [1].

400 BC—Egyptian medicine held a dominant position in the ancient world for 2500 years, until Hippocrates, in 400 BC, proposed the Humoral Theory of Medicine, according to which the body would be composed of four humors: phlegm, blood, yellow bile, and black bile, coming, respectively, from the heart, respiratory system, liver, and spleen. Any fluid imbalance could cause illness, with cancer being attributed to an excess of black bile. Hippocrates was the first to use the words *carcinos* and *carcinoma* to describe tumors, explaining the origin of the word "cancer," derived from *karkinos* ("crab" in Greek). He believed that it was better to leave cancer patients untreated, as treated patients did not survive for long. With the teachings of Hippocrates, the art of medicine in the ancient world reached its zenith in Greece [2]. The influence of Asclepius (or Aesculapius), God of medicine in Greek mythology, is still seen today in the symbol represented by the serpent wrapped around the rod of Asclepius. According to legend, Asclepius was ripped from his dead mother's womb and given to a centaur who would teach him the art of healing. During a visit to a patient, a snake climbed, wrapped itself around his rod, and remained there. Aesculapius' staff represents the tree of life and the snake the cycle of death and rebirth, in addition to wisdom and power [3]. The term "surgery" derives from the Greek word *cheiro*, which means hand, and from *ergon*, which means work, so literally surgery was the art of working with the hands.

400 BC—The first evidence of the existence of melanoma in the ancient world was found in skeletons of mummies originating in Chancay and Chongos, Peru, affected by diffuse metastases, dating back 2400 years. Metastatic bone damage was observed especially in the skull and extremities and rounded melanin masses in the skin [4–6].

25 BC—Ancient doctors and surgeons knew that cancer would usually come back after it was surgically removed. Aulus Cornelius Celsus, a Roman physician, wrote in his work "De Medicina": "after the excision, even when a scar formed, the disease nevertheless returned." Celsus uses the word "cancer" in his references to malignant diseases [7].

1 BC—In addition to the development of medicine in Egypt and Greece, there is evidence of surgical practice in other geographic regions before the Christian era. In Peru, contributions to the progress of surgery occurred with the intensive practice of trephination. Plastic surgery was practiced for over 2000 years in ancient India, using surgical instruments, hemostatic powders, and bandages. These records can be found in the ancient Indian text "Sushruta-samhita," written in Sanskrit, and attributed to the great Indian surgeon Sushruta, founder of Ayurvedic Medicine (traditional Indian medicine, which introduced remarkable innovations in the field of surgery) [8].

146 AD—Claudius Galenus (Galen of Pergamon) also believed in the Humoral Theory, however, he considered that cancer could be cured in early stages and that advanced tumors should be operated on by cauterizing or cutting around the affected area. His theories have dominated and influenced Western medical science

for over a millennium. Under the multidisciplinary approach, Galen of Pergamon gave rise to the idea that patients should be treated "as a whole," inspiring the paths of modern medicine, which made him known as "the man who built the foundations of modern medicine in antiquity." Galen strongly advocated surgery for the treatment of breast cancer. He instructed surgeons to "cut out a pathological tumor with a circle where it borders the scar tissue." Galen's teachings were accepted as dogmas and practiced for over 1500 years [2]. He was the first to use the word *oncos* ("swelling" in Greek) to describe tumors, giving rise to the term "oncology."

865 AD—The preservation of ancient Greco-Roman knowledge during the Middle Ages is due to the medieval Arabs. The leaders of Arab medicine were the Persians, Rhazes, and Avicenna (865–925 AD). Their teachings were highly regarded for many centuries. During the golden age of Muslim medicine, Avicenna was known as the "Prince of Physicians." His works were exemplary, including texts about general medicine, medicines, pathology, the science of fever, pharmacology, and surgery. He left many works, the most important of which was the "Canon of Medicine", a 50-volume treatise on medical theory, the most influential of subsequent centuries. In this work, Avicenna addressed cancer surgery and the usefulness of quarantine [9].

1190 AD—Moses Maimonides, a prominent physician, scientist, and philosopher, born in Cordoba, Spain, had to flee to Egypt due to the expulsion of Jews who had not converted to Islam. Maimonides wrote ten medical treatises, including surgical aphorisms on cancer treatment. He described that the treatment of large tumors would involve excising the tumor and its contours to the point of healthy tissue, unless the tumor contained large vessels or was located close to vital organs, when he warned that excision is dangerous [10].

1325 AD—Guy de Chauliac (Montpellier, France) studied the works of Greek and Arab Jewish physicians on anatomy. At that time, the Monastic Medicine was the predominant thought, where diseases were considered sins and the monks were considered healers. The distance between the "brain and the hands" gave reasons to call the surgeons as "barber surgeons." Guy de Chauliac became the most eminent surgeon of the fourteenth century, revolutionizing the medical mind of his time, becoming the "Father of Scholarly Surgery." The work "Chirurgia Magna," made for doctors who practiced surgery, became the base textbook for four centuries for surgeons in Europe, being the first treatise where a complete overview of all medical and surgical knowledge of the fourteenth century is observed, which would serve as a reference until the eighteenth century [11].

1550–1750—Among the theories that would replace the Humoral Theory of Cancer was the origin of cancer by the lymph, another bodily fluid. Stahl and Hoffman theorized that cancer was composed of lymph in fermentation and degeneration, varying in density, acidity, and alkalinity. The "Lymph Theory" gained rapid support [12]. Ambroise Paré, a surgeon in the French army, in 1552 abandoned the cauterizers used to stop bleeding in amputations and reintroduced the technique of ligatures to tie blood vessels. During his life, Paré served as a surgeon to four French kings and won the title of "Father of surgery" [13]. William Harvey, an English physician, used demonstrations to prove his revolutionary theory of blood circulation. His book, *De Motu Cordis*, published in 1628, disturbed Galen's traditional followers and brought up entirely new concepts of circulation and anatomy [14]. In 1731, Jean Louis Petit, Director of the French Academy of Surgery, is considered responsible for developing the first unified concept for the surgical treatment of breast cancer. In his writings, Petit suggests that the roots of the cancer were the enlarged "lymphatic" glands, which should be removed, including the pectoral fascia and muscle fibers itself, rather than leaving any suspicious tissue without removal [15].

Scientific surgery truly begins in 1750 with John Hunter, a supporter of Stahl and Hofman's Lymph Theory of Cancer. John Hunter, a Scottish surgeon, agreed that tumors grew from lymph constantly expelled from the blood. Hunter also believed that cancer could be removed if it hadn't already spread to nearby tissues and suggested that some cancers could be cured through surgery. He even described how the surgeon could decide which types of cancer should be operated on: "if the tumor has not invaded neighboring tissues and is mobile, there is no impediment to removing it." He was responsible for the first detailed description of a progression of malignant disease, identifying a case of osteosarcoma with lung metastases from the study of one of his patients during life and after death [3]. The first published report of a melanoma patient was also made by Hunter in 1787, although he never described the disease as such. It was a metastasis of melanoma in the jaw of a young patient. The lesion was removed, but it recurred locally after 3 years. Hunter reported that the original tumor was white, but contained a dark black part, like what was called a fungal cancerous outgrowth. In 1968, a microscopic study of the piece was made, confirming its melanocytic and secondary character [16].

1771—Giovanni Battista Morgagni, in Padua, Italy, was the first to systematically perform autopsies and correlate the disease with pathological findings after death, which served as the basis for the progress of scientific oncology and the in-depth study of cancer [17].

1775—Percival Pott of St. Bartholomew's Hospital in London described the occupational hazard in chimney sweeps through the correlation between cancer and soot collected in the skin folds of the scrotum. Subsequently, the discovery of several other tumors resulting from occupational exposures led to the institution of public health measures to reduce the risk of cancer [1].

1804—In the history of melanoma, Guillaume Dupuytren, anatomist, and surgeon, is considered by some to be responsible for the term *black cancer*, first used in 1804. However, René Laennec was the first to describe melanoma as a disease in 1806, in a presentation entitled "Sur les mélanôses," the article being published in 1812, in Paris. He individualized the disease as a pathological entity and proposed the name *melánosi*, from the Greek *melas*: black. Laennec observed metastases in the mediastinal and hilar lymph nodes and described melanomas involving other organs in research carried out in conjunction with Gaspard-Laurent Bayle. The controversy between Laennec and his professor Dupuytren over who was the first to describe "melanomatous" metastases to the lungs continued, each describing a similar pathological classification system [18, 19].

1809—Surgical treatment of intracavitary tumors in the preanesthetic era begins in 1809, with Ephraim McDowell, who performed the first successful oophorectomy for an ovarian tumor, performed on Mrs. Jane Todd Crawford in Danville, Kentucky, USA. This feat revolutionized the practice of surgery. Most academic physicians believed that operating on the abdomen would inevitably result in peritonitis and death. McDowell proved them wrong and performed several oophorectomies with an acceptable complication rate for the time [20].

1817—Jean-Louis Alibert illustrated melanoma under two names: anthracene cancer and melanoma cancer. In the description, "it is manifested by a very black and itchy spot; its color, which is the special attribute that distinguishes it, is generally very dark in the center of the tumor and does not have the same intensity at the edges. Another important characteristic is the surface of the skin, which is covered with granulations. When operating with a cutting instrument, the disease reappears sometime after the extirpation and, despite the care to make it disappear to the smallest traces, the patient eventually succumbs" [18].

1820—William Norris described the first case of melanoma recorded in the English literature, a fair-haired, fair-skinned man with a dark brown tumor on the abdominal wall. When the patient died, Dr. Norris himself performed the autopsy. Metastases were found in the sternum and throughout the abdomen, which contained ascitic fluid, with the liver enlarged and "speckled" from great masses. The lungs were involved, as was the dura. Norris was the first to study melanoma in depth. In 1857 he published eight cases of "melanosis" with pathological and therapeutic observations [21].

1826–1938—Thomas Fawdington published a case of melanosis in which he described an ocular melanoma. In 1827, Pierre Rayer included plantar involvement, producing in 1835 the first pathological analyses of melanoma. At the same time, Jean Cruveilhier published in his work *Anatomy Pathologique du Corps Humain* several observations on "melanoma cancer." Among these descriptions are the first cases of melanomas of the hand, sole, vulva and metastatic melanomas to the heart, and small intestine, mentioned by Pemberton in 1858 [18]. In 1828, the Scottish physician and draftsman Robert Carswell began his work *Pathological Anatomy: Illustrations of the Elementary Forms of Disease*, with more than 2000 color drawings, published in 1838, when the name "melanoma" is introduced in place of "melanoma cancer." He classified melanomas into two groups: true melanosis and false melanosis (of the lungs), the four aspects of true melanosis being the punctiform, tuberculous, stratiform, and liquid forms [22].

1829—Joseph-Claude-Anthelme Récamier, a French gynecologist, in his treatise on cancer treatment, created the term *metastasis* as a definition for the spread of cancer—in Greek, "moving from one place to another" [23].

1833—Johannes Müller was appointed professor and chairman of the Department of Anatomy, Physiology, and Pathology at the University of Berlin. Müller and the doctors in his laboratory were familiar with the work of botanists and plant physiologists such as Robert Brown, who in 1831 established the concept of nucleated cells, and Matthias Schleiden, who collaborated with Schwann to establish the cell theory in 1838. Müller demonstrated that cancer is composed of cells and not of lymph, but he believed that cancer cells did not come from normal cells. Müller proposed that cancer cells developed from sprouts (blastema) between normal tissues. Tumors and cancers were described and defined in a medical dictionary. In his monograph on cancer, Müller provided a systematic analysis of the microscopic features of benign and malignant neoplasms in humans [24].

1842—A fundamental new step would forever change the paths of medicine, the discovery of anesthesia. Ether was inhaled at meetings with the purpose of causing relaxation and well-being in the so-called ether parties. In one of these meetings at his home, Crawford Williamson Long realized the sensation of analgesia produced, as he did not feel pain when he was injured. Then, he had the idea of using ether in performing minor surgeries. The first surgical act was the removal of two small tumors from the back of a friend's neck in March 1842. Long worried about the consequences and dangers of prolonged inhalation for longer procedures. He used ether in eight surgeries; however, due to the risk of unconsciousness, he abandoned the technique and did not publish his work [25].

1844—William Thomas Green Morton entered Harvard Medical School, where he was introduced to the anesthetic properties of ether. Morton, a dentist and medical student tackled the subject of analgesia. On September 30, 1846, he performed the painless extraction of a tooth under ether anesthesia. After publicizing this event, the surgeon Henry Jacob Bigelow organized a demonstration of the application of ether on October 16, 1846, in the amphitheater of the Massachusetts General Hospital, when John Collins Warren removed a tumor from the cervical region of a patient anesthetized by Morton [26].

1853—Regarding melanoma, in 1853, Sir James Paget, consultant surgeon at St. Bartholomew's Hospital in London, reported 25 cases of "melanoid cancer" and described the passage from the horizontal growth phase to the vertical phase [18]. In 1857, Sir Jonathan Hutchinson described a melanoma on the hallux, discovered together with an inflammation of the nail. In 1858, Oliver Pemberton described the first case of melanoma on the side of the foot of a black man, originally from Madagascar. Later, in 1886, Hutchinson described the subungual melanoma. At this time, he warned of a diagnostic sign: the presence of "a small charcoal-black border" on top of the inflamed nail, the "Hutchinson's sign." In 1894, Hutchinson described "lentigo melanosis"in a 56-year-old man with a large black spot on his left cheek, which had been present for several years [27].

1858—Müller's student, Rudolph Virchow determined that all cells, including cancer cells, were derived from other cells. Creating the scientific basis for the modern study of cancer pathology by correlating microscopic findings with disease, Virchow became the founder of cell pathology, ensuring a better understanding of cancer biology and contributing to the development of cancer surgery [28].

1860—The German surgeon Karl Thiersch demonstrated that cancers metastasize through the spread of malignant cells rather than through some unidentified fluid [29].

1872—Christian Albert Theodor Billroth, one of the greatest German surgeons in the history of medicine, performed the first esophagectomy for cancer (1872) and the first gastrectomy for cancer (1878). He was also responsible for performing total laryngectomy, salivary glands surgeries, and developing the thyroid surgery. Billroth introduced the concept of palliative surgery based on the premises of prolonging life, considering as essential the need to maintain the quality of life [2].

1875—The German pathologist Friedrich Sigmund Merkel demonstrated on the snout skin of pigs and moles that some cells were sensitive to touch and that they functioned as receptors for mechanical stimuli in all animals, including man. The "Merkel cells" acted as receptors and were stimulated by touch, associated with sensory nerves [30]. In 1972, Cyril Toker described Merkel cell carcinoma, initially under the name "trabecular skin carcinoma" [31].

1881—The experiments on the "microbial theory of disease" carried out by Louis Pasteur [32], associated with the antisepsis principles advocated by Joseph Lister, including the use of carbolic acid to wash hands, and the use of proper clothing would transform surgical practice for the next 100 years [33].

1889—Over the years, the reasoning focused on the biological behavior of the disease gained strength with the theory of "seed and soil," proposed by the English surgeon Stephen Paget. Paget analyzed more than 1000 autopsy records from women with breast cancer and found that the patterns of metastasis were not random. Thus, he proposed that tumor cells (the seeds) would have specific affinity for specific organs (the soil), and metastases would only occur if the seed and soil were compatible, a highly sophisticated hypothesis, confirmed almost a hundred years later by modern techniques of cell and molecular biology [35, 36].

1890—Once the techniques of anesthesia, antisepsis, and new discoveries in the field of physiology have been mastered, surgery has made great progress in general, including cancer surgery. An important new concept would appear in the coming years. The general concept of radical mastectomy was established by the German surgeon Lorenz Heisen in 1819, but its technical standardization is attributed to William Stewart Halsted, whose work was based in part on the studies of Willian Sampson Handley. Handley discovered that the extent of breast cancer occurred through dissemination by lymphatic vessels. Based on these premises, Halsted believed that proper local removal would provide healing and that, in cases of metastases, they would be the consequence of a new process. This belief led to the development of the radical mastectomy technique for breast cancer in 1890 and became the basis for cancer surgery for nearly a century, establishing the concept of resection *en bloc*. Halsted was responsible for numerous achievements, including the creation of residency programs in surgery, which greatly contributed to the structuring of educational centers around the world [34].

1892—Following Halsted concepts, in London 1892, the surgeon Herbert Snow recommended the treatment of melanoma by excision of the primary lesion and preventive lymph node excision. He believed that the removal of primary melanoma alone would not be effective, recommending, whenever possible, the excision of the "lymph glands" that first received the "infectious protoplasm" [37].

1894—William Dubreuilh, in Bordeaux, described the "lentigo maligna in elderly people," referring to the article by Hutchinson, reporting some aspects: beginning with a black macula variable in shape and extension, in the vicinity of which a tumor may appear, malignant; the color may vary from "sepia to black" and there is a risk of reappearing after excision. Later, the term "lentigo maligna melanoma" was coined [38].

1895—A new discovery would forever change the paths of medicine and oncology. On November 8, 1895, in the laboratory of the University of Wurzburg, Germany, Wilhelm Conrad Röntgen discovered the X-ray. At his first public performance, on the evening of January 23, 1896, Röentgen completed his demonstration by X-raying the hand of Albert von Kölliker, professor of anatomy. This act quickly led to an understanding of the discovery's possible medical applications. Before long, the X-ray equipment would be used worldwide as a diagnostic tool [39].

1896—After noticing the peeling of his hands exposed to X-rays, Emil Grubbe, a medical student in Chicago, convinced one of his professors to allow irradiation of a patient with locally advanced breast cancer. Historically, in doing so, Grubbe became the first "radio-oncologist." He subsequently assembled the first X-ray machine in Chicago in 1896. By 1960, Grubbe had instructed more than 7000 physicians in the medical use of X-rays [40].

1896—Parallel discoveries contributed to drive the development of cancer treatment. Thomas Beatson found that castration of the ovaries stopped milk production in rabbits. The results were published in 1896, demonstrating the "control" of an organ over the secretion of another organ at a distance. Beatson pioneered the use of hormonal therapies to treat breast cancer. Oophorectomy would become the standard treatment for advanced breast cancer over the next few years. He discovered estrogen's stimulating effect on breast cancer even before the hormone itself was discovered. His work has provided the foundation for the modern use of hormone therapy for breast cancer [41].

1897—Two years after the discovery of X-rays, Henri Becquerel, a professor at the Polytechnic School of Paris, discovered natural radioactivity in his studies with uranium salts. At the end of 1897, Maria Skolodowska and her husband Pierre Curie verified that the uranium mineral had a very high radioactivity, not explained by its uranium content. In 1898, undergoing a series of chemical separations, they proposed the name "polonium," in honor of Maria Skolodowska's Polish origins, to designate the isolated element, about 400 times more radioactive than uranium. Later that year, they announced the existence of another radioactive chemical element, which they named "radio." She herself was one of the promoters of the use of radium in the treatment of cancer. It was the beginning of radiotherapy as a modality of cancer treatment. Later, the couple's daughter, Irene Curie, discovered the production of a radioactive element in the laboratory and called it radio-phosphorus. These three fabulous achievements of science—the discovery of X-rays, the discovery of natural radioactivity, and the production of artificial radioactive elements—together with the in-depth knowledge of atomic and nuclear structures—determined the evolution of radiotherapy throughout the century. It was the beginning of cancer radiotherapy [42].

1899—With the availability of radiation as a therapeutic weapon against cancer, Tage Anton Ultimus Sjogren, in 1899 in Stockholm, Sweden, successfully demonstrated the treatment of skin cancer of the eyelid in a patient treated with X-rays. At the same time, Thor Stenbeck treated a case of skin cancer of the nose, also successfully cured. In the international literature, both are among the first to successfully treat skin cancer patients using X-rays [43]. In 1900, Sjogren created the X-ray laboratory at Sabbatsberg Hospital. The first signs of cancer as a secondary effect of the use of radiation appeared in Sjogren himself in 1905, who later underwent amputation of his fingers [44].

1900—Halstedian thinking prevailed and led to the performance of radical resections for tumors of other organs, including radical prostatectomy (Hugh, 1904), radical hysterectomy (Ernest Wertheim, 1906), and abdominoperineal resection of the rectum (Ernest W. Miles, 1908). A historical milestone in Brazilian surgery was the publication by Prof. Arnaldo Vieira de Carvalho on the report of the fourth total gastrectomy performed in the world, in 1900 [45]. Until 1900, brain surgery was rarely performed, when surgical techniques were developed by Harvey W. Cushing at Johns Hopkins. Dr. Cushing removed nearly 2000 brain tumors and spread the knowledge to students in many countries.

1907—Scotsman William Sampson Handley, during the autopsy of a patient with melanoma, established what he called anatomical dissemination via the "centrifugal lymphatic route." He also established surgical rules, recommending a circular incision around the tumor at a safe and practicable distance (one inch), deep enough to expose subcutaneous fat, amputation for fingers' melanoma, initial systematic removal of lymph nodes, and described that regression episodes could happen [46].

1910—Studies aimed at understanding tumorigenesis have led to a better understanding of the biology of cancer. Francis Peyton Rous was able to prove that some chicken tumors were caused by viruses. In 1910, Rous scientifically demonstrated the formation of sarcomas in chickens injected with cell fluids from other chickens with sarcomas, giving rise to the idea that viruses could cause cancer [47].

1910—Parallel to the development of cancer surgery and radiotherapy, the systemic treatment of cancer has its roots in the work of the German researcher Paul Ehrlich. For many years he searched for substances that would bind to "specific receptors" that would act as "magic bullets"that would kill only the germs they bind to, leaving the body's host cells intact. In his laboratory at the Frankfurt Institute for Experimental Therapy, Ehrlich and his assistant Sahachiro Hata, announced in 1910 the "chemical bullet" for the treatment of syphilis. The success with the chemical synthesis of the drug gave impetus to a new medical science, "chemotherapy," originating the term used today as a modality of cancer treatment [48].

1912—A new way of looking at cancer patients would emerge to forever influence the pathways of modern oncology. In 1912, Dr. James Stephen Ewing was named a pathologist at Memorial Hospital, created in 1884 as a refuge for patients with advanced cancer. For 10 years, he focused his time and efforts on preparing a treatise called "Neoplastic Diseases," published in 1919, the book that became a reference in cancer pathology around the world. James Ewing was a supporter of cancer treatment alternatives beyond surgery, valuing the use of radiotherapy and the use of medication. The training imposed by Ewing laid the foundations for the modern concept of a multidisciplinary approach to cancer patients [49].

1913—The surgery was progressing. On March 14, 1913, German Franz Torek performed the first successful resection of a carcinoma of the thoracic esophagus. There was no other successful resection until 1921, when extrapleural esophagectomy was reported by Howard Lilienthal in New York. In addition to transthoracic esophagectomy, other feats contributed to Torek's prestige, such as the surgery to correct cryptorchidism and the first resection of intrathoracic metastasis, in 1930 [50].

1925—In the history of melanoma, Jean Darier was the first to make the correlation between equine melanocytic disease and certain tumors in humans. He called it "malignant mesenchymal melanoma" or "melanosarcoma,"what Wallace Clark later called "animal-type melanoma"(1990), Carney "epithelial blue nevus" (1996), and Zembowsky "epithelial melanocytoma pigmented" (2004) [51].

1928—The discovery of penicillin happened accidentally. The Scottish physician and bacteriologist Alexander Fleming, in 1928, forgot his study material on the table while on vacation. Upon returning, he noted that his Staphylococcus aureus cultures were contaminated with mold and that, where the fungus was, there were clear halos around them, indicating that it might contain some bactericidal substance. When studying the properties of this fungus identified as belonging to the *Penicillium genus*, Fleming realized that it provided a substance capable of eliminating several bacteria. The substance was called "penicillin" [52].

1933—With the advancement of anesthesiology techniques, the first successful pneumonectomy performed for the treatment of lung cancer was done by Evarts Ambrose Graham and Jacob Jesse Singer, in 1933, in the United States [53]. In the same year, Edward Archibald, at the Royal Victoria Hospital in Montreal, Canada, successfully performed the first pneumonectomy with hilar lymph node dissection [54].

1935—Allen Oldfather Whipple was an American surgeon who became known, among other accomplishments, for the pancreatic cancer operation that bears his name, as well as the triad for diagnosing insulinoma. Whipple began working on the procedure for resection of pancreatic tumors in 1935. In 1940, he performed the pancreatoduodenectomy procedure in one step. Among the great contributions, perhaps the most relevant is the concern with the clinical preparation of the surgical patient. During his lifetime, Whipple performed 37 pancreatoduodenectomies [55, 56].

1939—Charles Brendon Huggins, a Canadian physiologist working in the United States, postulated that prostate cancer was influenced by androgenic activity; therefore, disseminated prostate carcinoma would be inhibited by eliminating androgens through castration or neutralization using estrogens. The knowledge of hormonal dependence of some types of cancer and the possibility of using systemic therapy and surgical therapy through orchiectomy for the systemic control of prostate cancer were strengthened [57].

1942—During World War II, pharmacologists Louis Goodman and Alfred Gilman were searching for chemical agents under US government protection with the goal of discovering an antidote to the mustard agent. They found that when injected into rats and rabbits, the nitrogen mustard, a chemical derivative of the mustard gas, was capable to slow tumor's growth. In 1942, a patient with lymphoma, relapsed after surgical procedures and radiotherapy sessions, seems to have been the first patient treated with daily injections of nitrogen mustard. A month later, the lymph nodes shrunk. For some, this narrative represents the embryo of the development of clinical oncology. That's why it is said that the chemical warfare gave rise to modern chemotherapy. This experience led to the clinical use of nitrogen mustard in patients with hematologic malignancies, including Hodgkin's disease and lymphocytic lymphomas [58].

1947—Leukemia was a symbol of the impotence of medicine. For the American pathologist Sidney Farber, leukemia was a disease of the leukocyte cell tissue that involved the bone marrow. At that time, the folic acid was already known to stimulate bone marrow growth and maturation. Farber believed that if a drug chemically blocked folic acid, it might be possible to stop the abnormal bone marrow production associated with leukemia. In November 1947, he experienced a drug on a group of 16 seriously ill children with leukemia and temporary remissions were achieved in 10 of them [59]. In 1952, Dr. Farber described the complete remission of leukemia in 50 treated children (1% of treated children). Throughout the 1950s and 1960s, he continued to make advances in cancer research, with the discovery that the antibiotic actinomycin D and radiotherapy could lead to Wilms' tumor remission [60]. He was also responsible for introducing the concept of "total care" and was of great importance in raising funds for cancer research [61].

1948—Sophie Spitz and Arthur Allen, staff pathologists at Memorial Hospital in New York, described a form of nevus in children that could be confused with melanoma, a fusiform epithelioid cell nevus, initially called "benign juvenile melanoma" [62]. Benign melanocytic proliferation was later called Spitz's Nevus, a designation first used by McGovern in 1967. Allen and Spitz were also the first to recognize the importance of ulceration as an important adverse prognostic factor in melanoma [63].

1950—In the radiotherapy, the invention of the cobalt-60 teletherapy unit by H.E. Johns took place in Canada in the early 1950s, placing the cobalt unit at the forefront of radiotherapy for several years [64]. With technological development, linear accelerators would soon replace the cobalt unit and have become the most used radiation source in modern radiotherapy.

1953—James Dewey Watson, American molecular biologist, geneticist, and zoologist, and Francis Harry Compton Crick, British molecular biologist, biophysicist, and neuroscientist proposed the "double helix model" for the structure of the DNA molecule [65]. With the knowledge of the structure of DNA, the understanding of the mechanisms of tumor dissemination and the development of drugs with specific antineoplastic purposes, the fight against cancer would proceed in a different way [66].

1956—Metastatic cancer was first cured in 1956, when Methotrexate was used to treat a patient with choriocarcinoma. Long-term remissions and even cures of many patients with Hodgkin's disease and acute lymphoblastic leukemia treated with chemotherapy were first reported in the 1960s. Cures for testicular cancer were seen over the next decade [67].

1963—In surgery, Francis Daniels Moore was responsible for the in-depth study of the surgical patient's metabolism, body composition, and pre- and postoperative care, which contributed definitively to the reduction of operative mortality rates, which provided to Moore the recognition as the surgeon of the twentieth century [68].

1960—On the story of melanoma, in the early 1960s, Gerald W. Milton founded the Sydney Melanoma Unit (SMU). Recognizing the importance of data collection, he established a prospective database under the direction of Dr. Helen M. Shaw, which became the largest single-center melanoma database in the world. Milton pioneered the involvement of clinical oncologists, radio-oncologists, pathologists, and cancer surgeons in the care of patients with advanced melanoma [69]. In 1966, the American Wallace Clark proposed a classification scale based on the extent of invasion at five levels in the skin and subcutaneous tissue. In 1969, together with Martin C. Mihm, Jr. and colleagues, the "Clark invasion levels" were defined, as well as a description of a form of superficial spread of melanoma and in 1978, Clark et al. described the B-K mole syndrome (named after the initials of the first two families described) as a precursor and marker of increased risk in the context of familial melanoma [70], described simultaneously by Henry Lynch et al. such as familial atypical soft melanoma syndrome [71]. Thomas B. Fitzpatrick was a pioneer in early diagnosis and in establishing the natural history and risk factors for melanoma. In 1966, along with Wallace H. Clark, Jr. (pathologist), Martin C. Mihm, Jr. (dermatologist and pathologist), and John S. Raker (surgical oncologist), Fitzpatrick established the first multidisciplinary pigmented lesion clinic at Massachusetts General Hospital to study and treat patients with cutaneous melanoma. This unit has become the model for similar centers around the world [72].

1970—The American Alexander Breslow, professor of pathology at the George Washington University, observed that the prognosis of cutaneous melanoma was correlated with the size of the tumor and the level of invasion, with the thickness of invasion being the most significant parameter [73, 74]. Vincent McGovern, a pathologist in Sydney, in addition to numerous publications on cutaneous melanoma, had a large participation in organizing international consensus meetings and in attempting to delineate the histopathological features that were directly related to the prognosis in melanoma, including the prognostic significance of ulceration of lesions primary to the staging system, in addition to other histopathological features such as thickness, ulceration, mitotic rate, and regression [75]. McGovern and Lane Brown were also among the first to draw attention to the epidemiological and genetic characteristics of melanoma. The pioneering studies of immunotherapy to combat melanoma, in particular BCG therapy, are attributed to the American Donald L. Morton, in the early 1970s [76].

1977—The American surgeon Bernard Fisher expressed his thoughts by saying that "surgery has its contribution to cancer treatment in conjunction with other modalities and that advances in treatment will derive from better orchestration with other treatment modalities, and not from best isolated operative technique" [77].

1990—A new technical procedure with a biological rationale would make a great contribution to cancer surgery. Donald L. Morton and colleagues introduced intraoperative lymphatic mapping and sentinel lymph node biopsy to be used in patients with melanoma. A feline model was used by Morton's group to investigate the use of vital dyes for intraoperative lymphatic mapping. Patent blue V and isosulfan blue were considered the best agents, allowing easy identification of each lymphatic channel and its path to the sentinel lymph node [78, 79].

1990–2021—Modern technical and technological innovations have continued to expand the resources of the oncology surgeon. Recent examples include the development of microsurgical techniques, the evolution of automatic staplers and sophisticated endoscopic equipment, and the emergence of video laparoscopy and robotic surgery. The last 20 years of the surgical oncology practice were marked by the idea that oncologist surgeons should have skills in different fields of oncology. They should (1) be able to perform different operations, especially in special and unusual situations of patients with complex or recurrent neoplasms; (2) have expertise in diagnosing and treating rare or uncommon tumors; (3) have knowledge and experience to choose treatment options, in addition to having extensive knowledge of the modalities (radiotherapy, chemotherapy, immunotherapy, and hormone therapy); (4) understand the potential complications of multimodal therapy, surgical and non-surgical palliation techniques, in-depth knowledge of epidemiology, carcinogenesis, pathology, and tumor biology. As stated in the surgical training program guidelines of the Society of Surgical Oncology (SSO), "the oncologist surgeon is understood to be a well-qualified surgeon who has obtained additional training and experience in the multidisciplinary approach for the prevention, diagnosis, treatment and rehabilitation of cancer patients, and dedicates most of his professional practice to these activities and to research."

General Concepts

General Considerations

About 90% of patients with solid tumors will need the surgeon's participation at some point in the course of the disease, whether in guiding therapeutic planning, effectively through surgical interventions (diagnostics, treatment, acquisition of vascular access, or pain control), or through psychological support to the patient and their families [80]. Surgery represents the treatment of choice for 90–95% of the cases in the stage of localized disease. In cases with advanced disease, it can contribute to improving survival, relief of symptoms, and improvement of quality of life.

To idealize a therapeutic proposal, it is essential to know the disease's natural history. Cancer can progress from different ways: continuity, contiguity, limph vessels, hematogenously, and by implants. In the form of continuity progression, the invasion of organs or structures adjacent to the tumor occurs. In contiguity form, progression occurs by invasion of organs and/or structures adjacent to the host organ of the primary tumor. In lymphatic dissemination, tumor cells reach the intratumoral lymphatic capillaries and migrate through the lymphatic stream reaching the regional lymph nodes. Later, they can progress and compromise distant-chains lymph nodes. In hematogenous dissemination, tumor cells reach the intratumoral venous capillaries, enter the bloodstream, reach the systemic circulation, and can give rise to metastases. Dissemination by implants occurs from the detachment of neoplastic cells from the surface of the tumor in an "environment" conducive to cell proliferation and growth, such as in the peritoneal and pleural cavities.

Another concern of the surgeon should be focused on investigating the family history, with the aim of classifying the patient as having sporadic cancer or suspected of having a hereditary predisposition. This aspect has assumed growing importance and should be part of the investigation routine, as the therapeutic approach can be modified depending on the existence of an inherited genetic predisposition.

Based on the clinical suspicion of cancer, it is imperative to establish an investigation sequence. Thus, the choice of the type of biopsy and types of complementary exams must respect a logic based on the expected progression according to the primary tumor. Correct diagnosis and proper staging are fundamental steps to establish therapeutic planning, without wasting resources and without submitting the patient to unnecessary procedures.

Biopsies

Biopsies are procedures intended to obtain material for histological or cytological study to allow an accurate and definitive diagnosis; therefore, the quantity and quality of material must be adequate. In excisional biopsies, the complete removal of the lesion is performed. In general, excisional biopsies are reserved for skin lesions and small, superficial soft tissue tumors. In cutaneous lesions, excisional biopsies must be performed without definitive margins (1–2 mm), promoting complete resection of the lesion, and covering the entire depth of the skin. Incisional or punch biopsies are reserved for specific skin areas and/or extensive lesions, whose complete removal would imply the need for flap detachment and/or more elaborate reconstructions to close the resection area, which should be avoided. Thus, incisional biopsies are used for larger tumors (superficial or deep). In this case, a representative fragment of the lesion is removed. Needle biopsies are divided into fine-needle aspiration (FNAB—obtaining an aspirate of cells for cytological examination) or thick needle biopsy ("Trucut"; "Core biopsy"—obtaining tissue fragments for histological examination).

The choice of the type of biopsy and the technical precautions for its performance must be respected to avoid damage to the definitive approach. If surgical biopsies are performed, they must be done along the axis of future resection (longitudinal in limbs), avoiding the central portion of the tumor due to the chance of necrosis and hemorrhage. Dissection should be minimal, with careful hemostasis. The choice of the type of biopsy depends on the clinical rationale and considerations about the advantages and disadvantages of each method. For the diagnosis of intraluminal lesions, fragment biopsies can be performed using endoscopic procedures (upper digestive endoscopy, colonoscopy, bronchoscopy, cystoscopy). In soft tissue tumors, after adequate imaging, the preference is for an image-guided thick needle, which offers the following advantages: it can be performed under local anesthesia, does not require hospitalization, allows choosing the intralesional area to be biopsied, and minimizes the errors of improper incisions.

In some situations, the biopsy should ideally be performed with the presence of the pathologist for immediate assessment of the quality of the material, avoiding the need to repeat the procedure. In the definitive evaluation, the material should be directed to a specialized pathologist who has access to auxiliary diagnostic techniques (immunohistochemistry, in situ hybridization, molecular studies, etc.).

Staging

Another key step is staging. "Staging" consists of evaluating the extent of the disease in relation to the primary site of injury, locally and at a distance. In all patients, it is essential to consider the clinical history, physical examination, and natural history of the disease according to the suspected primary tumor. Complementary tests are important to assess the extent of the primary tumor, as well as the involvement of lymph node chains and possible metastases. Due to technological evolution, it is difficult to establish a tight suggestion regarding the tests to be performed, and the choice depends on the host organ of the primary lesion, the target organs to be studied, the correlation with clinical and laboratory data, and the biological behavior of the primary tumor. There are different proposals for standardization of staging, each one with its own particularities. The TNM system, adopted by the International Union Against Cancer (UICC), is the most used. This system is based on the determination of three components to describe the anatomical extent of the disease: T—size of the primary tumor or depth of invasion, N—presence or absence of regional lymph nodes, and M—presence or absence of distant metastases. Some entities provide for the determination of the degree of malignancy and add one more component to the classification (G—degree of histological malignancy), as in the staging of soft tissue sarcomas. In the case of non-seminomatous testicular tumors, the value of serum markers was incorporated into the staging. In other situations, specific classifications established by daily practice and effectiveness in distinguishing different risk groups continue to be used. This is the case of the Breslow and Clark classifications for the staging of cutaneous melanoma and the International Federation of Gynaecology and Obstetrics (FIGO) for the staging of gynecological tumors, among others. Combinations of TNM components allow the grouping of patients into categories that are related to the prognosis. For this reason, using the TNM classification becomes important for standardizing conduct and analyzing results, so that information can be universally compared [81].

Fundamental Concepts

With the anatomopathological diagnosis and the staging in hand, the surgeon can establish the therapeutic sequence to be proposed, including the possibility of neoadjuvant treatment and the prediction of adjuvant treatment. For patients diagnosed with advanced disease, it is sought to determine whether the treatment has curative or palliative intent, and then the treatment strategy can be delineated and may involve the use of non-surgical therapeutic resources in the phases that precede and/or succeed the operation.

The concepts of curative and palliative surgery must be separated as to the intention of the operative act and its definitive character. Curative intent portrays the surgeon's opinion regarding the absence of disease at the end of the operation. If the pathology reveals that the resection margins are compromised, the designation of curative intent surgery is maintained (surgeon's opinion based on the macroscopic findings and procedures performed); however, it is understood that the character was palliative, as the diagnosis of compromised microscopic margin is considered to imply the presence of residual disease. In general, when a palliative operation is indicated, surgical solutions with low morbidity should be sought, since the purpose of the surgical procedure is to create conditions to continue the treatment, resolve acute conditions, and improve quality of life. Sometimes, however, more complex operations can be indicated in patients with a favorable clinical condition.

Radical surgery is the procedure of complete removal of the tumor, with an adequate margin, associated with the removal of the area of locoregional lymphatic drainage, when indicated. Surgery is defined as radical-extended when, in addition to classic surgery, part or totality of one or more organs and/or structures which are assumed to be macroscopically compromised by the tumor are removed in one piece. Another concept that should be mentioned is cytoreductive surgery, which is more often performed to treat the peritoneal dissemination of neoplasms and implies the removal of disseminated macroscopic implants and is sometimes associated with hyperthermic intraperitoneal chemotherapy (HIPEC).

Prophylactic surgeries and risk-reducing surgeries are also part of the oncologic surgeon's range of work, with indications generally related to genetic predisposition syndromes. This is the case of total proctocolectomy for patients with polypoid syndromes to prevent colon carcinoma and mastectomy, and bilateral oophorectomy in the context of *BRCA1* and *BRCA2* pathogenic mutations, among others.

Regarding skin tumors, some specific techniques have individual concepts. Micrographically controlled surgery (Mohs surgery) requires well-defined steps: (1) initial excision of the visible part of the tumor; (2) systematic marking of the surgical specimen regarding the topographical situation of the affected site in the patient; (3) we await the result of the micrographic analysis of the surgical specimen; (4) in pathology, the part is systematically marked with special inks, maintaining the original topographical orientation and transformed into histological sections; exam of all surgical edges and evaluation whether there is involvement by the tumor; (5) if the edges are free, surgery moves to the reconstruction phase. If there is involvement of the surgical edge, the micrographic examination points exactly to the location. As the topographic orientation is maintained in both macro- and microscopy, it is possible to locate, in the patient, exactly where the residual tumor is; (6) return to the operating room and a new cycle is repeated. In the affected site indicated by the micrographic examination, a new ampliatio is performed. The part goes through the same process described above; (7) the excision proceeds in this way (by cycles or stages), successively, ending only after the micrographic examination proves that the entire surgical margin is free from tumor involvement. In micrographically controlled surgery known as "slow Mohs," a modified variant of Mohs, the knowledge of a dermatopathologist rather than the surgeon is incorporated to assess the status of the margin, which is assessed on formalin-fixed, paraffin-embedded tissue. The piece must be identified for circumferential evaluation, like a "watch." The surgical wound is maintained with a dressing and definitive closure is performed in the second surgical stage if all the margins are free or after ampliatio of the compromised margin properly identified in the piece. Another modality has been referred to as "Complete circumferential peripheral and deep margin assessment" (CCPDMA). This technique follows these steps: (1) The entire marginal surface of the surgical specimen is viewed microscopically and histopathologically analyzed for the presence of cancer. The marginal surface includes the deep and complete peripheral margins. (2) The surgical piece is oriented relative to the surgical site and marked so that any positive margin identified on histopathological analysis can be accurately located and re-excised. (3) The surgical margin of any re-excised tissue is again fully visualized and oriented as above. This process is repeated until cancer is no longer identified at the surgical margin or until a new excision is not anatomically possible or is not in the patient's best interest. (4) The time interval between steps in this process is fast enough to avoid significant changes in size or shape in the wound bed (i.e., granulation, contraction) that would decrease the accuracy of orientation. CCPDMA can be obtained with freezing cuts or fixation with formalin and embedding in paraffin. Although it is often helpful for the surgeon to examine the specimen histologically, he is not required to examine the specimen histopathologically to obtain CCPDMA; a trained pathologist or dermatopathologist can communicate the results to the surgeon. If a pathologist or dermatopathologist analyzes the specimen, a consistent communication system must be in place to designate the marginal surfaces for examination and to ensure that the three-dimensional orientation of the marginal surfaces and tissue blocks relative to the wound bed is maintained and communicated to the surgeon to allow accurate localization of the residual tumor within the wound bed.

In every oncologic operation, technical approach is important to minimize the risk of dissemination during the surgical act: surgical wound protection, minimum necessary manipulation (avoid fragmentation), "en bloc" resection if there are signs of invasion of adjacent organs and/or structures.

Surgical Margins

The ideal margin of resection depends on the primary tumor site, the histological type, and TNM staging. For this reason, it is impossible to establish a single rule with precise measures for establishing the ideal margin. For each specific neoplasm, safety margins have been established from studies over the years and must be respected to maintain the oncological safety, minimizing the risk of increasing in locoregional recurrence rates. The first intervention is the one that offers the best opportunity for curative treatment. Therefore, performing a marginal resection to preserve function can be disastrous. It is worth remembering that the multidisciplinary approach can allow to avoid some mutilating operations without violating oncological principles, with function preservation.

Thus, the definition of adequate margin varies and must be respected as defined by clinical trials. R0 resection indicates complete removal, with clear margins in pathology analysis. R1 resection indicates the presence of tumor cells in the margins and therefore a chance of residual microscopic disease. R2 resection indicates macroscopic compromised margins and, therefore, a residual macroscopic tumor after surgical resection.

Lymphadenectomies

The indication of lymphadenectomy as part of cancer surgical treatment depends on four fundamental aspects: biological behavior, histological type, staging, and location of the primary tumor. If the procedure is indicated to treat clinically detected lymph node disease or confirmed by anatomopathological examination, it is called "necessity lymphadenectomy." A "primary lymphadenectomy" is defined as the condition in which there is a presumptive risk of involvement of the lymph node chains, which must be included in the extension of the surgical procedure. In situations where the primary tumor is on a lymphatic drainage station, without evidence of lymph node involvement, an "opportunity lymphadenectomy" is considered.

In general, a lymphadenectomy of necessity has a therapeutic role, in addition to determining the pathological staging regarding the lymph node status. Primary and opportunity lymphadenectomies are intended to define the pathological staging;

however, when the examination reveals lymph nodes involvement, they may also have a therapeutic role. These statements must be interpreted according to the primary tumor in question.

To reduce the indication of unnecessary lymphadenectomies, different techniques were tested to study the condition of higher-risk lymph node that could predict the status of the lymphatic basis, giving rise to a procedure known as "sentinel lymph node biopsy," already incorporated into guidelines of patients with cutaneous melanoma, breast cancer, and Merkel cell carcinoma among others.

Sentinel node biopsy, established from studies on melanoma carried out by Donald L. Morton and published in 1992, is a dynamic methodology performed through the injection of radiotracer and dye (patent blue) in sites related to the primary tumor, with high staging accuracy of lymph node disease [78]. The sentinel node represents the first lymphatic drainage station from a particular primary tumor site. Once identified, the lymph node must be removed and carefully analyzed under specific recommendations for each type of tumor. Its involvement by neoplastic cells defines the risk condition of the lymph node chain, allowing the selection of patients who are candidates for more extensive lymphadenectomies and avoiding unnecessary ones.

Minimally Invasive Surgery and Cancer

The inclusion of laparoscopic surgery in the arsenal of surgical techniques used in cancer surgery deserves some considerations. The three main concerns are: (1) maintenance of the integrity of oncologic resection principles (resection margins, lymphadenectomy pattern, cavity inventory); (2) real demonstration of the advantages without putting the patient at risk (decreased hospital stay, less pain, faster return to work), and (3) no negative impact on survival. At the present time, randomized studies that have already been completed have shown the effectiveness of the method on the aforementioned questions, but in other areas they are still under evaluation.

Final Considerations

It is interesting to analyze the principles of cancer treatment from the perspective of skills that the oncologic surgeon must domain, inserted in the context of oncology in the broadest sense. It is expected from the training of surgical oncology specialists the acquisition of experience, knowledge, and development of clinical and surgical skills to provide comprehensive care to cancer patients.

The greatest evidence that the principles of oncologic treatment should be focused on the concept of a multidisciplinary approach is expressed in the results of randomized clinical trials of phase III, in which, in most cases, the combined treatment modalities offer higher rates of survival when compared to results obtained in the exclusive surgical treatment groups.

The current moment is clear in the sense that the oncologic surgeon must worry about refined staging and with the possibilities of multimodal treatment, whose sequence and therapeutic planning deserve priority. This statement is of the utmost importance, since outside specialized cancer treatment centers, the idea of surgery in the first instance still prevails. Decisions motivated by the lack of structure and multidisciplinary integration can lead the surgeon to deviate from scientific evidence with the aim of help; however, the deviation often leads to irreparable damage. How to solve the problem is not an easy task. In our opinion, the initial step depends on the joint effort of professionals working in oncology with the objective of spreading the idea that the treatment of cancer patients has as a cornerstone the multidisciplinary approach, where the cancer surgeon should be inserted.

References

1. Morton L, Moore RJ. A chronology of medicine and related sciences. Aldershot: Scolar Press; 1997. https://doi.org/10.1017/S0025727300064590.
2. https://www.cancer.org/content/dam/CRC/PDF/Public/6055.00.pdf.
3. Rezende JM. À sombra do plátano: crônicas de história da medicina. São Paulo: Editora Fap-Unifesp; 2009. https://doi.org/10.7476/9788561673635. Available from: http://books.scielo.org.
4. Urteaga O, Pack GT. On the antiquity of melanoma. Cancer. 1966;19(5):607–10. https://doi.org/10.1002/1097-0142(196605)19:5<607::aid-cncr2820190502>3.0.co;2-8.
5. Davis NC, McLeod GR. The history of melanomas from Hunter to Handley. In: Balch CM, Milton GW, editors. Cutaneous melanoma. Philadelphia: Lippincott; 1985. p. 1–19. https://doi.org/10.1007/978-3-319-46029-1_69-1.
6. Rebecca VW, Sondak VK, Smalley KS. A brief history of melanoma: from mummies to mutations. Melanoma Res. 2012;22(2):114–22. https://doi.org/10.1097/CMR.0b013e328351fa4d.
7. Puigbó JJ. Aulus Cornelius Celsus (25 a.C.–50 d.C.) "De Medicina". Gac Méd Caracas. 2002;110(4):517–39.
8. Loukas M, Lanteri A, Ferrauiola J, Tubbs RS, Maharaja G, Shoja MM, et al. Anatomy in ancient India: a focus on the Susruta Samhita. J Anat. 2010;217(6):646–50. https://doi.org/10.1111/j.1469-7580.2010.01294.x.
9. Shoja MM, Tubbs RS. The history of anatomy in Persia. J Anat. 2007;210(4):359–78. https://doi.org/10.1111/j.1469-7580.2007.00711.x.
10. Rosner F. Moses maimonides: biographic outlines. Rambam Maimonides Med J. 2010;1(1):e0002. https://doi.org/10.5041/RMMJ.10002.
11. Tsoucalas G, Karamanou M, Laios K, Markatos K, Androutsos G. Oncologic conceptions in the work of the surgeon Guy de Chauliac (c. 1300-1368). J BUON. 2019;24(1):410–4.
12. Sudhakar A. History of cancer, ancient and modern treatment methods. J Cancer Sci Ther. 2009;1(2):1–4. https://doi.org/10.4172/1948-5956.100000e2.
13. Paget S. Ambroise Paré and His Times, 1510–1590. New York: G. P. Putnam's Sons; 1897.
14. Haas LF. William Harvey 1578-1657. J Neurol Neurosurg Psychiatry. 1992;55(2):111. https://doi.org/10.1136/jnnp.55.2.111.
15. Jatoi I, Kaufmann M, Petit J. Atlas of breast surgery. Berlin: Science & Business Media; 2005.
16. Bodenham DC. A study of 650 observed malignant melanomas in the south-west region. Ann R Coll Surg Engl. 1968;43(4):218–39.
17. Androutsos G. Giovanni-Battista Morgagni (1682-1773): creator of pathological anatomy. J BUON. 2006;11(1):95–101.

18. Chevallier J. Histoire du mélanome cutané: de la mélanose de Laennec à la fin du XXe siècle [History of cutaneous melanoma: from Laennec's melanosis to the end of 20th century]. Ann Dermatol Venereol. 2017;144(8–9):545–57. French. https://doi.org/10.1016/j.annder.2017.03.022.
19. Lane-Brown M, Roxanas MG. Laennec's melanosis: the first published description of metastatic melanoma. Australas J Dermatol. 2017;58(3):234–5. https://doi.org/10.1111/ajd.12492.
20. Ikard RW. Ephraim McDowell's Ovariotomy on General Overton's Wife. Am Surg. 2016;82(4):291–4.
21. Davis NC. William Norris, M.D.: a pioneer in the study of melanoma. Med J Aust. 1980;1(2):52–4. https://doi.org/10.5694/j.1326-5377.1980.tb134622.x.
22. Karamanou M, Liappas I, Stamboulis E, Lymperi M, Kyriakis K, Androutsos G. Sir Robert Carswell (1793-1857): coining the term "melanoma". J BUON. 2012;17(2):400–2.
23. Androutsos G, Karamanou M, Stamboulis E, Tsoucalas G, Kousoulis AA, Mandelenaki D. Joseph-Claude-Anthelme Récamier (1774-1852): forerunner in surgical oncology. J BUON. 2011;16(3):572–6.
24. Classics in oncology: Johannes Müller (1801–1858). CA Cancer J Clin. 1973;23(5):305–12.
25. Anaya-Prado R, Schadegg-Peña D. Crawford Williamson long: the true pioneer of surgical anesthesia. J Investig Surg. 2015;28(4):181–7. https://doi.org/10.3109/08941939.2015.1061826.
26. Haridas RP, Bause GS. A newly discovered manuscript of Charles T. Jackson, MD: "History of the patenting of the application of sulphuric ether for the production of insensibility". J Anesth Hist. 2017;3(2):37–46. https://doi.org/10.1016/j.janh.2017.02.004.
27. Hutchinson J. Lentigo melanosis. Arch Surg. 1894;5:253–6.
28. van den Tweel JG, Taylor CR. A brief history of pathology: preface to a forthcoming series that highlights milestones in the evolution of pathology as a discipline. Virchows Arch. 2010;457(1):3–10. https://doi.org/10.1007/s00428-010-0934-4.
29. Schwokowski CF. Erinnerungen an Carl Thiersch—Zum 100. Todestag [In memory of Carl Thiersch—on the 100th anniversary of his death]. Zentralbl Chir. 1996;121(5):426–9. German.
30. Halata Z, Grim M, Bauman KI. Friedrich Sigmund Merkel and his "Merkel cell", morphology, development, and physiology: review and new results. Anat Rec A Discov Mol Cell Evol Biol. 2003;271(1):225–39. https://doi.org/10.1002/ar.a.10029.
31. Erovic I, Erovic BM. Merkel cell carcinoma: the past, the present, and the future. J Skin Cancer. 2013;2013:929364. https://doi.org/10.1155/2013/929364.
32. Bordenave G. Louis Pasteur (1822-1895). Microbes Infect. 2003;5(6):553–60. https://doi.org/10.1016/s1286-4579(03)00075-3.
33. Morson AC, Morson BC. Memories of Lord Lister. Proc R Soc Med. 1971;64(10):1060–3.
34. Halsted MP. William Stewart Halsted: his life and contributions to surgery. Lancet Oncol. 2007;8(3):256–65. https://doi.org/10.1016/S1470-2045(07)70076-1.
35. Paget S. The distribution of secondary growths in cancer of the breast. Lancet. 1889;133(3421):571–3.
36. Fidler IJ, Poste G. The "seed and soil" hypothesis revisited. Lancet Oncol. 2008;9(8):808. https://doi.org/10.1016/S1470-2045(08)70201-8.
37. Neuhaus SJ, Clark MA, Thomas JM. Dr. Herbert Lumley Snow, MD, MRCS (1847-1930): the original champion of elective lymph node dissection in melanoma. Ann Surg Oncol. 2004;11(9):875–8. https://doi.org/10.1245/ASO.2004.02.031.
38. Soulard R. Thank you, William! Arch Dermatol. 2012;148(7):843. https://doi.org/10.1001/archdermatol.2012.1252.
39. Reed AB. The history of radiation use in medicine. J Vasc Surg. 2011;53(1 Suppl):3S–5S. https://doi.org/10.1016/j.jvs.2010.07.024.
40. Hodges PC. Dr. Emil H. Grubbe, Pioneer Chicago Radiologist. Postgrad Med. 1964;35:A85–7.
41. Stockwell S. Classics in oncology. George Thomas Beatson, M.D. (1848-1933). CA Cancer J Clin. 1983;33(2):105–21. https://doi.org/10.3322/canjclin.33.2.105.

42. Mould RF. Marie and Pierre Curie and radium: history, mystery, and discovery. Med Phys. 1999;26(9):1766–72. https://doi.org/10.1118/1.598680.
43. Knutsson F. Thor Stenbeck—svensk röntgenpionjär [Thor Stenbeck—Swedish radiology pioneer]. Nord Medicinhist Arsb. 1970:219–32. Swedish.
44. Mould RF. A century of X-rays and radioactivity in medicine: with emphasis on photographic records of the early years. Philadelphia: Taylor & Francis; 2018.
45. Cameron JL. William Stewart Halsted. Our surgical heritage. Ann Surg. 1997;225(5):445–58. https://doi.org/10.1097/00000658-199705000-00002.
46. Handley WS. The pathology of melanotic growths in relation to their operative treatment. Lancet. 1907;1:927–33, 996–1003.
47. Peyton Rous (1879–1970). CA Cancer J Clin. 1972;22(1):21–2. https://doi.org/10.3322/canjclin.22.1.21.
48. Kasten FH. Paul Ehrlich: pathfinder in cell biology. 1. Chronicle of his life and accomplishments in immunology, cancer research, and chemotherapy. Biotech Histochem. 1996;71(1):2–37. https://doi.org/10.3109/10520299609117128.
49. Huvos AG. James Ewing: cancer man. Ann Diagn Pathol. 1998;2(2):146–8. https://doi.org/10.1016/s1092-9134(98)80052-x.
50. Dubecz A, Schwartz SI. Franz John A. Torek. Ann Thorac Surg. 2008;85(4):1497–9. https://doi.org/10.1016/j.athoracsur.2007.10.106.
51. Darier J. Le melanome malin mesenchymateaux ou melano-sarcome. Bull Assoc Fr Cancer. 1925;14:221–49.
52. Fleming A. La penicillina. Recent Prog Med. 2015;106(6):285–90. Italian. https://doi.org/10.1701/1884.20558.
53. D'Amico TA. Historical perspectives of The American Association for Thoracic Surgery: Evarts A. Graham (1883-1957). J Thorac Cardiovasc Surg. 2011;142(4):735–9. https://doi.org/10.1016/j.jtcvs.2011.06.028.
54. Archibald E. The technic of total unilateral pneumonectomy. Ann Surg. 1934;100(4):796–811. https://doi.org/10.1097/00000658-193410000-00020.
55. Are C, Dhir M, Ravipati L. History of pancreaticoduodenectomy: early misconceptions, initial milestones and the pioneers. HPB (Oxford). 2011;13(6):377–84. https://doi.org/10.1111/j.1477-2574.2011.00305.x.
56. Fuhrman GM. The legacy of Allen Oldfather Whipple. Curr Surg. 2005;62(2):275–6. https://doi.org/10.1016/j.cursur.2004.04.001.
57. Huggins C. How Charles Huggins made his Nobel prize winning discovery—in his own words: an historic audio recording. Interviewed by Willard Goodwin and Elmer Bell. Prostate. 2012;72(16):1718. https://doi.org/10.1002/pros.22524.
58. Goodman LS, Wintrobe MM, Dameshek W, Goodman MJ, Gilman A, McLennan MT. Landmark article Sept. 21, 1946: Nitrogen mustard therapy. Use of methyl-bis(beta-chloroethyl) amine hydrochloride and tris(beta-chloroethyl) amine hydrochloride for Hodgkin's disease, lymphosarcoma, leukemia and certain allied and miscellaneous disorders. By Louis S. Goodman, Maxwell M. Wintrobe, William Dameshek, Morton J. Goodman, Alfred Gilman and Margaret T. McLennan. JAMA. 1984;251(17):2255–61. https://doi.org/10.1001/jama.251.17.2255.
59. Farber S. Some observations on the effect of folic acid antagonists on acute leukemia and other forms of incurable cancer. Blood. 1949;4(2):160–7. Blood. 2016 Jan 21;127(3):271. https://doi.org/10.1182/blood-2015-12-685586.
60. Farber S, D'Angio G, Evans A, Mitus A. Clinical studies of actinomycin D with special reference to Wilms' tumor in children. 1960. J Urol. 2002;168(6):2560–2; discussion 2563. https://doi.org/10.1097/01.ju.0000042140.76846.d9.
61. Craig J. Sidney Farber (1903-1973). J Pediatr. 1996;128(1):160–2. https://doi.org/10.1016/s0022-3476(96)70455-9.
62. Gianluca N. The men or women behind nevi: Sophie Spitz. JAMA Dermatol. 2014;150(1):24. https://doi.org/10.1001/jamadermatol.2013.8431.

63. Fraitag S, Vignon-Pennamen MD. La tumeur de Spitz et le mélanocytome épithélioïde pigmenté: de nouveaux cadres nosologiques pour des tumeurs souvent mal définies [Spitz tumor and pigmented epithelioid melanocytoma: new nosological frameworks for commonly ill-defined tumors]. Ann Dermatol Venereol. 2009;136(2):133–44. French. https://doi.org/10.1016/j.annder.2008.11.011.
64. Leung PM, Rider WD, Webb HP, Aget H, Johns HE. Cobalt-60 therapy unit for large field irradiation. Int J Radiat Oncol Biol Phys. 1981;7(6):705–12. https://doi.org/10.1016/0360-3016(81)90461-2.
65. Watson JD, Crick FH. Molecular structure of nucleic acids; a structure for deoxyribose nucleic acid. Nature. 1953;171(4356):737–8. https://doi.org/10.1038/171737a0.
66. Watson JD. Molecular biology of the gene. New York: W.A. Benjamin; 1965.
67. Hertz R, Li MC, Spencer DB. Effect of methotrexate therapy upon choriocarcinoma and chorioadenoma. Proc Soc Exp Biol Med. 1956;93(2):361–6. https://doi.org/10.3181/00379727-93-22757.
68. Brennan MF. Francis Daniels Moore. Surgery. 2003;133(1):112–3. https://doi.org/10.1067/msy.2003.52.
69. Thompson JF, Shaw HM, Stretch JR, McCarthy WH, Milton GW. The Sydney Melanoma Unit—a multidisciplinary melanoma treatment center. Surg Clin North Am. 2003;83(2):431–51. https://doi.org/10.1016/S0039-6109(02)00090-7.
70. Clark WH Jr, From L, Bernardino EA, Mihm MC. The histogenesis and biologic behavior of primary human malignant melanomas of the skin. Cancer Res. 1969;29(3):705–27.
71. Lynch HT, Frichot BC 3rd, Lynch JF. Familial atypical multiple mole-melanoma syndrome. J Med Genet. 1978;15(5):352–6. https://doi.org/10.1136/jmg.15.5.352.
72. Parrish JA, Thomas B. Fitzpatrick, 1919-2003. J Am Acad Dermatol. 2004;51(2):323–4. https://doi.org/10.1016/j.jaad.2004.03.037. Erratum in: J Am Acad Dermatol. 2005 Jan;52(1):156.
73. Breslow A. Thickness, cross-sectional areas and depth of invasion in the prognosis of cutaneous melanoma. Ann Surg. 1970;172(5):902–8. https://doi.org/10.1097/00000658-197011000-00017.
74. Breslow A, Macht SD. Optimal size of resection margin for thin cutaneous melanoma. Surg Gynecol Obstet. 1977;145(5):691–2.
75. Finckh E, Jelihovsky T. Vincent John McGovern as researcher and medical author. Pathology. 1985;17(2):152–5. https://doi.org/10.3109/00313028509063750.
76. Morton DL, Eilber FR, Holmes EC, Hunt JS, Ketcham AS, Silverstein MJ, et al. BCG immunotherapy of malignant melanoma: summary of a seven-year experience. Ann Surg. 1974;180(4):635–43. https://doi.org/10.1097/00000658-197410000-00029.
77. Fisher B. Biological research in the evolution of cancer surgery: a personal perspective. Cancer Res. 2008;68(24):10007–20. https://doi.org/10.1158/0008-5472.CAN-08-0186.
78. Morton DL, Wen DR, Wong JH, Economou JS, Cagle LA, Storm FK, et al. Technical details of intraoperative lymphatic mapping for early stage melanoma. Arch Surg. 1992;127(4):392–9. https://doi.org/10.1001/archsurg.1992.01420040034005.
79. Balch CM, Donald L. Morton, MD…a living legend in surgical oncology. J Surg Oncol. 2011;104(4):338–40. https://doi.org/10.1002/jso.21860.
80. Hickey R, Vouche M, Sze DY, Hohlastos E, Collins J, Schirmang T, et al. Cancer concepts and principles: primer for the interventional oncologist-part II. J Vasc Interv Radiol. 2013;24(8):1167–88. https://doi.org/10.1016/j.jvir.2013.04.023.
81. Amin MB, Edge S, Greene F, Byrd DR, Brookland RK, Washington MK, et al. AJCC cancer staging manual. 8th ed. Chicago: Springer International Pu; 2017.

Chapter 10
Principles of Radiation Oncology

Alice Roxo Nobre de Souza e Silva, Fernanda Hayashida Yoshimoto, João Luis Fernandes da Silva, Letícia Hernandes de Brito, and Samir Abdallah Hanna

Key Points

- Many aspects of the **history** of radiation in medicine are told by the authors.
- General concepts about **radiation physics** and **radiobiology** are exposed and defined that are two forms of ionizing radiations: corpuscular and electromagnetic.
- **Biological effects** of ionizing radiation can range from DNA damage to genetic mutations, chromosomal aberrations, cell death, disturbances in the cycle and proliferation of cells, neoplastic transformations, and carcinogenesis.
- Radiotherapy is the term used to designate medical treatment that uses ionizing radiation, which is produced by devices or emitted by natural or artificial radioisotopes. Basically, there are two forms of treatment modality: **teletherapy**, in which there is a source of radiation distant from the patient, and **brachytherapy**, in which radioisotopes are placed in contact or close to the area that will be treated.

A. R. N. de Souza e Silva · J. L. F. da Silva
Radiation Oncology Department, Hospital Sírio-Libanês, São Paulo, Brazil

F. H. Yoshimoto · L. H. de Brito
Radiation Oncology Medical Residency Program, Hospital Sírio-Libanês, São Paulo, Brazil

S. A. Hanna (✉)
Radiation Oncology Department, Hospital Sírio-Libanês, São Paulo, Brazil

Radiation Oncology Medical Residency Program, Hospital Sírio-Libanês, São Paulo, Brazil
e-mail: samir.hanna@hsl.org.br

C. M. Z. Abdalla et al. (eds.), *Oncodermatology*,
https://doi.org/10.1007/978-3-031-29277-4_10

- The use of **radiotherapy in cutaneous tumors** is discussed on BCC, SCC, Merkel, and melanoma, analyzing the different aspects for suitable use.
- Important topics are discussed, such as the **interaction of radiotherapy** and other imaging modalities, such as MRI and PET-CT, useful for the planning CT scan, as well as the interaction with other kinds of systemic therapies.

History of Radiations in Medicine

The use of radiation as a cancer treatment, as well as to treat other diseases, emerged in the late nineteenth century. This therapeutic modality became possible due to the discovery of X-rays by the German physicist Wilhelm Röntgen, in 1985 (Fig. 10.1), and of radioactivity by the French physicist Antoine Henri Becquerel,

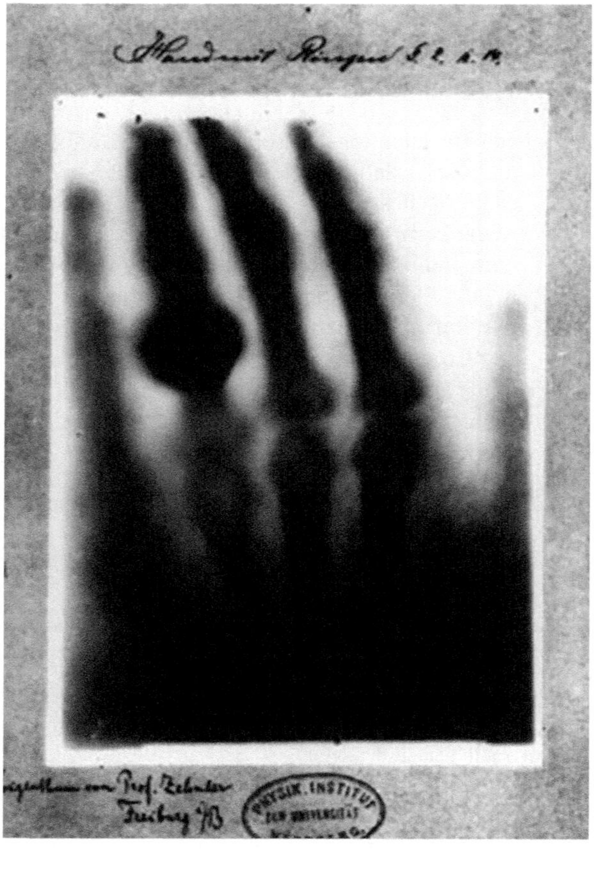

Fig. 10.1 The first X-ray (X-ray of the hand of Anna Bertha Röntgen)

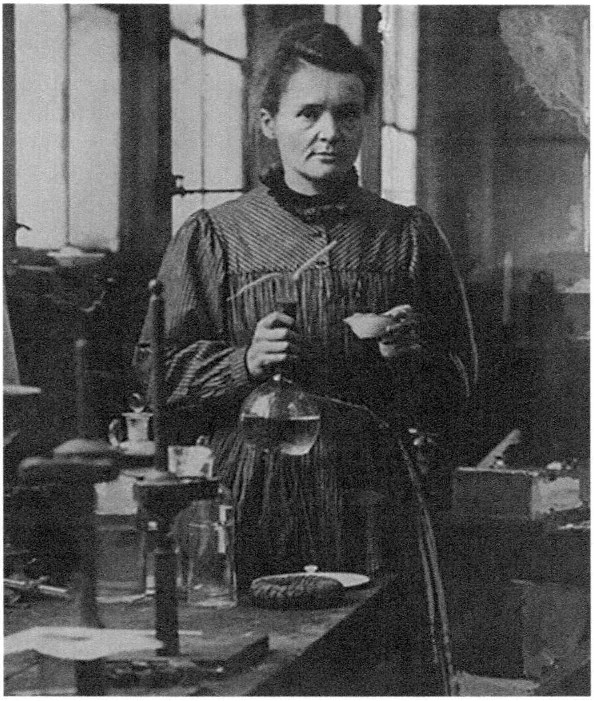

Fig. 10.2 Marie Curie in her laboratory

in 1986 [1]. Using a cathode ray tube, which consisted of a vacuum glass tube in which a warm metallic conductor emitted electrons in the direction of another conductor, Röntgen noticed that a paper covered with barium platinocyanide material became illuminated when positioned near the tube. This also occurred when, in a dark room, the tube was covered with black paper. This still-unknown radiation that produced the phenomenon of fluorescence was called X-rays. The following year, Becquerel revealed photographic plates that were previously placed under samples of a double sulfate of uranium and potassium, thus identifying the radioactive property of certain elements. The works of the couple Pierre and Marie Curie, in 1898 (Fig. 10.2), led to the discovery of two new radioactive elements: polonium and radium. This made it possible to perform the first cancer treatments using radioactive isotopes [1].

Several reports emerged in the early twentieth century describing the use of X-rays and radio-226 in medicine. The most frequent therapeutic applications were for skin tumors due to low radiation penetration. Later, higher-energy equipment was developed allowing the irradiation of deeper lesions. However, at that time, the treatments still had important side effects. Since then, radiotherapy has evolved considerably, both in its technologies and in the understanding of its biological effect, becoming a safer tool for patients who can benefit from it.

General Concepts of Radiation Physics

Radiation is classified as being ionizing or nonionizing. Nonionizing radiation does not have enough energy to eject electrons from biologically important atoms, while ionizing radiation ejects electrons from the atomic orbitals, producing ions. The radiation's ability to penetrate deep into tissues is directly proportional to its energy [2, 3].

Radiotherapy uses ionizing radiation, which is classified into two kinds:

- **Corpuscular radiations**: characterized by the presence of mass and/or electric charge, such as electrons, protons, alpha particles, neutrons, and heavy ions. Charged particles are considered directly ionizing because they have enough kinetic energy to interact with atoms of the absorbing medium and produce chemical and biological changes. Neutrons, which have no charge, are considered indirectly ionizing and produce protons, alpha particles, and heavy nuclear fragments after interacting with matter.
- **Electromagnetic radiations (Fig. 10.3)**: consist of waves with different wavelengths that travel at the speed of light. The shorter the wavelength, the greater its frequency and energy and, therefore, the greater its ability to penetrate deep into the tissues. X-rays and gamma rays are examples of electromagnetic radiation. X-rays are produced due to the deceleration of electrons when they hit a tungsten target. Gamma rays are emitted from the nucleus of natural or artificial radioactive elements during radioactive decay. Both can be considered as energy packages, which are called photons. Electromagnetic radiation is considered indirectly ionizing because it does not produce chemical and biological changes by itself. After the radiation is absorbed by the environment, they release energy and move charged particles that produce these changes.

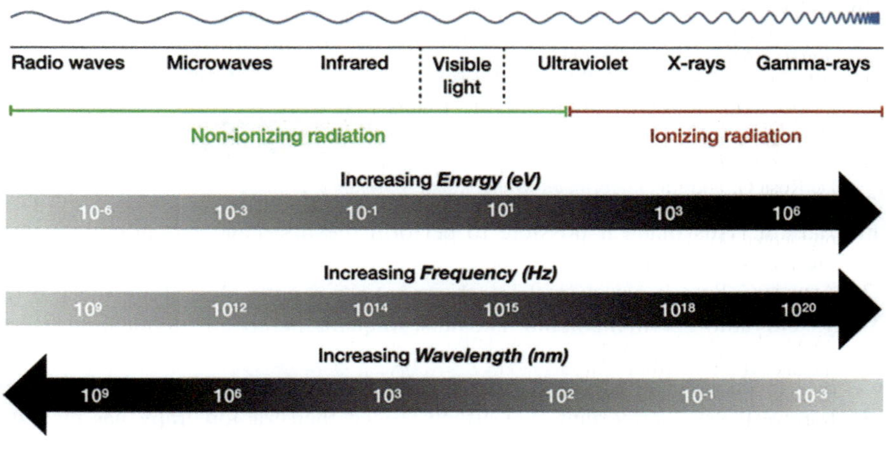

Fig. 10.3 Electromagnetic spectrum

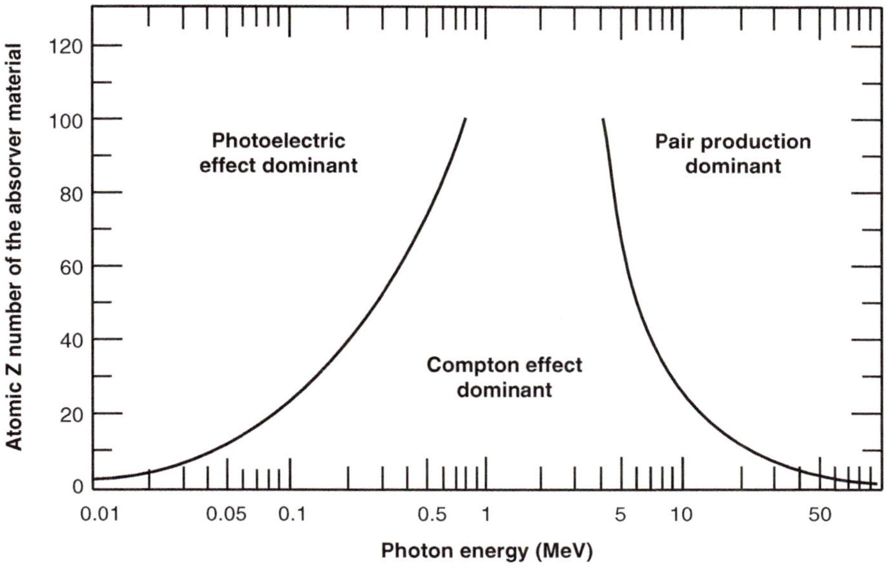

Fig. 10.4 Interactions of photons with matter

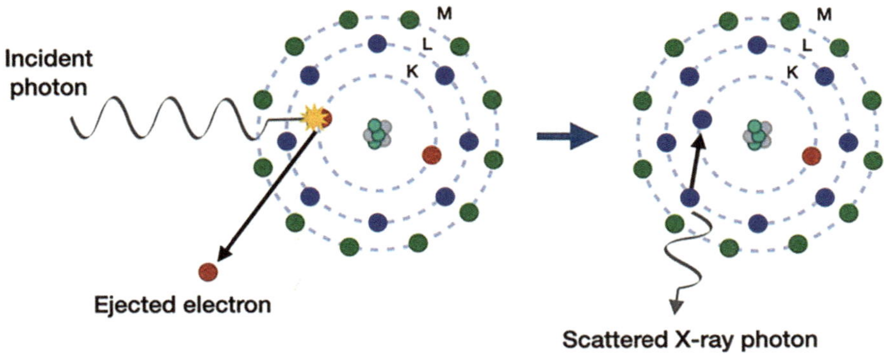

Fig. 10.5 Photoelectric effect

The photons absorption depends on the radiation energy and chemical composition of the matter, resulting in the photoelectric effect, Compton effect, and pair production [1, 3, 4] (Fig. 10.4):

- **Photoelectric effect (Fig. 10.5)**: the incident photon interacts with electrons of the inner shells of atoms and gives up all of its energy to these electrons, which thus acquire kinetic energy and are ejected from the atom. The vacancy is filled by another electron from an outer shell. Because of these changes of levels by the

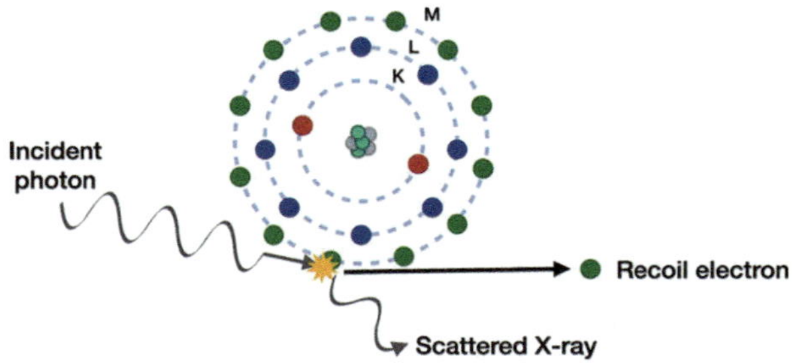

Fig. 10.6 Compton effect

electron, the difference in energy is emitted as a photon of characteristic X-ray. The photoelectric effect is dominant with low energies, depends strongly on atomic number, and is especially important for diagnostic imaging.

- **Compton effect (Fig. 10.6)**: photons interact with electrons that have very low binding energy, much lower than those of the incident photons. Part of this energy is given to the electron as kinetic energy, and photons deflect from the original direction with reduced energy. Thus, the scattered photon and the ejected electrons can ionize other electrons and finally cause chemical and biological changes. This effect is dominant with energies used in radiotherapy (megavoltage) and is independent of the atomic number of the absorbing matter.
- **Pair production**: photons with energy greater than 1022 MeV interact with electrons from internal shells and disappear. In this interaction, two electrons, one negative and the other positive (positron), are formed in opposite directions and, at a given moment, interact and annihilate each other. This produces electromagnetic radiation with energy equivalent to the mass of the two particles. This effect is important in positron emission tomography (PET).

General Concepts of Radiobiology

Radiobiology is the study of the biological effects of ionizing radiation, which can range from DNA damage to genetic mutations, chromosomal aberrations, cell death, disturbances in the cycle and proliferation of cells, neoplastic transformations, and carcinogenesis [1].

Radiobiology related to radiotherapy focuses on electromagnetic waves or subatomic particles with enough energy to cause the ionization of atoms. The radiation can be sparsely ionizing, such as X-rays and gamma rays, or densely ionizing, such as neutrons and alpha particles [1]. This process leads to the breakage of chemical bonds and damage to biomolecules, which results in the most significant effect of ionizing radiation: cell death [1].

DNA damage occurs through direct or indirect action of radiation on the DNA molecules [5, 6] (Fig. 10.7):

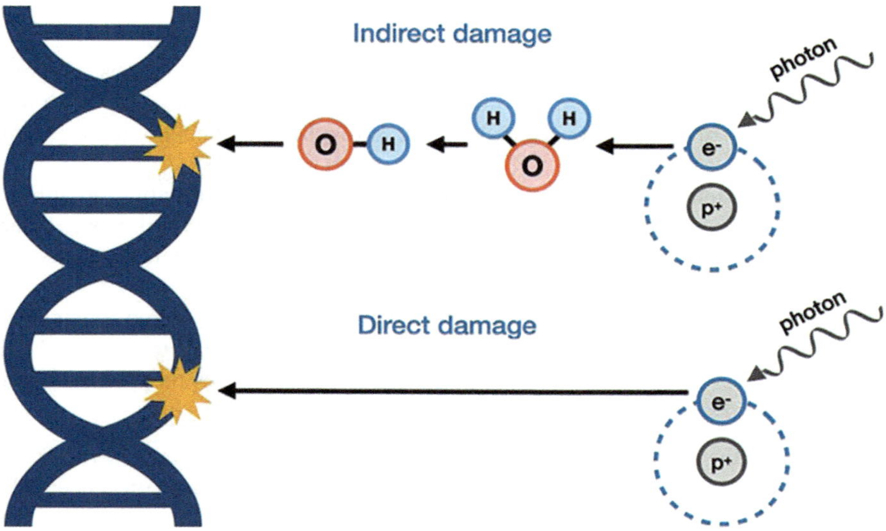

Fig. 10.7 Indirect and direct damage

- **Direct damage**: the energy of the radiation is absorbed by cells and tissues, and electrons are ejected, producing a direct break to the DNA. It is the dominant mechanism in high-LET (linear energy transfer) radiation.
- **Indirect damage**: the electron will interact with the water molecule and produce a hydroxyl radical (OH^-), which in the presence of oxygen induces the formation of free radicals. These radicals react with the DNA producing damage.

Some physical characteristics of radiation can interfere with the biological effect:

- **LET (linear energy transfer)**: rate of energy released per unit of the path traveled by the radiation. Typical values of LET are 0.3 keV/μm for cobalt-60 gamma rays, 2 keV/μm for 250 kV X-rays, and 100–200 keV/μm for heavy particles [4].
- **Dose rate**: quantity of radiation delivered per unit time (Gy/min). It is one of the main factors that determine the biological effect of a certain absorbed dose [4].
- **Oxygen effect**: it is the ratio between radiation doses in the absence and presence of oxygen, as O_2 interacts with free radicals from the radiolysis of water and generates additional free radicals. In addition, O_2 "fixes" the radio-induced lesion by blocking the original chemical structure [4].

The fundamental principles of radiobiology are known as the 4Rs of radiobiology—initially described in the 1950s—which are redistribution, reoxygenation, repair of sublethal injury, and repopulation [5]:

- **Redistribution**: cells with great proliferative capacity have a high rate of redistribution, ensuring that cells that were in more resistant phases migrate to more

sensitive phases (G2/M) of the cell cycle. This redistribution occurs mainly in early responding tissues.
- **Sublethal lesion repair**: it occurs more effectively in normal tissues, as tumor cells have a greater amount of mitosis than normal cells, associated with loss of control of the cell cycle and of the activation of checkpoints for damage repair.
- **Repopulation**: it is the increase in cell division at some point after radiation is delivered. Early responding tissues demonstrate this proliferative capacity earlier, making it even more important to complete radiotherapy before accelerated proliferation begins.
- **Reoxygenation**: phenomenon by which hypoxemic cells become oxygenated during fractionated radiotherapy. This happens because radiation first induces the death of well-oxygenated tumor cells and, thus, reduces their oxygen consumption, leaving a greater offer for the hypoxic cells.

Later, **radiosensitization** was incorporated, when the association of radiotherapy with other treatment modalities can increase its cytotoxic action on cancer cells or protect healthy cells from its action, and, more recently, the **reactivation of the immune response**—when radiotherapy treatments allow the body to recognize tumor antigens and enhance the immune response, especially in patients undergoing immunotherapy [6].

Cell Survival Curves

Cell survival curves describe the relationship between the fraction of cells that retain their reproductive integrity after irradiation, as cell death is defined as the loss of reproductive integrity [5, 6]:

- **Multitarget model (Fig. 10.8)**: one of the oldest models and used for many years. Cells would have one or more targets that could be damaged or inactivated by radiation. For low-LET radiation, the survival curve would present a "shoulder" in the low-dose region and then become exponential, representing events that occur exclusively by single impacts in the shoulder region, and the final decline represented by multiple impacts in the region exponential curve. If the number of "n" targets that must be inactivated is large, the "shoulder" is larger, and if the "n" is small, the "shoulder" will also be smaller. The shoulder represents the repair of sublethal lesions. As for high-LET radiation, the survival curve is a straight line from its origin with a low capacity to repair sublethal lesions.
- **Linear quadratic model (Fig. 10.9)**: currently most used model. It proposes that radiation-induced lethal events are the consequence of two components, the linear (alpha) and the quadratic (beta). In the linear component, the number of lethal events is proportional to the radiation dose. In the quadratic component, the number of lethal events is proportional to the square of the dose, in which two sublethal events interact and produce a lethal event. The alpha/beta ratio corresponds to the dose at which the alpha and beta cell killing components are equal and character-

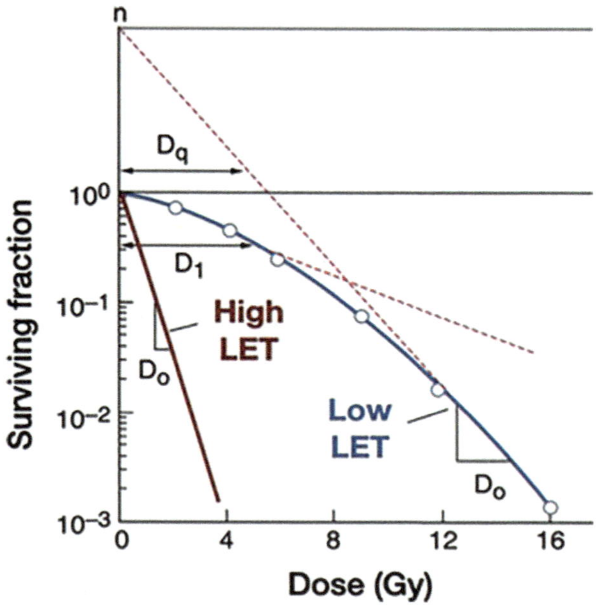

Fig. 10.8 Multi-target model

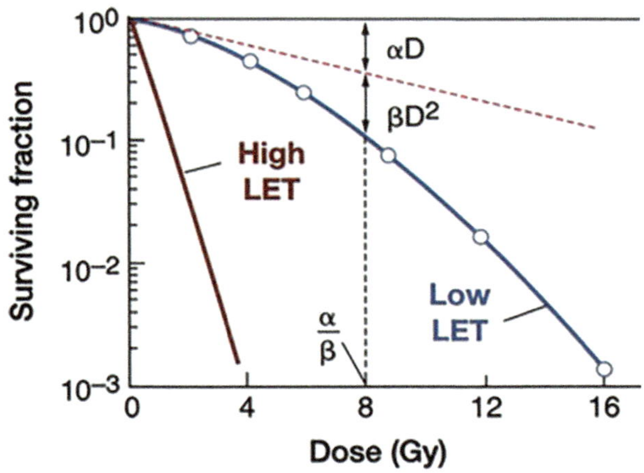

Fig. 10.9 Linear quadratic model

izes the survival curve for each tissue type. Tissues that early respond to radiation, such as skin, mucous membranes, and hematopoietic tissue, have a high alpha component, with a greater linear response at lower doses, and fractionation has little influence on these tissues. On the other hand, tissues that late respond to radiation, such as nervous tissue and lungs, have a high beta component. As a result, their survival curve quickly becomes more curved at low doses, and dose fractionation is beneficial for these tissues, allowing repair of the radio-induced lesion.

The response of cells and tissues to radiation can lead to different mechanisms of cell death [6]. In clonogenic death, irradiated cells go through mitosis without repairing chromosomal aberrations and produce daughter cells with the same changes. These new cells become non-clonogenic, that is, lost their reproductive capability [5, 6]. In programmed cell death, the main radiation-related mechanism, the signaling pathway occurs predominantly through the p53 protein. The protein is activated when DNA breaks are identified, and the apoptosis process begins [6]. Low radiation doses induce an apoptotic effect, while higher doses favor a non-apoptotic effect.

The concept of **relative biological effectiveness (RBE)** is related to the absorbed dose of one radiation type required to produce the same biological effect as the 250 kV X-ray dose [6]. For high-LET radiation, the RBE increases for low doses and for lower doses per fraction. This is due to the lack of repair of high-LET radiation, different from what happens in low-LET radiation. Thus, a higher RBE indicates a greater potential of high-LET radiation in inducing cell death [5, 6].

Principles of Radiotherapy

Radiotherapy is the term used to designate medical treatment that uses ionizing radiation, which is produced by devices or emitted by natural or artificial radioisotopes. It can be used for both benign and malignant pathologies. The main goal is to deliver an accurate dose of radiation in a certain volume, to promote control or eradication of the disease while preserving the adjacent normal tissues [1, 4]. The use of ionizing radiation from unsealed natural sources—such as iodine therapy in patients with thyroid cancer—is the focus of nuclear medicine. It is interesting to point out that the name of the radiotherapy specialist is "radio-oncologist" and that of the nuclear medicine specialist is "nuclear doctor" [1].

The clinical use of radiation involves a multidisciplinary team composed of physicians, physicists, dosimetrists, technicians, and nurses [2]. The purpose of the treatment is curative or palliative, and radiotherapy can be used alone, combined with systemic therapies, preoperatively or neoadjuvant, to promote a tumor reduction and/or improve resectability, or even adjuvant, to increase local control and/or survival. The choice of which approach to use is based on the histological tumor type, the staging of the disease, and the patient's clinical condition [1, 2, 4].

Once indicated, it is necessary to determine the volume to be treated and the most suited technique. The **ICRU 50** and **ICRU 62** (International Commission on Radiation Units and Measurements), published in 1993 and 1999, respectively, introduced nomenclatures and rules for dose prescription, which allowed the standardization of the methodology to be used [7, 8]. The main terms are (Fig. 10.10):

- **GTV (Gross Tumor Volume)**: gross, palpable, visible, or clinically demonstrable location and extent of tumor
- **CTV (Clinical Target Volume)**: tissue that contains the GTV and possibly subclinical disease
- **PTV (Planning Target Volume)**: surrounds the CTV with an additional margin to compensate for positioning or setup errors and CTV inter- and intrafraction movement

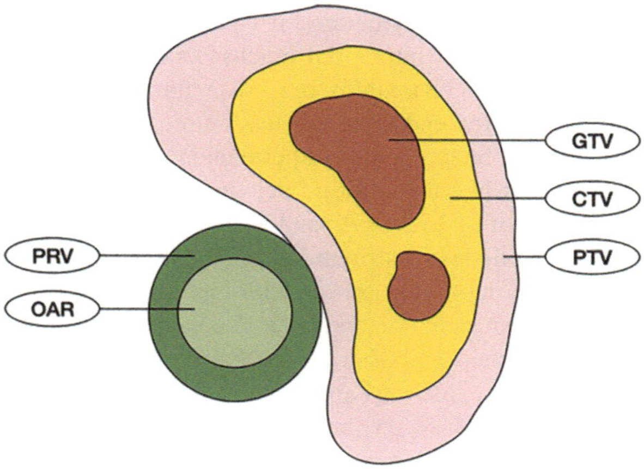

Fig. 10.10 Definition of volumes

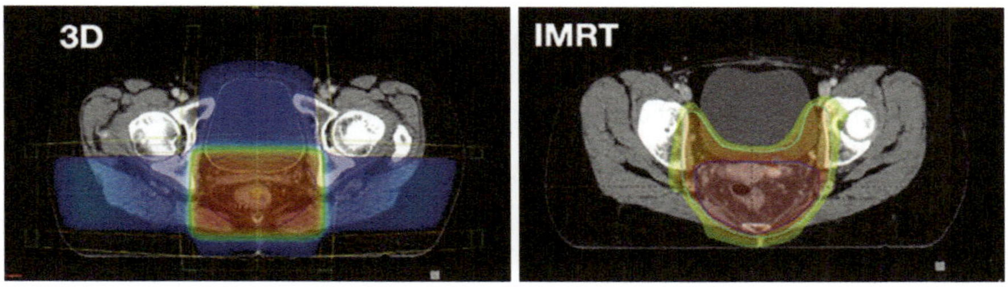

Fig. 10.11 Comparison of a 3D planning treatment with a IMRT treatment

- **OAR (Organ at Risk)**: critical normal structures close to the CTV which should be protected when possible
- **PRV (Planning Organ at Risk Volume)**: margins added to the OAR, using the same principles as for the PTV

To define these volumes, the radio-oncologist, in addition to defining the tumor volume visible on clinical and imaging examination, must also have knowledge about the patterns of dissemination of the neoplasm, such as the risk of lymph node dissemination and micro- or macroscopic invasion of adjacent organs [1, 2, 4].

Radiotherapy techniques involve the treatment modality in which there is a source of radiation distant from the patient, called teletherapy, and brachytherapy, in which radioisotopes are placed in contact or close to the area that will be treated. These modalities can be used together or isolated [1, 2, 4].

For external radiotherapy, planning can be done in two dimensions (2D), in three dimensions (3D), and with an intensity-modulated beam (IMRT), the latter one being the most modern technique, introduced in the 1990s [1]. With the use of IMRT, it is possible to obtain better dose distribution in the target volume, leading to greater local control and less toxicity to normal tissues (Fig. 10.11).

Regarding brachytherapy, it can be divided into interstitial, intracavitary, and endoluminal. For interstitial brachytherapy, the radiation source is placed directly on the tissue to be treated; for intracavitary, the source is positioned inside a cavity; and finally, for endoluminal, the source is placed inside the organ's lumen. The implant can be temporary or permanent. Brachytherapy is classified as HDR (high-dose rate) when using dose rates greater than 12 Gy/h; LDR (low-dose rate), with dose rates of up to 2 Gy/h; and MDR (medium-dose rate) [1, 2, 4].

The depth dose distribution in tissue is related to the beam energy. In general, the percentage depth dose raises with increasing energy used (Fig. 10.12). The choice of the type of radiation and energy to be used depends on factors such as lesion size, proximity to normal tissues, and their sensitivity to radiation. Among the corpuscular radiations, electrons are the most frequently used, as they manage to reasonably distribute the dose on the surface, decaying rapidly from a certain depth. Other types of radiation are gamma rays with 1.25 MeV of energy; linear accelerators, with photon energy ranging from 4 to 25 MV; and proton beam. The last one consists of positively charged particles that are accelerated at high speed in equipment more complex than linear accelerators [1, 4]. The interaction of protons with tissues starts sparsely, and, as the depth increases, they slow down and release most of the energy where they stop, in the region called "Bragg peak." This characteristic interaction allows conformable radiotherapy planning, significantly sparing healthy tissues [6].

The radiation dose to be delivered depends on factors such as treatment objective, lesion size, proximity, tolerance of surrounding normal tissues, and tumor radiosensitivity. Regarding radiosensitivity, germ cell tumors and lymphomas are considered the most radiosensitive, and sarcomas and melanomas are considered the least sensitive [6].

Complications related to radiation therapy are classified as acute or late effects. Acute toxicities occur during the treatment or up to 3 months after its completion,

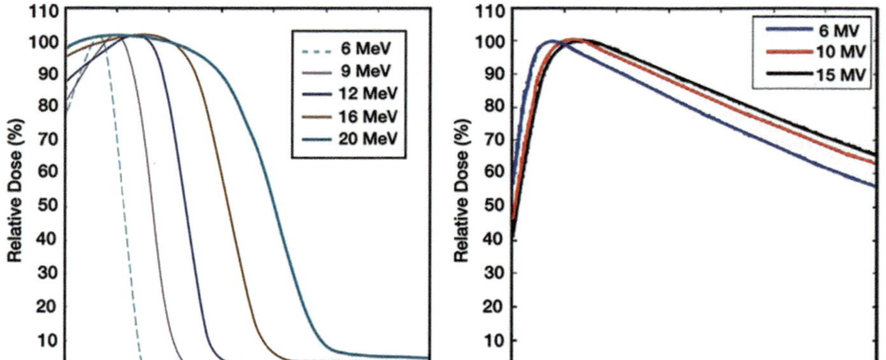

Fig. 10.12 PDP of electron and photon beams

while late complications emerge only 3 months after the end of the exposure [6]. It is important for radio-oncologists to be aware of these toxicities to minimize their occurrence. There are several variables that can interfere with the onset of complications, such as factors related to radiation itself (e.g., total radiation dose, dose per fraction, total treatment time, energy used, association with chemotherapy or radiation protection) or factors related to patient's clinical condition (e.g., patient's age, comorbidities) [1, 4].

Principles of Radiation Therapy for Skin Cancers

Radiotherapy is a useful treatment for melanoma and non-melanoma skin cancers [1].

Regarding non-melanoma tumors, **basal cell carcinoma (BCC)** is most often treated with definitive surgery, while radiotherapy is the second most used modality. Radiotherapy provides excellent control rates and great cosmetic and functional results, especially for lesions on the eyelids, nose, and ears [1]. As an adjuvant treatment, it is usually indicated for close or positive margins; the impossibility of re-excision; the presence of perineural invasion; and invasion of the skeletal muscle, cartilage, or bone [9].

Treatment volumes should include any palpable and visible lesion or surgical bed as GTV, adding clinical margins to the CTV, and usually a 5 mm margin for PTV [1]. The dose and fractionation consider the size of the lesion, and the prescribed doses for conventional fractionation are summarized ahead in Table 10.1.

Radiotherapy is discouraged for patients with nevoid basal cell carcinoma syndrome (Gorlin syndrome), xeroderma pigmentosum, and poorly controlled connective tissue disorders, such as scleroderma. Patients under 50 years old, with lesions in areas most susceptible to mechanical traumatic injuries (e.g., bony prominences) or in low-vascular areas, are relative contraindications, and the risks and benefits should be discussed. Furthermore, for patients with recurrent disease after radiotherapy, re-irradiation can be indicated with caution [1].

For **squamous cell carcinoma (SCC)**, radiotherapy treatment depends on some high-risk factors shown in Table 10.2.

Primary radiotherapy should be indicated in situations where surgery is contraindicated and the patient's option or surgery with adequate reconstruction is not feasible.

Table 10.1 Dose prescription for conventional fractionation

	Dose prescription
Lesions <2 cm	60 Gy in 30 fractions
Lesions >2 cm	66 Gy in 33 fractions
Bone or cartilage invasion	65 Gy in 35 fractions
Post-operatory with negative margins	60 Gy in 30 fractions

Table 10.2 Clinical and pathologic high-risk factors for squamous cell carcinoma

Clinical	Pathologic
Location/size: Area $L \geq 20$ mm; area $M \geq 10$ mm; area H	Poorly differentiated
Recurrent disease	High-risk histologic subtype (adenoid, adenosquamous, desmoplastic, metaplastic)
Site of prior radiation therapy	Clark IV–V
Rapidly growing tumor	Depth ≥2 mm
Borders poorly defined	Lymph node involvement
Immunosuppression	Perineural invasion (nerve diameter >0.1 mm)
Site of chronic inflammatory process	Vascular involvement
Neurological symptoms	

Adjuvant radiotherapy is supported for high-grade, recurrent, deep lesions (>6 mm), tumors larger than 4 cm, bone or muscle invasion, desmoplastic tumors, perineural invasion, or positive margins. It is important to emphasize the role of radiosensitizers, such as platinum-based chemotherapy and targeted therapy, that increase the sensitivity of hypoxic cells when treatment is combined with radiotherapy [1, 9].

Irradiation of regional lymph nodes is recommended for tumors with the involvement of parotid lymph nodes, multiple positive lymph nodes, lymph nodes larger than 3 cm, and extranodal extension. Palliative radiotherapy can be indicated for refractory cases or patients with poor performance status, with a total dose of 20–30 Gy, in 1–5 fractions. Contraindications to treatment are the same as those for BCC [1].

Regarding **Merkel carcinoma** treatment, primary radiotherapy is considered for unresectable lesions, with a dose of 60–66 Gy. For adjuvant radiotherapy, doses from 50–56 Gy to 60–66 Gy can be used for surgical free margins, while 60–66 Gy is the dose recommended for tumors resected with positive margins. It is noteworthy that immunocompetent patients with tumors smaller than 1 cm, without lymph-vascular invasion, and with negative surgical margins can be observed, without adjuvant irradiation [1].

Radiotherapy is a useful treatment option for patients with **melanoma** in some settings. It can be indicated for inoperable tumors or patients who refuse surgery. Adjuvant radiotherapy is reserved for stages I and II, especially in desmoplastic and mucosal melanomas, and for early recurrences after resection with positive margins [1]. Stereotactic ablative radiotherapy can be effective in ablating oligometastatic lesions, while conventional radiotherapy is an option for the palliative treatment of painful metastasis, bleeding, or obstruction [1, 10, 11].

Interaction of Radiotherapy with Other Spheres of Medicine

Radiotherapy planning evolved considerably in the last 30 years [1]. Using the 3D technique, the anatomical information from the planning tomography is transferred to a system, in which the images are segmented into millimeter sections to delimit the tumor, which must be treated, and healthy tissues, which must be protected [1, 4].

Modern technologies enable using other imaging modalities, such as MRI and PET-CT, to overlay with the planning CT scan. This allows a better anatomical definition of organs at risk and tumors, improving treatment targets delineation and maximizing the therapeutic benefit [1, 12].

With the use of IGRT (image-guided radiotherapy) modality, which is the incorporation of imaging during radiotherapy, added to new techniques, such as IMRT (intensity-modulated radiotherapy), SRS (stereotactic radiosurgery), and SABR (stereotactic ablative radiotherapy), it is possible to deliver radiation to cancer cells much more accurately and safely, significantly decreasing the toxicity by protecting healthy tissues from radiation doses [1, 13].

Radiation therapy treatment modalities may include external beam radiotherapy; brachytherapy, mentioned earlier in this chapter; and intraoperative radiation therapy [1].

Intraoperative radiotherapy (IORT) is the treatment where radiation is delivered during the surgical procedure. It can be performed with electron beam techniques, high-dose rate and low-dose rate brachytherapy and can be used in combination with EBRT (external beam radiotherapy) [1]. The great advantage of this modality is the ability to deliver higher effective doses of radiation at the tumor, or at the surgical bed, protecting healthy tissues by surgical procedures or lead plates [4, 14]. IORT requires a multidisciplinary team, with surgical oncologists, radio-oncologists, physicists, and trained and qualified nurses. In addition, it's important the appropriate patient selection for this treatment modality, considering the limitation of each anatomical region to be treated [1, 4].

Radiotherapy Interaction with Systemic Therapies

The combined use of systemic therapies with radiotherapy is a tool that modulates the biological response of tissues to radiation to improve the results of treatment, causing greater damage to the tumor and less damage to healthy tissues.

Both radiation and chemotherapy are cytotoxic to tumor cells and normal tissue, with increased damage when the two agents are combined. The effectiveness against the tumor and the severity of damage to normal tissue increase as doses are increased [5] (Fig. 10.13). With this, a therapeutic index is obtained, which consists of the ratio between the probabilities of tumor control and damage to healthy tissue according to doses of medication or radiation. To be a beneficial treatment, the combination of agents must be more effective against tumors than normal tissues, which is seen in therapeutic indices greater than 1.

The combination of radiotherapy and chemotherapy has advantages in cancer treatment, which has been shown in several clinical trials with a positive impact on disease control and overall survival. This treatment can further improve the positive therapeutic outcome of individual treatments through specific strategies:

- **Spatial cooperation (Fig. 10.14)**: refers to radiation and chemotherapy being directed toward different anatomical sites. Systemic chemotherapy is probably

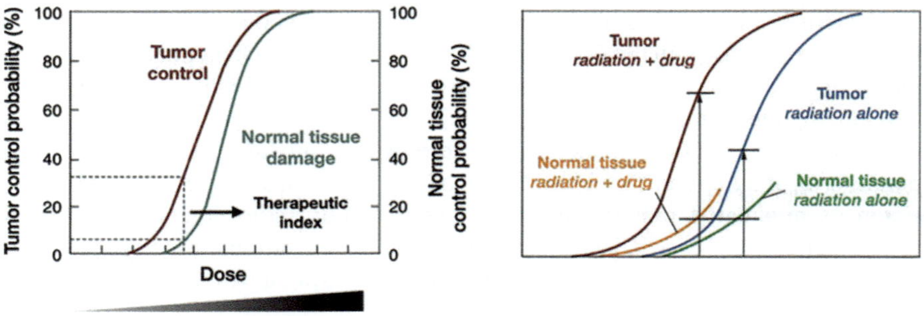

Fig. 10.13 Tumor control probability (TCP) and normal tissue control probability (NTCP)

Fig. 10.14 Spatial cooperation

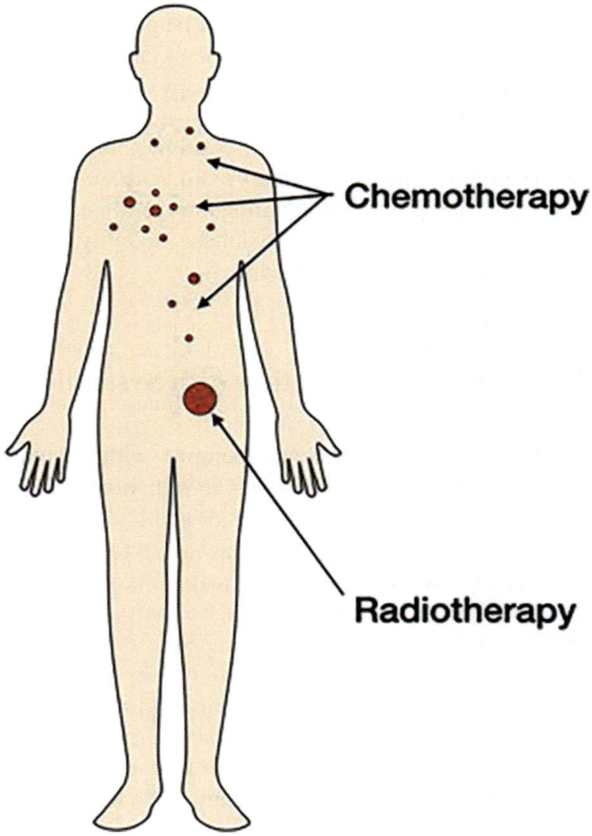

more effective in eradicating subclinical micrometastases, while radiation targets localized larger tumors. This way, the cooperation between chemotherapy and radiation occurs through the independent action of two agents. This strategy is the main justification for adjuvant treatment [1, 4].

- **Independent toxicity**: radiotherapy and chemotherapy have different dose-limiting toxicities, so the selection of combinations of the two treatment modalities should be done so that the toxicity of one drug for specific tissues does not overlap the radiation toxicity [1, 4].
- **Enhanced tumor response**: it is related to the ability of chemotherapy to increase the tumor's response to radiation, decreasing its radioresistance. This is the basis for concomitant radiotherapy and shows that drugs and radiation interact at the molecular, cellular, or metabolic level [1, 4].
- **Protection of normal tissues**: it can be achieved with the use of technical improvements in radiotherapy or through radioprotective agents. This protection should be performed to deliver higher doses of radiation to the tumor [1, 4].

Chemotherapy agents can interact with radiation by altering cell radiosensitivity so that the combination results in an increase or decrease in the effect, depending on whether cell death is greater or less than the sum of cell deaths produced by the individual agents. Cell survival curves are usually expressed by plotting the fraction of surviving cells on a logarithmic scale and the dose of radiation or drugs on a linear scale. Drugs can alter the survival curve, inhibiting cellular repair from radiation damage. A shallower slope indicates protection from radiation, while a steeper slope indicates greater sensitization.

The DNA molecule is the main target of radiation, which causes different types of injuries, such as single-strand breaks (SSBs) and double-strand breaks (DSBs), that can result in cell death. Any agent that makes DNA more susceptible to radiation damage can increase cell death. Among the synergistic mechanisms between radiation and chemotherapy, we have the following:

- **Inhibition of cellular repair**: some of the damage caused by radiation can be repaired. The sublethal damage repair (SLDR) is completed in 4–6 h after irradiation, which is the time required between two radiation fractions for the repair of DSBs. Potential lethal damage repair (PLDR) occurs when environmental conditions prevent cell division for several hours, making it possible to repair DNA lesions that would have been lethal if the DNA had replicated within a few hours of irradiation. PLDR is probably the main responsible for radioresistance in some tumors, such as melanomas. The repair can be accomplished through enzymes that mediate this process or through the renovation of damaged molecules by some oxidation-reduction reactions. Some agents, such as halogenated pyrimidines and nucleoside analogues (e.g., gemcitabine), when used in combined treatment, inhibit repair and increase tissue response to radiation [1, 4].

- **Inhibition of tumor cell repopulation**: tumors are characterized by an imbalance between cell production and cell death. After a loss of cells due to radiation, tumors, as well as healthy tissues, respond in a compensatory way with accelerated repopulation. This accelerated proliferation has a positive impact on normal tissues because it saves them from radiation damage. On the other side, repopulation has a detrimental impact on tumor control by treatment agents. Chemotherapy can increase treatment effectiveness when administered concomitantly with radiotherapy by reducing the rate of proliferation. This occurs because of its cytotoxic and cytostatic activity [1, 4].
- **Cell cycle redistribution**: the sensitivity to radiation depends on the phase of the cell cycle in which the cells are when irradiated (Fig. 10.15). Cells are more sensitive when they are in phases G2 and M and more resistant in late S and early G1. This variability also occurs with chemotherapeutic agents. Taxanes are agents that can block cell transition through mitosis, accumulating cells in radiosensitive phases of the cell cycle. Nucleoside analogues are agents that eliminate radioresistant S-phase cells by inducing apoptosis. Furthermore, they induce surviving cells to move on the cell cycle and accumulate in G2 and M phases [1, 4].
- **Neutralization of hypoxia-associated resistance**: tumor hypoxia occurs due to its defective vascularization, often leading to the appearance of regions of tumor necrosis. The presence of hypoxia causes the appearance of more aggressive tumor cells and stimulates metastatic dissemination, making tumors more resistant to radiation. The combination of chemotherapy with radiotherapy can reduce the detrimental effect of hypoxia on the tissue response to radiation. Destruction of tumor cells by chemotherapeutic agents in the regions close to blood vessels induces an increased oxygen supply to the hypoxic areas. Therefore, hypoxic tumor cells are reoxygenated. With tumor volume reduction, previously hypoxic areas get closer to the capillaries and access oxygen more easily. This mechanism of tumor reoxygenation is the main strategy to increase radiation response by taxanes [1, 15].

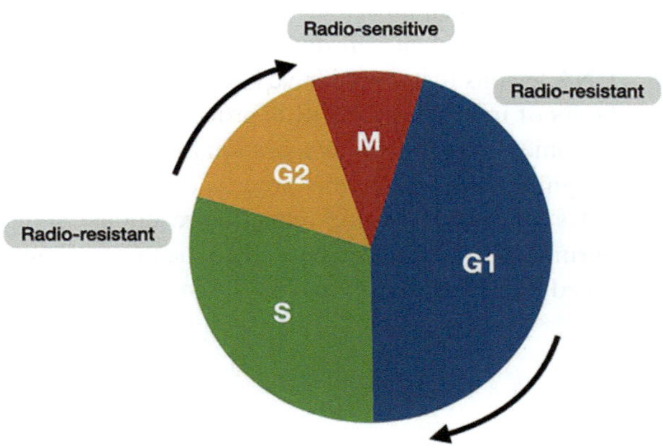

Fig. 10.15 Radiosensitivity in the cell cycle

The emergence of molecular target therapies led to the study of the interaction of these new medications with radiotherapy, and it was observed that the selective cytotoxic effect also presents synergism with ionizing radiation. However, as observed in the combination of chemotherapy and radiotherapy, the association with target therapies can lead to an increase in the toxicity of the treatment. The spectrum of radiotherapy interaction with other therapies is summarized ahead [15] (Fig. 10.16).

Combining immunotherapy with radiotherapy is also a growing field of research in recent years. The understanding of molecular signals involved in immunogenic cell death has increased significantly. Previously, radiotherapy was considered to have an immunosuppressive effect, especially if significant amounts of bone marrow were in the field of treatment. However, studies suggest that radiation can enhance the innate and adaptive immune response to increase the effects on tumor cells that have escaped immunosurveillance.

This effect occurs with the modulation of the immunogenic mechanism of cell death with radiation. Ionizing radiation acts on several stages of the immunological process, enhancing each one of them. Initially, it promotes the release of inflammatory cytokines that increase immunosurveillance and inhibit tumor growth. It also induces local inflammation, the release of tumor-specific antigens, maturation of dendritic cells (antigen-presenting cell—APC), increased initiation and activation of T cells, and elimination of tumor cells via cytotoxic T lymphocytes (CD8+ T) [5].

Due to the immune response to local radiation, the irradiated tumor works as a source of tumor antigens that stimulate the immune system, which acts in a systemic way, reaching distant metastases. This phenomenon is known as the abscopal effect and is what explains the research on the association of high-dose radiotherapy and immunological therapy.

The ideal time to administer immunotherapy in relation to radiotherapy is still widely studied. When the medication is used before the start of radiotherapy, the

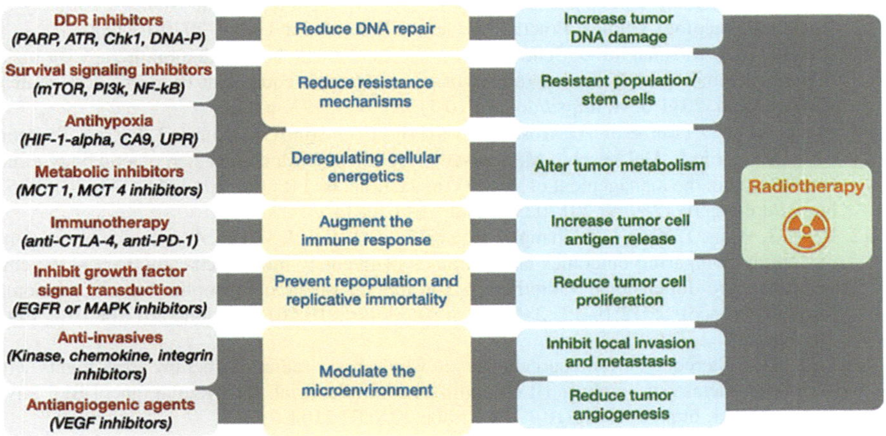

Fig. 10.16 Spectrum of radiotherapy interaction with other therapies

effect observed is the initiation of the host's immune response, without the intensification of toxicities. When performing a concomitant treatment, radiosensitization of tumor cells occurs, maximum availability of tumor antigens, and induction of effector T cell chemotaxis by radiotherapy. Finally, the sequential administration of immunotherapy strengthens "immunosurveillance," avoiding the toxicity of concomitant treatments [16].

With the study of the effects of the association of radiotherapy with numerous cancer therapies, it is possible to safely indicate modern treatments, while maintaining caution and multidisciplinary care for the patient, so that side effects are minimized and controlled.

References

1. Halperin EC, Fazer DE, Perez CA, Brady LW. Perez & Brady's principles and practice of radiation oncology. 7th ed. Philadelphia: Wolters Kluwer; 2019.
2. Salvajoli JV, Souhami L, Faria SL. Radioterapia em oncologia. 2nd ed. São Paulo: Atheneu; 2013.
3. Khan FM. The physics of radiation therapy. 6th ed. Baltimore: William & Wilkins; 2020.
4. Tepper JE, Foote RL, Michalski JM. Gunderson & Tepper's clinical radiation oncology. 5th ed. Philadelphia: Elsevier; 2021.
5. Segreto HRC, Held KD, Michael BD, Segreto RA. Radiobiologia—Da Bancada à Clínica. 2nd ed. São Paulo: Scortecci; 2016.
6. Hall EJ, Giaccia AJ. Radiobiology for the radiologist. 8th ed. Philadelphia: JB Lippincott; 2019.
7. ICRU. Prescribing, recording and reporting photon beam therapy, Report 50, Bethesda, 1993.
8. ICRU. Prescribing, recording and reporting photon beam therapy (supplement to ICRU report 50), Report 62, Bethesda, 1999.
9. Likhacheva A, Awan M, Barker CA, Bhatnagar A, Bradfield L, Brady MS, Buzurovic I, Geiger JL, Parvathaneni U, Zaky S, Devlin PM. Definitive and postoperative radiation therapy for basal and squamous cell cancers of the skin: executive summary of an American Society for Radiation Oncology Clinical Practice Guideline. Pract Radiat Oncol. 2020;10(1):8–20.
10. Stinauer MA, Kavanagh BD, Schefter TE, et al. Stereotactic body radiation therapy for melanoma and renal cell carcinoma: impact of single fraction equivalent dose on local control. Radiat Oncol. 2011;6:34. https://doi.org/10.1186/1748-717X-6-34.
11. Franceschini D, Franzese C, De Rose F, Navarria P, D'Agostino GR, Comito T, Tozzi A, Tronconi MC, Di Guardo L, Del Vecchio M, Scorsetti M. Role of extra cranial stereotactic body radiation therapy in the management of stage IV melanoma. Br J Radiol. 2017;90(1077):20170257. https://doi.org/10.1259/bjr.20170257. Epub 2017 Jul 14.
12. Peng G, Wang T, Yang KY, Zhang S, Zhang T, Li Q, Han J, Wu G. A prospective, randomized study comparing outcomes and toxicities of intensity-modulated radiotherapy vs. conventional two-dimensional radiotherapy for the treatment of nasopharyngeal carcinoma. Radiother Oncol. 2012;104(3):286–93. https://doi.org/10.1016/j.radonc.2012.08.013. Epub 2012 Sep 17.
13. Li J, et al. Stereotactic radiosurgery versus whole-brain radiation therapy for patients with 4-15 brain metastases: a phase III randomized controlled trial. Int J Radiat Oncol Biol Phys. 2020;108:S21. https://doi.org/10.1016/j.ijrobp.2020.07.2108.

14. Zangouri V, Nasrollahi H, Taheri A, et al. Intraoperative radiation therapy for early stage breast cancer. BMC Surg. 2022;22:26. https://doi.org/10.1186/s12893-021-01427-5.
15. Sharma R, Plummer R, Stock J, et al. Clinical development of new drug–radiotherapy combinations. Nat Rev Clin Oncol. 2016;13:627–42.
16. Williamson CW, Sherer MV, Zamarin D, Sharabi AB, Dyer BA, Mell LK, Mayadev JS. Immunotherapy and radiation therapy sequencing: state of the data on timing, efficacy, and safety. Cancer. 2021;127(10):1553–67.

Chapter 11
Principles of Clinical Oncology and Systemic Treatments

Beatriz Mendes Awni, Marcello Moro Queiroz, Gustavo dos Santos Fernandes, and Mauricio Fernando Silva Almeida Ribeiro

Key Points

- Systemic therapies such as chemotherapy, targeted therapy, and immunotherapy play an important role in the multidisciplinary management of high-risk cutaneous malignancies.
- Understanding their mechanisms of action, potential benefits and adverse events may be useful to understand how to best integrate them with other treatment modalities.

Chemotherapy

History of Chemotherapy

Surgery remained the main cancer treatment modality for many years until the advent of radiotherapy, when both dominated the scenario, especially before the 1950s [1, 2]. Drug discovery was essentially limited to the first half of the twentieth

Beatriz Mendes Awni and Marcello Moro Queiroz are co-first authors.

B. M. Awni · M. M. Queiroz
Oncology Center, Hospital Sírio-Libanês, São Paulo, SP, Brazil

G. dos Santos Fernandes
DASA Oncology, Brasília, DF, Brazil

Mauricio Fernando Silva Almeida Ribeiro (✉)
Oncology Center, Hospital Sírio-Libanês, São Paulo, SP, Brazil

Division of Medical Oncology and Hematology, Princess Margaret Cancer Center - University of Toronto, Toronto, Canada
e-mail: mauricio.ribeiro@uhn.ca

C. M. Z. Abdalla et al. (eds.), *Oncodermatology*,
https://doi.org/10.1007/978-3-031-29277-4_11

century due to two main difficulties: (1) the development of models that could predict which few chemicals of the vast repertoire available at that time could have any activity against human cancer and (2) access to clinical facilities that could test such agents [3]. At a certain point, it started to become obvious that surgery and radiotherapy would not be enough to cure cancers, especially in the metastatic setting, rising up the necessity of systemic therapies [4].

The first milestone of chemotherapy development was the discovery of nitrogen mustard as an effective treatment for cancer [1]. Such discovery was related to military efforts to identify toxic agents, and, even though gases were not used in World War II (different from the first one), many studies were conducted on vesicant war gases in this period [5, 6]. To exemplify, after an observation that both bone marrow and lymph nodes were markedly depleted in humans exposed to mustard gas in an accidental spill of sulfur mustards in Bari Harbor (World War II) [7, 8], Louis Goodman and Alfred Gilman carried some experiments in this area [9–11]. After their first conclusions, they convinced a thoracic surgeon named Gustaf Lindskog to administer nitrogen mustard in the bloodstream of a non-Hodgkin's lymphoma patient. Dr. Lindskog testified short-lived tumor shrinkage, but enough to definitely change the paradigm of cancer treatment [4, 12].

Soon after that, in 1937, based on the observation that folic acid administration was able to accelerate leukemia cells growth, Drs. Sidney Farber, Heinle, and Welch developed folate analogs, especially the one known today as methotrexate [13, 14]. Acting as a folate antagonist, these substances were later tested in children with acute lymphoblastic leukemia (ALL) and, in 1948, showed suppression of malignant cell proliferation and unquestionable remissions [15]. Regarding solid tumors, methotrexate was later proved to have antitumor activity in breast, ovarian, bladder, and head and neck cancers [4]. However, it was in two uncommon histologies that its remarkable effects were described: choriocarcinoma (which became the first solid tumor to be cured by drug therapy alone) [16] and osteosarcoma, in which the administration of this agent proved to be effective in reducing recurrence after surgery, establishing the concept of adjuvant treatment [17, 18].

From that on, chemotherapy advanced with the creation of programs and specialized centers around the world, like the Cancer Chemotherapy National Service (CCNSC) at the National Cancer Institute (NCI) in 1955, focused on the discovery, development, toxicological testing, and clinical evaluation of cancer treatment [19–21]. Soon after that, with the discovery of the antitumor effect of vinca alkaloids by Eli Lilly Company (a substance from *Catharanthus roseus*) and procarbazine by Brunner, Young, and DeVita, combination therapy strategies were developed, and the concept of cure was finally established in the 1960s [3, 22–24]. For example, in the late 1960s, Vincent DeVita, George Canellos, and colleagues at the NCI proved that they could cure patients with Hodgkin's and non-Hodgkin's lymphoma with a chemotherapy regimen called MOPP (nitrogen mustard, vincristine, procarbazine, and prednisone) [25, 26].

Cancer treatment grew exponentially after that, being leveraged by the interest of the pharmaceutical industry. Concepts developed throughout chemotherapy development set the stage for another modality of systemic treatment, known as targeted therapy [3, 4].

Classes of Chemotherapy

Chemotherapies can be divided into many subgroups based on their mechanism of action to interfere in the cellular cycle: microtubule inhibitors, alkylating agents, platinum compounds, antimetabolites, topoisomerase inhibitors, and antibiotics with anticancer activities. Here we will discuss their main characteristics, examples, and adverse effects.

Alkylating Agents

Alkylating agents are characterized for the alkyl halide in their structure, which can promote covalent reaction with nucleophilic intracellular components and was the first nonhormonal therapy to show positive results in cancer treatment. As described previously, the effects of this class of chemotherapy were first described during the World War I. The action of nitrogen mustards was later studied against lymphoid and other tissues, especially after the World War II, culminating in a wide range of new substances being synthesized [8, 12].

This group can be divided into six subgroups, based on their pharmacological and structural characteristics: (1) alkyl sulfonate (busulfan), (2) aziridine (thiotepa), (3) triazene (dacarbazine and temozolomide), (4) nitrogen mustard (mechlorethamine, cyclophosphamide, ifosfamide, melphalan, and chlorambucil), (5) nitrosourea (carmustine, lomustine, fotemustine, streptozotocin), and (6) nonclassified (procarbazine and altretamine).

These drugs act basically by binding with nucleophilic sites in many different biologic molecules, especially DNA and RNA. Bindings between DNA and RNA or DNA and proteins, linked due to the alkylation reaction, are responsible for the lethal damage to their structure, and inhibition of DNA and RNA synthesis, resulting in apoptosis and cellular death. This class of chemotherapy depends on cellular proliferation for their activity, but is not restricted to any cell cycle phase [27, 28].

Main adverse effects related to these drugs can vary depending on the subgroup, but some are more common than others, such as myelosuppression, hepatotoxicity, cardiotoxicity, and nausea/vomiting [27, 29].

Platinum Agents

Barnett Rosenberg was a biophysicist at the University of Michigan and had decided to examine whether electrical currents played a role in cellular division. This was prompted by Rosenberg's feeling that the mitotic spindles in a dividing cell appeared similar to the classic school science experiment, where magnetic field lines are formed by scattering iron filings on paper over a magnet. He tested his hypothesis by putting platinum electrodes into a solution containing *Escherichia coli* and seeing that the bacteria cell division stopped [30, 31]. At first, he thought that the reason for this was the electric field, but some years later discovered that the cell division block was occurring because of the platinum compound released by the electrodes. He eventually called it the "accidental discovery that led eventually to cisplatin." So, the first drug of this class was cisplatin, first synthesized in 1847 and proven to have antitumoral activity only in the 1960s, by Rosenberg et al., with the experiment cited above [32–34]. This is the most potent and toxic drug of this class, used mainly in gastrointestinal, head and neck, testicular, and genitourinary tumors. There are two more platinum agents with antitumor activity widely used nowadays: carboplatin, created in the 1980s, which is usually correlated with less nephrotoxicity, and oxaliplatin, approved to be used as chemotherapy in 2004, especially against colorectal cancer [35].

The cytotoxic effect of platinum agents comes from their covalent bonds to DNA and RNA, preventing their duplication and impairing their function [36, 37]. Adverse effects can vary depending on the drug, but nausea, vomiting, and myelosuppression are common. Besides, cisplatin is usually associated with nephrotoxicity, while carboplatin with drug hypersensitivity, and oxaliplatin with neurotoxicity. Despite this range of adverse effects, their incidence oftentimes can be prevented by using specific symptomatic medications before infusion [38–41].

Antimetabolites

These drugs act inhibiting DNA and RNA synthesis and function in many ways. The three main subgroups are pyrimidine analogs (fluorouracil, capecitabine, cytarabine, and gemcitabine), folic acid analogs (methotrexate, pemetrexed, and raltitrexed), and purine analogs and related inhibitors (6-mercaptopurine, cladribine, fludarabine, and pentostatin).

Pyrimidine analogs are characterized by alterations in the pyrimidine ring when compared to the physiologic nitrogen bases or by alterations in the sugar bound to the nitrogen base. This subgroup is represented mainly by fluorouracil (5-FU), a drug synthesized in 1957 by Heidelberger after the report of a vital enzyme inhibition with this drug, resulting in efficacy against transplanted tumors in rats [42]. This drug is a uracil analog and interferes in the cell cycle during the S phase. Briefly, 5-FU targets and inhibits the thymidylate synthase (TS), an enzyme that catalyzes the enzymatic reaction responsible for the production of thymidylate, essential precursor in the synthesis of the DNA. This inhibition prevents the correct synthesis, DNA function, and repair [43].

Adverse effects are myelosuppression, cardiotoxicity (only anthracyclines are more cardiotoxic agents), mucositis, and diarrhea. It is important to consider dihydropyrimidine dehydrogenase (DPD) deficiency in patients with intense adverse effects, as they can no longer be exposed to 5-FU [44–47].

Another subgroup is the oral fluoropyrimidines, for instance, capecitabine, which is a prodrug that results in 5-FU following liver enzymatic conversion. The mechanism of action is similar to 5-FU, and the main adverse effects are palmar-plantar erythrodysesthesia, diarrhea, mucositis, nausea, vomiting, and myelosuppression [48].

The folic acid analogs, represented by methotrexate, were the first drugs associated with leukemic remission in history [49]. Methotrexate acts in the S phase of the cell cycle by enzymatic inhibition, interfering in the nucleotide's purine and thymidylate synthesis. As a conclusion, methotrexate acts in DNA synthesis and repair, as well as in cell replication. Toxicity is associated with dose intensity, drug administration route, and the amount of time of drug use. Main adverse effects are myelosuppression, mucositis, nausea, and vomiting [50, 51].

Topoisomerase Inhibitors

As topoisomerase works separating DNA strands for replication and transcription, this class of drugs is formed by enzymes that change the structure (or topology) of the DNA. This results in impairment of replication, transcription, recombination, and repair of the DNA, culminating in DNA damage and apoptosis, apparently via p53 pathway [52, 53].

Some examples of this group include irinotecan, topotecan, anthracyclines (doxorubicin and daunorubicin), and epirubicin. These drugs can vary on their mechanism of action (especially depending on the enzyme that they inhibit), but the main mechanism of topoisomerase inhibition is the same. Irinotecan is highly associated with diarrhea (acute or chronic) and myelotoxicity. On the other hand, anthracyclines are correlated with cardiotoxicity, depending on the cumulative dose used, infusion time, and preexistent risk factors [54]. Myocardial damage occurs through many mechanisms, but the most important is the generation of reactive species of oxygen [55]. Dexrazoxane is a metal chelator that reduces anthracycline-associated myocardial toxicity, mostly because of its interference in reduction and oxidation reactions [56, 57].

Another important anthracycline adverse effect is the intense damage correlated to drug overflow, because these subgroups of drugs can rapidly accumulate in affected cells. When suspected of extravasation, the best initial conduct is to vacuum any fluid from the subcutaneous site, which limits the amount of drug available. Other local treatments are also indicated, like cooling the area, but others do not have strong evidence (like thiosulfate and topical steroids) [58, 59].

Anti-Microtubules

Microtubules are protein filaments that make part of the cell cytoskeleton, participate in intracellular transport, and are essential to cell motility and division. Vinca alkaloids and taxanes are the main classes that inhibit microtubules, and some less common are estramustine phosphate and epothilone [60].

Vinca alkaloids are natural or semisynthetic compounds obtained from vinca (*Catharanthus roseus*), and, although their chemical structure is similar, the toxicity profile of each drug is distinct. The main examples of drugs consist of vincristine and vinblastine (first generation) and vinorelbine, vindesine, and vinflunine (semisynthetic second generation) [22]. These drugs bind to the beta-tubulin, a microtubule subunit, and their action depends on their dose concentration [61]. In low doses they can inactivate the microtubules and impair the mitotic fuse formation, blocking the metaphase-anaphase transition and resulting in cell apoptosis. In high concentrations, these drugs act by stimulating conformational changes in tubulin structure, resulting in microtubules depolymerization [62]. Neurotoxicity is an important adverse effect for all drugs in this class; however, other toxicities like leucopenia and alopecia are also commonly related [63].

Paclitaxel and docetaxel represent the class of taxanes and are used to treat several types of cancer. Paclitaxel strongly binds to the beta-tubulin subunit, stabilizing the microtubule and consequently interfering with its function [64]. Some studies also describe a second mechanism of action of this drug, by inactivating anti-apoptotic proteins like Bcl-xL/Bcl-2. Neutropenia is the most common adverse effect of this class, but patients can also present with peripheral neuropathy, myalgia, alopecia, cutaneous alterations, arthralgia, and acute hypersensitivity reactions [63, 65].

Antibiotics with Anticancer Activity

The main example of this class is bleomycin. This drug is a compound of glycopeptides antibiotics with cytotoxic activities extracted from a fungus called *Streptococcus verticillus*. The cytotoxic effect results from the oxidative damage in nucleotides induced by this drug, leading to DNA damage, mainly in the G2 and M phases from the cell cycle. The lung toxicity is bleomycin's more common side effect, occurring in approximately 10% of the patients, and can cause permanent lung impairment. Other common adverse effects are fever (in almost 50%), hypersensitivity reaction, and mucocutaneous toxicities. Other examples of antibiotics with anticancer activity are dactinomycin, hydroxyurea, L-asparaginase, and mitomycin C [66]. Figure 11.1 illustrates cytotoxic agents' mechanisms of action according to their classes.

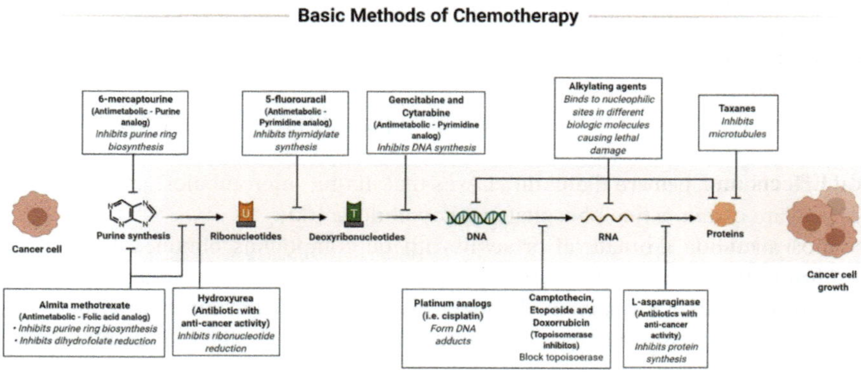

Fig. 11.1 Summary of chemotherapy agents' mechanisms of action. (Reprinted from "Basic methods of chemotherapy," by BioRender.com (2021). Retrieved from https://app.biorender.com/biorender-templates)

Targeted Therapy

General Concepts

In recent decades, the growing knowledge in the field of precision medicine enabled the identification of specific molecular alterations responsible for promoting growth of diverse subtypes of malignancies, with consequent development of targeted therapies that considerably changed the paradigm of cancer treatment [67]. Unlike conventional cytotoxic chemotherapy, modern targeted therapies tend to be more effective and selective, with a distinct safety profile, acting on specific targets involved in proliferation and differentiation of cancer cells, with less activity in normal cells [68, 69].

Protein tyrosine kinases are enzymes responsible for catalyzing the transfer of a phosphoryl group from a nucleoside triphosphate donor to the hydroxyl group of tyrosine residues in protein substrates, using ATP as its donor, and triggering the activation of downstream signaling. Abnormal activation of tyrosine kinases due to mutations, translocations, or amplifications is implicated in tumorigenesis, progression, invasion, and metastasis [70].

There are 518 encoded kinases in the human genome, and these enzymes phosphorylate up to a third of the proteome. At least 58 receptor tyrosine kinases (RTKs) and 32 non-receptor tyrosine kinases (NRTKs) are already known. Molecules that control cell proliferation and death, such as receptor tyrosine kinases (RTKs), are among the best targets for this type of therapeutic approach. Two classes of compounds targeting RTKs are currently used in clinical practice: monoclonal antibodies (macromolecules) and tyrosine kinase inhibitors (small molecules [71, 72]).

Monoclonal antibodies (mAbs) and tyrosine kinase inhibitors (TKIs) employ different strategies to interfere with RTK activity. The mAbs are directed against the extracellular domain of receptors or against ligands and do not need to enter the tumor cell to exert their activity; small inhibitors bind to the protein's intracellular kinase domain and need to cross the plasma membrane [73].

Tyrosine Kinase Inhibitors

Vascular endothelial growth factor receptor (VEGFR), epidermal growth factor receptor (EGFR), platelet-derived growth factor receptor (PDGFR), insulin receptor family (InsR), and fibroblast growth factor receptor (FGFR) are examples of receptor tyrosine kinases (RTKs). RTKs belong to the family of cell surface receptors that transduce a response by attaching themselves to a ligand. They usually have an extracellular domain that binds to a specific ligand, a transmembrane region, and an intracellular kinase domain that selectively binds to and phosphorylates the substrate. RTK can bind to ligands, phosphorylate tyrosine residues of target proteins, and transduce information through PI3K-AKT-mTOR, RAS-RAF-MEK-ERK, or other signaling pathways to activate a series of important biochemical reactions associated with cell proliferation and survival [74].

Non-receptor tyrosine kinases (NRTKs), on the other hand, are located within the cytosol and activated by binding to an already activated RTK. They are responsible for activating the receptor by phosphorylation without the presence of a ligand. Rous sarcoma virus (v-SRC) and Bcr-Abl (Abelson protooncogene breakpoint cluster region) are examples of this class [73].

TKIs are small molecules derived from pyridines, pyrimidines, quinolones, quinazolines, or carboxamides that exert their activity in the intracellular compartment. These drugs inhibit their corresponding kinases from playing their role of catalyzing phosphorylation and activating the downstream signaling cascade, with consequent impairment in tumor progression. TKIs can be designed to target one specific alteration or block a broader range of targets concurrently. These drugs are orally administered, and their toxicity profile can vary significantly depending on which kinase is the target and the role played by the enzyme in overall cell function [75, 76].

Monoclonal Antibodies

Unlike TKIs, mAbs are agents that are too large to passively enter cell membranes, so they are designed to bind selectively and specifically to epitopes expressed on the surface of cancer cells, that is, they require complex biotechnology production models. When used as monotherapy, mAbs against RTKs approved for clinical use are associated with modest antitumor activity; for this reason, they are most often combined with conventional cytotoxic chemotherapy [73, 76]. Figure 11.2 illustrates differences between TKI and mAbs mechanisms of action.

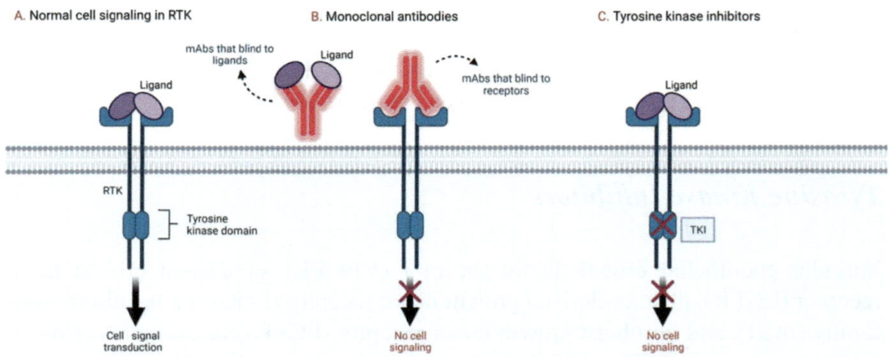

Fig. 11.2 Comparison of the activity between monoclonal antibodies (mAbs) and tyrosine kinase inhibitors (TKIs) on receptor tyrosine kinases (RTKs). (**a**) Normal RTK cell signaling. When ligands bind to RTKs, activation of the tyrosine kinase domain by phosphorylation occurs. This phosphorylation initiates intracellular cell signaling and therefore cellular activities, including proliferation and growth. (**b**) Monoclonal antibodies. mAbs prevent the ligand from binding to RTKs, avoiding dimerization, phosphorylation, and cell signaling. (**c**) TKI. TKIs inhibit RTK phosphorylation. The signaling transduction cascade is not initiated, interrupting cell signaling. (Created with BioRender)

These drugs have a longer half-life than TKIs and are usually given intravenously. They can interfere with cell surface signal transduction, act in a stimulant way to induce cellular events such as apoptosis, or elicit an immune response against targeted cancer cells, possibly interfering with proteins that are necessary for the growth of cancer cells [76].

The HER receptor family was the first to be correlated with cancer onset and progression. It includes four receptors, namely, HER1 (also referred to as EGFR), HER2, HER3, and HER4, which have the particularity of forming homo- and heterodimers that induce reciprocal activation. Gene amplification and overexpression of HER1 and HER2, leading to constant activation of downstream pathways, are involved in some epithelial cancers, such as lung, colon, and breast carcinomas [77].

Target Therapy Approvals Evolution

The era of targeted therapy began with the approval of trastuzumab (a monoclonal antibody against HER2) for the treatment of metastatic breast cancer and imatinib (a small tyrosine kinase inhibitor targeting BCR-Abl) in chronic myeloid leukemia. Since then, we have testified a huge increase in approvals of small molecules and mAbs by the US Food and Drug Administration (FDA) for the treatment of cancer [78]. However, despite the initial excitement related to the effectiveness of these new agents, drug resistance oftentimes associated with activation of alternative signaling pathways turned out to be a big challenge in patients' management [79, 80].

The first FDA-approved TKI was imatinib, in 2001, which changed the perception of protein kinases as therapeutic targets and became known as the "magical bullet" due to its remarkable antitumor activity [81]. The Philadelphia (Ph) chromosome, a hallmark of chronic myelogenous leukemia (CML), was first identified in 1959 by David Hungerford and Peter Nowell. This chromosome is the result of a reciprocal translocation between the long arms of chromosomes 9 and 22. The molecular consequence of this translocation is the formation of fusion-gene BCR and ABL, generating the chimeric BCR-ABL protein with a constitutively activated tyrosine kinase present in practically all patients with CML. According to mutational analysis seen in in vitro studies and in animal models, the protein tyrosine kinase activity is necessary for its oncogenic activity. The pioneer drug, imatinib, is an oral drug that inhibits the ABL tyrosine kinase, having revolutionized the treatment of CML [82–85]. Later, it was also seen that this TKI also inhibits c-KIT and platelet-derived growth factor receptor alpha (PDGFRA), being important in the treatment of steroid-refractory chronic graft-versus-host disease and gastrointestinal stromal tumor (GIST) [81]. Shortly after this approval, EGFR inhibitors gefitinib and erlotinib were approved for the treatment of non-small cell lung cancer (NSCLC) [69].

Since 2001, several potent and well-tolerated TKIs targeting EGFR, ALK, ROS1, HER2, NTRK, VEGFR, RET, MET, MEK, FGFR, PDGFR, and KIT have been discovered and approved for clinical use in a variety of cancers, contributing to a remarkable advance in the clinical oncology scene [67, 72]. In addition, several of the specially designed humanized or chimeric mAbs have recently been approved by the FDA, with the most clinical applicability being those that act on EGFR, VEGF, CTLA-4, PD-1, CD20, and HER-2.

Milestone Approvals for Cutaneous Oncology

A major milestone in the history of cutaneous oncology was the understanding of BRAF role in a subset of cutaneous metastatic melanomas, in 2002. The year of melanoma, 2011, commemorated the FDA approval of both the BRAF inhibitor vemurafenib [86] and the anti-CTLA4 antibody ipilimumab, forever changing the way we would treat melanoma patients with advanced disease [87]. Monoclonal antibodies such as ipilimumab are able to directly amplify the antitumor immune response by inhibiting the control mechanisms of cellular immunity, and tyrosine kinase inhibitors such as vemurafenib can directly influence the signaling pathways that control tumor growth [88]. *BRAF* gene mutation is present in approximately 40–50% of metastatic melanomas (more than 90% of V600E-type mutations, where valine is replaced by glutamic acid at position 600) and has been described in other cancers, including colorectal cancer, papillary thyroid cancer, anaplastic thyroid cancer, serous ovarian cancer, non-small cell lung cancer, gastric cancer, and cholangiocarcinoma [89, 90]. However, despite solid data on progression-free survival gains with BRAF inhibitor versus conventional chemotherapy, targeting BRAF alone derives short-lived disease control due to acquired resistance via bypass signaling, also contributing to the development of secondary cutaneous squamous cell carcinomas (SCC) owing to paradoxical MAPK activation [91].

In an attempt to delay or prevent the onset of resistance without increasing the development of secondary cancers, preclinical and clinical studies combined BRAF and MEK inhibitors, and the results met high expectations: increased response, progression-free, and overall survival rates, when compared to single-agent BRAF inhibitor.

Unlike melanomas, non-melanoma skin cancers (NMSC), such as basal cell carcinomas (BCCs) and cutaneous squamous cell carcinomas (cSCC), usually have an indolent clinical course and rarely metastasize. However, metastatic forms of these tumors often lead to poor outcomes for patients, and recent advances in precision medicine have facilitated the development of new agents to treat these morbid conditions as well [92]. Over the past decade, the US FDA has approved several agents capable of modifying the disease course, comprising Hedgehog inhibitors and anti-PD1 for BCCs, along with anti-PD1 antibodies for cSCC [93]. Apart from targeted agents, another crucial class of antitumor drugs with immunomodulatory properties (and capable of inducing prolonged remissions) was being developed, which would change forever the way we understand the treatment of some otherwise hard-to-treat solid tumors. The next paragraphs are dedicated to discuss the historical background and how immunotherapeutic agents act against tumor cells.

Immunotherapy

Historical Background

Attempts to promote immune system activation to fight cancer date to the eighteenth century. In the 1890s, Dr. William B. Coley was the first researcher to investigate the effects of the immune system against tumor cells while treating patients diagnosed with advanced malignancies with repeated intralesional administration of extracts containing *Streptococcus pyogenes* and *Bacillus prodigious*, the so-called Coley's toxin. The rationale for those experiments was based on occasional observations of patients with inoperable tumors achieving spontaneous remission after recovering from severe bacterial infections. Likewise, Coley has been able to reproduce and report several cases of advanced tumors developing shrinkage following induction of local and systemic inflammation with intralesional administration of his toxin.

Nevertheless, the idea of pursuing tumor remission by inducing life-threatening infections has definitely not gained many supporters in the academia; the high number of treatment-related deaths, a limited (and unknown) subgroup of patients deriving benefit, difficulties regarding reproducibility of Coley's data among other physicians, and advances in the field of radiation therapy have collectively discouraged further development of strategies to modulate antitumor immune response for the following decades [94].

General Concepts of Antitumor Immunity

As previously mentioned, our immune system is able to respond to a broad spectrum of organisms considered as "nonself," irrespective of their nature. This is a stepwise process in which T cells (cellular immunity) play a central role in both initiation and maintenance, aiming to overcome transformed cells. Tumors cells harbor a variety of genomic alterations (e.g., non-synonymous point mutations, insertions/deletions—"indels"—etc.) with potential to generate aberrant peptides called "neoantigens." A neoantigen may ultimately be expressed on the cell surface attached to a major histocompatibility complex class I (MHC-I) molecule, an event that makes tumor cells susceptible to recognition by CD4+ ("helper") and CD8+ ("cytotoxic") T-lymphocytes that, eventually, had already been programmed to recognize these specific peptide sequences. A brief summary of the process of generating antitumor immune response follows below.

Cellular destruction in the tumor microenvironment occurs as a result of local therapies or of natural cell turnover. The release of abnormal peptides—neoantigens—in the tumor bed is the first step to generate the immune response. Neoantigens are captured, processed, and exposed on the surface of antigen-presenting cells—APCs (e.g., dendritic cells)—associated with MHC classes I and II. Subsequently, dendritic cells return to lymphoid structures and present a given neoantigen associated with MHC-I/MHC-II to the T-cell receptor (TCR) of resident T cells. The recognition, a process called "priming," and activation of specialized T CD4+ and T CD8+ lymphocytes culminate in interleukin-2-mediated exponential increase in the number of "programmed" T cells, a phenomenon known as clonal expansion.

Subsequently, T cells travel via blood vessels to tumor sites and infiltrate malignant lesions. Lastly, by recognizing the complex neoantigen-MHC-I using their TCR, T cells generate amplified responses with the release of pro-inflammatory cytokines such as interleukin-1 (IL-1), interferon-α (IFN-α), tumor necrosis factor-α (TNF-α) (mostly T CD4+), and cancer cell destruction through direct secretion of proteases such as perforins and granzymes by T CD8+ lymphocytes (effector phase). Figure 11.3 illustrates this process in a summarized fashion.

However, in order to avoid exacerbated and harmful immune system activation, this process is tightly regulated in different steps called "immune checkpoints," and the final balance between several stimulatory and inhibitory signals defines the direction of the immune response. For instance, priming and activation phases that occur within lymphoid structures depend not only on the interaction between TCR and peptide-MHC but also on a variety of co-stimulatory/inhibitory signals coming from an interaction among molecules, such as B7, CTLA-4, and CD28, all spatially located beside TCR-MHC-peptide complex, in a molecular region known as "immunologic synapse." Another well-known immune checkpoint is present in the effector

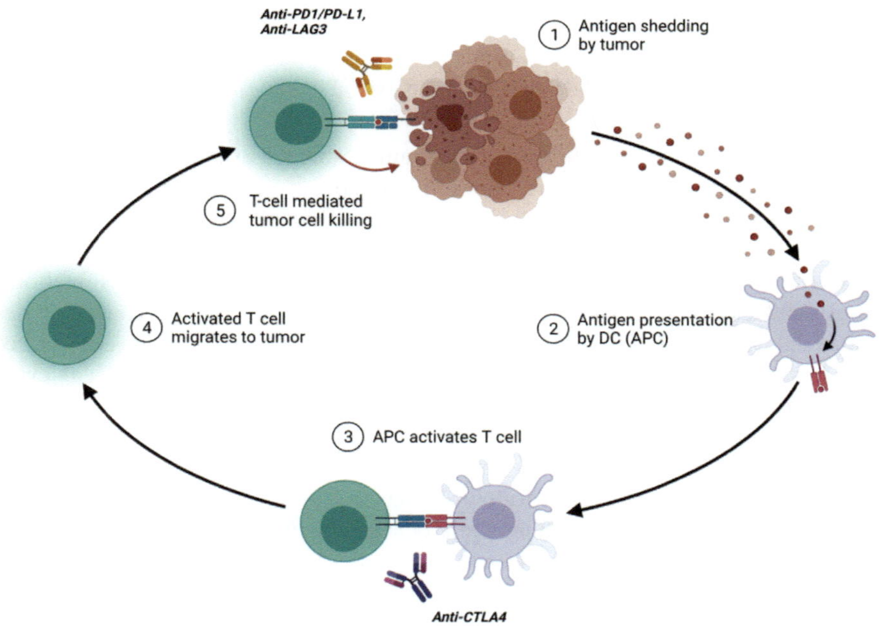

Fig. 11.3 Overview of the antitumor immune response. (Created with BioRender)

phase, when T-lymphocytes directly interact with tumor cells. Inhibitory signals coming from the interaction between PD-1 (on T-cell surface) and its ligand PD-L1 (on tumor surface) may be sufficient to suppress tumor destruction regardless of a nonself antigen recognition. In addition, another important group of immunosuppressive cells, for instance, regulatory T cells (Tregs), myeloid-derived suppressor cells (MDSCs), and tumor-associated macrophages (TAMs), has been implicated in downregulation of tumor-related inflammation, contributing to immune exhaustion and malignant cell evasion.

In summary, a balance between co-stimulatory and co-inhibitory signals is crucial to define how the immune system will behave in relation to an already identified cancer cell. Once some cancer cells develop the ability to disrupt these interactions, evading from immune recognition and destruction, a novel class of immunotherapeutic agents that modulate signals in immune checkpoints, unleashing immunologic antitumor activity, have been developed. The following section provides a brief overview of some immunotherapy agents commonly used in clinical practice and under investigation in prospective clinical studies [95].

Immunotherapy Modalities

Cytokine Therapy

(a) **Interleukin-2 (IL-2)**: produced mainly by CD4+ T cells, IL-2 is a pro-inflammatory cytokine with pleiotropic effects in the immune system. Through binding to IL-2 receptors (IL-2R), via activation of JAK-STAT signaling pathway, it plays a critical role in CD4+ T-cell differentiation and modulation in response to antigens, as well as enhances the cytotoxic activity of both CD8+ T cells and NK cells. Therapeutic intravenous infusion of IL-2 to treat metastatic cancer had its first US FDA approval in 1992 to treat renal cell carcinomas; 6 years later, its second FDA approval was granted to treat metastatic melanoma. Despite presenting durable benefits in less than 10% of the treated patients in both scenarios, this is the modality of immunotherapy with the longest follow-up among survivors. Clark and colleagues [96] published a series of long-term metastatic melanoma and renal cell carcinoma survivors who had been treated with high-dose IL-2 (HD-IL2), with a median follow-up time of 10 years; interestingly, this publication reported patients who had achieved complete response in the setting of advanced melanoma and renal cell carcinoma alive after 15+ and 30+ years, respectively. However, the administration of therapeutic doses of IL-2 has its drawbacks, namely, severe manifestations of systemic inflammation (e.g., fever, chills, arthralgia, acute kidney injury, increased vascular permeability with cardiopulmonary overload), which makes patients' selection stricter [97]. IL-2 has also been studied in combination with other treatment modalities, such as chemotherapy (biochemotherapy) and ICIs, being an important tool in adoptive-cell therapies as well.

(b) **Interferon-α (IFN-α)**: similar to IL-2, this cytokine displays a pleiotropic effect and has extensively been used to treat malignancies in both metastatic and adjuvant settings. IFN-α effects have already been linked to a higher activity of T helper and NK cells and increased number of tumor-infiltrating lymphocytes (TILs) and tumor-specific CD8+ T cells in peripheral blood. More importantly, this cytokine has been constantly associated with rapid differentiation and enhanced MHC-I expression by dendritic cells, which allows for increased immune recognition of cancer cells. IFN-α has been approved for the treatment of a broad range of hematologic and solid malignancies, most of them at advanced stages. It had also played an important role in the adjuvant treatment of melanoma patients until the development of ICIs [95, 98, 99].

Immune Checkpoint Inhibitors (ICIs)

(a) **Anti-CTLA-4**: anti-CTLA-4 antibodies, mainly represented by ipilimumab, have a historical importance in the treatment of metastatic melanoma and for cancer immunotherapy as a whole. Based on the overall survival advantage demonstrated over chemotherapy in previously untreated metastatic melanoma patients, this monoclonal antibody was approved by the US FDA in 2011, being the first ICI to receive approval by a regulatory agency. By binding to CTLA-4, these antibodies block the inhibitory signals arising from the interaction between CTLA-4 (T cell) and B7 (APCs) in the priming phase. Through disrupting this interaction, anti-CTLA-4 antibodies allow the interaction of B7 with the co-stimulatory molecule expressed by T cells known as CD28. The CD28/B7 interaction stimulates the recognition of neoantigens presented by APCs, as well as activation of T-lymphocytes to fight cancer cells (Fig. 11.4). Since these drugs tend to act in early steps of the immune response cycle, adverse events (AEs) are more frequently observed then with other ICIs, a phenomenon that occurs regardless of combination with other drugs [95, 100, 101]. These ICIs are approved for a diversity of malignancies, such as melanoma, malignant mesothelioma, lung cancer, specific subtypes of colorectal carcinomas, etc. [102].

(b) **Anti-PD-1 and anti-PD-L1**: antibodies blocking the interaction between PD-1 and PD-L1 usually act in the priming/activation and effector phases of the immune response (especially in the later checkpoint). In the effector phase, PD-1 binding to its ligand PD-L1 provides a strong inhibitory signal to CD8+ T cells that allows cancer cells to evade despite the successful recognition of a given tumor neoantigen-MHC-I complex by the TCR. By blocking PD-1/PD-L1 interaction, these monoclonal antibodies are able to unleash cytotoxicity coming from T cells (Fig. 11.5). PD-1 antibodies are represented mostly by nivolumab, pembrolizumab, spartalizumab, and cemiplimab, while atezolizumab, durvalumab, and avelumab are among PD-L1 antibodies routinely used in clinical practice. These drugs are currently approved for a great variety of

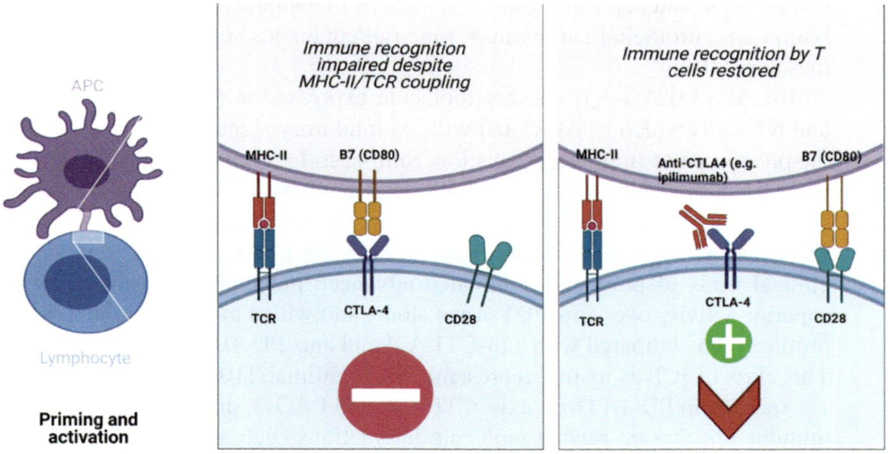

Fig. 11.4 A simplified immune synapse illustrates interactions between MHC-II/TCR and CTLA-4/B7 in the priming and activation phase. By binding to B7, CTLA-4 prompts strong inhibition of neoantigen recognition/lymphocyte activation. Disruption of this interaction using a monoclonal antibody unleashes MHC-II/neoantigen recognition and lymphocyte activation, generating antitumor immune response. (Created with BioRender)

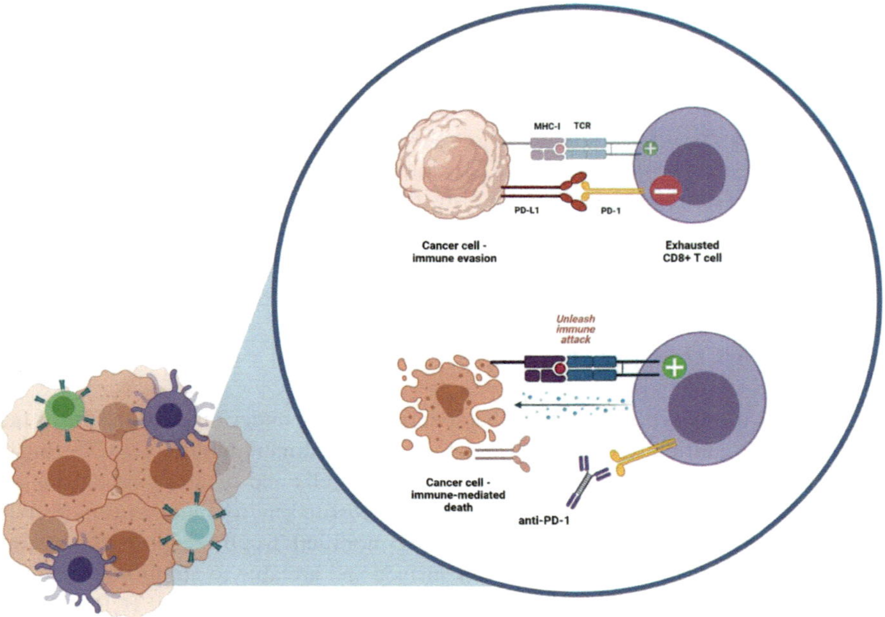

Fig. 11.5 A simplified immune synapse illustrates interactions between TCR/MHC-I and PD-1/PD-L1 in the effector phase. PD-1/PD-L1 interaction sends a strong inhibitory signal to T CD8+ lymphocytes, avoiding cancer cell killing. Disruption of this interaction using a monoclonal antibody unleashes T-lymphocyte-mediated cancer cell destruction. (Created with BioRender)

hematologic and solid malignancies, such as melanoma, lung cancer, Hodgkin lymphoma, urothelial carcinomas, mucosal/cutaneous squamous cell carcinomas, etc. [102].

(c) **Anti-LAG-3**: LAG-3 is another molecule expressed in CD4+, CD8+ T cells and NK cells which is associated with co-inhibitory signals and, consequently, the phenotype of immune exhaustion. Similar to PD-1, it is frequently upregulated in chronic inflammation as well as in malignancies, figuring among the mechanisms of immune evasion displayed by tumor cells. Anti-LAG-3 and PD-1 antibodies in combination have recently been prospectively evaluated in clinical trials of previously untreated advanced melanoma patients, showing superior activity over anti-PD1 drugs alone, and with a more favorable toxicity profile when compared with anti-CTLA-4 and anti-PD-1/PD-L1 combinations. This class of ICIs is mainly represented by relatlimab [103, 104].

Apart from PD-1/PD-L1 axis, CTLA-4, and LAG-3, drugs that disrupt other immune checkpoint-related molecule interactions such as TIM-3, TIGIT, and VISTA are under development and promise to broaden therapeutic arsenal, adding even more complexity to the use of ICIs [105].

Immune-related adverse events (irAEs) associated with the treatment with ICIs can affect almost every structure in the body (causing uveitis, thyroiditis, pneumonitis, hepatitis, colitis, myositis, and so on), being fatigue and cutaneous toxicities the most common ones. The profile of irAEs can vary according to the ICI in use; for instance, anti-CTLA-4 may offer a higher risk of hypophysitis and colitis, when compared to anti-PD1/PD-L1 drugs, which, in turn, are frequently associated with thyroiditis. Additionally, the combination of ICIs usually relates to increased rates of severe AEs; for example, data from the combination of ipilimumab and nivolumab in the treatment of advanced melanoma disclosed roughly 60% of the patients experiencing grades 3/4 AEs, while in the nivolumab monotherapy arm, this occurred in 23% of them [106]. A thorough discussion on ICIs efficacy and safety is out of the scope of this chapter, being addressed later in this book.

Adoptive-Cell Therapy (ACT)

Regardless of the type of immunotherapeutic strategy under discussion, it is a fact that T cells are ultimately the main weapon in this treatment modality. ACTs consist in a subtype of immunotherapy in which both T cells and patient's organisms are manipulated to generate an immunologically hostile environment to tumor cells. This could be achieved through engineering-modified T-cell receptors that recognize specific neoepitopes on tumor cell surface and are able to amplify signals that ultimately lead to lymphocyte activation (genetically engineered TCR cells, or TCR-T, and chimeric antigen receptor—CAR—T cells) or by collecting tumor-infiltrating lymphocytes (TILs), promoting their ex vivo expansion, and infusing them into the patient's body. Both strategies require the administration of non-myeloablative chemotherapeutic regimens to promote reduction in patients' lymphocyte counts after TILs collection and prior to their infusion. Following the infusion of TILs, patients undergo treatment with HD-IL-2 to stimulate lymphocytes' clonal expansion, a step that is not required for TCR-T products. Even though data coming from both strategies are promising, they are not yet approved for the treatment of solid malignancies outside clinical trials [107, 108]. As an example of the great potential of these strategies, we can briefly mention the preliminary results of the global phase II study C-144-01 evaluating the efficacy and safety of lifileucel (LN-144), a cryopreserved autologous TIL therapy to treat patients diagnosed with advanced melanoma resistant to ICIs. This study enrolled patients with high-volume disease who had progressed to anti-PD1/PD-L1 (99%) and CTLA-4 (77%), showing an objective response rate of 36% and disease control rate of 80%. In a median follow-up of 33 months, the duration of response was not reached, suggesting that even patients with poor prognosis who respond to this therapy tend to remain in response for long periods of time. Toxicities usually observed with this modality of treatment are usually related to the lymphodepleting chemotherapy regimen and cytokine release syndrome, including pyrexia, chills, cytopenias, fatigue, hypotension, tachycardia, etc, which can restrict potential candidates for this treatment based on age and comorbidities [109].

Final Considerations

Despite the fact that several systemic treatment subtypes are available to treat cutaneous malignancies, as illustrated in this chapter, one must always have in mind that their appropriate selection and the adequate time to start any of them should be ideally discussed in multidisciplinary boards. Since patients diagnosed with cutaneous malignancies require a complex management, the expertise of other specialties, whenever possible, are always warmly welcome.

References

1. Papac RJ. Origins of cancer therapy. Yale J Biol Med. 2001;74:391–8.
2. DeVita VT. The evolution of therapeutic research in cancer. N Engl J Med. 1978;298:907–10. https://doi.org/10.1056/NEJM197804202981610.
3. DeVita VT, Chu E. A history of cancer chemotherapy. Cancer Res. 2008;68:8643–53. https://doi.org/10.1158/0008-5472.CAN-07-6611.
4. Chabner BA, Roberts TG. Chemotherapy and the war on cancer. Nat Rev Cancer. 2005;5:65–72. https://doi.org/10.1038/nrc1529.
5. Goldin A, Schepartz SA, Venditti JM, DeVita VT. Historical development and current strategy of the National Cancer Institute Drug Development Program. In: Busch H, DeVita VT, editors. Methods in cancer research, vol. 16. New York: Academic Press; 1979. p. 165–245.
6. Zubrod CG, Schepartz S, Leiter J, Endicott KM, Carrese LM, Baker CG. The chemotherapy program of the National Cancer Institute: history, analysis and plans. Cancer Chemother Rep. 1966;50:349–540.

7. Marshall EK. Historical perspectives in chemotherapy. Adv Chemother. 1964;13:1–8. https://doi.org/10.1016/B978-1-4831-9929-0.50006-1.
8. Krumbhaar EB, Krumbhaar HD. The blood and bone marrow in Yelloe Cross gas (mustard gas) poisoning: changes produced in the bone marrow of fatal cases. J Med Res. 1919;40:497–508.3.
9. Gilman A. Symposium on advances in pharmacology resulting from war research: therapeutic applications of chemical warfare agents. Fed Proc. 1966;1946(5):285–92.
10. Goodman LS, Wintrobe MM, Dameshek W, Goodman MJ, Gilman A, McLennan MT. Landmark article Sept. 21, 1946: Nitrogen mustard therapy. Use of methyl-bis(beta-chloroethyl)amine hydrochloride and tris(beta-chloroethyl)amine hydrochloride for Hodgkin's disease, lymphosarcoma, leukemia and certain allied and miscellaneous disorders. JAMA. 1984;251:2255–61. https://doi.org/10.1001/jama.251.17.2255.
11. Gilman A, Philips FS. The biological actions and therapeutic applications of the B-chloroethyl amines and sulfides. Science. 1946;103:409–15.
12. Gilman A. The initial clinical trial of nitrogen mustard. Am J Surg. 1963;105:574–8. https://doi.org/10.1016/0002-9610(63)90232-0.
13. Wills L, Clutterbuck PW, Evans BD. A new factor in the production and cure of macrocytic anaemias and its relation to other haemopoietic principles curative in pernicious anaemia. Biochem J. 1937;31:2136–47. https://doi.org/10.1042/bj0312136.
14. Farber S. Some observations on the effect of folic acid antagonists on acute leukemia and other forms of incurable cancer. Blood. 1949;4:160–7.
15. Farber S, Diamond LK, Mercer RD, Sylvester RF, Wolff JA. Temporary remissions in acute leukemia in children produced by folic acid antagonist, 4-aminopteroyl-glutamic acid (aminopterin). N Engl J Med. 1948;238:787–93. https://doi.org/10.1056/NEJM194806032382301.
16. Li MC, Hertz R, Bergenstal DM. Therapy of choriocarcinoma and related trophoblastic tumors with folic acid and purine antagonists. N Engl J Med. 1958;259:66–74. https://doi.org/10.1056/NEJM195807102590204.
17. Jaffe N, Frei E, Traggis D, Bishop Y. Adjuvant methotrexate and citrovorum-factor treatment of osteogenic sarcoma. N Engl J Med. 1974;291:994–7. https://doi.org/10.1056/NEJM197411072911902.
18. Jaffe N, Link MP, Cohen D, Traggis D, Frei E, Watts H, et al. High-dose methotrexate in osteogenic sarcoma. Natl Cancer Inst Monogr. 1981;56:201–6.
19. Frei E. The National Cancer Chemotherapy program. Science. 1982;217:600–6. https://doi.org/10.1126/science.7046055.
20. Driscoll JS. The preclinical new drug research program of the National Cancer Institute. Cancer Treat Rep. 1984;68:63–76.
21. Grever MR, Schepartz SA, Chabner BA. The National Cancer Institute: cancer drug discovery and development program. Semin Oncol. 1992;19:622–38.
22. Johnson IS, Armstrong JG, Gorman M, Burnett JP. The vinca alkaloids: a new class of oncolytic agents. Cancer Res. 1963;23:1390–427.
23. Brunner KW. A methylhydrazine derivative in Hodgkin's disease and other malignant neoplasms: therapeutic and toxic effects studied in 51 patients. Ann Intern Med. 1965;63:69. https://doi.org/10.7326/0003-4819-63-1-69.
24. DeVita VT, Serpick A, Carbone PP. Preliminary clinical studies with ibenzmethyzin. Clin Pharmacol Ther. 1966;7:542–6. https://doi.org/10.1002/cpt196674542.
25. Moxley JH, De Vita VT, Brace K, Frei E. Intensive combination chemotherapy and X-irradiation in Hodgkin's disease. Cancer Res. 1967;27:1258–63.
26. Devita VT, Serpick AA, Carbone PP. Combination chemotherapy in the treatment of advanced Hodgkin's disease. Ann Intern Med. 1970;73:881–95. https://doi.org/10.7326/0003-4819-73-6-881.
27. Tew KH. Alkylating agents. In: De Vita VTH, Rosenberg S, editors. Cancer principles & practice of oncology. 8th ed. Philadelphia: Lippincott Williams & Wilkins; 2007. p. 408–19.

28. Doroshow JH. Princípios de oncologia médica. In: Pollock RED, Khayat JH, Nakao D, et al., editors. Manual de oncologia clínica da UICC. Hoboken: John Wiley & Sons; 2004. p. 243–60.
29. Bastos DA, Jardim DLF. Agentes Alquilantes. In: Hoff PMG, Katz A, et al., editors. Tratado de Oncologia. Editora Atheneu; 2006. p. 707–21.
30. Kelland L. The resurgence of platinum-based cancer chemotherapy. Nat Rev Cancer. 2007;7:573–84. https://doi.org/10.1038/nrc2167.
31. Chabner BA. Barnett Rosenberg: in Memoriam (1924–2009). Cancer Res. 2010;70:428–9. https://doi.org/10.1158/0008-5472.CAN-09-4146.
32. Rosenberg B, Van Camp L, Krigas T. Inhibition of cell division in Escherichia coli by electrolysis products from a platinum electrode. Nature. 1965;205:698–9. https://doi.org/10.1038/205698a0.
33. Rosenberg B, Vancamp L, Trosko JE, Mansour VH. Platinum compounds: a new class of potent antitumour agents. Nature. 1969;222:385–6. https://doi.org/10.1038/222385a0.
34. Williams CJ, Whitehouse JM. Cis-platinum: a new anticancer agent. Br Med J. 1979;1: 1689–91. https://doi.org/10.1136/bmj.1.6179.1689.
35. Capdevila J, Elez E, Peralta S, Macarulla T, Ramos FJ, Tabernero J. Oxaliplatin-based chemotherapy in the management of colorectal cancer. Expert Rev Anticancer Ther. 2008;8:1223–36. https://doi.org/10.1586/14737140.8.8.1223.
36. Reed E. Cisplatin, carboplatin, and oxaliplatin. In: Chabner BA, Longo DL, editors. Cancer chemotherapy & biotherapy: principles & practices. 4th ed. Philadelphia: Lippincott Williams & Wilkins; 2006. p. 332–43.
37. De Vita VT Jr, Hellman S, Rosenberg SA. Cancer: principles and practice of oncology. 8th ed. Philadelphia: Lippincott Williams & Wilkins; 2008.
38. Bastos DA, Jardim DLF. Cisplatina e Seus Análogos. In: Hoff PMG, Katz A, et al., editors. Tratado de Oncologia. Editora Atheneu; 2006. p. 723–31.
39. BC cancer drug manual. Drug name: Cisplatin. 1994.
40. BC cancer drug manual. Drug name: Carboplatin. 1994.
41. BC cancer drug manual. Drug name: Oxaliplatin. 2001.
42. Heidelberger C, Chaudhuri NK, Danneberg P, Mooren D, Griesbach L, Duschinsky R, et al. Fluorinated pyrimidines, a new class of tumour-inhibitory compounds. Nature. 1957;179:663–6. https://doi.org/10.1038/179663a0.
43. Grem JL. 5-Fluorouracil: forty-plus and still ticking. A review of its preclinical and clinical development. Investig New Drugs. 2000;18:299–313. https://doi.org/10.1023/a:1006416410198.
44. Ezzeldin H, Diasio R. Dihydropyrimidine dehydrogenase deficiency, a pharmacogenetic syndrome associated with potentially life-threatening toxicity following 5-fluorouracil administration. Clin Colorectal Cancer. 2004;4:181–9. https://doi.org/10.3816/ccc.2004.n.018.
45. McEvoy GK, Snow EK, Kester L. AHFS 2006 drug information. Bethesda: American Society of Health-System Pharmacists; 2006.
46. Rubenstein EB, Peterson DE, Schubert M, Keefe D, McGuire D, Epstein J, et al. Clinical practice guidelines for the prevention and treatment of cancer therapy-induced oral and gastrointestinal mucositis. Cancer. 2004;100:2026–46. https://doi.org/10.1002/cncr.20163.
47. Floyd JD, Nguyen DT, Lobins RL, Bashir Q, Doll DC, Perry MC. Cardiotoxicity of cancer therapy. J Clin Oncol. 2005;23:7685–96. https://doi.org/10.1200/JCO.2005.08.789.
48. Miwa M, Ura M, Nishida M, Sawada N, Ishikawa T, Mori K, et al. Design of a novel oral fluoropyrimidine carbamate, capecitabine, which generates 5-fluorouracil selectively in tumours by enzymes concentrated in human liver and cancer tissue. Eur J Cancer. 1998;34:1274–81. https://doi.org/10.1016/s0959-8049(98)00058-6.
49. Meyer LM, Miller FR, Rowen MJ, Bock G, Rutzky J. Treatment of acute leukemia with amethopterin (4-amino, 10-methyl pteroyl glutamic acid). Acta Haematol. 1950;4:157–67. https://doi.org/10.1159/000203749.

50. Longo-Sorbello GS, Bertino JR. Current understanding of methotrexate pharmacology and efficacy in acute leukemias. Use of newer antifolates in clinical trials. Haematologica. 2001;86:121–7.
51. Mayne Pharma (Canada) Inc. Methotrexate injection product monograph. Montreal, Quebec; 2003.
52. Berger JM, Fass D, Wang JC, Harrison SC. Structural similarities between topoisomerases that cleave one or both DNA strands. Proc Natl Acad Sci. 1998;95:7876–81. https://doi.org/10.1073/pnas.95.14.7876.
53. Ruiz-Ruiz C, Robledo G, Cano E, Redondo JM, Lopez-Rivas A. Characterization of p53-mediated up-regulation of CD95 gene expression upon genotoxic treatment in human breast tumor cells. J Biol Chem. 2003;278:31667–75. https://doi.org/10.1074/jbc.M304397200.
54. Chanan-Khan A, Srinivasan S, Czuczman MS. Prevention and management of cardiotoxicity from antineoplastic therapy. J Support Oncol. 2004;2:251–6; discussion 259–61, 264–6.
55. Simůnek T, Stérba M, Popelová O, Adamcová M, Hrdina R, Gersl V. Anthracycline-induced cardiotoxicity: overview of studies examining the roles of oxidative stress and free cellular iron. Pharmacol Rep. 2009;61:154–71. https://doi.org/10.1016/s1734-1140(09)70018-0.
56. Cvetković RS, Scott LJ. Dexrazoxane : a review of its use for cardioprotection during anthracycline chemotherapy. Drugs. 2005;65:1005–24. https://doi.org/10.2165/00003495-200565070-00008.
57. van Dalen EC, Caron HN, Dickinson HO, Kremer LCM. Cardioprotective interventions for cancer patients receiving anthracyclines. Cochrane Database Syst Rev. 2008:CD003917. https://doi.org/10.1002/14651858.CD003917.pub3.
58. Dahlstrøm KK, Chenoufi HL, Daugaard S. Fluorescence microscopic demonstration and demarcation of doxorubicin extravasation. Experimental and clinical studies. Cancer. 1990;65:1722–6. https://doi.org/10.1002/1097-0142(19900415)65:8<1722::aid-cncr2820650810>3.0.co;2-e.
59. Andersson AP, Dahlstrøm KK. Clinical results after doxorubicin extravasation treated with excision guided by fluorescence microscopy. Eur J Cancer. 1993;29A:1712–4. https://doi.org/10.1016/0959-8049(93)90110-2.
60. Jordan MA, Wilson L. Microtubules as a target for anticancer drugs. Nat Rev Cancer. 2004;4:253–65. https://doi.org/10.1038/nrc1317.
61. Jordan MA, Thrower D, Wilson L. Mechanism of inhibition of cell proliferation by Vinca alkaloids. Cancer Res. 1991;51:2212–22.
62. Lobert S, Fahy J, Hill BT, Duflos A, Etievant C, Correia JJ. Vinca alkaloid-induced tubulin spiral formation correlates with cytotoxicity in the leukemic L1210 cell line. Biochemistry. 2000;39:12053–62. https://doi.org/10.1021/bi001038r.
63. Machado KK, Braghirolli MI, Rêgo JFM, Hoff PMG. Agentes Antimicrotúbulos. In: Hoff PMG, Katz A, et al., editors. Tratado de Oncologia. Editora Atheneu; 2006. p. 767–77.
64. Schiff PB, Fant J, Horwitz SB. Promotion of microtubule assembly in vitro by taxol. Nature. 1979;277:665–7. https://doi.org/10.1038/277665a0.
65. Ganansia-Leymarie V, Bischoff P, Bergerat J-P, Holl V. Signal transduction pathways of taxanes-induced apoptosis. Curr Med Chem Anticancer Agents. 2003;3:291–306. https://doi.org/10.2174/1568011033482422.
66. Medeiros RB, Nebuloni DR, Toloi DA. Outros Agentes Quimioterápicos. In: Hoff PMG, Katz A, et al., editors. Tratado de Oncologia. Editora Atheneu; 2006. p. 779–89.
67. Huang L, Jiang S, Shi Y. Tyrosine kinase inhibitors for solid tumors in the past 20 years (2001–2020). J Hematol Oncol. 2020;13:143. https://doi.org/10.1186/s13045-020-00977-0.
68. Ferguson FM, Gray NS. Kinase inhibitors: the road ahead. Nat Rev Drug Discov. 2018;17:353–77. https://doi.org/10.1038/nrd.2018.21.
69. Cohen P, Cross D, Jänne PA. Kinase drug discovery 20 years after imatinib: progress and future directions. Nat Rev Drug Discov. 2021;20:551–69. https://doi.org/10.1038/s41573-021-00195-4.

70. Ardito F, Giuliani M, Perrone D, Troiano G, Muzio LL. The crucial role of protein phosphorylation in cell signaling and its use as targeted therapy (review). Int J Mol Med. 2017;40:271–80. https://doi.org/10.3892/ijmm.2017.3036.
71. Metibemu DS, Akinloye OA, Akamo AJ, Ojo DA, Okeowo OT, Omotuyi IO. Exploring receptor tyrosine kinases-inhibitors in cancer treatments. Egypt J Med Hum Genet. 2019;20:35. https://doi.org/10.1186/s43042-019-0035-0.
72. Zhong L, Li Y, Xiong L, Wang W, Wu M, Yuan T, et al. Small molecules in targeted cancer therapy: advances, challenges, and future perspectives. Signal Transduct Target Ther. 2021;6:201. https://doi.org/10.1038/s41392-021-00572-w.
73. Gharwan H, Groninger H. Kinase inhibitors and monoclonal antibodies in oncology: clinical implications. Nat Rev Clin Oncol. 2016;13:209–27. https://doi.org/10.1038/nrclinonc.2015.213.
74. Cocco E, Scaltriti M, Drilon A. NTRK fusion-positive cancers and TRK inhibitor therapy. Nat Rev Clin Oncol. 2018;15:731–47. https://doi.org/10.1038/s41571-018-0113-0.
75. Ling Y, Liu J, Qian J, Meng C, Guo J, Gao W, et al. Recent advances in multi-target drugs targeting protein kinases and histone deacetylases in cancer therapy. CMC. 2020;27:7264–88. https://doi.org/10.2174/0929867327666200102115720.
76. Giordano S, Petrelli A. From single- to multi-target drugs in cancer therapy: when aspecificity becomes an advantage. CMC. 2008;15:422–32. https://doi.org/10.2174/092986708783503212.
77. Trikha M, Yan L, Nakada MT. Monoclonal antibodies as therapeutics in oncology. Curr Opin Biotechnol. 2002;13:609–14. https://doi.org/10.1016/S0958-1669(02)00348-8.
78. Chang JC. HER2 inhibition: from discovery to clinical practice: Fig. 1. Clin Cancer Res. 2007;13:1–3. https://doi.org/10.1158/1078-0432.CCR-06-2405.
79. Jiao Q, Bi L, Ren Y, Song S, Wang Q, Wang Y. Advances in studies of tyrosine kinase inhibitors and their acquired resistance. Mol Cancer. 2018;17:36. https://doi.org/10.1186/s12943-018-0801-5.
80. Arora A, Scholar EM. Role of tyrosine kinase inhibitors in cancer therapy. J Pharmacol Exp Ther. 2005;315:971–9. https://doi.org/10.1124/jpet.105.084145.
81. Iqbal N, Iqbal N. Imatinib: a breakthrough of targeted therapy in cancer. Chemother Res Pract. 2014;2014:1–9. https://doi.org/10.1155/2014/357027.
82. Nowell PC. Discovery of the Philadelphia chromosome: a personal perspective. J Clin Invest. 2007;117:2033–5. https://doi.org/10.1172/JCI31771.
83. Kang Z-J, Liu Y-F, Xu L-Z, Long Z-J, Huang D, Yang Y, et al. The Philadelphia chromosome in leukemogenesis. Chin J Cancer. 2016;35:48. https://doi.org/10.1186/s40880-016-0108-0.
84. Agrawal M, Garg RJ, Cortes J, Quintás-Cardama A. Tyrosine kinase inhibitors: the first decade. Curr Hematol Malig Rep. 2010;5:70–80. https://doi.org/10.1007/s11899-010-0045-y.
85. Druker BJ, Talpaz M, Resta DJ, Peng B, Buchdunger E, Ford JM, et al. Efficacy and safety of a specific inhibitor of the BCR-ABL tyrosine kinase in chronic myeloid leukemia. N Engl J Med. 2001;344:1031–7. https://doi.org/10.1056/NEJM200104053441401.
86. Kim A, Cohen MS. The discovery of vemurafenib for the treatment of BRAF-mutated metastatic melanoma. Expert Opin Drug Discovery. 2016;11:907–16. https://doi.org/10.1080/17460441.2016.1201057.
87. Bollag G, Tsai J, Zhang J, Zhang C, Ibrahim P, Nolop K, et al. Vemurafenib: the first drug approved for BRAF-mutant cancer. Nat Rev Drug Discov. 2012;11:873–86. https://doi.org/10.1038/nrd3847.
88. Popescu A, Anghel RM. Tyrosine-kinase inhibitors treatment in advanced malignant melanoma. Maedica (Bucur). 2017;12:293–6.
89. Cheng L, Lopez-Beltran A, Massari F, MacLennan GT, Montironi R. Molecular testing for BRAF mutations to inform melanoma treatment decisions: a move toward precision medicine. Mod Pathol. 2018;31:24–38. https://doi.org/10.1038/modpathol.2017.104.
90. Smalley KSM, Sondak VK. Targeted therapy for melanoma: is double hitting a home run? Nat Rev Clin Oncol. 2013;10:5–6. https://doi.org/10.1038/nrclinonc.2012.215.

91. Ribas A, Flaherty KT. BRAF targeted therapy changes the treatment paradigm in melanoma. Nat Rev Clin Oncol. 2011;8:426–33. https://doi.org/10.1038/nrclinonc.2011.69.
92. Tanese K, Nakamura Y, Hirai I, Funakoshi T. Updates on the systemic treatment of advanced non-melanoma skin cancer. Front Med. 2019;6:160. https://doi.org/10.3389/fmed.2019.00160.
93. Spallone G, Botti E, Costanzo A. Targeted therapy in nonmelanoma skin cancers. Cancers. 2011;3:2255–73. https://doi.org/10.3390/cancers3022255.
94. Sell S. Cancer immunotherapy: breakthrough or "deja vu, all over again"? Tumour Biol. 2017;39(6):1010428317707764. https://doi.org/10.1177/1010428317707764.
95. Chen DS, Mellman I. Oncology meets immunology: the cancer-immunity cycle. Immunity. 2013;39(1):1–10. https://doi.org/10.1016/j.immuni.2013.07.012.
96. Clark JI, Curti B, Davis EJ, Kaufman H, Amin A, Alva A, et al. Long-term progression-free survival of patients with metastatic melanoma or renal cell carcinoma following high-dose interleukin-2. J Investig Med. 2021;69:888. https://doi.org/10.1136/jim-2020-001650.
97. Jiang T, Zhou C, Ren S. Role of IL-2 in cancer immunotherapy. Onco Targets Ther. 2016;5(6):e1163462. https://doi.org/10.1080/2162402X.2016.1163462.
98. Motzer RJ, Hutson TE, Tomczak P, Michaelson MD, Bukowski RM, Rixe O, et al. Sunitinib versus interferon alfa in metastatic renal-cell carcinoma. N Engl J Med. 2007;356(2):115–24. https://doi.org/10.1056/NEJMoa065044.
99. Ives NJ, Suciu S, Eggermont AMM, Kirkwood J, Lorigan P, Markovic SN, et al. Adjuvant interferon-alpha for the treatment of high-risk melanoma: an individual patient data meta-analysis. Eur J Cancer. 2017;82:171–83. https://doi.org/10.1016/j.ejca.2017.06.006.
100. Robert C, Thomas L, Bondarenko I, O'Day S, Weber J, Garbe C, et al. Ipilimumab plus dacarbazine for previously untreated metastatic melanoma. N Engl J Med. 2011;364(26):2517–26. https://doi.org/10.1056/NEJMoa1104621.
101. Larkin J, Hodi FS, Wolchok JD. Combined nivolumab and ipilimumab or monotherapy in untreated melanoma. N Engl J Med. 2015;373(13):1270–1. https://doi.org/10.1056/NEJMc1509660.
102. Oliveira LJC, Gongora ABL, Jardim DLF. Spectrum and clinical activity of PD-1/PD-L1 inhibitors: regulatory approval and under development. Curr Oncol Rep. 2020;22(7):70. https://doi.org/10.1007/s11912-020-00928-5.
103. Puhr HC, Ilhan-Mutlu A. New emerging targets in cancer immunotherapy: the role of LAG3. ESMO Open. 2019;4(2):e000482. https://doi.org/10.1136/esmoopen-2018-000482.
104. Lipson EJ, Tawbi HA-H, Schadendorf D, Ascierto PA, Matamala L, Gutiérrez EC, et al. Relatlimab (RELA) plus nivolumab (NIVO) versus NIVO in first-line advanced melanoma: primary phase III results from RELATIVITY-047 (CA224-047). J Clin Oncol. 2021;39(15_Suppl):9503. https://doi.org/10.1200/JCO.2021.39.15_suppl.9503.
105. Qin S, Xu L, Yi M, Yu S, Wu K, Luo S. Novel immune checkpoint targets: moving beyond PD-1 and CTLA-4. Mol Cancer. 2019;18(1):155. https://doi.org/10.1186/s12943-019-1091-2.
106. Larkin J, Chiarion-Sileni V, Gonzalez R, Grob JJ, Rutkowski P, Lao CD, et al. Five-year survival with combined nivolumab and ipilimumab in advanced melanoma. N Engl J Med. 2019;381(16):1535–46. https://doi.org/10.1056/NEJMoa1910836.
107. Kirtane K, Elmariah H, Chung CH, Abate-Daga D. Adoptive cellular therapy in solid tumor malignancies: review of the literature and challenges ahead. J Immunother Cancer. 2021;9(7):e002723. https://doi.org/10.1136/jitc-2021-002723.
108. Morotti M, Albukhari A, Alsaadi A, Artibani M, Brenton JD, Curbishley SM, et al. Promises and challenges of adoptive T-cell therapies for solid tumours. Br J Cancer. 2021;124(11):1759–76. https://doi.org/10.1038/s41416-021-01353-6.
109. Larkin J, Sarnaik A, Chesney JA, Khushalani NI, Kirkwood JM, Weber JS, et al. Lifileucel (LN-144), a cryopreserved autologous tumor infiltrating lymphocyte (TIL) therapy in patients with advanced melanoma: evaluation of impact of prior anti-PD-1 therapy. J Clin Oncol. 2021;39(15_Suppl):9505. https://doi.org/10.1200/JCO.2021.39.15_suppl.9505.

Chapter 12
Imaging Assessment of Cutaneous Tumors

Luciana Carmen Zattar, Isabela dos Santos Alves, Marcelo Araújo Queiroz, and Antônio Sérgio Zafred Marcelino

Key Points

- Carefully revision was made in imaging technology, describing noninvasive modalities useful for practice in skin malignancies.
- Consultation with a radiologist is strongly encouraged to determine the best study or combination of imaging studies, optimizing the use of them, using these tools more efficiently for any given patient.
- Different imaging modalities address specific clinical questions, as we can see in the next paragraph.
  - **Plain films** currently play no significant role in the workup of cutaneous malignancies.
  - **Computed tomography (CT)** scans are most useful for cortical bone evaluation and potentially for nodal staging, with a significant role in the evaluation of pulmonary metastases.
  - **Magnetic resonance imaging (MRI)** is best for the evaluation of bone barrow, deep soft tissues, nerves, and the central nervous system.
  - **High-frequency ultrasound (HFUS)** can be used to noninvasively evaluate primary lesions, micrometastases, and lymph nodes and to guide biopsy procedures.
  - **Positron emission tomography (PET)** combined with CT (PET-CT) provides both morphologic information and data on tumor metabolic activity, ideal for the evaluation of regional nodes, distant metastases, and therapeutic response assessment and potentially for postoperative surveillance.

L. C. Zattar (✉) · I. dos Santos Alves · M. A. Queiroz · A. S. Z. Marcelino
Department of Radiology, Hospital Sírio-Libanês, São Paulo, SP, Brazil
e-mail: luciana.czattar@hsl.org.br

C. M. Z. Abdalla et al. (eds.), *Oncodermatology*,
https://doi.org/10.1007/978-3-031-29277-4_12

General Concepts

Evaluation of the skin and its pathologies can sometimes be difficult with only physical and dermatologic examinations. Due to recent advances in imaging technology, now we have emerging tools for the diagnosis and management of skin lesions and cancer: the noninvasive radiological imaging modalities that allow visualization of skin and provide optimal in vivo anatomical information and cutaneous detailing in submillimetric range and real time, without the need of a traditional biopsy [1, 2].

Imaging examinations have many advantages and promising features not available through routine histology: examination of the whole lesion rather than a section of the biopsied tissue, temporal management and surveillance of lesions, monitoring growth or regression, and the effectiveness of treatments by tracking their changes over time. These tools can save time, decrease costs, and ensure complete tumor removal [1, 3, 4].

Radiological imaging devices help in detecting, diagnosing, and even treating skin cancer and aid in baseline tumor staging, preoperative planning, and assessment of response to treatment. Studies may be indicated (Table 12.1) to assess the extent of the primary tumor, refine the assessment of local spread, assist in determining regional nodal and distant metastatic involvement as well as follow up for recurrence, and provide whole-body staging for cutaneous malignancies [1, 3–6].

The choice of imaging modality will not only be based on the suspected tumor biology and location but also on patient characteristics, depending on the clinical scenario and indications; each case must be considered individually [4, 6]. While many different devices are available and certain generalizations can be made regarding the utility of these modalities, each one provides optimal diagnoses under certain conditions, has limitations on their uses, and varies in its resolution depth, clarity of image, applicability in a clinical setting, accuracy, sensitivity, and specificity [1]. Consultation with a radiologist is strongly encouraged to determine the best study or combination of imaging studies for any given patient for more positive outcomes and timely treatments and to optimize the use of imaging resources, using

Table 12.1 Indication of radiologic imaging examination in skin cancers

Differentiation of skin tumors
Assessment of the measures and extent of the primary tumor
Tracking invasion in skin layers and soft tissues
Local staging detecting tissues and lymph node metastasis
Determining regional and distant metastatic involvement
Possible bony, orbital, or perineural spread
Surveillance and follow-up for recurrence

these tools more efficiently and effectively when evaluating patients with skin cancer [1, 4, 6].

In general, **plain films** currently play no significant role in the workup of cutaneous malignancies; **computed tomography (CT)** scans are most useful for cortical bone evaluation and potentially for nodal staging, with a significant role in the evaluation of pulmonary metastases; contrast-enhanced **magnetic resonance imaging (MRI)** is best for the evaluation of bone marrow, deep soft tissues, nerves, and the central nervous system; **high-frequency ultrasound (HFUS)** can be used to noninvasively evaluate primary lesions, micrometastases, and lymph nodes and to guide biopsy procedures; **positron emission tomography (PET)** combined with CT (PET-CT) provides both morphologic information and data on tumor metabolic activity, ideal for the evaluation of regional nodes, distant metastases, and therapeutic response assessment and potentially for postoperative surveillance [4–6].

In addition to streamlining patient care, an understanding of these different imaging modalities, its findings, advantages, and disadvantages in patients with skin cancer will facilitate the use of cost-effective imaging resources [7].

Methods

Plain Films

Medical X-rays for diagnostic imaging have been used since the published discovery by Roentgen in 1896. The basis for medical applications depends on the differential attenuation of X-rays when interacting with the human body. A uniform X-ray beam incident on the patient interacts with the tissues of the body, where a portion of the X-rays are either absorbed or scattered by the internal structures, producing a variable transmitted X-ray flux that produces a superimposed "shadow" of the internal anatomy, captured to an X-ray-sensitive detector and converted into a visible projection image to provide anatomic information to a medical practitioner [8]. The relative attenuation of the X-ray beam is responsible for the areas of relative brightness or darkness on the image. The X-ray technique should be suitable for evaluating soft tissues that appear dark or in shades of gray and black, rather than bone and calcifications that appear bright or white [9].

Radiographs may be considered an interesting historical footnote with currently no significant role in the workup of cutaneous tumors, except perhaps for bone invasion evaluation (remodeling, periosteal reaction, or overt osseous invasion and destruction) or screening chest radiographs for metastatic lung disease when CT is not possible [4, 10]. Plain films may help in differential diagnosis of a palpable lesion caused by an underlying skeletal deformity (such as exostosis) and reveal soft-tissue calcifications, which can suggest certain diagnoses, especially in soft-tissue sarcomas [10]. Generally, CT is more sensitive than plain films and preferred for all these potential indications.

Computed Tomography

In the early 1970s, computed tomography (CT) revolutionized the use of ionizing radiation (radiography) in diagnostic medical imaging providing a true three-dimensional representation of the anatomy by the acquisition of multiple, angular-dependent projections synthesized with computer algorithms in the computer [7, 10]. Modern CT scanners employ a circular rotating X-ray tube head and detector array in combination with a continuously movable patient gantry to permit rapid scanning of a contiguous anatomic segment [4, 11]. As the X-ray beam travels through the body or tissue being imaged, the beam is attenuated, and the detector registers the resulting changed radiation level. The degree of beam attenuation reflects tissue density, which is expressed in Hounsfield units (HUs), and is responsible for the areas of relative brightness or darkness on the image [4, 7]. HUs represent an arbitrarily defined scale of attenuation, by definition CT value of air is −1000 HUs and the value of water is 0 HU, fat has negative values (−100 HUs), soft tissues and muscle range from 10 to 50 HUs, and bone, calcium, and metal range from 200 to greater than 1000 HUs. Intrinsic differences between tissues often provide substantial resolution [4, 7, 11, 12].

Tumor imaging is significantly improved by intravenous contrast administration. Contrast is utilized to highlight normal and abnormal structures, increasing the physical density of blood, enhancing the tissue contrast of vascular structures, organs, and neoplasms. The use of intravenous iodinated contrast may precipitate acute renal injury or increase renal insufficiency in at-risk patients with borderline renal function. In addition, hypersensitivity to iodine may be a relative contraindication to the use of contrast, although premedications may permit its use. True allergy is uncommon, but more serious reactions, including hypertension and airway compromise, should prompt strong consideration for withholding contrast [4, 7].

Computed tomography imaging can be improved by using tailored reconstruction algorithms that limits the monitor display to a specific spectrum of the gray scale for specific tissues evaluation (i.e., soft tissue, lung, or bone windows). For this reason, CT scans offer great spatial resolution and excellent visualization of bony structures, frequently used for showing the soft-tissue extent of tumor, to evaluate tumor invasion of cortical bone, permitting assessment for subtle sclerotic change or superficial bony erosion, and nodal metastases. Lymph nodes measuring more than 1.0 cm can be identified as metastatic if they show necrosis or abnormal enhancement.

CT is often the initial technique used to image skin cancers with potential extracutaneous involvement because it delivers excellent spatial resolution and is fast, relatively inexpensive, and widely available, but involves exposure to ionizing radiation. Cumulative exposure with repeat studies can be significant especially in radiation-sensitive tissues, such as the thyroid and eye, may pose a relative contraindication in children, and must be carefully considered and discussed with a pregnant patient because of the potential threat of radiation to the developing fetus [7, 12].

The main advantages of computed tomography include speed, intermediate cost, easy accessibility or wide availability at most institutions compared with MRI. In addition, CT can be routinely performed on patients with implanted metal devices, intravenous pumps, or monitors, but is generally less sensitive for subtle intracranial disease, perineural spread, and imaging of soft-tissue tumors [4, 7].

Positron Emission Tomography (PET): Nuclear Medicine

PET imaging uses the pathway of normal glucose metabolism in cells to detect areas or tissues of high or increased metabolic activity by injecting intravenously radiolabeled 18-fluorodeoxyglucose (18-FDG), taken up by cells and incorporated into metabolic pathways. In particular, malignancies with high rate of cellular turnover take up greater amounts of the radiotracer, as the initial glycolytic metabolite becomes trapped within the cell after initial phosphorylation. The detection of positrons emitted by areas of high FDG uptake in tissue identifies enhanced metabolic activity of neoplastic cells. The intensity of the signal is measured in standard uptake values (SUVs) and can be displayed as a color heat map; higher SUVs generally indicate a greater likelihood of pathology [4, 7].

PET scanning alone provides moderate-resolution metabolic cross-sectional information. Anatomic detail and localization is provided by using a PET detector ring merged on the same gantry with a multidetector CT scanner. This fusion combines form and function, providing both structural and functional data displayed in an overlayed image. The preimaging protocol for PET-CT scans requires that patients fast for 4–6 h before radiotracer injection followed by a 1-h rest period to allow distribution, resulting in greater preparation time [4, 7, 13].

Positron emission tomography with computed tomography is an excellent technique for the detection of hypermetabolic skin tumors, such as squamous cell (SCC) and Merkel cell carcinomas (MCC), but the utility is limited for tumors with low metabolic activity or slowly growing tumors, such as basal cell carcinoma (BCC), and infiltrating tumors, such as dermatofibrosarcoma protuberans (DFSP) that may also be less vascular. Staging sensitivity may also be reduced for tumor volumes less than 1.0 cm^3, and false negatives can occur with nodes and distant metastases that are smaller than 1.0 cm in diameter. PET-CT is more sensitive in detecting tumor response to therapy and recurrence and occult local, nodal, and distant tumor metastases, in areas of necrosis, scarring, and fibrosis secondary to radiotherapy [4, 7].

Because PET-CT detects all types of increased glucose uptake, false positives can be seen in areas of infection and inflammation. PET-CT is not able to assess for cerebral metastasis, often necessitating a separate MRI scan, because of the high metabolic demand (and 18-FDG uptake) of the brain, particularly the gray matter [7]. It is possible to use hybrid PET-MRI scanners, not widely available, which would improve soft-tissue resolution and reduce the total ionizing radiation to patients [4].

Magnetic Resonance Imaging

MRI devices use magnetic fields and radiofrequency waves to generate images. Scanners apply very strong magnetic fields which align protons or hydrogen in organic molecules and water that behave as small dipole magnets. Within the static main magnetic field, these protons precess rapidly about the vertical axis of gravity. This steady-state equilibrium is modified by applying a short-duration radiofrequency pulse, which causes these protons to be deflected from the main magnetic field axis and also causes the protons to precess in phase **with one another rather** than the usual random precession. This brief change yields a weak but measurable signal, providing the data that is ultimately reconstructed to form an MR image. When the radiofrequency (RF) pulse ends, a rapid realignment of the protons with the main magnetic field and a rapid return to random precession occur. Although this is a simplistic description, these two phenomena define T1 and T2 relaxation.

In general, high signal (bright images) on a T1-weighted scan includes acute blood, highly proteinaceous material, fat, and paramagnetic gadolinium contrast. A high signal (bright images) on T2-weighted scan primarily reflects free fluid and tissues with high free water content, such as edema, cysts, vitreous and aqueous humor, intraluminal contents (hepatobiliary, gastrointestinal, and genitourinary tracts), and tumors with moderate/high intracellular fluid and cerebrospinal fluid [4, 12].

Manipulation of these technical parameters of each individual scan yields the image characteristics specific for that particular pulse sequence. Application of an additional pulse sequence can be employed to null the high signal from fat (fat suppression technique) and improve the visualization of normal structures or pathology exhibiting gadolinium enhancement. Short tau inversion recovery (STIR) sequence suppresses all substances with short T1 relaxation, such as acute blood, fat, pus, and certain valent states of calcium [4, 9, 12].

The use of contrast is critical for tumor visualization and typically consists intravenously administered chelated gadolinium compounds. Enhancement is increased in the presence of highly vascularized tissues and in particular tissues with incomplete blood/tissue barrier as in many tumors and in active inflammation. Because gadolinium compounds are renally excreted, renal insufficiency is a relative contraindication. Nephrogenic sclerosing dermopathy, also known as nephrogenic systemic fibrosis (NSF), has been associated with the use of gadodiamide in the setting of poor renal function. The concern is related to release and accumulation of free gadolinium in tissues. Relative contraindications to the use of contrast also include pregnant or breastfeeding women, children, chronic liver function impairment, and hepatorenal syndrome. Premedication with steroids and antihistamines can be used in patients with known hypersensitivity reactions [4, 7].

MRI is contraindicated in patients with pacemakers and automated implanted cardiac defibrillators, ferromagnetic aneurysm clips, and spine stimulators. An exhaustive reference of implanted devices and relative safety at various field strengths is available online at www.mrisafety.com [4]. In addition high cost, longer imaging time, and sensitivity to motion and magnetic interference can also be drawbacks for MRI scans [7].

Magnetic resonance imaging scans have superior soft-tissue contrast, especially stronger magnets (at least 1.5–3.0 T), with excellent visualization of bone marrow changes and soft tissues distinguish between benign and malignant lymph nodes, when compared to computed tomography scans, and do not involve ionizing radiation. MRI is the most sensitive imaging modality for detecting central nervous system disease and perineural invasion and is superior to assess the skull-base foraminal contents or intracranial spread of disease [4, 7, 9].

High-Frequency Ultrasound

Ultrasound consists of obtaining images through the transformation of electrical energy into acoustic energy by a transducer with piezoelectric crystal array, which generates sound waves (above the threshold of the human ear) within a narrow frequency spectrum. The wave formed interacts in different ways (reflected or refracted) with each tissue and structure. A returning wave from the body reaches the transducer and is processed by a computer system to generate diagnostic ultrasound images. Changes in voltage and different time of returning detected by the transducer are interpreted and converted into images, with different shades of gray (B mode image or brightness), according to the "echo" that returns to the transducer.

In general, hypoechoic structure absorbs more ultrasound waves and appears gray or darker than the surrounding tissue and includes muscles, fibrous connective tissue, and fat. Hyperechoic structure reflects more ultrasound waves and appears lighter or brighter than surrounding tissue and includes keratin and bone or calcified lesions. Anechoic lesion appears black and generally includes fluid-filled lesions.

Imaging parameters and the frequency of the acoustic energy released from the transducer can be adjusted; however, as the frequency increases, the depth to which it penetrates decreases. In dermatology, the most useful ultrasound transducer frequencies are up to 15 mHz (high frequency), which aids in visualizing the depth of skin tumors, and the 7.5–14 mHz, which can be used to visualize lymph nodes. For better images acoustically conductive gel is used to move the face of the transducer away from the surface of the skin.

Imaging is in real time and can include measurements of vascularity and quantitative blood flow because of the Doppler effect created by the moving blood through the vasculature included in the field of view. Blood flow evaluation and specific parameters are related to high metastatic rates and angiogenesis of skin tumors. Ultrasound can identify areas of tumor extension/invasion and is also useful for assessment of regional lymph node groups and is significantly more sensitive than CT alone to evaluate suspicious nodes and guide minimally invasive needle sampling.

Advantages include not only the real-time images reconstructions but also the lack of ionizing radiation. The procedure is entirely noninvasive, is painless, does not require confinement or immobilization of the patients, has no risk of adverse reaction to contrast agents, and allows for positioning, dynamic maneuvers, wide survey examination, easy contralateral comparison, and interaction with the patient. HFUS is the least costly modality, mobile, and suitable for use with ancillary equipment, such as needle guides and cryogenic probes, good for intraprocedural imaging and image-guided procedures.

A common problem encountered with ultrasound is an overestimation of the tumor thickness mainly due to an inflammatory infiltration seen under the melanoma that produces a hypoechoic area that cannot be differentiated from the hypoechoic area generated by the melanoma itself [1, 2, 4, 12, 14].

Current Applications

Knowing the functioning bases, advantages, and disadvantages of noninvasive imaging exams, it is then possible to have precise indications and applications at different stages in the evaluation of skin tumors. This includes diagnosis or "first" diagnosis (identification of the lesion and therefore its topographical position, characterization or differential diagnosis of the lesion, in the sense of nontumor vs. tumor, benign vs. malignant, and primary vs. metastatic), staging (evaluation of the spread of the disease, not only for the purposes of completing the diagnosis but also for treatment and prognosis), treatment planning (including an evaluation of operability), the evaluation of response during and after treatment (both in the short term for the judgment of radicality, the identification of residual tumor, and the exclusion of complications and in the long term for follow-up), and the identification of recurrence [14, 15].

Diagnosis and Pretreatment Assessment

Appropriate pretreatment assessment of tumor extent can help choosing the best therapeutic option and reducing the extent of surgical defects. This includes diagnosis or "first" diagnosis with identification and evaluation of the lesion and therefore its measurements (submillimetric and in three dimensions), topographical position in skin layers or tissues/structures, and characterization or differential diagnosis of the lesion, in the sense of nontumor vs. tumor, benign vs. malignant, and primary vs. metastatic. Staging is also included this time with evaluation of tissue invasion and the spread of the disease, not only for the purposes of completing the diagnosis but also for treatment and prognosis [15].

Tumor-Type Differentiation

There are some characteristics observed in radiological noninvasive imaging exams that allow the characterization and differential diagnosis of the most probable histological type of skin tumor.

Basal Cell Carcinoma (BCC)

The non-melanoma skin cancers (NMSCs) have been described on contrast-enhanced CT imaging as infiltrative soft-tissue lesions that exhibit heterogeneous enhancement (Fig. 12.1). On MRI, these show hypointense signal intensity on T1-weighted images compared with muscle, heterogeneously hyperintense signal intensity on T2-weighted images, and enhancement after IV gadolinium-based contrast agent administration (Fig. 12.2). NMSCs are usually non-FDG-avid lesions on PET-CT, except in cases of locally aggressive behavior with perineural spread or soft-tissue involvement (Fig. 12.3) [5].

On B mode ultrasound, BCCs often appear as oval, bulging, or band-like hypoechoic dermal and/or hypodermal lesion with slightly irregular borders that commonly presents hyperechoic spots (Fig. 12.4). These spots are correlated to the presence of compact nests of neoplastic cells, and the presence of seven or more hyperechoic spots (Fig. 12.5) within the lesion has been associated with BCC histologic subtypes having a high risk of recurrences, such as micronodular, sclerosing, infiltrating, morpheiform, and metatypical subtypes. The low risk of recurrence histologic subtypes include macronodular or nodular, superficial, adenoid cystic, and

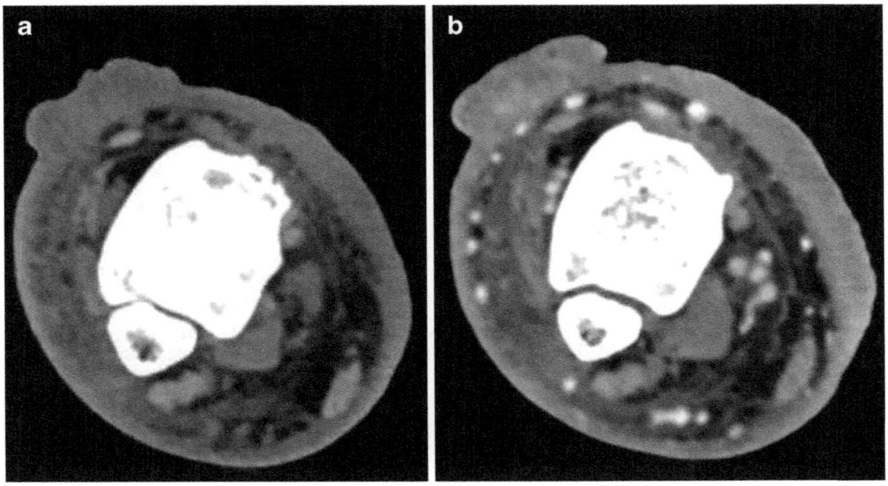

Fig. 12.1 Axial CT images (soft tissue) before (**a**) and after (**b**) intravenous injection of contrast showing a basal cell carcinoma in the left leg that appears as a soft-tissue lesions that exhibit heterogeneous enhancement, similar to the others non-melanoma skin cancers

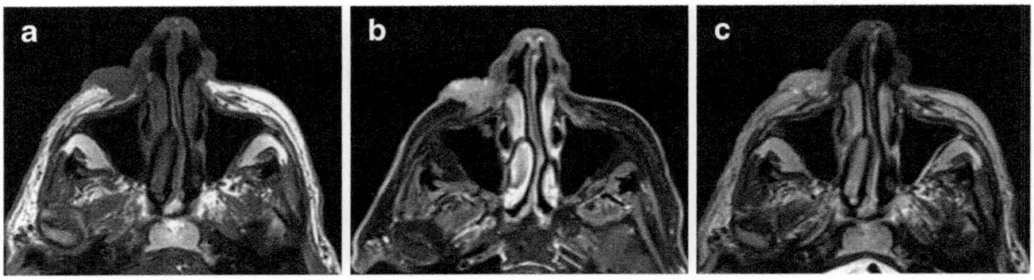

Fig. 12.2 Axial MRI images showing a basal cell carcinoma in the right nasolabial fold, with hypointense signal intensity on T1-weighted images (**a**) compared with muscle, heterogeneously hyperintense signal intensity on T2-weighted images (**b**), and enhancement after IV gadolinium-based contrast agent administration (**c**), similar to the others non-melanoma skin cancers

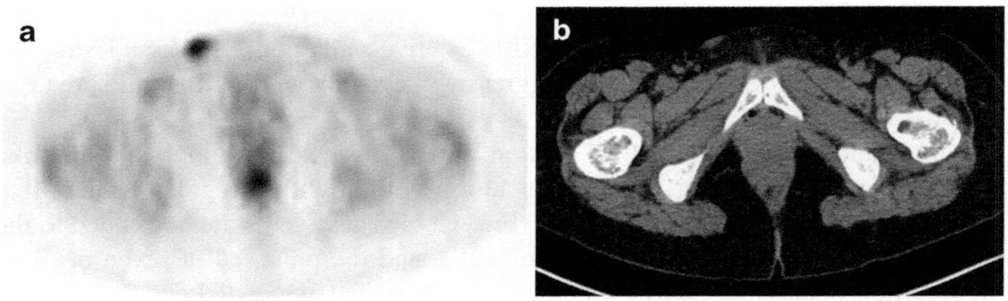

Fig. 12.3 Axial PET/FDG (**a**) and CT (**b**) image of a basal cell carcinoma in pubic region that appears as FDG-avid lesions on PET/FDG with an average standardized uptake value (SUV) of 5.7

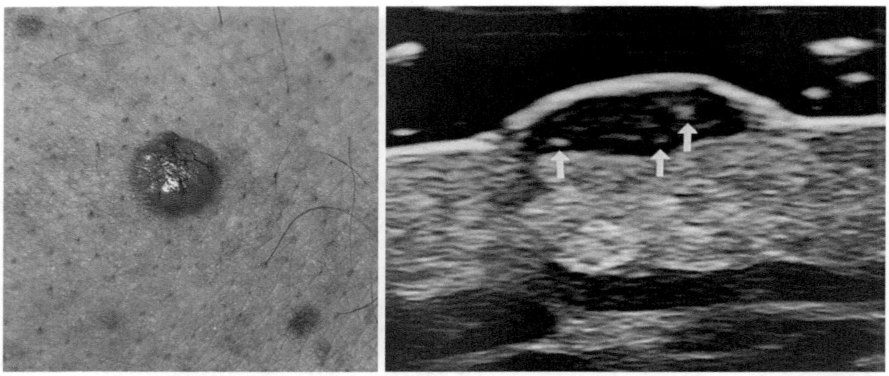

Fig. 12.4 Clinical and B mode HFUS (24 MHz) image of a basal cell carcinoma, that appears as oval/hypoechoic dermal lesion with presents hyperechoic spots (arrows)

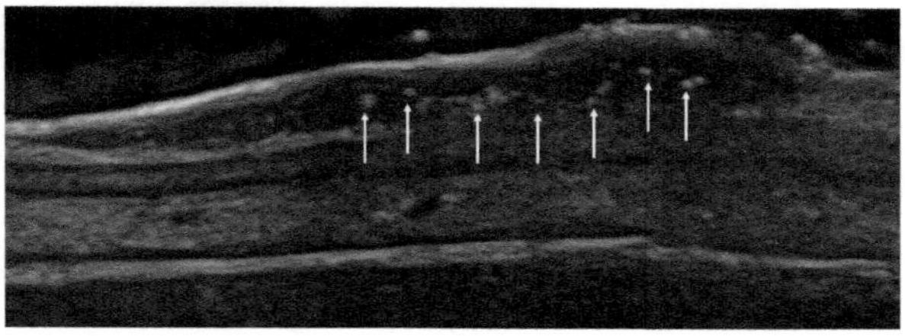

Fig. 12.5 B mode HFUS (33 MHz) image of a basal cell carcinoma, that appears as oval/hypoechoic dermal lesion with more than seven hyperechoic spots within the lesion (arrows), that is been associated with BCC histologic subtypes having a high risk of recurrences

Pinkus fibroepithelioma. There are mixed types of BCC with the high and low risk of recurrence subtypes in the same lesion. Knowledge of this can support the choice of the site of biopsy and/or the type of surgery. On color Doppler ultrasound, there is low to moderate vascularity within or at the bottom of the lesion, with low-velocity arterial and/or venous vessels.

Ultrasound is the best method to evaluate primary NMSCs lesions, with measurements and invasion detection. BCCs rarely metastasize (0.1%) and usually have slow growth and indolent behavior; therefore, it is generally not necessary to perform other imaging exams, unless there is suspicion of local invasion, with infiltration of cartilage, fascia, and periosteum; in these cases, resonance may be indicated [2, 14, 16–25].

Squamous Cell Carcinoma (SCC)

In general, SCCs have been described in the same way of BCC on contrast-enhanced CT (Fig. 12.6) and MR imaging (Fig. 12.7) and on PET-CT but with higher FDG uptake (Fig. 12.8) as NMSCs [5].

On B mode ultrasound, SCCs often appear as hypoechoic dermal and/or hypodermal structure, generally more exophytic or with deep layers involvement. On color Doppler ultrasound, a moderate increase in the blood flow may be detected within and at the periphery of the lesion (Fig. 12.9) [2, 18].

SCC also has a low chance of metastasis (2–6%), but greater than BCC. Scar lesions and in immunosuppressed patients have a greater chance of metastasis. Imaging examinations are indicated in thick lesions (up to 2–6 millimeters (mm)) and diameter greater than 2.0 centimeters (cm). Sonography may be considered the initial modality of choice for local staging and assessment of regional lymph nodes. Tumor depth is of critical importance in identifying high-risk cutaneous squamous cell carcinoma and should be reported in all cases. CT, MRI, and PET-CT are helpful for surgical staging, especially to detect neural or bone invasion [2, 5, 14, 26–32].

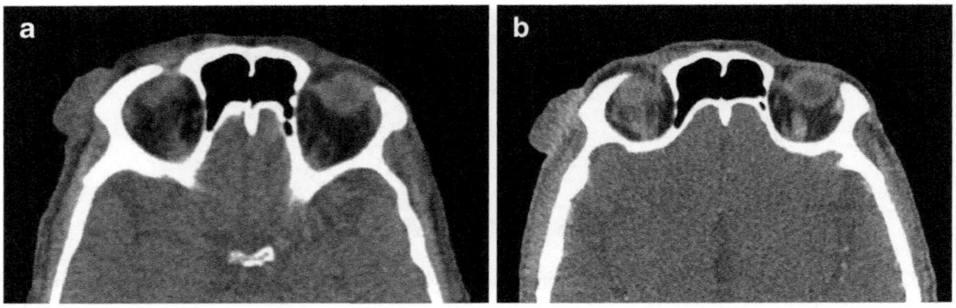

Fig. 12.6 Axial CT images (soft tissue) before (**a**) and after (**b**) intravenous injection of contrast showing a squamous cell carcinoma in right frontotemporal region that appears as infiltrative soft-tissue lesions that exhibit heterogeneous enhancement, similar to the others non-melanoma skin cancers. Same patient in Figs. 12.8 and 12.9

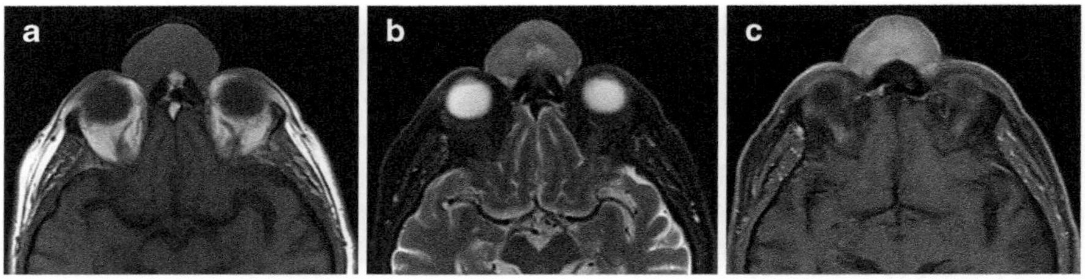

Fig. 12.7 Axial MRI images showing a nasal squamous cell carcinoma with hypointense signal intensity on T1-weighted images (**a**) compared with muscle, heterogeneously hyperintense signal intensity on T2-weighted images (**b**), and enhancement after IV gadolinium-based contrast agent administration (**c**), similar to the others non-melanoma skin cancers

Merkel Cell Carcinoma (MCC)

Merkel cell carcinoma lesions have been described on contrast-enhanced CT as isoattenuating to hyperattenuating cutaneous and subcutaneous masses relative to adjacent skeletal muscle with avid enhancement (Fig. 12.10). On MRI, they usually appear as homogeneous lesions with slight hyperintense signal intensity on T1-weighted images, hyperintense signal intensity on T2-weighted images as compared with skeletal muscle, and enhancement on gadolinium-enhanced images. Reported findings in MCC include numerous subcutaneous lymphatic nodular metastases in a typical row configuration, reticular subcutaneous fat stranding from lymphatic spread, and enlarged draining metastatic lymph nodes with compressed thin fatty hila. On PET-CT, Merkel cell carcinomas are usually FDG avid and may be used for detection of primary tumor and whole-body staging of nodal and distant metastases.

On B mode ultrasound, SCCs often appear as ill-defined hypoechoic dermal and/or hypodermal tumor that shows intense hypervascularity on color Doppler and can invade deeper layers (Fig. 12.11).

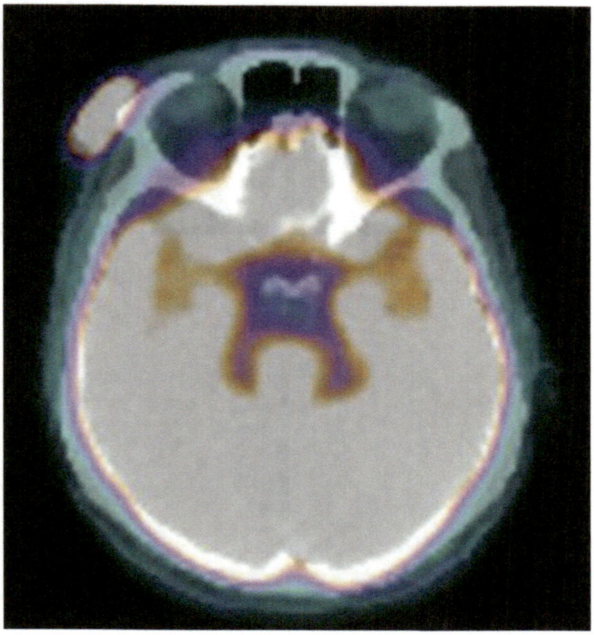

Fig. 12.8 Axial PET-CT image of a squamous cell carcinoma in right frontotemporal region that appears as FDG-avid lesions on with an average standardized uptake value (SUV) of 12.6. Same patient in Figs. 12.6 and 12.9

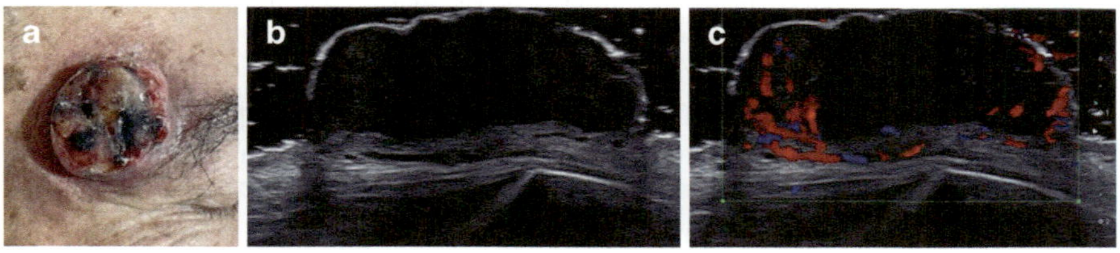

Fig. 12.9 Clinical aspect (**a**) of a squamous cell carcinoma in the right frontotemporal region. HFUS (24 MHz) images showing hypoechoic exophytic dermal structure on B mode (**b**) and a moderate increase in the blood flow at the periphery of the lesion on Doppler ultrasound (**c**). Same patient in Figs. 12.6 and 12.8

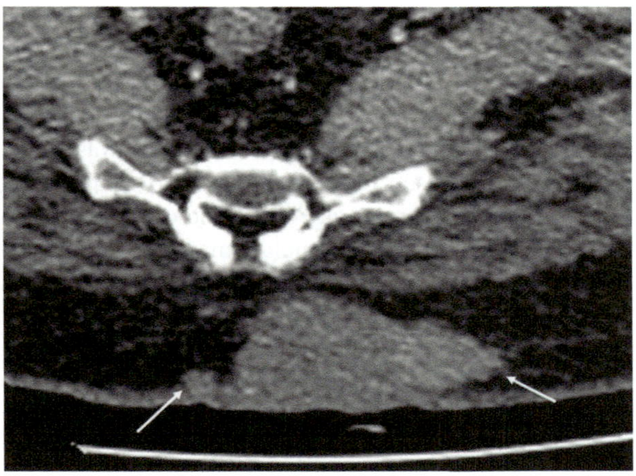

Fig. 12.10 Axial enhanced-CT image (soft tissue window) of a Merkel cell carcinoma (arrows) that appears as isoattenuating cutaneous and subcutaneous mass relative to adjacent skeletal muscle with contrast enhancement

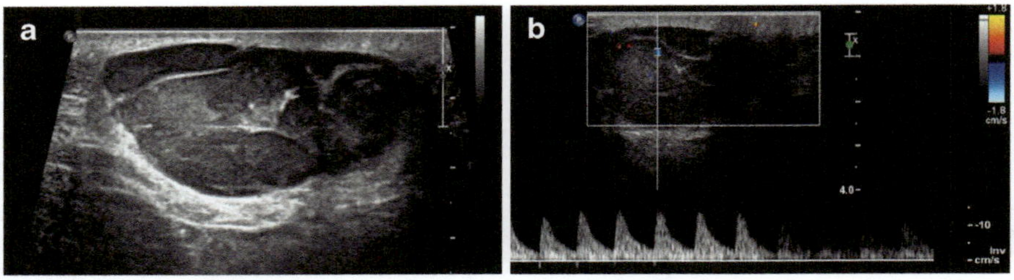

Fig. 12.11 Ultrasound (12 MHz) images of a Merkel cell carcinoma that appears as ill-defined hypoechoic hypodermal tumor on B mode (**a**) that shows internal arterial vascularity on Doppler (**b**)

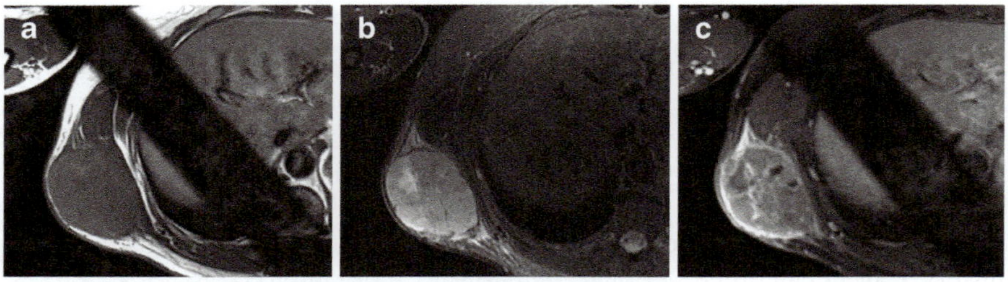

Fig. 12.12 Axial MRI images showing a dorsal melanoma that appears as slightly hyper/isointense lesion on T1-weighted image (**a**), heterogeneous sign on T2-weighted image (**b**) and enhancement after gadolinium-based contrast agent administration (**c**)

CT, MRI, and PET-CT are helpful for surgical staging and posttreatment follow-up of MCC. MRI is particularly useful for local staging and to evaluate for metastases to the brain, spine, bone marrow, and liver. PET-CT is currently the imaging modality of choice for the evaluation of Merkel cell carcinoma in both primary staging and restaging. Sonography is also considered to be the initial modality of choice for local staging and assessment of regional lymph nodes [2, 5, 14, 18, 33].

Melanoma

On MRI, melanoma generally appears as hyperintense lesions on T1-weighted images because of melanin, with restricted diffusion on diffusion-weighted imaging and enhancement after gadolinium-based contrast agent administration (Fig. 12.12). CT is not often used for skin melanoma evaluations, but can show bigger lesions (Fig. 12.13). Melanomas are FDG avid on PET-CT (Fig. 12.14).

On B mode ultrasound, melanoma often appears as hypoechoic and commonly fusiform-shaped dermal and/or hypodermal structure with prominent hypervascularity that is within and at the periphery of the tumors on color Doppler (Fig. 12.15). Melanoma metastasis commonly shows hypervascularity on color Doppler. Satellite (metastatic lesions within 2.0 cm from the primary tumor) and in-transit metastases usually follow the path of the lymphatic and venous drainage of the tumor and appear as oval-shaped, hypoechoic hypodermal structures commonly surrounded by hyperechoic hypodermal fatty tissue (Fig. 12.16).

Although it is an uncommon tumor, melanoma is the most lethal skin cancer and is considered to be very aggressive because of its ability to metastasize in early stages of the disease. The choice for the use of imaging tests in the staging of patients undergoing surgery or newly diagnosed should take into account the risk of synchronous metastatic disease. The evaluation of the primary tumor, considering

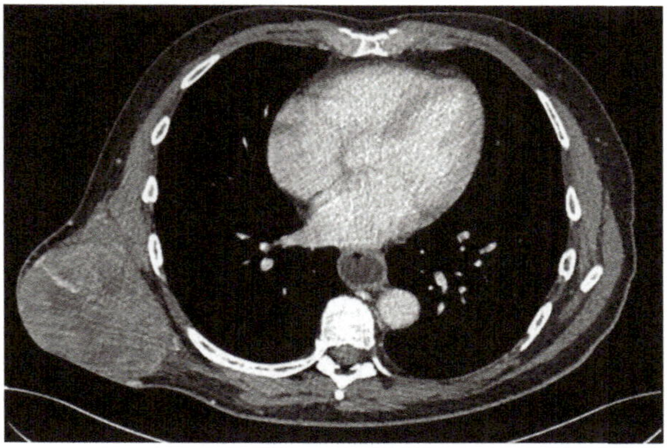

Fig. 12.13 Axial enhanced-CT image (soft tissue window) of dorsal melanoma that appears as heterogeneous cutaneous and subcutaneous mass with contrast enhancement

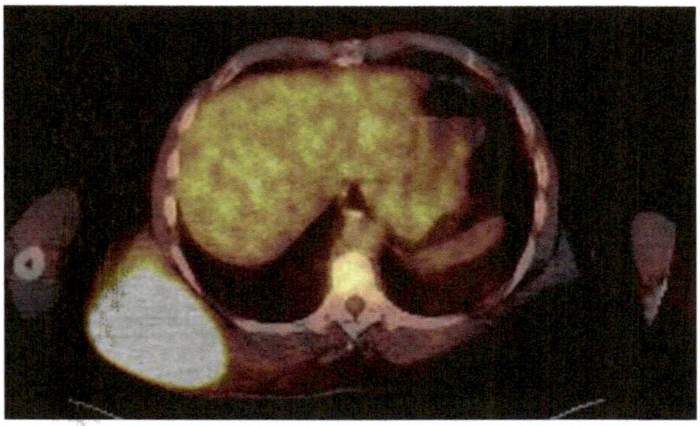

Fig. 12.14 Axial PET-CT image of a dorsal melanoma that appears as FDG-avid lesions on with an maximum standardized uptake value (SUV) of 14.3

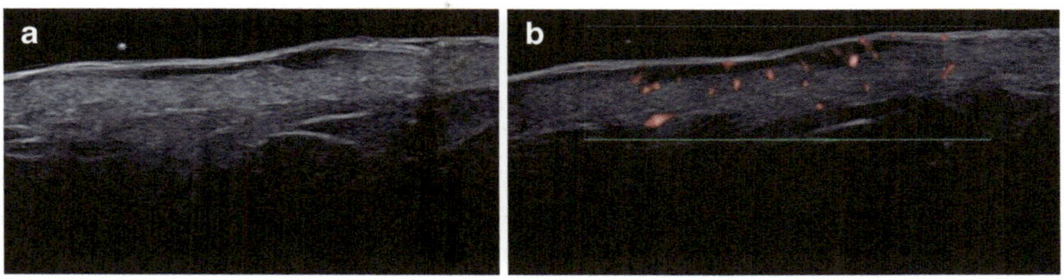

Fig. 12.15 Ultrasound (33 MHz) images of a melanoma that appears as appear as hypoechoic fusiform-shaped dermal structure on B mode (**a**) with prominent hypervascularity is within and at the periphery of the tumors on Doppler (**b**)

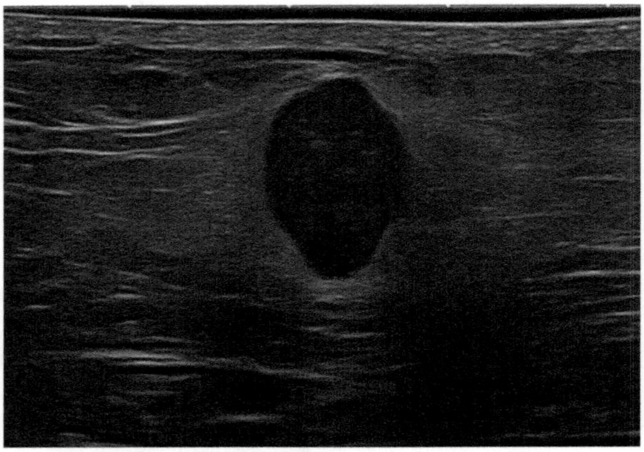

Fig. 12.16 B mode HFUS (24 MHz) image showing in-transit metastases of melanoma that appear as oval-shaped, hypoechoic hypodermal structures surrounded by hyperechoic hypodermal fatty tissue

Breslow, ulceration, and nodal involvement (including the measurement of tumor extension), among other variables, allows an estimation of the risk. Thoracic, abdominal, and head and neck CT must be considered in initial evaluation. In patients with high risk of synchronous metastases, PET-CT is indicated, because it is more sensitive than CT or MRI for the detection of nodal and distant metastases. As melanoma lesions are strongly avid to FDG, PET-CT may be the imaging of choice for primary staging with high sensitivity to detect occult lesions, and for therapeutic response assessment, especially in the era of immunotherapy and targeted drugs.

Ultrasound may be used to evaluate the primary lesion. Measurement of thickness is related to Breslow and can help in surgical planning and staging. HFUS is also indicated to detect satellite and locoregional metastasis and can support guided fine-needle aspiration and biopsy for melanoma. Surveillance can avoid sentinel node biopsy or completion lymph node dissection [2, 5, 14, 18, 34–49].

Dermatofibrosarcoma Protuberans (DFSP)

Both CT and MRI are beneficial in evaluating the size, shape, and extent of DFSP. Primary DFSP usually appears as a well-defined noncalcified isoattenuating to hypoattenuating mass on CT (Fig. 12.17) and has nonspecific signal-intensity characteristics on MRI (Fig. 12.18), but with homogeneous enhancement on CT and MRI, with larger tumors revealing heterogeneity due to internal necrosis or degeneration. DFSP has in general low FDG uptake on PET-CT, which may not be considered in the imaging workup.

On B mode ultrasound, DFSP often appears as ill-defined, mixed-echogenicity mass with a hypoechoic dermal and/or hypodermal superficial part and a hyperechoic hypodermal region with convex borders or pseudopod-like areas. On color Doppler lesions tend to show a moderate presence of low-velocity arterial and venous vessels (Fig. 12.19).

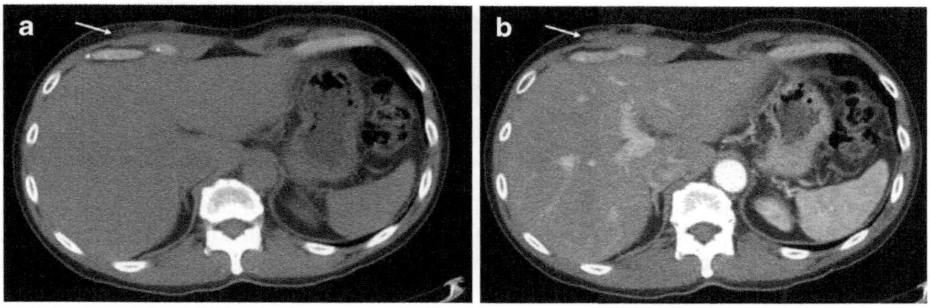

Fig. 12.17 Axial CT images (soft tissue) before (**a**) and after (**b**) intravenous injection of contrast showing a dermatofibrosarcoma protuberans in the right thoraco-abdominal wall that appears as ill-defined noncalcified hypoattenuating cutaneous and subcutaneous mass with contrast enhancement (arrow)

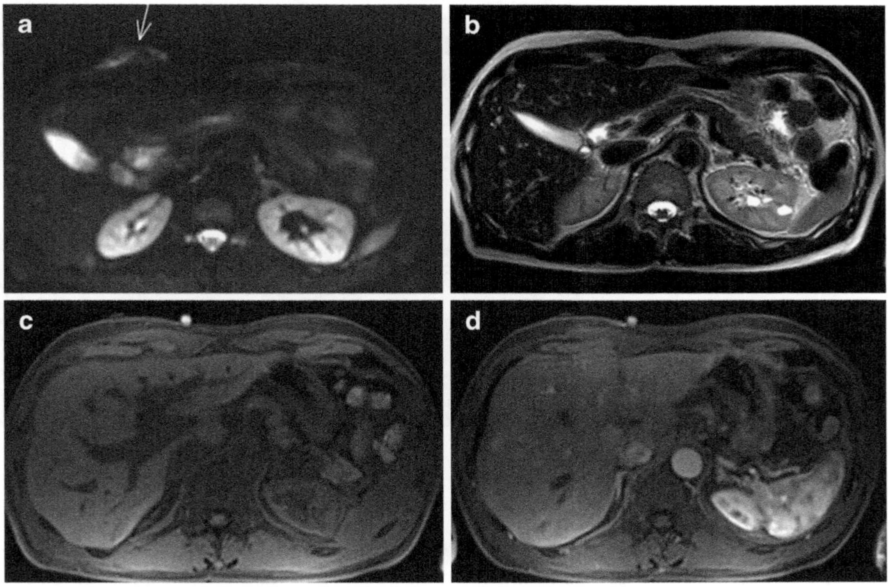

Fig. 12.18 Axial MRI images showing a dermatofibrosarcoma protuberans in the right thoraco-abdominal wall that appears as ill-defined lesion with high signal on diffusion (**a**: arrow), difficult to be characterized in other sequences (**b**: T2-weighted image; **c**: T1-weighted fat suppressed image), even after gadolinium-based contrast agent administration (**d**)

Despite uncommon regional nodal and distant metastases, DFSP exhibits a high predisposition for subcutaneous fat infiltration and local recurrence, can involve the fascial and muscular layers, and may present satellite metastases, thereby making preoperative imaging useful for adequate wide radical excision of the tumor [2, 5, 14, 18, 50–53].

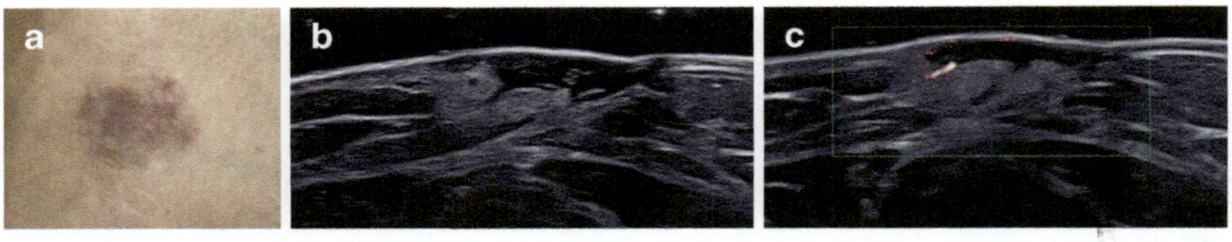

Fig. 12.19 Clinical image of a dermatofibrosarcoma protuberans (**a**). On B mode ultrasound (24 MHz) DFSP appears as ill-defined, mixed-echogenicity mass with a hypoechoic dermal and hypodermal superficial part and a hyperechoic hypodermal region with convex borders or pseudopods-like areas (**b**). On Doppler lesions show a moderate presence of vascularity (**c**)

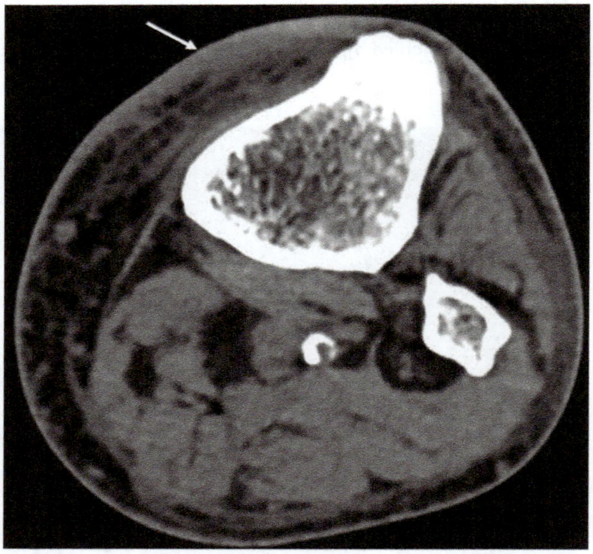

Fig. 12.20 Axial CT image (soft tissue) showing a cutaneous lymphoma in the left leg that appears as plaque like lesion characterized as skin thickening forming plaques (arrow)

Lymphoma

Primary cutaneous lymphoma (PCL) is an uncommon form of extranodal non-Hodgkin's lymphoma. CT scan shows cutaneous nodules and plaque-like lesions (Fig. 12.20), but the papular lesions could not be clearly demarcated. Although the clinical findings are difficult to assess with imaging and may be characterized as skin thickening in a nodular-like pattern or forming plaques, the extent of skin thickening or a skin mass can be evaluated in detail with CT, MRI, or PET-CT, and a comparison with previous imaging allows assessment of treatment response. These methods can also provide important information regarding tumor thickness, size, local extent, and visceral and nodal involvement. In most types of PCL, the ability of FDG PET-CT to detect cutaneous involvement is poor, but it may demonstrate nodal and extranodal disease activity (Fig. 12.21).

On B mode ultrasound, cutaneous papules were seen as focal infiltrative lesions, and few of them coalesced later to form ill-defined pseudonodules. The cutaneous nodules appear as pseudonodules and nodules, and the cutaneous plaques as

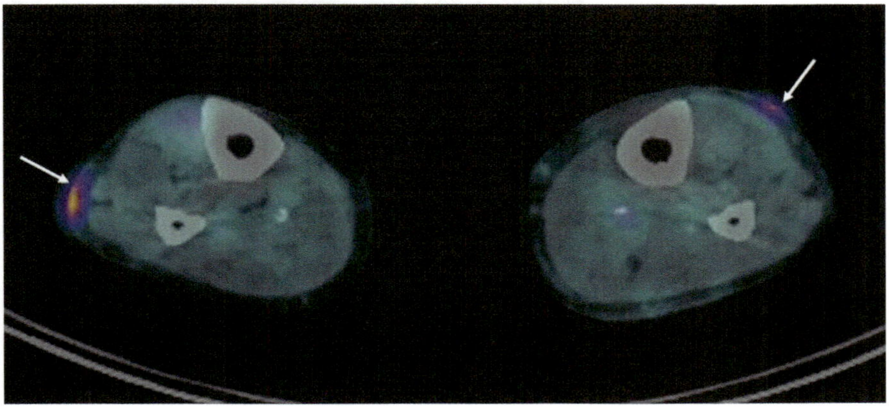

Fig. 12.21 Axial PET-CT image of a cutaneous lymphoma in the legs that appears as FDG-avid superficial cutaneous and subcutaneous lesions (arrows) with an maximum standardized uptake value (SUV) of 7.6

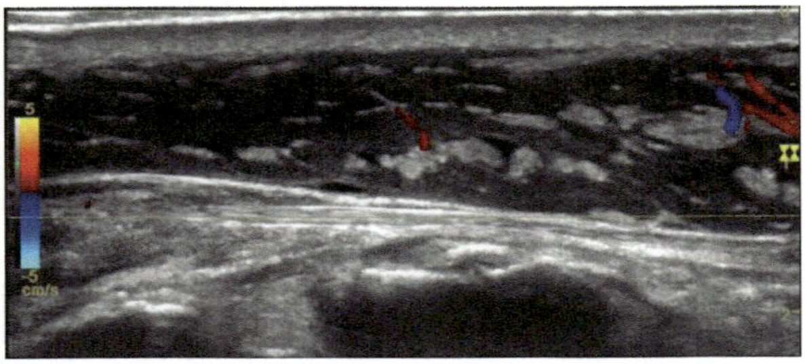

Fig. 12.22 Color Doppler (12 MHz) image of cutaneous lymphoma in the right leg that appears as thickening of dermis and diffusely infiltrate hypoechoic lesion in subcutaneous tissue with moderate vascularization

hypoechoic, diffusely infiltrative lesions. HFUS also reveals thickening of the dermis in all the cases. On color Doppler, the initial focal infiltrative lesions may be avascular, but the nodular, pseudonodular, and diffusely infiltrative lesions are highly vascular (Fig. 12.22).

The detection of extracutaneous involvement by imaging is crucial for therapy planning, because the 5-year survival rate decreases considerably with systemic dissemination. CT is useful in assessing pulmonary involvement and determining the benign nature of fatty hilum-containing lymph nodes. However, CT can be less accurate in assessing extracutaneous lymphomatous involvement in normal-sized lymph nodes, bone marrow, the spleen, and extranodal tissues [2, 5, 14, 18, 54].

Skin Metastasis

Cutaneous metastases are uncommon, occurring in 0.7–10% of internal malignancies and representing 2% of skin cancers; however these often indicate underlying widespread metastatic disease and a poor prognosis. Among women the common sites of origin are the breast, whereas in men is the lung. Cutaneous metastases can

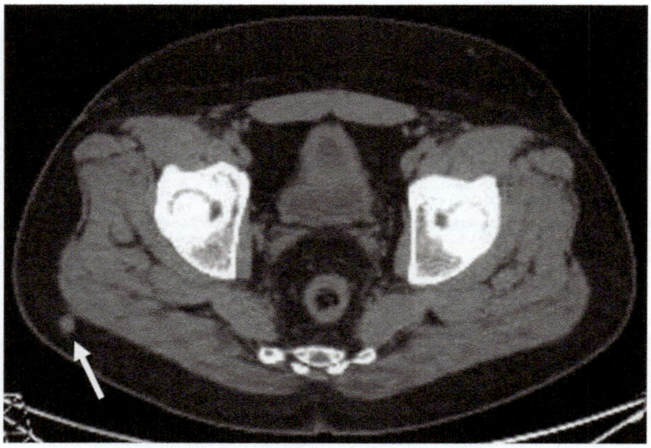

Fig. 12.23 Axial CT image (soft tissue) showing a cutaneous metastasis in the left dorsal subcutaneous tissue (arrow) and appears as small isoatenuating nodule to the muscle

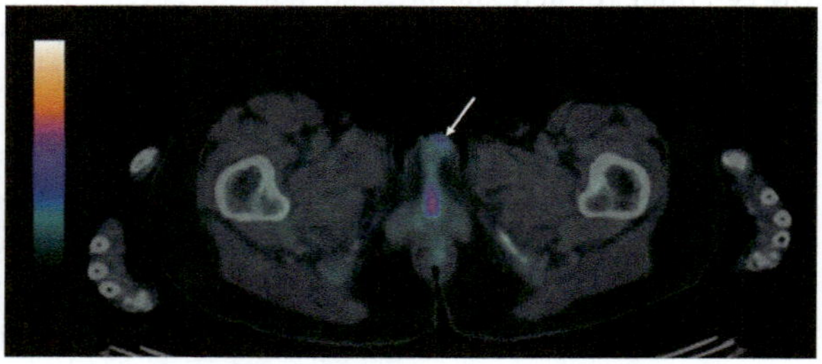

Fig. 12.24 Axial PET-CT image of a leiomyosarcoma cutaneous metastasis in the vulva that appears as FDG-avid superficial subcutaneous lesions (arrow) with an maximum standardized uptake value (SUV) of 5.2

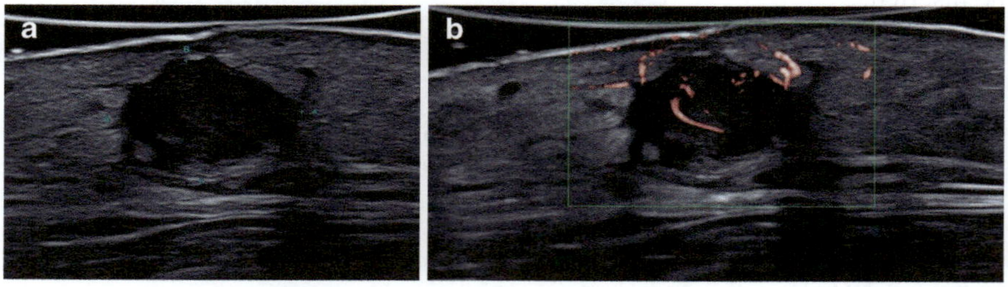

Fig. 12.25 Ultrasound imagens of cutaneous metastasis of melanoma that appears as on B mode ultrasound (24 MHz) as ill-defined hypoechoic hypodermal nodule (**a**) with peripheral and internal vascularity (**b**)

be from hematogenous spread, lymphatic spread, or tumor seeding from a previous surgical incision site.

Cutaneous and subcutaneous metastases most commonly present as multiple small (<2.0 cm) nodules or as an infiltrative mass with homogeneous or heterogeneous contrast enhancement on both CT and MRI (Fig. 12.23). On PET-CT, these manifest as FDG-avid skin thickening or subcutaneous nodules. PET-CT has higher sensitivity (Fig. 12.24) than CT and MRI in detecting metastases, but false-positive uptake may also be present. HFUS can be used to define the lesion and to guide biopsy (Fig. 12.25) [2, 5].

Treatment Planning and Staging

Imaging is an indispensable tool for the detection of local, nodal, and distant disease and staging of aggressive cutaneous neoplasms. Preoperative or pretreatment imaging of skin tumors should be considered for large, recurrent tumors with suspected subcutaneous involvement or in critical anatomic locations. HFUS and MRI are the modality of choice for imaging soft tissue because of its superior resolution. Imaging can play an important role in planning for reconstruction, particularly when muscle or other critical structures are involved.

Treatment planning depends on characteristics of the primary lesions and evidence of local, regional, or distant metastasis. Staging is made with evaluation of tissue invasion and the spread of the disease also for treatment planning and prognosis. CT, MRI, PET-CT, and HFUS can add information [2, 5, 6].

Margins and Size

Imaging scans can be used preoperatively to determine the tumor size, margins, and depth of extension or invasion of the skin tumors, parameters that will greatly impact in clinical (adjuvant or neoadjuvant therapy) and/or surgical planning, but results can be different when compared to histologic margins obtained at the time of surgery. HFUS has optimal and submillimetric resolution to evaluate skin tumors margins and size (Fig. 12.26), and even depth similar to Breslow, when performed with high-frequency transducers up to 22 MHz [2, 5, 6].

Invasiveness

BCC is rarely metastatic, but large or aggressive tumors can infiltrate critical anatomic structures, such as cartilage, vessels, nerves, and the orbit, most often in lesions located on the face. SCC can be more aggressive than BCC, with subcutaneous and bone invasion and lymph node metastasis. DFSP can also be more invasive

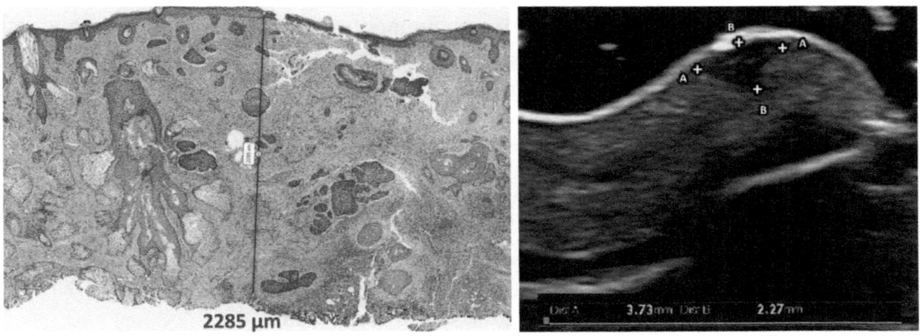

Fig. 12.26 B mode ultrasound imaging (33 MHz) measuring a cutaneous tumor thickness (2.27 mm) similar to biopsy findings (2.28 mm) in in the anatomopathological study

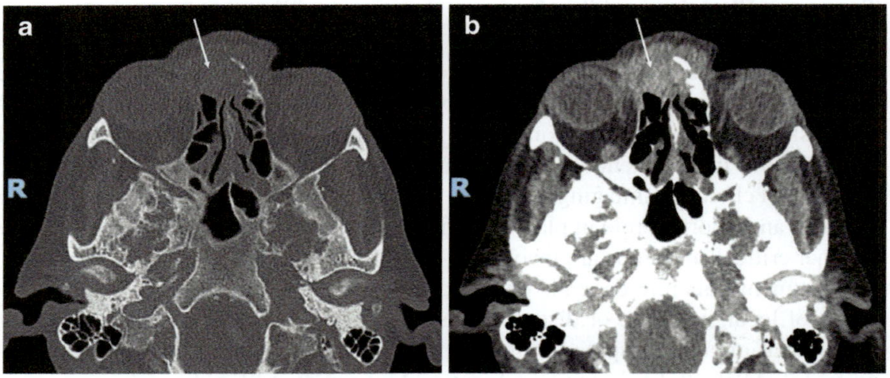

Fig. 12.27 Axial CT-enhanced images (**a**: bone; **b**: soft tissue) showing a nasal squamous cell carcinoma with bone invasion with loss of the expected architecture of cortical bone and bone destruction (arrows)

with skeletal muscle invasion. MCC is associated with a high rate of nodal and distant metastasis.

Infiltration of relevant anatomic structures, including fascia, muscles, cartilages, and bone cortex, can be effectively recognized using noninvasive imaging methods and help the surgeon for choosing a more aggressive approach [14].

Bone Invasion/Erosion

The presence of a firm, fixed tumor mass or focal tenderness over a bony margin is suspicious for bony invasion, and an imaging study is indicated in these cases. A CT scan is indicated when bony invasion by tumor is suspected, and it is the study of choice for the evaluation of cortical bone. Cortical invasion of the skull is typically manifested by loss of the expected architecture of cortical bone (Fig. 12.27). MRI scans provide better evaluation of the bone marrow and can detect abnormal enhancement or replacement of marrow fat by tumor, typically with lower T1 signal in tumor. Contrast-enhanced MRI can make tumor infiltration of bone less conspicuous, as the enhancing tumor is closer in signal to fatty marrow (Fig. 12.28) [4, 6]. Particularly in the head, where the subcutaneous layer is very thin, there is risk of bony involvement, and HFUS is an effective alternative to CT and MRI in establishing the presence of calvarium infiltration (Fig. 12.29) [14].

Neural Invasion/Nerve Spread

Detection of perineural pathology on imaging is relevant to overall staging and treatment planning and currently is optimally detected with MRI that is also most sensitive and superior to CT to identify perineural spread and subtle intracranial extension of the tumor, including meningeal involvement.

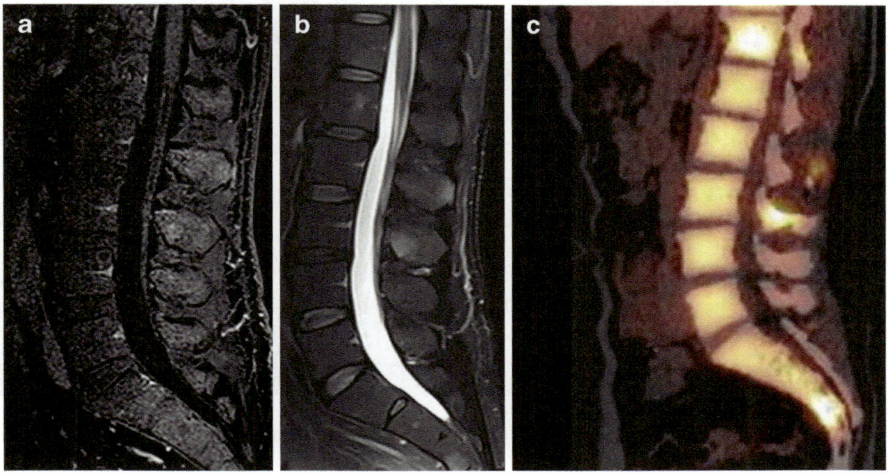

Fig. 12.28 Sagittal T1 + Gd (**a**), T2 + fat sat (**b**) and PET/CT (**c**). Patient with melanoma and bone infiltration tumor with contrast enhancement on posterior elements of L2 and L3 (**a**) with high signal on T2WI (**b**) and hypermetabolism on PET/CT (**c**)

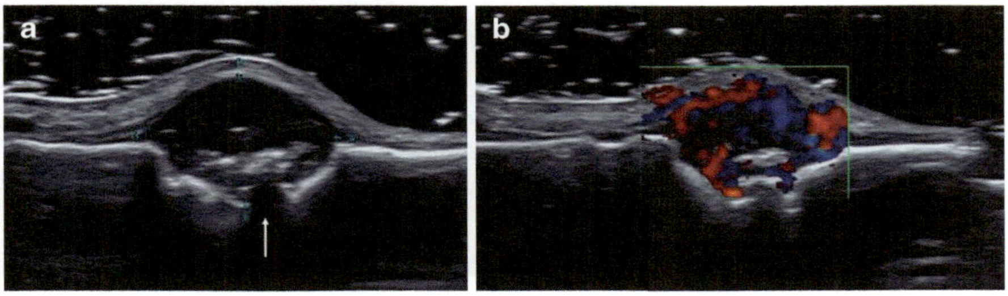

Fig. 12.29 Ultrasound images B mode (**a**) and color Doppler (**b**) showing signs of bone invasion with loss of the expected architecture of cortical bone and bone erosion/destruction (arrow)

In addition to defining tissue planes and determining depth of invasion, MRI is superior at identifying neurotropic tumors. MRI findings include direct (enlargement of the affected nerve or contrast enhancement along the nerve, enlargement or erosion of the associated bony foramina, loss of brightness in the perineural fat pads on the unenhanced T1-weighted image) and indirect findings (associated with muscle denervation) (Fig. 12.30). CT scan can also be useful in the detection of bony changes around the foramina or to evaluate the skull base. US-guided preoperative mapping of the lesion and the detection of relevant neurovascular structures close to the lesion can decrease the surgical risk and improve the cosmetic prognosis of the patient (Fig. 12.31) [4, 6, 14]. PET-CT may also play a role in detecting perineural spread of skin tumors, especially in those cases that the morphological change is subtle.

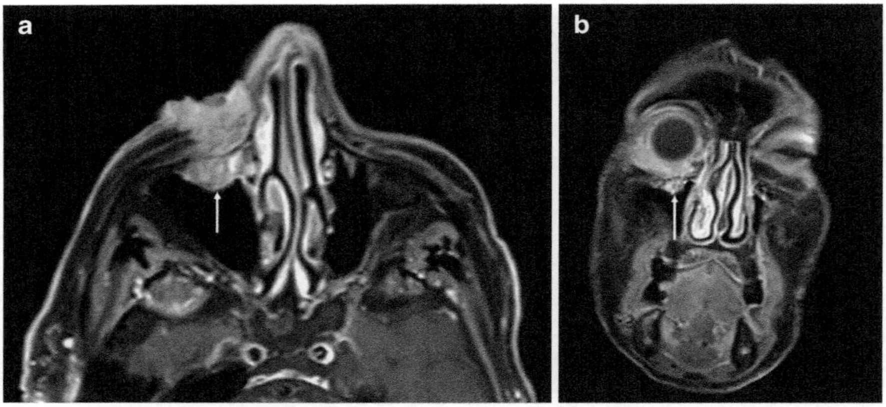

Fig. 12.30 Post-contrast MRI in axial (**a**) and coronal plane (**b**) showing signs of perineural spread/invasion of facial squamous cell carcinoma through right infraorbital nerve (arrows)

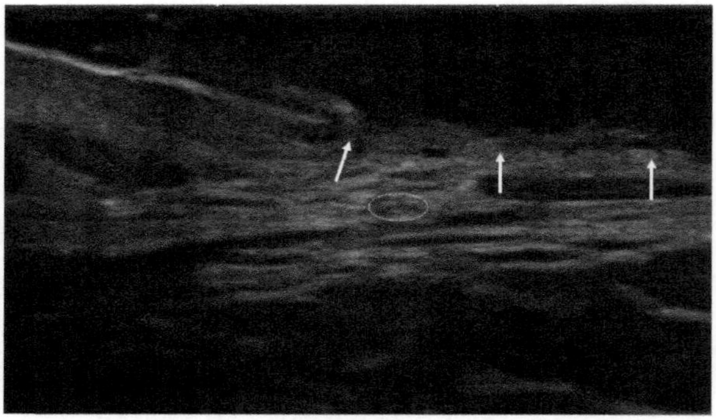

Fig. 12.31 Ultrasound B mode image showing detection of relevant neurovascular structure (dashed line), the temporal superficial nerve, close to the squamous cell carcinoma margins (arrows), without invasion

Orbital Invasion

BCC is the most common malignant periorbital skin tumor, and while orbital invasion is considered rare, it may occur in recurrent disease, incompletely excised medial canthal tumors, or less common, more aggressive histological subtypes. SCC is a less common periocular malignancy, but with regional involvement in between 1% and 24.3% of cases [55]. Accurate estimation for the presence of orbit invasion before surgery can help surgeons to choose appropriate surgical approach, involvement of the anterior portion of the orbit may be treated with excision and radiation therapy, while bulbar or extensive orbital invasion may require exenteration. Painful, fixed tumors involving the orbital rim or medial canthus or reduced ocular mobility and displacement of the globe should prompt imaging to evaluate orbital invasion. Aggressive skin cancers in the orbital region can invade the orbit by direct extension into orbital contents or retrograde perineural spread [6, 56].

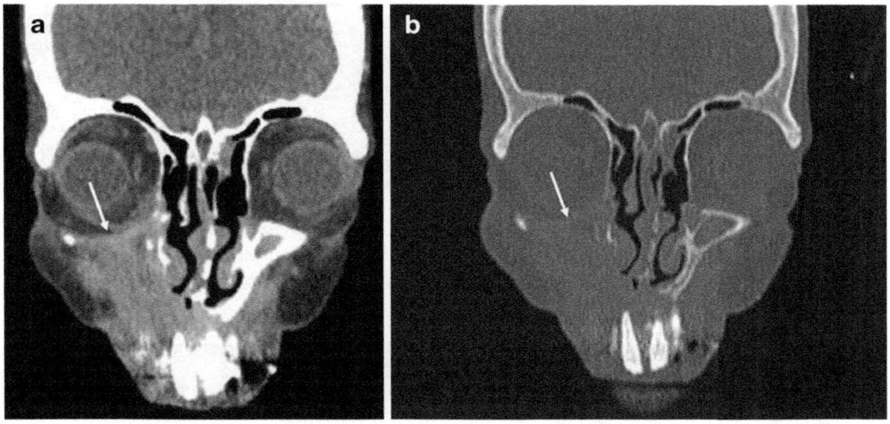

Fig. 12.32 Coronal CT images (**a**: soft tissue; **b**: bone) showing a nasal basal cell carcinoma with orbital bone invasion characterized by loss of the expected architecture of cortical bone and bone destruction (arrows)

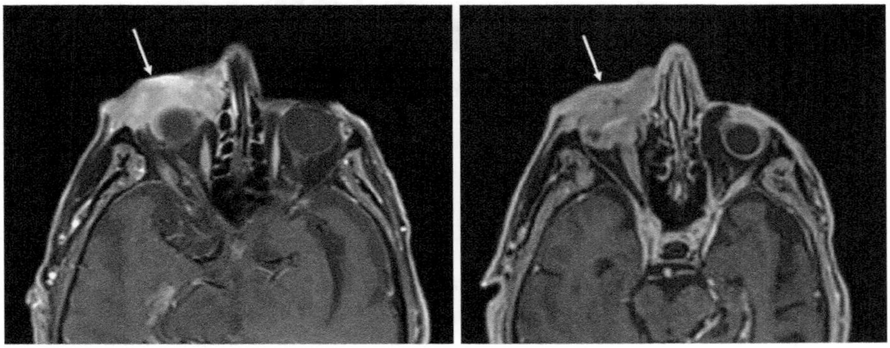

Fig. 12.33 Post-contrast MRI images of the same patient showing signs of orbital invasion of facial squamous cell carcinoma (arrows)

CT scans are appropriate for evaluating the bony margins of the orbit (Fig. 12.32), while soft-tissue invasion and perineural spread are better detected by a MRI scan (T1-weighted contrast-enhanced fat-suppressed images are performed for optimal visualization) (Fig. 12.33). PET-CT aids physiological and functional information that can be used to complement morphological findings obtained from conventional imaging, thereby aiding noninvasive tissue characterization. Because of the superficial location of the globe and its cystic nature, HFUS with Doppler allows accurate evaluation and enables noninvasive and cost-effective follow-up and can aid information with dynamic orbital evaluation (Fig. 12.34) [6, 55, 56].

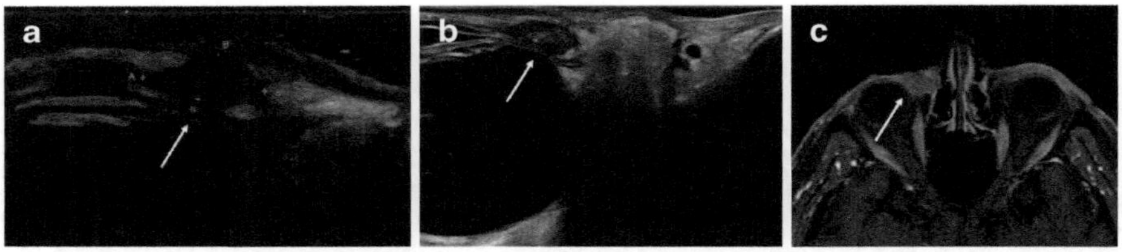

Fig. 12.34 HFUS imaging in sagittal (**a**) and axial (**b**) plane showing signs of orbital invasion of a basal cell carcinoma lesion in the medial cantus of the right eye (arrows). Post-contrast MRI image (**c**) of the same patient showing the same signs of orbital invasion (arrow)

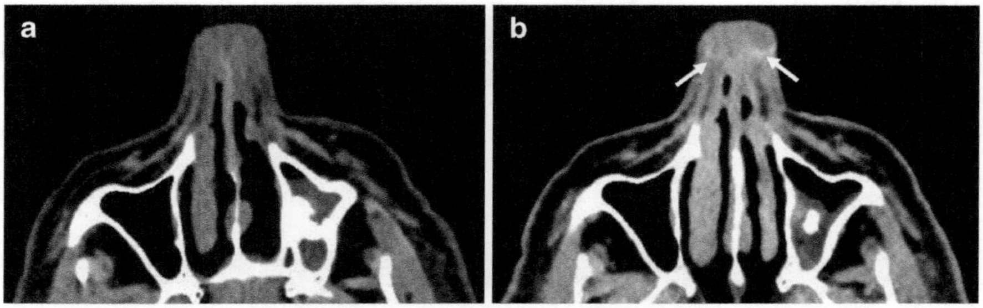

Fig. 12.35 Axial CT images (soft tissue) before (**a**) and after (**b**) intravenous injection of contrast showing a squamous cell carcinoma in the nose that appears as ill-defined hypoattenuating cutaneous and subcutaneous mass with contrast enhancement (arrow) and signs of cartilage invasion

Cartilage Invasion

The skin overlying the nose cartilage is a particularly frequent localization of skin carcinoma (about 25% of all carcinomas occurring on the head and neck). It is therefore of great practical interest diagnosing cartilage invasion for making treatment-related decisions, to best plan skin tumors therapy, able to combine effectiveness with a good cosmetic and functional result.

MR imaging has a high sensitivity and high negative predictive value for detecting cartilage invasion compared with conventional CT. Cartilage invasion was "positive" in cases in which the cartilage displayed signals similar to those of the adjacent tumor on all pre- and postcontrast T1- and T2-weighted images. When the cartilage had higher signal intensity than the adjacent tumor on T2-weighted images or when stronger enhancement was present on postcontrast T1-weighted images. On CT, the most sensitive criterion of neoplastic invasion of these cartilages is cartilage sclerosis. It is also possible to observe superficial irregularities, erosion or lysis of cartilage, and even transcartilaginous extension of tumors (Fig. 12.35). Destruction of cartilage is a significant risk factor for metastatic disease [57–62]. HFUS can also detect cartilage invasion especially in facial skin tumors, showing cartilage irregularities or transcartilaginous extension of tumors (Fig. 12.36) [2].

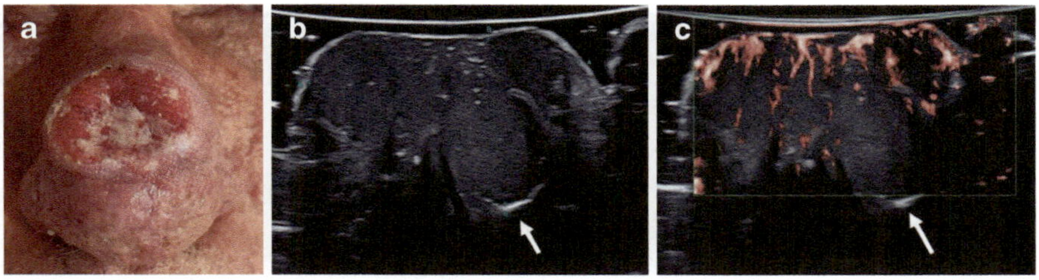

Fig. 12.36 Clinical image of a squamous cell carcinoma in the nose (**a**). Ultrasound (24 MHz) images showing hypoechoic dermal structure on B mode (**b**) and a moderate increase in the blood flow at the periphery of the lesion on Doppler ultrasound (**c**) with signs of cartilage invasion (arrow)

Metastasis

Cutaneous malignancies differ in their capacity for local invasion and metastases. Metastases can occur via hematogenous and lymphatic routes. BCCs rarely metastasize but rather tend to extend locally along the periosteum, perichondrium, or fascia. SCCs have a low rate of distant metastasis (2–6% of cases) to lungs, bones, and the brain. Locoregional metastasis of SCC may be detected and can involve the paths of lymphatic drainage of the tumor. This is also true of DFSP, with rare distant metastasis (less than 5% of cases), mostly to the lung and regional lymph nodes, and rarely with extensive metastases. MCC is an aggressive tumor that frequently metastasizes to regional nodes, mostly to cervical, inguinal, and pelvic nodes and distant sites, including distant nodes, the skin, lung, liver, brain, and bones. Melanoma commonly metastasizes via lymphatics to in-transit and satellite sites and regional lymph nodes. Cutaneous melanoma metastases are an important prognostic factor, and early recognition may be very beneficial for patients to access to new targeted therapies [5, 18].

Local

Local metastasis includes satellites and in-transit metastasis, common in melanoma. The lymphatic diffusion is termed "satellitosis," when the lesion develops within 2.0 cm from the primary cutaneous tumor (or its scar, if the tumor has already been excised), and as in-transit metastasis, when the lesion grows at a greater distance.

It is commonly seen in the subcutaneous and soft-tissue locations. On CT these appear as well-defined 0.5–2.5 cm isoattenuating mostly homogeneously enhancing subcutaneous nodules, with an occasional heterogeneous appearance after internal necrosis. On MRI, melanoma lesions generally appear as hyperintense lesions on T1-weighted images, with restricted diffusion and enhancement after IV gadolinium-based contrast agent administration. On HFUS these lymphatic metastases appear as solid, hypoechoic, and well-circumscribed or irregular contours nodules (Fig. 12.16), with posterior shadowing and internal vascular signals at

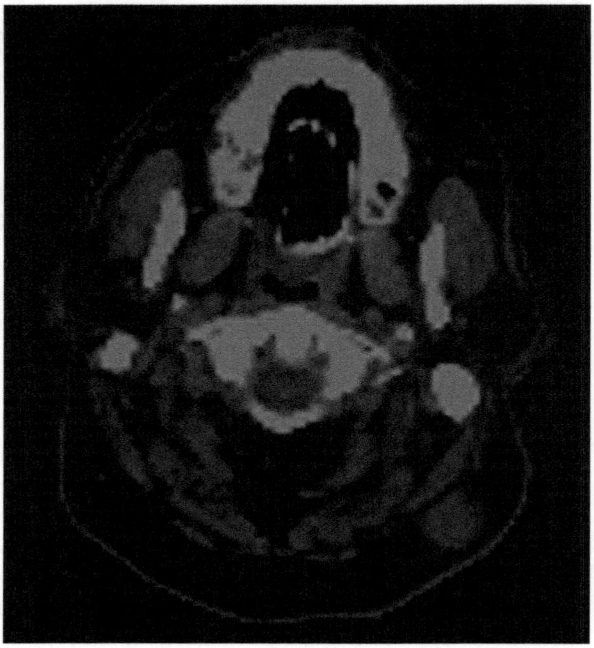

Fig. 12.37 Patient with scalp melanoma with an occipital lymph node with hypermetabolism on PET/CT suspect for satellite lesion

power-Doppler imaging. The presence of internal fluid areas appears to be related to necrosis and is therefore more common in larger lesions.

Satellite lesions are best evaluated with ultrasound or PET-CT (Fig. 12.37). PET-CT is superior to CT and MRI scans and may play a relevant role in the detection of the exact number, size, and location of in-transit metastases and may subsequently impact patient management and therapy-related decisions, but rarely detects metastatic disease smaller than 5.0 mm (the lower limit size resolution of PETs). US is capable of detecting a very significant number of in-transit or satellite metastases in subclinical/clinically negative patients, detecting small/submillimetric lesions, good for staging and better therapeutic planning [2, 45, 63–67].

Regional/Lymph Node

Computed tomography and magnetic resonance imaging scans are both used to evaluate lymph nodes (Fig. 12.38) and should be selected based on the imaging requirements of the primary site. Using a size cutoff of 1.0 cm, the sensitivity and specificity of CT and MRI scans are comparable. At subcentimeter sizes, irregular or intense enhancement, central necrosis, surrounding fat stranding, conglomerated nodes, and asymmetry can be used to suggest metastasis.

Overall, PET-CT is superior to other imaging modalities in the detection of nodal metastases, may detect smaller hypermetabolic nodes, and, thus, offers a more complete imaging evaluation of the regional spread (Fig. 12.39). We should be aware of

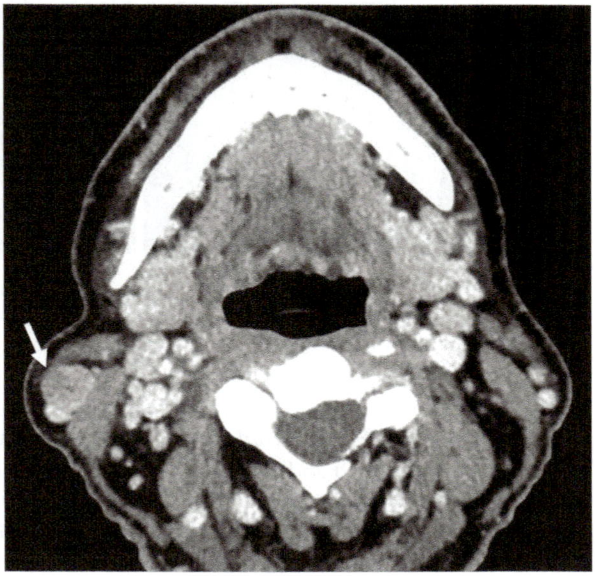

Fig. 12.38 Axial enhanced-CT image showing a small lymph node near, suspected for squamous cell carcinoma metastasis with an intense enhancement and central necrosis (arrow)

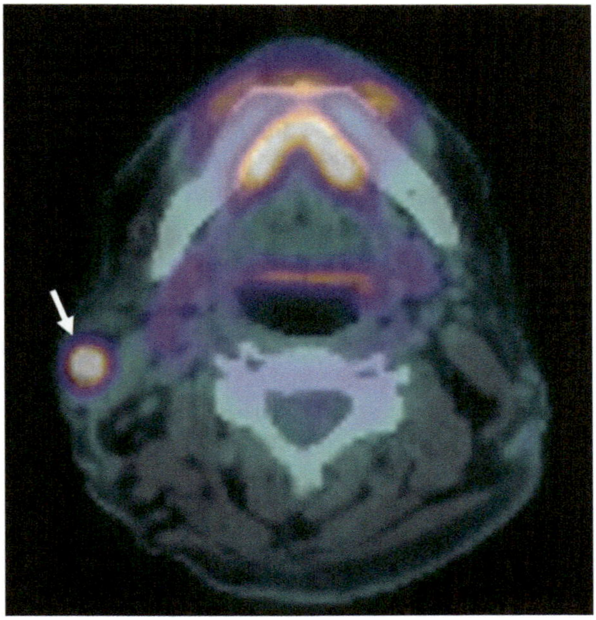

Fig. 12.39 Axial PET-CT image of a small hypermetabolic lymph node near right parotid gland, suspected for squamous cell carcinoma metastasis with an maximum standardized uptake value (SUV) of 11.2

false-positive lymph nodes, as FDG PET-CT presents high sensitivity and inflammatory/reactive lesions may appear.

Among the diagnostic imaging modalities for the assessments of lymph node metastasis, ultrasonography was superior to CT and PET-CT. US did have the

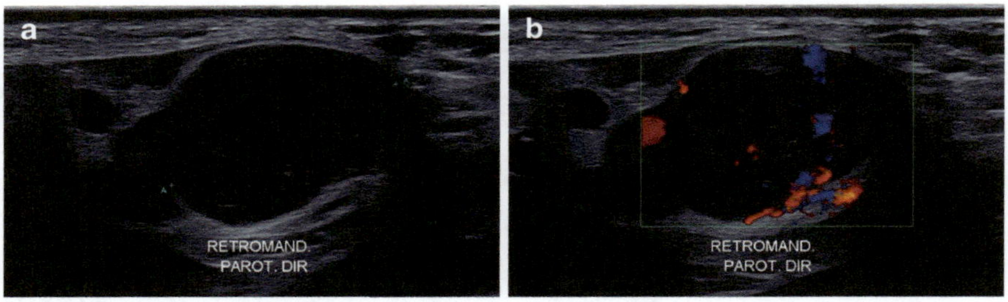

Fig. 12.40 HFUS (24 MHz) images of a intraparotid lymph node, suspected for squamous cell carcinoma metastasis, with round shape and loss of the echogenic hilum on B mode (**a**) and increased peripheral vascularity on Doppler (**b**)

highest sensitivity for screening of superficial regional lymph node basins. Benign lymph nodes are ovoid or flat in the long axis and typically display an echogenic hilum with bidirectional flow in the hilum. In contrast, malignant nodes tend to be larger (more than 1.0 cm), rounder in shape, and display necrosis, calcification, and increased peripheral vascularity (Fig. 12.40). Loss of the echogenic hilum and of regular architecture may be noted. When suspicious lymph nodes are identified, fine-needle aspiration biopsy (FNAB) with US guidance can be used to sample them. The combination of preoperative ultrasound and fine-needle biopsy in select high-risk patients can, however, eliminate the need for sentinel lymph node biopsy by preoperatively identifying lymph node metastases, which indicate the need for therapeutic lymph node dissection. One of the major limitations with regard to lymph node evaluation is that US requires an acoustic window that limits the depth of evaluation because of bone and cannot reliably visualize retropharyngeal or nodes deeper in the head and neck [5–7, 48, 67].

Distant

PET-CT had the highest positive predictive value for the detection of distant metastasis. Distant metastases from hematogenous spread of skin cancers can occur often to the skin, soft tissues, lung, liver, bone, and brain. MRI has a special role in evaluating intracranial (Fig. 12.41), bone marrow, liver, and soft-tissue metastases. Contrast-enhanced CT is superior in assessing small pulmonary metastases (Fig. 12.42). Typical imaging of patients with suspected advanced disease may include brain MRI with contrast-enhanced CT of the thorax or PET-CT.

In the staging of melanoma, both whole-body MRI and PET-CT are considered more accurate than whole-body CT, with PET providing the added value of detecting in-transit or satellite metastatic lesions. With the addition of diffusion to whole-body MRI, whole-body MRI appears more accurate. PET-CT can be limited because

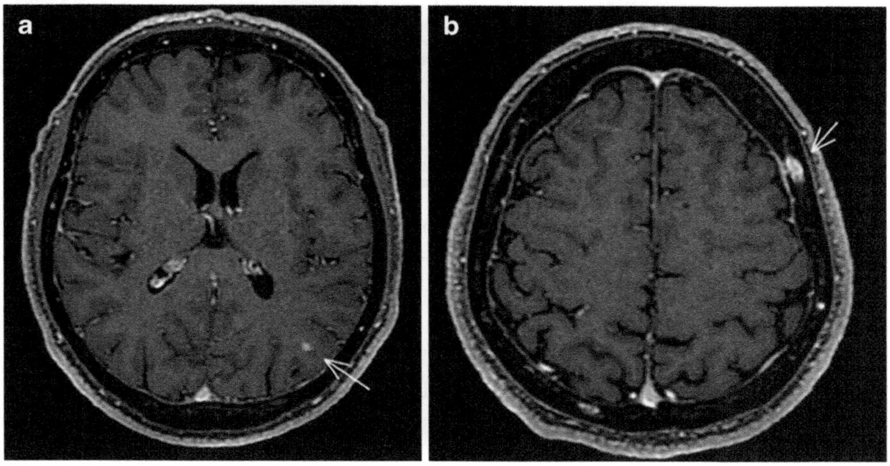

Fig. 12.41 Post-contrast brain MRI in a patient with melanoma showing an intracranial left parietal enhancing nodule (**a**) and a left parietal skull lesion (**b**) both suspicious for secondary involvement

Fig. 12.42 Lung CT in a patient with melanoma showing a pulmonary nodule with 1.0 cm suspicious for metastatic lesion (arrow)

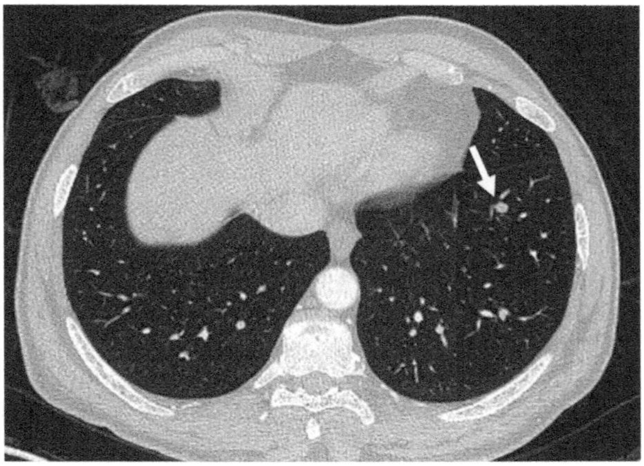

of false-positive findings from physiologic uptake and infective or inflammatory conditions [5, 48].

Posttreatment Assessment

Posttreatment assessment of high-risk cases allows an early detection of reminiscent lesions and of local or nodal recurrence. Clinical presentation and circumstances vary in each case, so the imaging workup should be carefully considered.

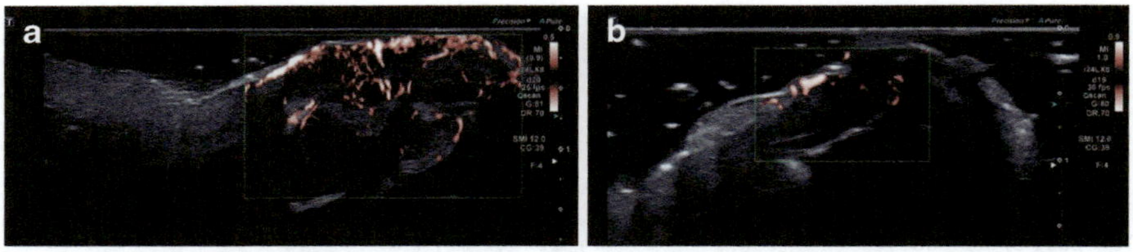

Fig. 12.43 HFUS (24 MHz) Doppler images of a basal cell carcinoma before (**a**) and after (**b**) immunotherapy, showing decrease of size and vascularity, signs of good response to treatment

Ultimately, it is critical to communicate clearly with your radiologist in order to choose the best imaging modality or combination of studies to best evaluate the patient. Appropriate evaluation can help choosing the best surveillance and therapeutic option [6, 24].

Responses

For the response to treatment evaluation, there are two fundamental rules: (1) a "baseline" examination should be available; (2) the same technique or combination of techniques used in the baseline study should also be used in the subsequent phases of evaluation between treatment rounds and restaging until the end of treatment. If possible, it would also be desirable that the baseline and follow-up examinations were always performed with the same scanner, the same examination technique, and the same operator, although this is clearly difficult to obtain in clinical practice.

The different types of treatment produce effects which can be detected with imaging modalities, including US, and reflect the combination of destructive and induced reparative phenomena. In general, lesions show changes in characteristics with size reduction and less vascularization (Fig. 12.43). On HFUS, hypoechoic lesions tend to become hyperechoic following treatment, particularly due to fibrosis. Lesions that are already hyperechoic tend to become heterogeneous, due to liquefactive necrosis. The reduction in vascularity is indubitably one of the most important effects. A typical reparative phenomenon that can be also detected is calcification.

PET is a highly effective technique for assessing response to chemotherapy or immunotherapy (Fig. 12.44), as metabolic changes precede morphologic changes detected by conventional techniques such as CT, MRI, and HFUS. It also helps to identify nonresponders and therefore avoids unnecessary, toxic treatments.

The response to treatment can be assessed according to size criteria as per the Response Evaluation Criteria in Solid Tumors (RECIST) [5, 20, 40, 68–70] and also by newer criteria, such as iRECIST.

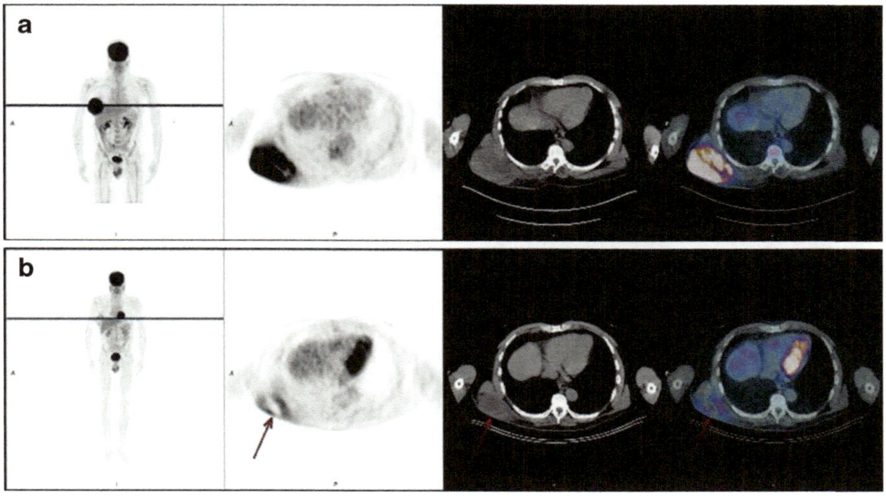

Fig. 12.44 Composed PET-CT images of melanoma before (**a**) and after (**b**) immunotherapy, showing decrease of size and vascularity, and also metabolic changes, signs of good response to treatment

Reminiscent

Reminiscent lesions refer to residual tumor, where there is a malignant component right from the beginning which has resisted treatment and which can further develop and spread and is common after limited surgical excision. Postsurgical changes can interfere with interpretation and mimic lesions.

HFUS is good for superficial scar tissues evaluation. It can detect residual nodular lesions or areas of abnormal vascularity (Fig. 12.45). PET is also useful in the follow-up of patients following surgical resection of tumor, most of whom have a complicating appearance at CT or MR imaging due to postoperative changes or scar tissue. The scarring, fibrosis, and altered anatomy can make detection difficult on MRI or CT scans.

Surgery is a form of tissue injury, and it elicits an inflammatory response, which can be visualized as an area of focal increased FDG activity. These changes usually resolve in a few weeks, and a PET scan is recommended 6–8 weeks after surgery to avoid misinterpretation. Although false-positive rates can be high in the immediate postoperative period because of inflammation and swelling, a PET-CT scan can be useful for detecting the reminiscent lesions and also the early recurrence after surgery. In malignant lesions, there is often a focal and intense FDG uptake, whereas inflammatory lesions present diffuse and mild metabolic uptake. It is valuable the knowledge of the patient history and an awareness of the different pitfalls of noninvasive imaging tools to achieve a correct diagnosis [6, 15, 71].

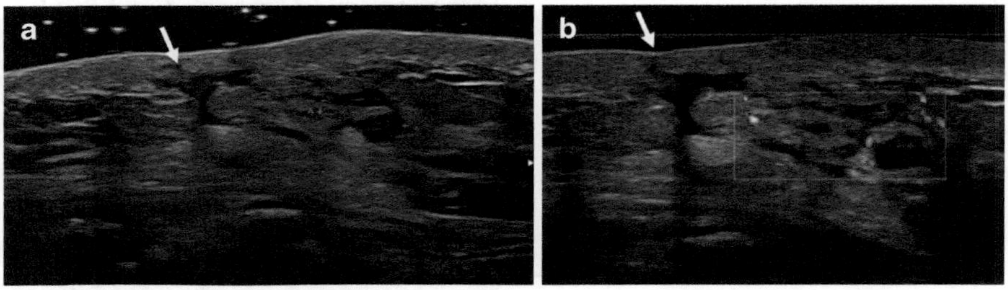

Fig. 12.45 HFUS (24 MHz) B mode (**a**) and Doppler (**b**) images of dermatofibrosarcoma protuberans showing reminiscent lesion (markers) near the surgical scar (arrow) after incomplete resection

Recurrence

Tumor recurrence refers to the reappearance of disease, identified clinically and/or instrumentally, after a variable length of time following radical surgery or complete response to systemic treatment. HFUS is useful for local recurrence assessment and guided biopsy of suspected lymph nodal metastases. The presence of postsurgical fibrosis and alteration of the normal anatomy may obscure local tumor recurrence on conventional CT or MRI scans. PET-CT is particularly useful in this scenario because it is still able to detect recurrent, metabolically active disease in areas with surgically altered anatomy. The main indication of PET-CT in cutaneous tumors, especially in melanoma, is to detect recurrence or to restage disease following the detection of recurrence, particularly in patients who are candidates for resection with curative intent [5, 6, 15, 70].

Surveillance

The purpose of staging and surveillance is to detect treatable tumors, monitor success of therapy, and provide reassurance and support to patients. Frequent follow-up examinations with ultrasound allow early detection of tumor recurrences and seem to lead to a prolonged overall survival. The primary function of US for the assessment of metastases in regional lymph nodes is for imaging surveillance, while PET-CT has the highest positive predictive value for the surveillance of distant metastasis, given the low positive predictive value of CT, PET, and PET-CT in the surveillance of patients at low risk of lymph node metastasis.

In summary, when diagnostic imaging is indicated for staging or surveillance, HFUS was the best diagnostic imaging test to detect lymph node metastases, and PET-CT was more suitable for the detection of distant metastases in patients at intermediate or high risk or when distant metastases are clinically indicated [48, 72].

References

1. Wassef C, Rao BK. Uses of non-invasive imaging in the diagnosis of skin cancer: an overview of the currently available modalities. Int J Dermatol. 2013;52(12):1481–9.
2. Zattar L, et al. In: Zattar L, Cerri G, editors. Ultrassonografia dermatológica. 1st ed. São Paulo: Manole; 2021.
3. Fan B, Neel VA, Yaroslavsky AN. Multimodal imaging for nonmelanoma skin cancer margin delineation. Lasers Surg Med. 2017;49(3):319–26.
4. Vidimos AT, Stultz TW. Imaging in cutaneous oncology: radiology for dermies. Dermatol Clin. 2011;29(2):243–60. https://doi.org/10.1016/j.det.2011.01.009.
5. Juan YH, Saboo SS, Tirumani SH, Khandelwal A, Shinagare AB, Ramaiya N, et al. Malignant skin and subcutaneous neoplasms in adults: multimodality imaging with CT, MRI, and 18F-FDG PET/CT. Am J Roentgenol. 2014;202(5):422–38.
6. Humphreys TR, Shah K, Wysong A, Lexa F, MacFarlane D. The role of imaging in the management of patients with nonmelanoma skin cancer: when is imaging necessary? J Am Acad Dermatol. 2017;76(4):591–607. https://doi.org/10.1016/j.jaad.2015.10.009.
7. MacFarlane D, Shah K, Wysong A, Wortsman X, Humphreys TR. The role of imaging in the management of patients with nonmelanoma skin cancer: diagnostic modalities and applications. J Am Acad Dermatol. 2017;76(4):579–88. https://doi.org/10.1016/j.jaad.2015.10.010.
8. Seibert JA. X-ray imaging physics for nuclear medicine technologists. Part 1: basic principles of x-ray production. J Nucl Med Technol. 2004;32(3):139–47. Available from: http://www.ncbi.nlm.nih.gov/pubmed/15347692.
9. Westbrook C, Roth CKTJ, editors. MRI in practice. 4th ed. West Sussex: Blackwell Publishing Ltd; 2011.
10. Kransdorf MJ, Murphey MD. Radiologic evaluation of soft-tissue masses. Am J Roentgenol. 2000;175(3):575–87. Available from: http://www.ajronline.org/doi/10.2214/ajr.175.3.1750575.
11. Hounsfield G. Computed medical imaging. Science. 1980;210(4465):22–8. Available from: http://www.ncbi.nlm.nih.gov/pubmed/6997993.
12. Zattar L, Viana PCC, Cerri GG, editors. Radiologia diagnóstica prática. Manual da residência do Hospital Sírio-Libanês. São Paulo: Manole; 2017.
13. Hany TF, Steinert HC, Goerres GW, Buck A, Von Schulthess GK. PET diagnostic accuracy: improvement with in-line PET-CT system: initial results. Radiology. 2002;225(2):575–81.
14. Catalano O, Roldán FA, Varelli C, Bard R, Corvino A, Wortsman X. Skin cancer: findings and role of high-resolution ultrasound. J Ultrasound. 2019;22(4):423–31. https://doi.org/10.1007/s40477-019-00379-0.
15. Catalano O, Nunziata A, Siani A. Fundamentals in oncologic ultrasound. 2nd ed. Springer; 2009.
16. Baheti AD, Tirumani SH, Giardino A, Rosenthal MH, Tirumani H, Krajewski K, et al. Basal cell carcinoma: a comprehensive review for the radiologist. AJR Am J Roentgenol. 2015;204(2):W132–40.
17. Barcaui EDO, Carvalho ACP, Valiante PMN, Barcaui CB. High-frequency ultrasound associated with dermoscopy in pre-operative evaluation of basal cell carcinoma. An Bras Dermatol. 2014;89(5):828–31. Available from: http://www.scielo.br/scielo.php?script=sci_arttext&pid=S0365-05962014000500828&lng=en&tlng=en.
18. Wortsman X. Atlas of dermatologic ultrasound. Cham: Springer International Publishing; 2018. Available from: http://link.springer.com/10.1007/978-3-319-89614-4.
19. Desai TD, Desai AD, Horowitz DC, Kartono F, Wahl T. The use of high-frequency ultrasound in the evaluation of superficial and nodular basal cell carcinomas. Dermatol Surg. 2007;33(10):1220–7.

20. Wang SQ, Liu J, Zhu QL, Zhao CY, Qu T, Li F, et al. High-frequency ultrasound features of basal cell carcinoma and its association with histological recurrence risk. Chin Med J (Engl). 2019;132(17):2021–6.
21. Hernández C, Del Boz J, De Troya M. Can high-frequency skin ultrasound be used for the diagnosis and management of basal cell carcinoma? Actas Dermosifiliogr. 2014;105(2):107–11.
22. Shin D, Williams J, Kurd SK, Gelfand JM. Test characteristics of high frequency ultrasound in the pre-operative assessment of margins of basal cell and squamous cell carcinoma in patients undergoing Mohs micrographic surgery. Dermatol Surg. 2009;35(1):9–16.
23. Bobadilla F, Wortsman X, Muñoz C, Segovia L, Espinoza M, Jemec GBE. Pre-surgical high resolution ultrasound of facial basal cell carcinoma: correlation with histology. Cancer Imaging. 2008;8(1):163–72.
24. Grajdeanu I-A, Vata D, Statescu L, Popescu I, Porumb-Andrese E, Patrascu A, et al. Use of imaging techniques for melanocytic naevi and basal cell carcinoma in integrative analysis (review). Exp Ther Med. 2020;20:78–86.
25. Wortsman X, Vergara P, Castro A, Saavedra D, Bobadilla F, Sazunic I, et al. Ultrasound as predictor of histologic subtypes linked to recurrence in basal cell carcinoma of the skin. J Eur Acad Dermatol Venereol. 2015;29(4):702–7.
26. Piłat P, Borzęcki A, Jazienicki M, Gerkowicz A, Krasowska D. High-frequency ultrasound in the diagnosis of selected non-melanoma skin nodular lesions. Postep Dermatol Alergol. 2019;36(5):572–80.
27. Burton KA, Ashack KA, Khachemoune A. Cutaneous squamous cell carcinoma: a review of high-risk and metastatic disease. Am J Clin Dermatol. 2016;17(5):491–508.
28. Que SKT, Zwald FO, Schmults CD. Cutaneous squamous cell carcinoma: management of advanced and high-stage tumors. J Am Acad Dermatol. 2018;78(2):249–61. https://doi.org/10.1016/j.jaad.2017.08.058.
29. Kawaguchi M, Kato H, Tomita H, Hara A, Suzui N, Miyazaki T, et al. MR imaging findings for differentiating cutaneous malignant melanoma from squamous cell carcinoma. Eur J Radiol. 2020;132:109212. https://doi.org/10.1016/j.ejrad.2020.109212.
30. Richards PS. The role of ultrasound in the detection of cervical lymph node metastases in clinically N0 squamous cell carcinoma of the head and neck. Cancer Imaging. 2007;7(1):167–78. Available from: https://www.ncbi.nlm.nih.gov/pmc/articles/PMC2151323/.
31. Newlands C, Currie R, Memon A, Whitaker S, Woolford T. Non-melanoma skin cancer: United Kingdom National Multidisciplinary Guidelines. J Laryngol Otol. 2016;130(S2):S125–32.
32. Stratigos AJ, Garbe C, Dessinioti C, Lebbe C, Bataille V, Bastholt L, et al. European interdisciplinary guideline on invasive squamous cell carcinoma of the skin: part 1. Epidemiology, diagnostics and prevention. Eur J Cancer. 2020;128:60–82. https://doi.org/10.1016/j.ejca.2020.01.007.
33. Lebbe C, Becker JC, Grob JJ, Malvehy J, Del Marmol V, Pehamberger H, et al. Diagnosis and treatment of Merkel cell carcinoma. European consensus-based interdisciplinary guideline. Eur J Cancer. 2015;51(16):2396–403.
34. Faries MB, Thompson JF, Cochran AJ, Andtbacka RH, Mozzillo N, Zager JS, et al. Completion dissection or observation for sentinel-node metastasis in melanoma. N Engl J Med. 2017;376(23):2211–22. Available from: http://www.nejm.org/doi/10.1056/NEJMoa1613210.
35. Coit D. The enigma of regional lymph nodes in melanoma. N Engl J Med. 2017;376(23):2280–1.
36. Goldberg BB, Merton DA, Liu J, Thakur M, Murphy GF, Needleman L, et al. Radiology sentinel lymph nodes in a swine model with melanoma: lymphatic US 1. Radiology. 2004;230:727–34.
37. Oxman M, Levin J, Johnson G, Schmader K, Straus S. Sentinel-node biopsy or nodal observation in melanoma. N Engl J Med. 2005;353(10):977–87.
38. Wortsman X. Sonography of the primary cutaneous melanoma: a review. Radiol Res Pract. 2012;2012:1–6. Available from: http://www.hindawi.com/journals/rrp/2012/814396/.
39. Gonzalez A. Sentinel lymph node biopsy: past and present implications for the management of cutaneous melanoma with nodal metastasis. Am J Clin Dermatol. 2018;19(s1):24–30. https://doi.org/10.1007/s40257-018-0379-0.

40. Bartlett EK, Lee AY, Spanheimer PM, Bello DM, Brady MS, Ariyan CE, et al. Nodal and systemic recurrence following observation of a positive sentinel lymph node in melanoma. Br J Surg. 2020;107(11):1480–8.
41. Srivastava A, Hughes LE, Woodcock JP, Laidler P. Vascularity in cutaneous melanoma detected by Doppler sonography and histology: correlation with tumour behaviour. Br J Cancer. 1989;59(1):89–91.
42. Machet L, Belot V, Naouri M, Boka M, Mourtada Y, Giraudeau B, et al. Preoperative measurement of thickness of cutaneous melanoma using high-resolution 20 MHz ultrasound imaging: a monocenter prospective study and systematic review of the literature. Ultrasound Med Biol. 2009;35(9):1411–20.
43. Quartuccio N, Siracusa M, Pappalardo M, Arnone A, Arnone G. Sentinel node identification in melanoma: current clinical impact, new emerging SPECT radiotracers and technological advancements. An update of the last decade. Curr Radiopharm. 2019;13(1):32–41.
44. Broman KK, Hughes T, Dossett L, Sun J, Kirichenko D, Carr MJ, et al. Active surveillance of patients who have sentinel node positive melanoma: an international, multi-institution evaluation of adoption and early outcomes after the multicenter selective lymphadenectomy trial II (MSLT-2). Cancer. 2021;127(13):2251–61. Available from: https://onlinelibrary.wiley.com/doi/10.1002/cncr.33483.
45. Ulrich J, van Akkooi AJC, Eggermont AMM, Voit C. New developments in melanoma: utility of ultrasound imaging (initial staging, follow-up and pre-SLNB). Expert Rev Anticancer Ther. 2011;11(11):1693–701.
46. Solivetti FM, Elia F, Guerrisi A, Desiderio F, Santaguida MG, Sperduti I, et al. Cutaneous melanoma follow-up: appropriateness of requests for ultrasound tests—the S. Gallicano national referral centre experience. J Exp Clin Cancer Res. 2013;32(1):1.
47. King DM. Imaging of metastatic melanoma. Cancer Imaging. 2006;6(1):204–8.
48. Xing Y, Bronstein Y, Ross MI, Askew RL, Lee JE, Gershenwald JE, et al. Contemporary diagnostic imaging modalities for the staging and surveillance of melanoma patients: a meta-analysis. J Natl Cancer Inst. 2011;103(2):129–42.
49. Dewing D, Emmett M, Pritchard JR. The roles of angiogenesis in malignant melanoma: trends in basic science research over the last 100 years. ISRN Oncol. 2012;2012:1–7.
50. Bergin P, Rezaei S, Lau Q, Coucher J. Dermatofibrosarcoma protuberans, magnetic resonance imaging and pathological correlation. Australas Radiol. 2007;51(Suppl. 1):64–6.
51. Lee RKL, Griffith JF, Ng AWH, Lai FMM. Ultrasound appearances of dermatofibrosarcoma protuberans. J Med Ultrasound. 2013;21(1):21–8. https://doi.org/10.1016/j.jmu.2013.01.009.
52. Riggs K, McGuigan KL, Morrison WB, Samie FH, Humphreys T. Role of magnetic resonance imaging in perioperative assessment of dermatofibrosarcoma protuberans. Dermatol Surg. 2009;35(12):2036–41.
53. Saiag P, Grob JJ, Lebbe C, Malvehy J, Del Marmol V, Pehamberger H, et al. Diagnosis and treatment of dermatofibrosarcoma protuberans. European consensus-based interdisciplinary guideline. Eur J Cancer. 2015;51(17):2604–8. https://doi.org/10.1016/j.ejca.2015.06.108.
54. Mandava A, Koppula V, Wortsman X, Catalano O, Alfageme F. The clinical value of imaging in primary cutaneous lymphomas: role of high resolution ultrasound and PET-CT. Br J Radiol. 2019;92(1096):1–6.
55. Gerring RC, Ott CT, Curry JM, Sargi ZB, Wester ST. Orbital exenteration for advanced periorbital non-melanoma skin cancer: prognostic factors and survival. Eye. 2017;31(3):379–88. Available from: http://www.nature.com/articles/eye2016218.
56. Xie M, Yu J, Li L, Jia R, Song X, Wang Y, et al. Nomogram for preoperative estimation of orbit invasion risk in periocular squamous cell carcinoma. Front Oncol. 2020;10:1–7.
57. Kuno H, Sakamaki K, Fujii S, Sekiya K, Otani K, Hayashi R, et al. Comparison of MR imaging and dual-energy ct for the evaluation of cartilage invasion by laryngeal and hypopharyngeal squamous cell carcinoma. Am J Neuroradiol. 2018;39(3):524–31.
58. Boisen J, Malone CH, Kelly B, Wagner RF. Cutaneous squamous cell carcinoma with invasion through ear cartilage. Case Rep Dermatol Med. 2016;2016:1–3.

59. Weselik L, Majchrzak E, Ibbs M, Lewandowski A, Marszałek A, Machczyński P, et al. Assessment of cartilage invasion in case of laryngeal cancer by means of longitudinal sectioning for histopathology—clinical implications. Rep Pract Oncol Radiother. 2019;24(5):443–9.
60. Çağli S, Öztürk M, Yüce I, Deniz K, Güney E. The value of routine clinical and radiologic studies in predicting neoplastic invasion of cricoarytenoid units. Am J Neuroradiol. 2009;30(10):1936–40.
61. Wegner I, Hooft L, Reitsma JB, Pameijer FA, de Bree R, Stegeman I. MRI versus CT for detecting cartilage invasion in patients with laryngeal and hypopharyngeal squamous cell carcinoma. Cochrane Database Syst Rev. 2016;2016(4)
62. Alfageme RF. Ultrasound skin imaging. Acta Dermosifiliogr (Engl Ed). 2014;105(10):891–9. Available from: https://linkinghub.elsevier.com/retrieve/pii/S1578219014002765.
63. Corvino A, Corvino F, Catalano O, Sandomenico F, Petrillo A. The tail and the string sign: new sonographic features of subcutaneous melanoma metastasis. Ultrasound Med Biol. 2017;43(1):370–4.
64. Liberini V, Messerli M, Husmann L, Kudura K, Grünig H, Maurer A, et al. Improved detection of in-transit metastases of malignant melanoma with BSREM reconstruction in digital [18F]FDG PET/CT. Eur Radiol. 2021;31:8011.
65. Solivetti FM, Di Luca Sidozzi A, Pirozzi G, Coscarella G, Brigida R, Eibenshutz L. Valutazione ecografica delle metastasi in transito e delle lesioni satelliti da melanoma maligno cutaneo clinicamente occulte. Radiol Med. 2006;111(5):702–8.
66. Solivetti FM, Desiderio F, Guerrisi A, Bonadies A, Maini CL, Di Filippo S, et al. HF ultrasound vs PET-CT and telethermography in the diagnosis of in-transit metastases from melanoma: a prospective study and review of the literature. J Exp Clin Cancer Res. 2014;33(1):1–7.
67. Neuschmelting V, Lockau H, Ntziachristos V, Grimm J, Kircher MF. Lymph node micrometastases and in-transit metastases from melanoma: in vivo detection with multispectral optoacoustic imaging in a mouse model. Radiology. 2016;280(1):137–50.
68. Moro R, González-Ramos J, Martínez-García S, Requena C, Traves V, Manrique-Silva E, et al. Locoregional lymph node recurrence of trunk melanoma in non-sentinel lymph node basins: an observational retrospective study. Acta Derm Venereol. 2020;100(17):adv00284.
69. Lassau N, Lamuraglia M, Koscielny S, Spatz A, Roche A, Leclere J, et al. Prognostic value of angiogenesis evaluated with high-frequency and colour Doppler sonography for preoperative assessment of primary cutaneous melanomas: correlation with recurrence after a 5 year follow-up period. Cancer Imaging. 2006;6(1):24–9.
70. Sánchez-Sánchez R, Serrano-Falcón C, ACR A. Diagnostic imaging in dermatology: utility of PET-CT in cutaneous melanoma. Actas Dermosifiliogr. 2015;106(1):29–34.
71. Shih GL, Shih W-J, Milan PP. FDG uptake in an abdominal surgical scar from an exploratory laparotomy. Br J Radiol. 2009;82(978):523–5. Available from: http://www.birpublications.org/doi/10.1259/bjr/33452580.
72. Rubaltelli L, Beltrame V, Scagliori E, Bezzon E, Frigo A, Rastrelli M, et al. Potential use of contrast-enhanced ultrasound (CEUS) in the detection of metastatic superficial lymph nodes in melanoma patients. Ultraschall der Medizin—Eur J Ultrasound. 2013;35(01):67–71. Available from: http://www.thieme-connect.de/DOI/DOI?10.1055/s-0033-1335857.

Chapter 13
Actinic Keratosis, Other Precursors, and Squamous Cell Tumors

Cristina Martinez Zugaib Abdalla, Renato Marchiori Bakos, Luiz Guilherme Cernaglia Aureliano de Lima, Beatrice Martinez Zugaib Abdalla, Luis Fernando Tovo, Francisco Aparecido Belfort, and Rodrigo Ramella Munhoz

Key Points

- Cutaneous squamous cell carcinoma (cSCC) is the second most common human cancer with over 250,000 new cases annually in the USA.
- Approximately 70% of all cSCCs occur on the head and neck.
- AK is considered a SCC precursor with 5–20% risk of developing into invasive neoplasia.
- Field cancerization is an important concept regarding the development of SCC with **clinically** imperceptible or incipient **lesions with** histopathology areas of dysplastic cells or even areas with SCC in situ.
- cSCC may be stratified into low, high, or very high risk for local recurrence, metastasis, or death from disease based on clinical and pathological parameters.
- Surgery is still the main goal for the best cSCC treatment. Radiotherapy and systemic therapy are reserved for local advanced or metastatic disease.
- Immunotherapy emerged as a novel systemic treatment and is considered a standard of care for patients with advanced disease, with promising results also in the perioperative setting.

C. M. Z. Abdalla (✉) · B. M. Z. Abdalla · L. F. Tovo · F. A. Belfort
Hospital Sírio-Libanês, São Paulo, Brazil

R. M. Bakos
Department of Dermatology, Hospital de Clínicas de Porto Alegre, Porto Alegre, Brazil

L. G. C. A. de Lima
NOCS - Hospital Sírio-Libanês, São Paulo, Brazil

R. R. Munhoz
Oncology Center, Hospital Sírio-Libanês, São Paulo, Brazil

C. M. Z. Abdalla et al. (eds.), *Oncodermatology*,
https://doi.org/10.1007/978-3-031-29277-4_13

Epidemiology and Pathogenesis

Cutaneous squamous cell carcinoma (cSCC) is the second most common human cancer with over 250,000 new cases annually in the USA. Squamous cell tumors (SCTs) arise from epidermal keratinocytes with locally invasive behavior, potential to metastasize and even progress to death, depending on tumor stage. cSCC typically manifests as a spectrum of progressively advanced malignancies, ranging from a precursor actinic keratosis (AK) to in situ and invasive cSCC. There is controversy in the literature regarding the classification of AKs as preneoplastic lesions or an intraepidermal neoplasia, especially when considering that AKs share many of the genetic alterations of cSCC [1–3]. AKs will either persist in the same stage or regress, while only a few will progress into cSCC [1–3].

Classically categorized as preneoplastic lesions, some authors suggest considering them as in situ neoplasms, since they derive from clonal DNA modifications in the keratinocyte. AK is a clear clinical indicator of intraepithelial actinic damage that can range from mild to severe, as well as be part of the field cancerization. Most cSCC arises directly from the field cancerization [4, 5].

Several risk factors have been reported for AK and cSCC, including individuals with lightly pigmented skin (Fitzpatrick types I and II), age, and outdoor occupation. For cSCC ionizing radiation, human papillomavirus (HPV), cutaneous genetically inherited skin diseases (albinism, recessive dystrophic epidermolysis bullosa, epidermodysplasia verruciformis, and xeroderma pigmentosum), immunosuppression, ultraviolet light exposure, and chemical carcinogens (arsenic, polycyclic aromatic hydrocarbons) are also important risk factors. However, the most important risk factor is represented by UV radiation and sunlight [6]. Risk factors for the development of cSCC in darkly pigmented individuals are chronic scarring and areas of chronic inflammation. Lesions that are associated with chronic scarring account for 20–40% of cSCCs in black patients. Organ transplant recipients also demonstrate an increased risk of developing AK and cSCC [7]. Solid-organ transplant recipients present 65–250 times the risk of cSCC. Heart and lung transplant recipients tend to have a higher risk of cSCC than renal transplant recipients because of intensive immunosuppression regimens and greater age. Patients with chronic lymphocytic leukemia have an eight- to tenfold increased risk for developing cSCC [8, 9].

AK and cSCC show high tumor mutation burden and mutation in several genes including TP53, NOTCH1, NOTCH2, FAT1, KMT2C, and CDKN2a. Progression of AK to cSCC involves among other mechanisms dysregulation of TGFb signaling [10–13]. cSCC carries more mutations than other common malignancies. Through the accumulation of these mutations and other cellular changes, epithelial cells can progress through increasing levels of dysplasia and transform into a cSCC. Mutations in the p53 gene are the most common genetic abnormalities found in actinic keratosis and in situ and invasive cSCC. The p53 mutations enable tumor cells to resist apoptosis and expand clonally to the neighbor cells. Other mutations involved are cyclin-dependent kinase inhibitor 2A mutations (CDKN2A), Ras mutations, and mutations of NOTCH1. The accumulation of mutations ultimately involves various signaling pathways including the activation of the NF-kB, MAPK, and PI3K/AKT/mTOR pathways which mediate epidermal growth factor receptor (EGFR) overexpression [8, 10, 11].

Oncogenic human papillomavirus (HPV) 16 and 18 are implicated in the development of cSCC, particularly periungual and anogenital cSCC. HPV is not transcriptionally active in cSCC; it is likely involved during the induction, not the maintenance of the tumor. HPV proteins E6 and E7 inhibit p53 and retinoblastoma genes, respectively, that prevents apoptosis. HPV types 8, 9, and 15 are involved in the pathogenesis of cSCC in solid-organ transplant recipients [8]. HPV plays an important role in the pathogenesis of cSCC in immunocompromised patients [8].

cSCC most commonly arises in sun-exposed areas but also develops on any cutaneous surface [7]. There are several clinical variants. Given its increasing incidence and potential for poor outcome, it is important to have an appropriate diagnosis workup and management of high-risk tumors [8].

Clinical Features and Histopathology

Approximately 70% of all cSCCs occur on the head and neck (most frequently involving the lower lip, external ear and periauricular region, or forehead and scalp). cSCCs also arise in non-photodamaged skin areas such as oral mucosa and periungual skin, and anogenital areas.

There are a great variety of cutaneous lesions that typically begin as a tender erythematous papule plaque or nodule that can be smooth, hyperkeratotic, or ulcerated. Pigmented cSCC is a variant particularly seen in high Fitzpatrick skin phototypes.

Dermoscopy and reflectance confocal microscopy may enhance the diagnostic accuracy of cSCC; however, skin biopsy is required to confirm the diagnosis (this will be presented in the chapter on Ancillary Tools in the Dermatologic Assessment). The clinical features of cSCC are extremely polymorphous, and they depend also on the anatomical site and subtype [4, 14].

Actinic Keratosis

AKs constitute a significant portion of dermatological practice, and they are considered the second cause for medical consultation with dermatologists in the USA. There is a cumulative chance of 5–20% of developing into invasive neoplasia, and the number of lesions maximizes this occurrence. On the other hand, it is estimated that up to 27–82% of the cSCCs evolve from AK and some 82–97% of the cSCCs have contiguous AK [15–17].

AKs present as single or multiple erythematous or brownish macules, papules, or plaques, usually with poorly defined borders, mostly covered by adherent dry scales (Fig. 13.1). Some authors divide the clinical presentation of the lesions into three levels: level I, visible and slightly palpable; level II, visible and palpable; and level III, frankly visible and hyperkeratotic (Fig. 13.2) [15–17]. They are usually asymptomatic although some patients may refer burning sensation or pruritus. Clinical inspection, dermoscopy, and palpation may be sufficient to identify most of them. Although clinical diagnosis is possible for most lesions, equivocal lesions should be biopsied [2, 17].

In actinic cheilitis there is a loss of the sharp border of the lip, rough scaly areas which become thick and may present focal ulceration as well as leukoplakia and would develop into cSCCs with a higher metastatic potential [15–17].

The histopathology features of AK are confined within the epidermis. Aggregates of atypical and pleomorphic keratinocytes which show nuclear atypia, dyskeratosis, and loss of polarity, hyperkeratosis, and parakeratosis are often seen. There are different subtypes including hypertrophic, atrophic, acantholytic, pigmented, proliferative, and bowenoid AK. In general, the hypertrophic and proliferative variants are associated with more aggressive biologic behaviors and have a higher malignant

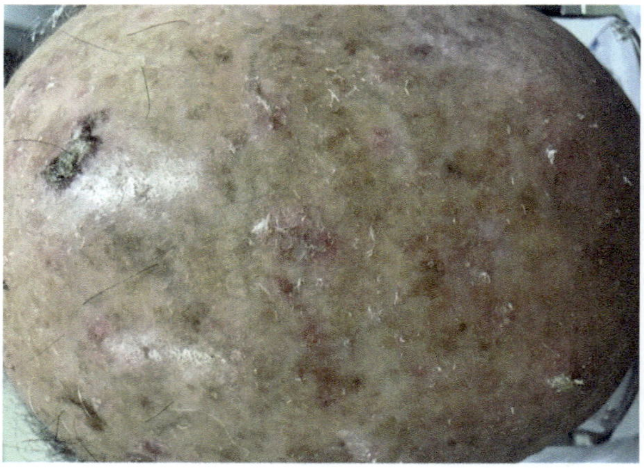

Fig. 13.1 Field cancerization on the scalp with multiple actinic keratoses and a squamous cell carcinoma on the occipital region (field cancerization—Courtesy of Renato M Bakos, MD)

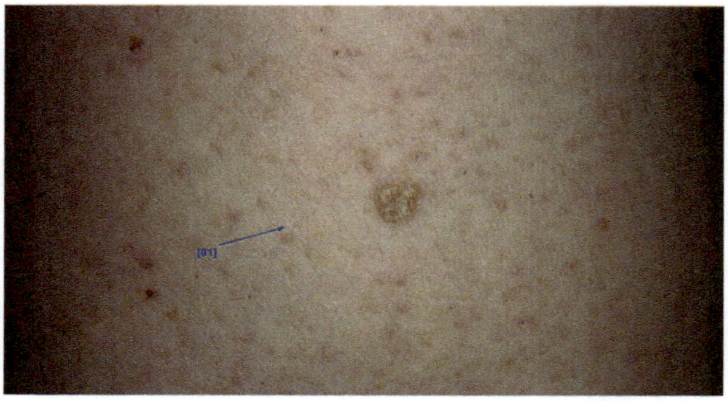

Fig. 13.2 Hyperkeratotic actinic keratosis (Courtesy of Renato M Bakos, MD)

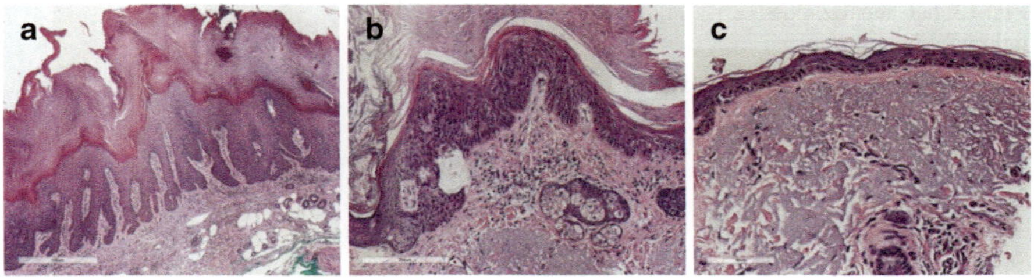

Fig. 13.3 Actinic keratoses (AKs) and its histopathological variants. (**a**) Hypertrophic AK. (**b**) Bowenoid AK. (**c**) Atrophic AK (Courtesy of Renato M Bakos, MD)

potential. Atypical keratinocytes from the basal cell layer will frequently extend into the granular and cornified layers; however, they will not spread to the full thickness of the epidermis. In bowenoid AK, which resembles Bowen's disease, keratinocytes are less disordered with less nuclear atypia and crowding. Lichenoid AKs show basal layer degeneration and the formation of Civatte bodies, as a result of an infiltrate with irregular acanthosis (Fig. 13.3) [18].

Field Cancerization

Field cancerization was a term first described in 1953 by *Slaughter et al.* that studied oropharyngeal squamous cell carcinomas that showed areas clinically appearing as normal tissue, and histopathology presenting areas of dysplastic cells or even areas with SCC in situ [19]. Therefore, areas with dysplastic changes could present multiple heterogeneous mutations from chronic carcinogenic stimuli that develop into independent tumors rather than being from the same single tumor [20]. In dermatology, field cancerization is described as the anatomical area including or adjacent to AKs with visibly photodamaged skin, characterized by pigmentary changes, rough texture, atrophy, or telangiectasia. This observation demonstrates how AK lesions develop and subsequently transform into cutaneous cSCC. Currently, there is no reliable method to discern which AKs will transform into cSCC from those that will either remain benign or resolve without treatment, complicating the treatment algorithm of AKs (Fig. 13.4) [21].

This concept has important clinical consequences, as it clarifies the existence of multiple areas of premalignant disease, multiple sites of synchronous primary tumors, and the presence of distant tumors. A genetically altered field increases the chances of local tumor recurrence developing and/or the appearance of a second tumor. Determining the risk of cSCC development from a single lesion as well as risk for a field may improve patient outcomes by identifying those patients who would benefit most from earlier treatment. Biopsy specimens of visible lesions and perilesional areas usually show distinct grades of cellular atypia and dysplasia. "Field cancerization" should be managed as a chronic and elapsing condition that usually requires repetitive treatment course for its remission [20, 22]. The goal of

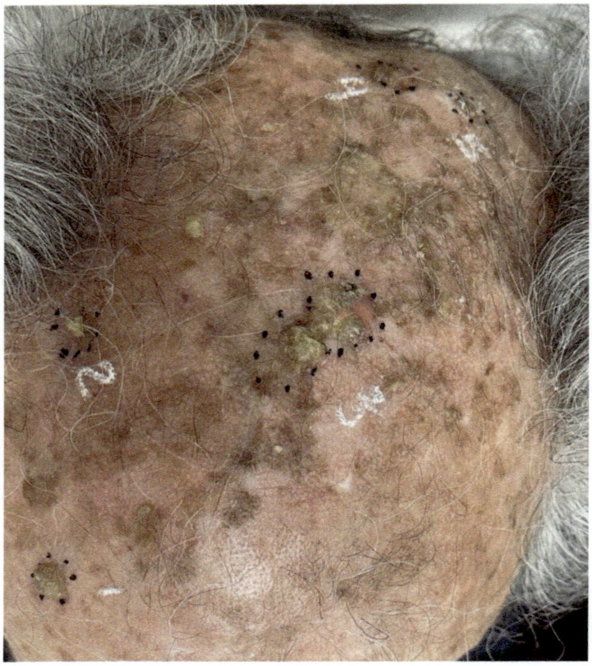

Fig. 13.4 Cancerization field with hypertrophic AKs and cSCC suspicious lesions programmed for biopsy (Courtesy of Cristina M. Z. Abdalla, MD)

treatment is to avoid the risk of progression to cSCC. When choosing a treatment, the number, location, and extension of AKs and cancerization field as well as the patient's age, comorbidities, immunosuppression (transplants), previous history of skin cancer, continuous sun exposure (rural workers, athletes), cost, and condition of treatment must be considered [21].

Squamous Cell Carcinoma "In Situ"

cSCC in situ appears as a skin color or an erythematous, well-demarcated, scaly patch or plaque. Bowen's disease is in situ cSCC of non-sun-exposed skin. These lesions tend to grow slowly, enlarging over the course of years. Invasive cSCC could develop in 3–5% in situ cSCC (Figs. 13.5, 13.6, 13.7 and 13.8) [8].

Histologically, keratinocyte atypia is present in full-thickness epidermis. Adnexal involvement by in situ cSCC may occur, and it brings a challenge in the precise margin's assessment [17].

Erythroplasia of Queyrat (EQ) is a variant that manifests as single or multiple erythematous plaques on the mucosa of the glans or prepuce, and genital Bowen's disease presents as a single, scaly plaque on keratinized skin, generally on the distal

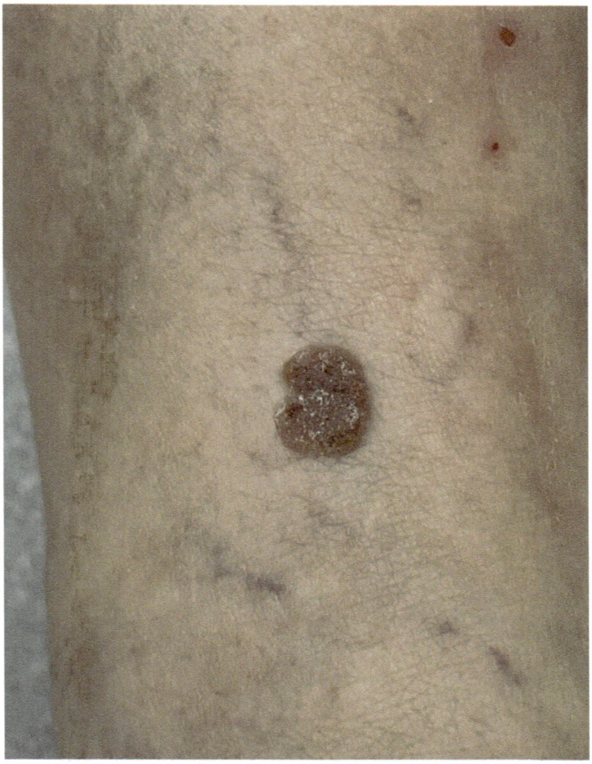

Fig. 13.5 Pigmented in situ cSCC (Courtesy of Francisco A. Belfort, MD)

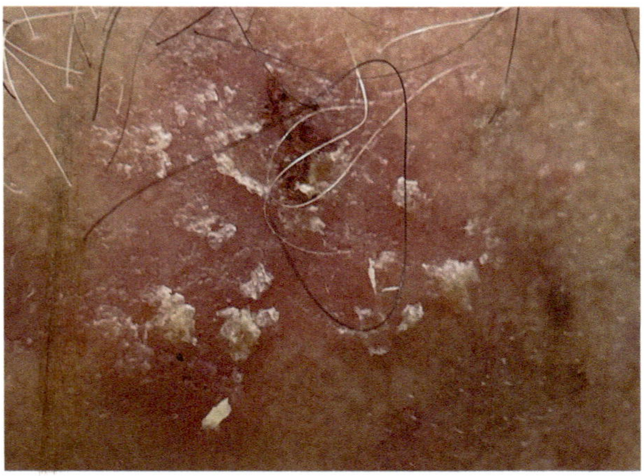

Fig. 13.6 In situ cSCC of the forehead (Courtesy of Cristina M. Z. Abdalla, MD)

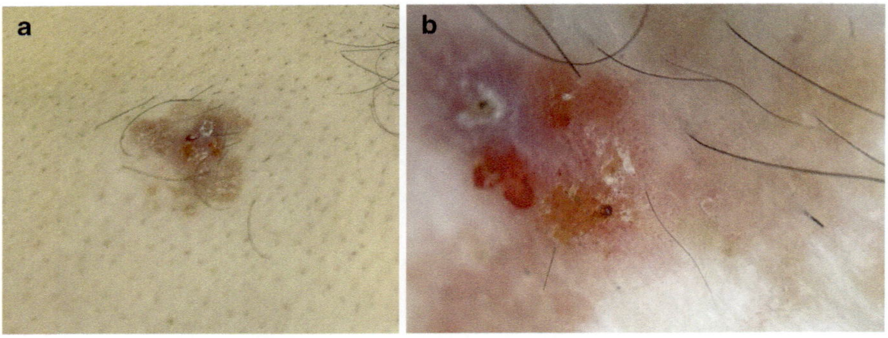

Fig. 13.7 Bowen's disease. (**a**) Clinical picture. (**b**) Noncontact polarized dermoscopy—crusts and irregular vessels (Courtesy of Cristina M. Z. Abdalla, MD)

Fig. 13.8 cSCC in situ dorsum of the hand (Courtesy of Cristina M. Z. Abdalla, MD)

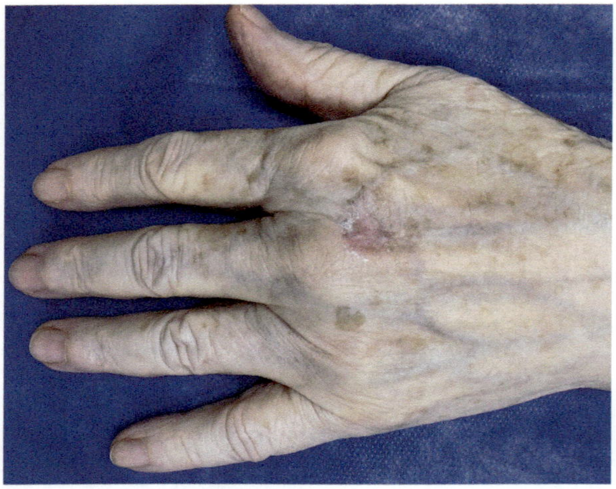

third of the penis. The risk of invasive carcinoma is estimated to be higher, approximately 10% of EQ.

Intraepidermal cSCC may start to grow under a nail when it results in a red streak (erythronychia) that later may destroy the nail plate. It is also classified as a high-risk cSCC [19].

The differential diagnoses are superficial basal cell carcinoma (BCC) and psoriasis.

Keratoacanthoma

Keratoacanthoma (KT), well-differentiated cSCC, or keratoacanthoma-like cSCC is a solitary, symmetrical dome-shaped or crateriform nodule with a central keratotic core. It is considered cSCC with clinical distinguished behavior, including rapid

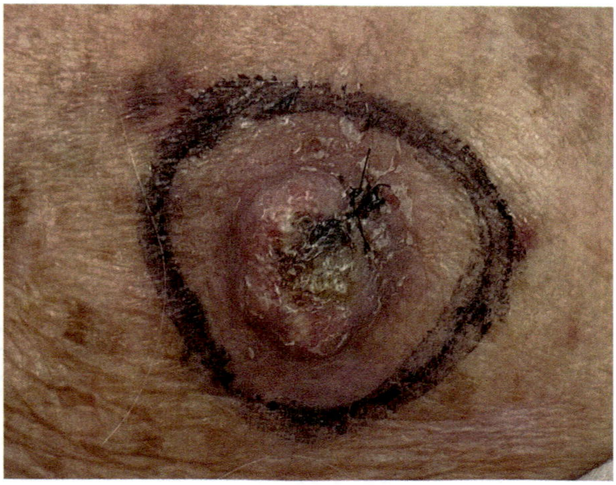

Fig. 13.9 KT before excision (after biopsy including the epidermis until reticular dermis) (Courtesy of Cristina Abdalla, MD and Francisco Belfort, MD)

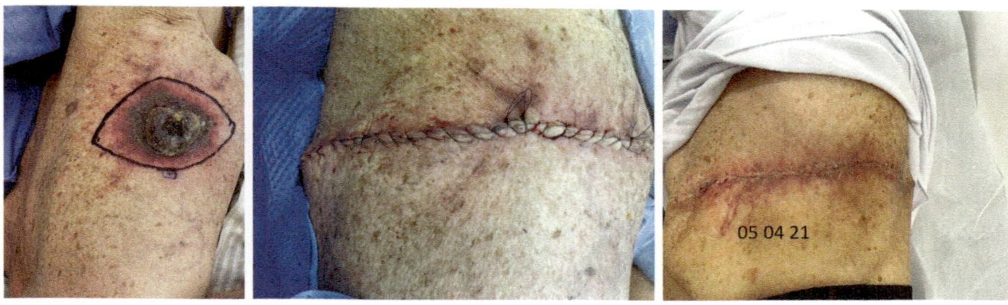

Fig. 13.10 Giant KT surgery (Courtesy of Francisco A. Belfort, MD)

growth (few days or weeks), sometimes with spontaneous regression and particular histological criteria (Figs. 13.9 and 13.10) [23].

KT's histopathology features are characterized by a symmetrical dome-shaped tumor filled with keratin. Its base may be well circumscribed or infiltrative, both likely representing a well-differentiated invasive cSCC. Invasive lobules and nests of tumor cells with low-grade nuclei and abundant, eosinophilic cytoplasm that mature toward the center are characteristic. KT usually shows a sharp delineation between the tumor nests and stroma and can entrap elastic fibers (Figs. 13.11 and 13.12) [24].

Invasive Cutaneous Squamous Cell Carcinoma

Early invasive cSCCs range from a small patch to erythematous-squamous papule or plaque, which may evolve into a hyperkeratotic lesion on an erythematous base.

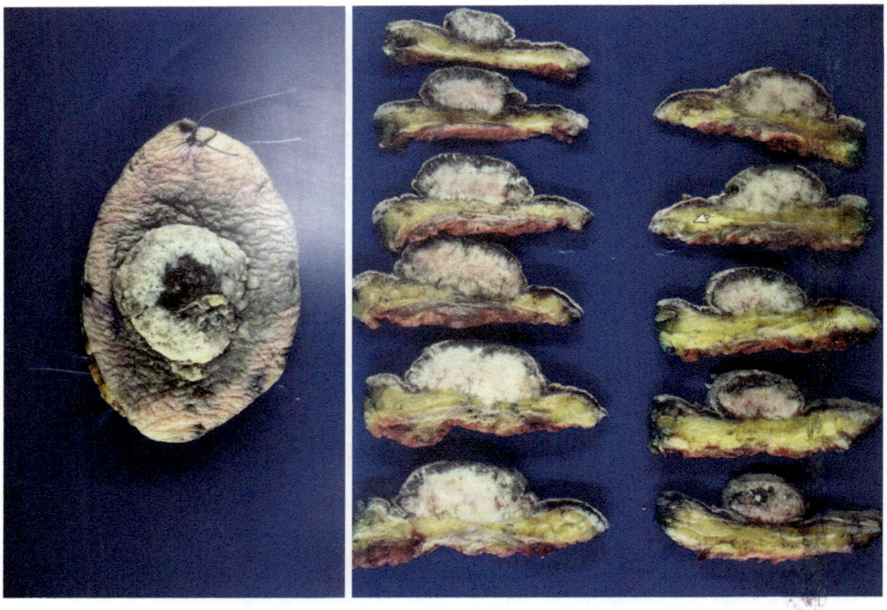

Fig. 13.11 Giant KT surgical specimen with well-circumscribed dome-shaped tumor filled with keratin (Courtesy of Francisco A. Belfort, MD and Mariana Macedo Petaccia, MD)

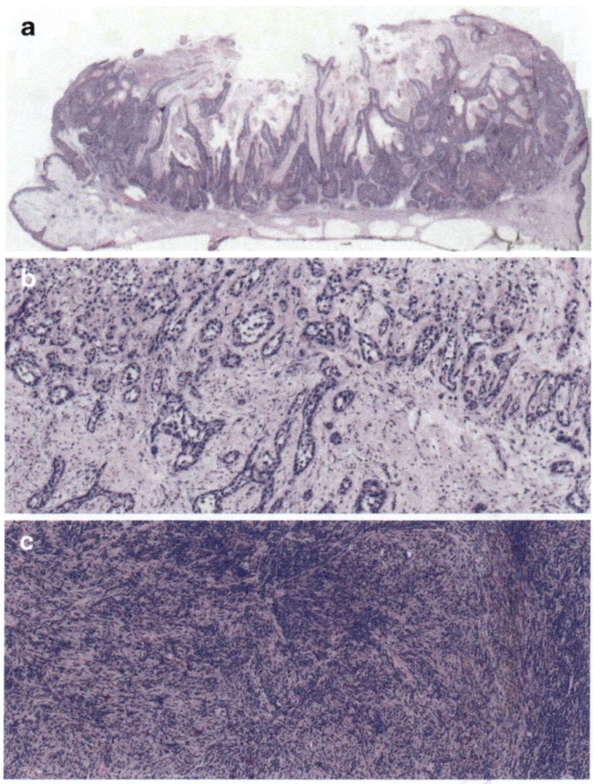

Fig. 13.12 Morphology of variants of cutaneous squamous cell carcinoma (cSCC) by hematoxylin and eosin (H&E). (**a**) Keratoacanthoma-type, symmetrical dome-shaped tumor filled with keratin, likely representing a well-differentiated invasive cSCC. (**b**) Acantholytic type characterized by acantholysis in the tumor lobules forming pseudoglandular spaces. (**c**) Spindle cell variant, dense proliferation of pleomorphic spindle cells, and no obvious squamous differentiation (Courtesy of Francisco Cernaglia, MD)

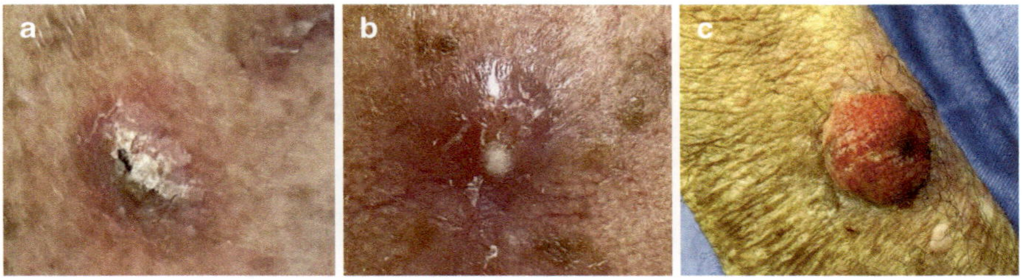

Fig. 13.13 SCC: (**a**) Clinically well-differentiated SCC. (**b**) Clinically moderately differentiated SCC. (**c**) Clinically non-differentiated SCC (Courtesy Cristina M. Z. Abdalla, MD and Francisco A. Belfort, MD)

At this stage, the most common differential diagnoses are hypertrophic AK and BCC [19].

Well-differentiated cSCCs are easier to diagnose, and they are usually hyperkeratotic and verrucous tumors or with a crateriform appearance (Fig. 13.13). Poorly differentiated cSCCs appear as non-keratotic, erythematous infiltrating tumors, with frequent ulceration and with greater difficulty in distinguishing between other neoplasms such as amelanotic melanoma, skin metastasis, Merkel cell carcinoma, or even BCC [19].

Invasive cSCCs are often asymptomatic but may be painful. High-risk cSCC with histologic perineural invasion may present local neurologic symptoms such numbness, stinging, burning, paresthesia, paralysis, or visual disturbance [19].

Histology of invasive cSCC will present close resemblance to their precursor AK and be distinguished from AK by the presence of infiltrative cells passing through the basement membrane into the dermis [25].

The invasive lesion may not have an associated in situ component and may present with a variable degree of differentiation and a diverse range of morphologic variants. The lesions might be classified as well, moderately, or poor differentiated based on cytologic atypia and degree of keratinization (Fig. 13.14).

The current classification of skin tumors of the *World Health Organization Skin Tumors* (2018) recognizes different histopathology variants of invasive cSCC, each one of them with a characteristic morphologic finding:

- Acantholytic cSCC is a subtype of invasive cSCC displaying acantholysis inside the squamous cells of the tumor lobules, forming empty spaces in the lobules and giving them a pseudoglandular aspect.
- Spindle cell variant is a dense proliferation of malignant squamous cells with pleomorphic spindle cells morphology and high mitotic activity and may lack obvious squamous differentiation by morphology.
- Adenosquamous cSCC is formed by mixed components of squamous and variable degree of glandular differentiation and a high cytologic atypia. Mucin production in these lesions might be verified by mucin staining.

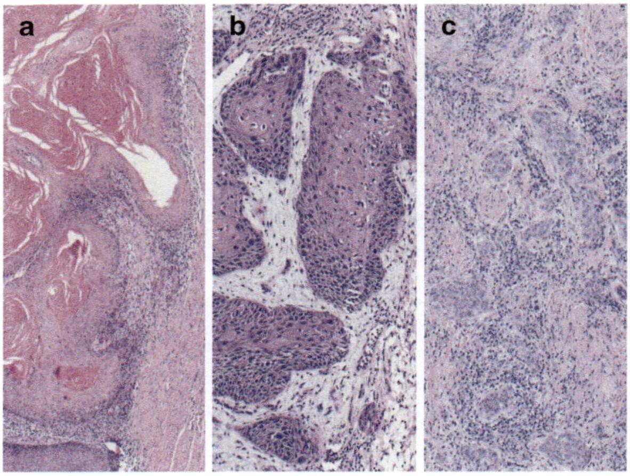

Fig. 13.14 Degree of differentiation of cutaneous squamous cell carcinoma (cSCC). (**a**) Well-differentiated cutaneous squamous cell carcinoma, with low cytologic atypia and well-formed squamous pearls with cell with abundant pink cytoplasm. (**b**) Invasive lobules of cSCC with moderate degree of cytologic atypia. (**c**) Poorly differentiated cSCC with high degree of high nuclear-to-cytoplasm ratio, marked atypia, and solid nests with no low degree of keratinization (Courtesy of Luis Cernaglia, MD)

- Clear cell cSCC variant displays "univacuolated" cytoplasm giving a clear cell appearance constituted of glycogen and thus positive for periodic acid-Schiff (PAS) staining.
- cSCC with sarcomatoid differentiation is also known for carcinosarcomatous cSCC or metaplastic cSCC, and it is composed by variable proportion of sarcomatous component and variable heterologous elements such as condroblastic, osteoblastic, myoid, or rhabdoid.
- Desmoplastic cSCC or also known as sclerosing cSCC characterizes a cSCC associated with an intense desmoplastic stroma and usually a more aggressive biologic behavior [25].

The differential diagnosis for cSCC is very diverse and depends on the morphological finding of each lesion. Many lesions such as benign keratoses and pseudoepitheliomatous hyperplasia may present as a differential diagnosis for well-differentiated and superficial cSCC. Other differential diagnosis includes metatypical BCC, a diverse range of adnexal tumors, sarcoma, melanoma, lymphomas, and metastatic carcinomas. Immunohistochemistry such as p63, p40, 34BE12, and Ck5/6 may aid in difficult cases for confirming the epithelial/squamous nature of the lesion, especially when facing some morphological challenging variants such as spindle cells, which may impair a wide range of differential diagnoses like sarcomas, melanoma, and lymphomas. Many other immunohistochemistry markers may also be used depending on the morphological finding and aim confirmation of primary sites or lineage differentiation [25].

Clinical Presentation of cSCC Variants

Verrucous Carcinoma

The term verrucous carcinoma (VC) was first described as an exogenous and well-differentiated variant of cSCC by Ackerman in 1948. It commonly arises in the sixth–seventh decade of life. This variant is characterized by well-defined, exophytic, cauliflower-like growths that resemble large warts [26].

Pathogenesis of VC remains largely unknown. VC is a differentiated, low-grade cSCC, locally aggressive with minimal dysplasia and a low incidence of metastasis. Human papillomaviruses (HPV), types 6 and 11, may play role in the pathogenesis, as also repeated microtrauma or chronic inflammatory may be related [19]. Other known risk factors for oral VC include chewing tobacco, poor oral hygiene, smoking, and frequent alcohol consumption [26].

Lesions are classified by anatomical site: **oral florid papillomatosis**, VC of the oral mucosa; **anogenital, also known as giant condyloma acuminatum of Buschke-Löwenstein,** involving the penis, scrotum, or perianal region; and **epithelioma cuniculatum**—VC on the plantar foot [26].

Histology of VC has demonstrated a well-differentiated cSCC characterized by endo- and exophytic outline of squamous proliferation with low cytologic atypia, hyperkeratosis, and deep tongues of intradermal growth [25].

Lymphoepithelioma-Like Carcinoma of the Skin (LELCS)

LELCS is a very rare variant of cSCC, generally seen in individuals over 50 years of age. The clinical presentation is an asymptomatic flesh-colored to red solitary firm dermal nodule, papule, or plaque, commonly found in the sun-exposed skin of the head, neck, and scalp, but trunk, arms, and penis involvement have also been reported. It is characterized by slow growth, from months to years. Histology shows islands of poorly differentiated epithelial cells with a dense lymphoid infiltrate, resembling undifferentiated nasopharyngeal carcinoma [27].

The differential diagnosis is undifferentiated nasopharyngeal carcinoma, lymphoepithelial-like carcinoma metastases from other sites, poorly differentiated squamous cell carcinoma, adnexal carcinomas, Merkel cell tumors, lymphoepithelial lesions, lymphomas, melanoma, and skin metastases [27].

Marjolin's Ulcer (MU)

Classically, the term MU is a cSCC arising in chronic wounds or scars. Malignant transformation may happen over a period generally greater than 10 years with an average of 30 years; however, this phenomenon of cancerization can also occur in young subjects, with rapid transformation (Fig. 13.15) [28].

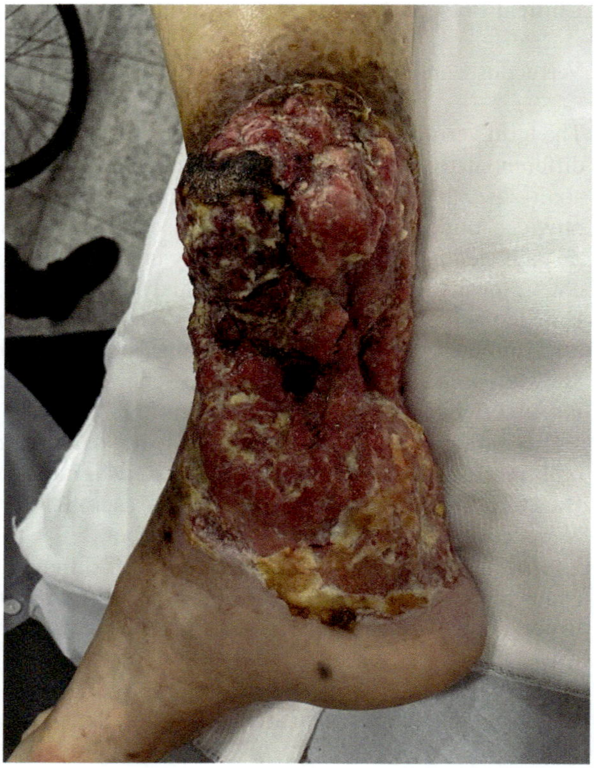

Fig. 13.15 MU is a cSCC arising in chronic wounds or scars (Courtesy of Francisco A. Belfort, MD)

MU has a more aggressive biological behavior compared to squamous cell carcinoma arising in photodamaged skin. The overall mortality is 21%. Metastasis is the most important prognostic factor; regional metastasis may affect 20–66% of cases, and distant metastasis around 14% (lung and brain) [28].

Lip cSCC and Oral cSCC

cSCC of the lip presents leukoplakic or erythroplakia showing scales or crusts, ulcerated lesion with infiltration at the base, usually in the lower lip. In advanced stages the ulcer shows indurated borders and infiltrated base that does not heal. It may present a bleeding, friable, verrucous, exophytic mass [16].

Oral cSCC is the most common oral malignancy, representing up to 80–90% of all malignant neoplasms of the oral cavity. Major predisposing factors include smoking and drinking habits, but several other factors such as human papillomavirus (HPV) and *Candida* infections, nutritional deficiencies, and genetic predisposition have been also associated. Oral cSCC is a disease of adults and elderly that arises on the tongue and floor of the mouth, in apparently normal mucosa, but others are preceded premalignant lesions, especially erythroplakia and leukoplakia.

Usually, it presents as a white ulcer with necrotic center, raised exophytic margins, and/or a lump [29, 30].

Evaluation for Locoregional and Distant Metastases in Cutaneous cSCC

Most cutaneous cSCC disease remains limited to the skin and is successfully managed with local therapy, such as excision, lesion destruction, or irradiation of the primary lesion. However, locoregional or distant metastases occur in 3–7% of patients, resulting in an increased risk for mortality. Lymph nodes are the most common sites for metastasis. All patients diagnosed with invasive cutaneous cSCC should undergo regional lymph node palpation at the time of diagnosis and during posttreatment follow-up. The lungs, liver, brain, and bone are the most frequent sites for distant metastases of cutaneous cSCC [31].

Principles of Pathology Report

According to NCCN Guidelines Version 2.2022 Squamous Cell Skin Cancer [32]:

Principles of Biopsy Reporting

Pathology evaluation of skin biopsy is ideally performed by a dermatologist, pathologist, or dermatopathologist experienced in interpreting cutaneous neoplasms (reporting of margins and elements below is not required for biopsy specimens).

Principles of Excision Report (Including Mohs Excisions)

- Specimens from intended complete surgical removal (e.g., shave excisions) should be labeled as such so that margin status is reported.
- Since depth of invasion (in mm) may not be ascertained on tangentially cut of Mohs specimens, anatomic level of invasion should be reported. Frozen or permanent section analysis of the clinical tumor specimen may be undertaken if needed for complete reporting of the features below to enable American Joint Committee on Cancer (AJCC) tumor staging.
- Immunohistochemistry may be utilized as needed to help identify lymphovascular or nerve invasion or to identify single tumor cells or small aggregates.

Recommended Elements for Pathology Reporting of Excisional Specimens (Including Mohs Excisions)

Tumors less than 2 cm in diameter without perineural invasion (as defined below) that are superficial (<6 mm in depth or confined to skin and fat) are AJCC T1 and do not require specific reporting of the histologic findings below except for grade. However, reporting the presence of any of the prognostic features below is strongly encouraged.

- *Elements reported by clinician submitting tissue*: anatomic location, clinical pre-excision diameter in cm, primary or recurrent tumor, clinical or radiologic nerve invasion, including name of nerve, other risk factors (optional), e.g., immunosuppression or prior radiation at site.
- *Elements reported by the physician reporting the histologic findings*: margin status (whether or not tumor is present at margins); well, moderate, or poor differentiation; depth of invasion (either Breslow depth in mm measured from granular layer of adjacent normal epidermis to the base of the tumor or tissue plane of deepest invasion, e.g., dermis, fat, fascia, muscle, perichondrium/periosteum, cartilage bone); perineural invasion (PNI) defined as tumor cells within the nerve sheath of a nerve deep to the dermis or with a caliber 0.1 mm or larger; lymphovascular invasion (LVI); high-risk histology, e.g., desmoplasia, adenomatous, sarcomatous, or spindle cell; low-risk histology (optional), e.g., verrucous, keratoacanthomatous.

Diagnosis

Early recognition and appropriate approach are the best opportunity for cure. Incorrect initial management of primary cSCC, especially aggressive type, can progress to relapses, locally advanced disease (LcSCC), or metastatic disease (McSCC). Special attention should be taken in larger tumors, regarding invasion to regional anatomical sites, such as orbits, sinuses, and auricular pavilion. In McSCC, metastasis can be in-transit, nodal, or distant (visceral). Palpation of the lymph nodes, especially those of primary drainage, is mandatory. Additional imaging should be considered for high-risk cSCC. Before appropriate treatment it is important to perform total body examination, photographic documentation, and measurement of the diameter of the lesion. Clinical assessment of tumor diameter is a critical parameter in the risk classification and staging of cSCC. Skin biopsy (saucerization, punch, incisional, or excisional) should include at least the reticular dermis [8].

Additional imaging may be necessary as an adjunct in the investigation of advanced stage cSCC. CT scanning or MRI can be helpful in defining the extent of disease. CT scanning is useful for determining the presence of bone or soft tissue invasion and for evaluating cervical lymph nodes at risk for metastasis. MRI is the preferred imaging modality for perineural invasion and orbital or intracranial extension evaluation [8].

Once the diagnosis of cSCC is confirmed, risk stratification is performed for staging, therapeutic approach, and follow-up.

Risk Stratification for cSCC

cSCC may be stratified into low, high, or very high risk for local recurrence, metastasis, or death from disease based on clinical and pathological parameters [32].

cSCC may be classified in risk groups based on both clinical and pathological features. Pathology may include degree of differentiation, type of cSCC, tumor size, and tumor invasion [32].

The NCCN Guidelines for Squamous Cell Skin Cancer provide recommendations for diagnostic workup, clinical stage, and treatment options for patients with cutaneous squamous cell carcinoma (Table 13.1). The version 1.2022 recommended three-tier risk stratification for cSCC based on local recurrence, metastasis, or death and divided into low-, high-, or very high-risk group. High-risk pathological features include the acantholytic, adenosquamous, carcinosarcomatous, or desmoplastic histology subtypes, depth of invasion greater than 6,0 mm (measured from the granular layer of the adjacent epidermis), depth of infiltration that extends beyond the subcutaneous fat, perineural invasion in nerves localized deeper than the dermis and measuring greater than or equal to 0,1 mm, and lymphatic or vascular involvement. Risk stratification should be based on the highest-risk factor present. The high-risk group has a high chance of local recurrence, and the very high-risk group, in addition to local recurrence, also has a high metastatic risk [32].

Clinical Staging and Preoperative Assessment

There are a small set of cSCCs classified as a high and very high risk of poor outcomes and about 8% of patients die of disease. Locoregional tumor burden is responsible for 70% death rates. The American Joint Committee on Cancer (AJCC) Tumor Classification, seventh edition (AJCC 7), for cutaneous cSCC introduced several prognostic factors besides tumor diameter [33, 34].

The Brigham and Women's Hospital (BWH) system is an alternative tumor classification system. An analysis of a single-institution cohort demonstrated that the BWH staging system offers improved distinctiveness, homogeneity, and monotonicity over AJCC 7 [33, 34].

Previous studies have shown that the AJCC 7 failed to stratify disease-related outcomes. The recently released eighth edition (AJCC 8) features a revised tumor classification for only head and neck cutaneous cSCC (Tables 13.2, 13.3, 13.4 and 13.5). Risk factors from these studies were incorporated into *AJCC 8* tumor classification with a marked expansion of criteria for T3. In *AJCC 8*, tumor size greater than 4 cm or the presence of another risk factor (e.g., minor bone erosion, large

Table 13.1 NCCN guidelines for squamous cell skin cancer

National Comprehensive Cancer Network (NCCN) risk stratification			
Risk group	Low risk	High risk	Very high risk
History and physical			
Location/size	Trunk, extremities ≤2 cm	Trunk, extremities >2 cm ≤ 4 cm	>4 cm (any location)
		Head and neck, hand, feet, pretibial, and anogenital (any size)	
Borders	Well-defined	Poorly defined	
Primary vs. recurrent	Primary	Recurrent	
Immunosuppression	(−)	(+)	
Site of prior radiotherapy or chronic inflammatory process	(−)	(+)	
Rapidly growing tumor	(−)	(+)	
Neurologic symptoms	(−)	(+)	
Pathology			
Degree of differentiation	Well or moderately differentiated		Poor differentiation
Histologic features: acantholytic, adenosquamous, or metaplastic subtypes	(−)	(+)	Desmoplastic cSCC
Depth, thickness, or level of invasion	≤6 mm or invasion beyond subcutaneous fat		>6 mm or invasion beyond subcutaneous fat
Perineural involvement	(−)	(+)	Tumor cells within the nerve sheath of a nerve lying deeper than the dermis or ≥0.1 mm
Lymphatic or vascular involvement	(−)	(−)	(+)

caliber or subdermal perineural invasion, or deep invasion past fat or >6 mm) classifies a tumor as T3. This shifted the classification from T2 (AJCC 7) to T3 (AJCC 8) of high-risk tumors that causes local recurrence, nodal metastasis, and disease-specific death. The change in inclusion criteria for *AJCC 8* T3 resulted in superior homogeneity and monotonicity, with greater separation of low- and high-risk tumors.

Although AJCC 8 captures mostly poor outcomes, twice the number of tumors are staged as a high tumor class by AJCC 8. Use of the BWH tumor classification may minimize the number of patients recommended for radiologic evaluation, close surveillance, and possible adjuvant therapy while still identifying most patients at risk for recurrence, metastasis, and death. Further studies are necessary for improvement of cSCC staging system [33, 34].

Table 13.2 Primary tumor—American Joint Committee on Cancer Staging Manual, eighth edition

Primary tumor (T)	
T category	T criteria
TX	Primary tumor cannot be assessed
Tis	Carcinoma in situ
T1	Tumor smaller than or equal to 2 cm in greatest dimension
T2	Tumor larger than 2 cm, but smaller than or equal to 4 cm in greatest dimension
T3	Tumor larger than 4 cm in maximum dimension or minor bone erosion or perineural invasion or deep invasion[a]
T4	Tumor with gross cortical bone/marrow, skull base invasion and/or skull base foramen invasion
T4a	Tumor with gross cortical bone/marrow invasion
T4b	Tumor with skull base invasion and/or skull base foramen involvement

[a]Deep invasion is defined as invasion beyond the subcutaneous fat or >6 mm (as measured from the granular layer of adjacent normal epidermis to the base of the tumor); perineural invasion for T3 classification is defined as tumor cells within the nerve sheath of a nerve lying deeper than the dermis or measuring 0.1 mm or larger in caliber or presenting with clinical or radiographic involvement of named nerves without skull base invasion or transgression

Table 13.3 Lymph node involvement—American Joint Committee on Cancer Staging Manual, eighth edition

Lymph nodes	
NX	Regional lymph nodes cannot be assessed
N0	No regional lymph node metastasis
N1	Metastasis in a single ipsilateral lymph node, 3 cm or smaller in greatest dimension and ENE(−)
N2	Metastasis in a single ipsilateral node larger than 3 cm but not larger than 6 cm in greatest dimension and ENE(−) Metastases in multiple ipsilateral lymph nodes, none larger than 6 cm in greatest dimension and ENE(−) In bilateral or contralateral lymph nodes, none larger than 6 cm in greatest dimension and ENE(−)
N2a	Metastasis in a single ipsilateral node larger than 3 cm but not larger than 6 cm in greatest dimension and ENE(−)
N2b	Metastases in multiple ipsilateral nodes, none larger than 6 cm in greatest dimension and ENE(−)
N2c	Metastases in bilateral or contralateral lymph nodes, none larger than 6 cm in greatest dimension and ENE(−)
N3	Metastasis in a lymph node larger than 6 cm in greatest dimension and ENE(−) Metastasis in any node(s) and clinically overt ENE [ENE(+)]
N3a	Metastasis in a lymph node larger than 6 cm in greatest dimension and ENE(−)
N3b	Metastasis in any node(s) and ENE(+)

Note: A designation of "U" or "L" may be used for any N category to indicate metastasis above the lower border of the cricoid (U) or below the lower border of the cricoid (L)
Similarly, clinical and pathological ENE should be recorded as ENE(−) or ENE(+)

Table 13.4 Distant metastasis—American Joint Committee on Cancer Staging Manual, eighth edition

Distant metastasis (M)	
M category	M criteria
M0	No distant metastasis
M1	Distant metastasis

Table 13.5 Prognostic stage groups—American Joint Committee on Cancer Staging Manual, eighth edition

Prognostic stage groups			
When T is...	And N is...	And M is...	Then the stage group is...
Tis	N0	M0	0
T1	N0	M0	I
T2	N0	M0	II
T3	N0	M0	III
T1	N1	M0	III
T2	N1	M0	III
T3	N1	M0	III
T1	N2	M0	IV
T2	N2	M0	IV
T3	N2	M0	IV
Any T	N3	M0	IV
T4	Any N	M0	IV
Any T	Any N	M1	IV

TNM tumor, node, metastasis, *AJCC* American Joint Committee on Cancer, *UICC* Union for International Cancer Control, *ENE* extranodal extension

Brigham and Women's Hospital Tumor Classification System for Cutaneous Squamous Cell Carcinoma

T1—0 high-risk factor[a]

T2a—1 high-risk factor

T2b—2 to 3 high-risk factors

T3—4 high-risk factors or bone invasion

[a]BWH high-risk factors include tumor diameter ≥2 cm, poorly differentiated histology, perineural invasion of nerve(s) ≥0.1 mm in caliber, or tumor invasion beyond subcutaneous fat (excluding bone invasion, which upgrades tumor to BWH stage T3) [34]

Treatment of cSCC

Surgical Treatment

Surgery is still the main goal for the best cSCC treatment. In low-risk tumors, curettage and electrodesiccation (C&E) could be performed to treat lesions, excluding terminal hair-bearing areas such as scalp, pubic, axillary regions, and beard area in male. C&E may be reserved for specific cases, and less aggressive treatment options may promote relapses under scar areas associated with future complications and morbidities.

If tumor appears to extend beyond the dermis, surgical excision should generally be performed rather than C&E. Standard excision should be performed with 4- to 6-mm clinical margins and postoperative margin assessment. Tissue rearrangement should not be undertaken until clear margins are identified. If positive margins after postsurgery margin assessment occur, standard re-excision or surgery with intraoperative total margin assessment is indicated (total margin assessment with Mohs micrographic surgery or other forms of peripheral and deep *en face* margin assessment (PDEMA) could be performed). Radiotherapy is reserved for nonsurgical candidates [32].

High-risk and very high-risk cSCC requires Mohs surgery or PDEMA or surgery with wider margins and postoperative margin assessment. If surgery with intraoperative controlled margins is positive, tumor board consultation would be necessary to discuss options: re-excision, if feasible, radiotherapy, or systemic therapy. In case of negative margins with extensive perineural or large nerve involvement or other poor prognostic features, consider radiotherapy [32].

Surgery for Regional Nodal Disease

Patients with nodal metastases from cSCC should be managed surgically similarly to patients with cutaneous melanoma or Merkel cell carcinoma.

Therapeutic regional lymph node dissection for lymph nodes clinically detected or following imaging is the preferred surgical treatment.

A radical lymph node dissection of the affected areas should be performed. The extent of surgical resection is determined by the interdisciplinary tumor board. The three levels of axillary lymph nodes should be removed in cases of axillary nodal disease. In the groin, the procedure should include the superficial and deep inguinal lymph nodes. If the nodal disease occurs on the neck, the five levels of nodes should be included in the dissection. Superficial parotidectomy should be discussed if the parotid gland is affected. It is unclear whether a more selective procedure will affect the disease-free survival and the overall survival [32].

Elective (prophylactic) lymph node dissection is not recommended in the management of lymph node-negative cSCC patients, due to the low rate of nodal metastasis and associated morbidity from the dissection.

A meta-analysis (17 studies) in patients with metastatic cSCC to the parotid with no clinically evident cervical disease reported that the overall prevalence of occult disease was 22.5%.

The authors suggested that elective neck dissection is recommended in patients with metastasis of cSCC to the parotid due to the prevalence of occult cervical disease. The extent of dissection is determined by the surgeon in collaboration with the interdisciplinary tumor board [35].

For all tumors not amenable to surgery (due to patient-related factors or when the intention of a R0 resectability cannot be achieved), nonoperative therapies should be considered by a multidisciplinary tumor board decision.

In-transit metastasis should be removed surgically if the number, size, and location allow complete removal of them. For multiple unresectable metastasis on the limbs, currently systemic and several local alternatives are available to prevent mutilation. Local options include radiotherapy, intralesional chemotherapy, interferon alpha, electrochemotherapy, or isolated limb perfusion or infusion.

It's important to note that either ENE (extranodal extension) or STM (soft tissue metastasis) occurs in most patients with head and neck squamous cell carcinoma regional metastasis, and both are adverse prognostic factors.

Until now, there is no consensus about the use of sentinel node biopsy in patients with cutaneous cSCC. NCCN (version 2022) [36] recommends a discussion and consideration prior to PDEMA for very high-risk group with normal draining nodal basin. Although small sample sizes and low rates of SLN positivity limit assessment of prognostic factors, a few studies suggest that risk factors for SLNB positivity include tumor diameter and thickness, LVI, PNI, and the presence of multiple high-risk factors.

Nonsurgical Treatments

Topical and Local Nonsurgical Treatments for AK and Cancerization Field

The appropriate and timely management of AK and cancerization field may translate into improved cosmetic and functional results and mitigate the risk of recurrence and progression to invasive lesions. Topical preparations and photodynamic therapy are usually classified as field approaches, while surgical resection or ablative procedures are the hallmark of the management of solitary or limited lesions. Nevertheless, oftentimes combinations of the sequential use of different techniques are necessary in the patient journey affected by actinic keratoses or cancerization field, and distinct alternatives are described below [37–42]:

- 5-Fluorouracil (5-FU) is a pyrimidine analogue that has been used for the treatment of AKs for many decades. It is usually used for patients with field cancerization or with multiple actinic keratoses. Frequently used regimens include topical formulations of 5-FU, applied once or twice a day for 2–4 weeks. If large areas are affected, 5-FU should be used sequentially in areas not exceeding 500 cm^2. Mild to moderate irritating side effects, such as erythema, crust formation, erosion, and pain, are common. A recent randomized double-blind controlled trial demonstrated the superiority of 5-FU over imiquimod, photodynamic therapy, and ingenol mebutate in the treatment of AKs [2, 37–39].
- Imiquimod is a topical immune response modifier that is also used for the treatment of non-hypertrophic AKs on the face and scalp and low risk. It is usually used three times a week for 4–16 weeks. The efficacy of imiquimod was demonstrated in several clinical trials showing complete response rates of approximately 50% in patients with AKs. Side effects are like those observed with 5-FU preparations [31, 32].
- Photodynamic therapy (PDT) is another treatment that may be useful in treating field cancerization. A photochemical reaction occurs by using a photosensitizing agent and a light source at a specific wavelength to produce reactive oxygen species, which then destroy target lesions. Photosensitizing agents include 5-aminolevulinic acid (5-ALA) and methylaminolevulinate (MAL). Several regimens are proposed for PDT. Conventional PDT for field cancerization or patients with multiple actinic keratoses is usually performed with one treatment, but occasionally a second course may be performed following a 4–8-week interval. A recent meta-analysis demonstrated that PDT may offer superior long-term control in comparison to other field cancerization treatment options. Pain during light irradiation is a major side effect. Daylight PDT is an alternative regimen to increase tolerance to the procedure, and its efficacy is generally non-inferior in comparison to conventional PDT for low-grade AK [2, 40].

Among ablative methods for isolated AK, cryotherapy with liquid nitrogen is the most frequently used alternative, as it offers an excellent tolerability and simple technique. Immediate side effects include burning sensation, edema/erythema, vesiculation, and residual hypopigmentation.

Especially hyperkeratotic lesions may require surgical methods, which can be performed by shaving, curettage, or excision. These methods are particularly important when treating lesions in which an invasive cSCC cannot be ruled out clinically [2].

Of note, ingenol mebutate has been reported to potentially relate to increased risk of cSCC, and the European Medicines Agency has recommended that the use be suspended until more investigations demonstrate the safety of the product [39].

Patients presenting with AK and cancerization field should be closely monitored, as the majority may present multiple recurrences and new primary lesions. The recommended frequency of clinic visits for low-risk patients (mild actinic keratoses level) is once or twice a year, while patients with severe photodamage and/or a significant history of cutaneous carcinomas should be monitored every 3–6 months [41, 42].

All patients should be advised regarding physical photoprotection and the use of sunscreens as an adjuvant to the treatment and to prevent the onset of new lesions, regardless the type of treatment proposed. Regular use of sunscreen with a sun protection factor (SPF) over 15 reduces the development of new actinic keratoses in immunocompetent patients, ranging from a 50% reduction in the number of new lesions in 1 year (study using SPF 29) and 37% in 2 years (study using SPF 16) ($p < 0.05$) [2].

Topical and Local Nonsurgical Treatments for cSCC

Surgery is the gold standard in the treatment of cSCC. The available data do not currently support the use of the topical modalities discussed for AK for the treatment of invasive cSCC. There are few exceptions for the recommendation of topical therapy when surgical therapy is not feasible to treat low-risk cSCC. Topical treatment as imiquimod, 5-FU, or cryotherapy should be reserved as an alternative therapy for patients with in situ cSCC [32].

Radiation therapy is an alternative in situations when a complete surgical resection cannot be performed and also in the adjuvant treatment of cSCC. The choice of this technique should consider functional and cosmetic results and potential long-term sequelae, including the possibility of radiation-induced malignancies. The advantages over an unwanted surgical procedure should be compared to the disadvantages of the technique, such as lack of margin control, poor long-term aesthetic result, and increased risk of skin cancer in the future. Radiation therapy is indicated in the adjuvant treatment of aggressive/high-risk cSCC, especially in the setting of perineural involvement or nodal metastases. Verrucous carcinomas, which are well differentiated, usually have contraindication for radiotherapy, because there is concern about a cell transformation with a worse prognosis [35, 43].

Systemic Treatments for Localized AK, Cancerization Field, and cSCC

Acitretin is an oral retinoid that is used for chemoprevention. It should be considered in patients with more than five non-melanoma skin cancers over the course of 2–3 years and having significant chronic field cancerization areas. Doses may range from 10 to 30 mg per day.

Nicotinamide, a vitamin B3 derivative, has been shown to present modest effects on AK reduction. It reduces ultraviolet-associated immunosuppression. Nicotinamide 500 mg twice daily seems to reduce the number of AKs compared with baseline by 13% at 12 months [42, 43].

For both treatments, the effects disappear shortly after cessation of the drugs.

In immunosuppressed patients, including solid-organ transplant recipients, the reduction, adjustment, or interruption of immunosuppressive therapy may be indicated in order to minimize doses of antimetabolites and calcineurin inhibitors in favor of mammalian target of rapamycin (MTOR) inhibitors. This strategy may be useful in patients with multiple lesions or in cases of metastatic disease. Changes in the immunosuppressive regimen should be made in a multidisciplinary approach with the medical team responsible for the immunosuppressive treatment [35].

Systemic Treatment of Advanced cSCC

Most of those affected by cSCC are cured by surgery and/or radiation therapy. Nevertheless, a proportion of patients may develop recurrent or locally advanced lesions, leading to significant morbidity and disability. In addition, metastases of cSCC can occur in 2–35% of newly diagnosed cases, initially to regional lymph nodes and, subsequently, to distant sites including the lungs, bones, and liver. In this setting, palliative systemic treatments should be considered.

Until recently, treatment options in cases of advanced/inoperable cSCC were limited, resulting in a poor prognosis and a median overall survival (OS) of less than 12 months (mo) [35, 44, 45]. Distinct cytotoxic-based regimens, wither as single agents or in combination, have shown variable degrees of activity and usually a marginal long-term efficacy in small, prospective trials or retrospective series, including platinum salts (cisplatin, carboplatin), taxanes (paclitaxel), antitumor antibiotics (bleomycin), and fluoropyrimidines (5-fluorouracyl) [35, 45–47]. Anti-epidermal growth factor receptor (EGFR) monoclonal antibodies and tyrosine kinase inhibitors (TKIs), including cetuximab, erlotinib, gefitinib, and panitumumab, have also demonstrated activity in patients with a cSCC, however with objective response rates below 20% and short-lived benefits [48–53].

Over the past years, the use of immunotherapy targeting receptors involved in the modulation of the immune response and the interaction of cancer cells and immune cells, of immune checkpoints, emerged as a novel systemic therapy and is now considered a standard of care. Indeed, underlying risk factors and mechanisms of carcinogenesis, which include UV radiation-induced DNA skin damage, chronic inflammation, ionizing radiation, immunosuppression, and familial cancer syndromes associated with increased photosensitivity or defective DNA repair [54], qualify cSCC as a potentially immunogenic tumor, which has been confirmed through the demonstration of a high tumor mutational burden and *programmed death 1 (PD-1)* ligand expression in both tumor cells and microenvironment inflammatory cells [55–57].

Distinct monoclonal antibodies targeting PD-1 (cemiplimab, pembrolizumab, and nivolumab) have demonstrated robust antitumor activity across several prospective studies, with objective response rates of approximately 50–60% and sustained responses, resulting in a median overall survival of over 20 months and median

Table 13.6 Overview of prospective studies investigating anti-PD-1 agents in cSCC

Intervention	Number of patients	Setting	Outcomes
Nivolumab	24	First line	ORR: 58.3% mPFS: 12.7 months mOS: 20.7 months
Pembrolizumab	39	First line	ORR: 41% mPFS: 6.7 months mOS: 25.3 months
Pembrolizumab	105	First or subsequent lines	ORR: 34.3% mPFS: 6.9 months mOS: NR
Cemiplimab	193	First or subsequent lines	ORR: 47.2% mPFS: 22.1 months mOS: NR

ORR objective response rate, *mPFS* median progression-free survival, *mOS* median overall survival, *NR* not reached

duration of response not reached [58–61]. As a result, both cemiplimab and pembrolizumab have been approved for clinical use for patients with advanced cSCC in the first and subsequent lines of therapy. The role of immune-checkpoint blockers in the perioperative setting (adjuvant and neoadjuvant treatment) is currently being evaluated in prospective studies and remains investigational (Table 13.6).

Despite the clinical activity and a better tolerability in comparison to cytotoxic compounds and targeted therapies, these agents are associated with the risk of immune-related adverse events, and immunosuppressed patients, those requiring chronic steroids, and solid-organ transplant recipients were excluded from most clinical trials. For these subgroups not eligible for immunotherapy, systemic chemotherapy and EGFR inhibitors are other options to be considered, accompanied by a careful reconsideration of the immunosuppressive therapy, as discussed above.

References

1. Werner RN, Sammain A, Erdmann R, Hartmann V, Stockfleth E, Nast A. The natural history of actinic keratosis: a systematic review. Br J Dermatol. 2013;169(3):502–18. https://doi.org/10.1111/bjd.12420.
2. Reinehr CPH, Bakos RM. Actinic keratoses: review of clinical, dermoscopic, and therapeutic aspects. An Bras Dermatol. 2019;94(6):637–57. https://doi.org/10.1016/j.abd.2019.10.004.
3. Criscione VD, Weinstock MA, Naylor MF, Luque C, Eide MJ, Bingham SF, et al. Actinic keratoses: natural history and risk of malignant transformation in the veterans affairs topical tretinoin chemoprevention trial. Cancer. 2009;115:2523–30.
4. Fernández-Figueras MT, Carrato C, Sáenz X, Puig L, Musulen E, Ferrándiz C, et al. Actinic keratosis with atypical basal cells (AK I) is the most common lesion associated with invasive squamous cell carcinoma of the skin. J Eur Acad Dermatol Venereol. 2015;29:991–7.
5. Heaphy MR, Ackerman AB. The nature of solar keratosis: a critical review in historical perspective. J Am Acad Dermatol. 2000;43:138–50.
6. Didona D, Paolino G, Bottoni U, Cantisani C. Non-melanoma skin cancer pathogenesis overview. Biomedicines. 2018;6(1):6. https://doi.org/10.3390/biomedicines6010006.

7. Adinarayan M, Krishnamurthy SP. Clinicopathological evaluation of nonmelanoma skin cancer. Indian J Dermatol. 2011;56(6):670–2. https://doi.org/10.4103/0019-5154.91826.
8. Orchado-Cobos R, García-Sancha N, González-Sarmiento R, Pérez-Losada J, Cañueto J. Cutaneous squamous cell carcinoma: from biology to therapy. Int J Mol Sci. 2020;21(8):2956. https://doi.org/10.3390/ijms21082956).
9. Velez NF, Karia PS, Schmults CD, et al. Association of advanced leukemic stage and skin cancer tumor stage with poor skin cancer outcomes in patients with chronic lymphocytic leukemia. JAMA Dermatol. 2014;150:280–7.
10. Thomson J, Bewicke-Copley F, Anene CA, Gulati A, Nagano A, Purdie K, Inman GJ, Proby CM, Leigh IM, Harwood CA, Wang J. The genomic landscape of actinic keratosis. J Invest Dermatol. 2021;141(7):1664–1674.e7. https://doi.org/10.1016/j.jid.2020.12.024.
11. Nelson MA, Einspahr JG, Alberts DS, Balfour CA, Wymer JA, Welch KL, Salasche SJ, Bangert JL, Grogan TM, Bozzo PO. Analysis of the p53 gene in human precancerous actinic keratosis lesions and squamous cell cancers. Cancer Lett. 1994;85(1):23–9. https://doi.org/10.1016/0304-3835(94)90234-8.
12. Que SKT, Zwald FO, Schmults CD. Cutaneous squamous cell carcinoma: incidence, risk factors, diagnosis, and staging. J Am Acad Dermatol. 2018;78(2):237–47. https://doi.org/10.1016/j.jaad.2017.08.059.
13. Ratushny V, Gober MD, Hick R, Ridky TW, Seykora JT. From keratinocyte to cancer: the pathogenesis and modeling of cutaneous squamous cell carcinoma. J Clin Invest. 2012;122(2):464–72. https://doi.org/10.1172/JCI57415.
14. Fania L, Didona D, Di Pietro FR, Verkhovskaia S, Morese R, Paolino G, Donati M, Ricci F, Coco V, Ricci F, Candi E, Abeni D, Dellambra E. Cutaneous squamous cell carcinoma: from pathophysiology to novel therapeutic approaches. Biomedicine. 2021;9(2):171. https://doi.org/10.3390/biomedicines9020171.
15. Schmitt JV, Miot HA. Actinic keratosis: a clinical and epidemiological revision. An Bras Dermatol. 2012;87:425–34.
16. Vieira RA, Ribeiro MA, et al. Actinic cheilitis and squamous cell carcinoma of the lip: clinical, histopathological and immunogenetic aspects. An Bras Dermatol. 2012;87(1):105–14. https://doi.org/10.1590/S0365-05962012000100013.
17. Schmitt JV, Miot HA, Schmitt JV, et al. Actinic keratosis: a clinical and epidemiological revision. An Bras Dermatol. 2012;87(3):425–34.
18. Yanofsky VR, Mercer SE, Phelps RG. Histopathological variants of cutaneous squamous cell carcinoma: a review. J Skin Cancer. 2011;2011:210813. https://doi.org/10.1155/2011/210813).
19. Lallas A, Pyne J, Kyrgidis A, Andreani S, Argenziano G, Cavaller A, Zalaudek I. The clinical and dermoscopic features of invasive cutaneous squamous cell carcinoma depend on the histopathological grade of differentiation. Br J Dermatol. 2015;172(5):1308–15.
20. Slaughter DP, Southwick HW, Smejkal W. Field cancerization in oral stratified squamous epithelium; clinical implications of multicentric origin. Cancer. 1953;6(5):963–8.
21. Christensen SR. Recent advances in field cancerization and management of multiple cutaneous squamous cell carcinomas. F1000Research. 2018;7:12837. https://doi.org/10.12688/f1000research.12837.1.
22. Huang A, Nguyen JK, Austin E, Mamalis A, Jagdeo J. Updates on treatment approaches for cutaneous field cancerization. Curr Dermatol Rep. 2019;8(3):122–32. https://doi.org/10.1007/s13671-019-00265-2.
23. Savage JA, Maize JC Sr. Keratoacanthoma clinical behavior: a systematic review. Am J Dermatopathol. 2014;36(5):422–9.
24. Ra S, Su A, Li X, et al. Keratoacanthoma and squamous cell carcinoma are distinct from a molecular perspective. Mod Pathol. 2015;28:799–806. https://doi.org/10.1038/modpathol.2015.5).
25. Elder DE, Massi D, Scoyler RA, Willemze R, editors. Who classification of skin tumors. 4th ed. Lyon: IARC; 2018.
26. Schwartz RA. Verrucous carcinoma of the skin and mucosa. J Am Acad Dermatol. 1995;32(1):1–21.

27. Welch PQ, Williams SB, Foss RD, Tomaszewski MM, Gupta A, Ojha J. Lymphoepithelioma-like carcinoma of head and neck skin: a systematic analysis of 11 cases and review of literature. Oral Surg Oral Med Oral Pathol Oral Radiol Endodontol. 2011;111(1):78–86.
28. Hahn SB, Kim DJ, Jeon C, cSCC. Clinical study of Marjolin's ulcer. Yonsei Med J. 1990;31(3):234–41.
29. Pires FR, Ramos AB, Oliveira JB, Tavares AS, Luz PS, Santos TC. Oral squamous cell carcinoma: clinicopathological features from 346 cases from a single oral pathology service during an 8-year period. J Appl Oral Sci. 2013;21(5):460–7. https://doi.org/10.1590/1679-775720130317.
30. Markopoulos AK. Current aspects on oral squamous cell carcinoma. Open Dent J. 2012;6:126–30.
31. Khan K, Mykula R, Kerstein R, et al. A 5-year follow-up study of 633 cutaneous cSCC excisions: rates of local recurrence and lymph node metastasis. J Plast Reconstr Aesthet Surg. 2018;71:1153.
32. National Comprehensive Cancer Network (NCCN) Guidelines Version 1.2021 Squamous Cell Skin Cancer. https://cSCC.nccn.org/professionals/physician_gls/pdf/squamous.pdf. Accessed 18 June 2021.
33. Karia PS, Morgan FC, Califano JA, Schmults CD. Comparison of tumor classifications for cutaneous squamous cell carcinoma of the head and neck in the 7th vs 8th edition of the AJCC cancer staging manual. JAMA Dermatol. 2018;154(2):175–81. https://doi.org/10.1001/jamadermatol.2017.3960).
34. Ruiz ES, Karia PS, Besaw R, Schmults CD. Performance of the American joint committee on cancer staging manual, 8th edition vs the Brigham and Women's hospital tumor classification system for cutaneous squamous cell carcinoma. JAMA Dermatol. 2019;155(7):819–25. https://doi.org/10.1001/jamadermatol.2019.0032.
35. Stratigos AJ, Garbe C, Dessinioti C, Lebbe C, Bataille V, Bastholt L, et al. European interdisciplinary guideline on invasive squamous cell carcinoma of the skin: part 2. Treatment. Eur J Cancer. 2020;128:83–102. https://doi.org/10.1016/j.ejca.2020.01.008.
36. Rotman A, Kerr SJ, Giddings CEB. Elective neck dissection in metastatic cutaneous squamous cell carcinoma to the parotid gland: a systematic review and meta-analysis. Head Neck. 2019;41:1131–9.
37. Dianzani C, Conforti C, Giuffrida R, Corneli P, di Meo N, Farinazzo E, Moret A, Magaton Rizzi G, Zalaudek I, Dianzani C, et al. Current therapies for actinic keratosis. Int J Dermatol. 2020;59(6):677–84.
38. Eisen DB, Asgari MM, Bennett DD, Connolly SM, Dellavalle RP, Freeman EE, Goldenberg G, Leffell DJ, Peschin S, Sligh JE, Wu PA, Frazer-Green L, Malik S, Schlesinger TE, Eisen DB, et al. Guidelines of care for the management of actinic keratosis: executive summary. J Am Acad Dermatol. 2021;85(4):945–55.
39. Ahmady S, Jansen MHE, Nelemans PJ, Kessels JPHM, Arits AHMM, de Rooij MJM, Essers BAB, Quaedvlieg PJF, Kelleners-Smeets NWJ, Mosterd K. Risk of invasive cutaneous squamous cell carcinoma after different treatments for actinic keratosis: a secondary analysis of a randomized clinical trial. JAMA Dermatol. 2022;158(6):634–40. https://doi.org/10.1001/jamadermatol.2022.1034.
40. Hadley G, Derry S, Moore RA, Hadley G, et al. Imiquimod for actinic keratosis: systematic review and meta-analysis. J Invest Dermatol. 2006;126(6):1251–5.
41. Steeb T, Wessely A, Petzold A, Brinker TJ, Schmitz L, Leiter U, Garbe C, Schöffski O, Berking C, Heppt MV, Steeb T, et al. Evaluation of long-term clearance rates of interventions for actinic keratosis: a systematic review and network meta-analysis. JAMA Dermatol. 2021;157(9):1066–77.
42. Cornejo CM, Jambusaria-Pahlajani A, Willenbrink TJ, Schmults CD, Arron ST, Ruiz ES, Cornejo CM, et al. Field cancerization: treatment. J Am Acad Dermatol. 2020;83(3):719–30.
43. Chen AC, Martin AJ, Choy B, Fernandez-Peñas P, Dalziell RA, McKenzie CA, Scoyler RA, Dhillon HM, Vardy JL, Kricker A, St George G, Chinniah N, Halliday GM, Damian DL. A

phase 3 randomized trial of nicotinamide for skin-cancer chemoprevention. N Engl J Med. 2015;373:1618–26.
44. Work Group Invited Reviewers, Kim J, Kozlow J, Mittal B, Moyer J, Olenecki T, Rodgers P. Guidelines of care for the management of cutaneous squamous cell carcinoma. J Am Acad Dermatol. 2018;78(3):560–78. https://doi.org/10.1016/j.jaad.2017.10.007.
45. Cranmer LD, Engelhardt C, Morgan SS. Treatment of unresectable and metastatic cutaneous squamous cell carcinoma. Oncologist. 2010;15:1320–8.
46. Sadek H, Azli N, Wendling JL, Cvitkovic E, Rahal M, Mamelle G, et al. Treatment of advanced squamous cell carcinoma of the skin with cisplatin, 5-fluorouracil, and bleomycin. Cancer. 1990;66:1692–6.
47. Jarkowski A, Hare R, Loud P, et al. Systemic therapy in advanced cutaneous squamous cell carcinoma. The Roswell Park experience and review of the literature. Am J Clin Oncol. 2016;39(6):545–8.
48. Maubec E, Petrow P, Scheer-Senyarich I, Skitzki JJ, Kane JM, May KS, et al. Phase II study of cetuximab as first-line single-drug therapy in patients with unresectable squamous cell carcinoma of the skin. J Clin Oncol. 2011;29(25):3419.
49. Joseph K, Alkaabi K, Warkentin H, Ghosh S, Jha N, Smylie M, et al. Cetuximab-radiotherapy combination in the management of locally advanced cutaneous squamous cell carcinoma. J Med Imaging Radiat Oncol. 2019;63(2):257–63.
50. Trodello C, Pepper JP, Wong M, Wysong A. Cisplatin and cetuximab treatment for metastatic cutaneous squamous cell carcinoma: a systematic review. Dermatol Surg. 2017;43(1):40–9.
51. Gold KA, Kies MS, William WM Jr, Johnson FM, Lee JJ, Glisson BS. Erlotinib in the treatment of recurrent or metastatic cutaneous squamous-cell carcinoma: a single-arm phase 2 clinical trial. Cancer. 2018;124(10):2169–73.
52. Foote MC, McGrath M, Guminski A, Hughes BGM, Meakin J, Thomson D, et al. Phase II study of single-agent panitumumab in patients with incurable cutaneous squamous cell carcinoma. Ann Oncol. 2014;25(10):2047–52.
53. William WN Jr, Feng L, Ferrarotto R, Ginsberg L, Kies M, Lippman S, et al. Gefitinib for patients with incurable cutaneous squamous cell carcinoma: a single-arm phase II clinical trial. J Am Acad Dermatol. 2017;77(6):1110–3.
54. Que SKT, Swald FO, Schmults C. Cutaneous squamous cell carcinoma: incidence, risk factors, diagnosis, and staging. J Am Acad Dermatol. 2018;78(2):237–47.
55. Corchado-Cobos R, Garcia-Sancha N, González-Sarmiento R, Pérez-Losada J, Canueto J. Cutaneous squamous cell carcinoma: from biology to therapy. Int J Mol Sci. 2020;21(8):2956.
56. Pickering CR, Zhou JH, Lee JJ, Drummond JA, Peng SA, Saade RE, et al. Mutational landscape of aggressive cutaneous squamous cell carcinoma. Clin Cancer Res. 2014;20(24):6582–92.
57. Chalmers ZR, Connelly CF, Fabrizio D, Gay L, Ali SM, Ennis R, et al. Analysis of 100,000 human cancer genomes reveals the landscape of tumor mutational burden. Genome Med. 2017;9(1):34.
58. Migden MR, Rischin D, Schmults CD, Guminski A, Hauschild A, Lewis KD, et al. PD-1 blockade with cemiplimab in advanced cutaneous squamous-cell carcinoma. N Engl J Med. 2018;379(4):341–51.
59. Grob JJ, Gozalez R, Basset-Seguin N, Vornicova O, Schachter J, Joshi A, et al. Pembrolizumab monotherapy for recurrent or metastatic cutaneous squamous cell carcinoma: a single-arm phase II trial (KEYNOTE-629). J Clin Oncol. 2020;38(25):2916–5.
60. Maubec E, Boubaya M, Petrow P, Baylot-Barry M, Basset-Seguin N, Deschamps L, et al. Phase II study of pembrolizumab as first-line, single-drug therapy for patients with unresectable cutaneous squamous cell carcinomas. J Clin Oncol. 2020;38(26):3051–61.
61. Munhoz RR, Nader-Marta G, Camargo VP, Queiroz MM, Cury-Martins J, Ricci H, de Mattos MR, de Menezes TAF, Machado GUC, Bertolli E, Barros M, de Souza CE, Franke F, Ferreira FO, Feher O, de Castro G Jr. A phase 2 study of first-line nivolumab in patients with locally-advanced or metastatic cutaneous squamous-cell carcinoma. Cancer. 2022;128(24):4223–31.

Chapter 14
Basal Cell Carcinoma

Beatriz Mendes Awni, Suzy Maria Rabello Ferrer, André Sapata Molina, Melissa Fugimori Lissae, Marina Sahade, Rodrigo Ramella Munhoz, and Cristina Martinez Zugaib Abdalla

Key Points
- Basal cell carcinoma (BCC) is the most common type of carcinoma worldwide.
- BCCs usually are indolent, slow-growing tumors, and the occurrence of metastases is extremely rare.
- BCC can be stratified as low risk or high risk of recurrence, based on clinical and pathological characteristics.
- The surgical treatment is the main approach with adequate surgical margins allied with satisfactory cosmetic and functional results.
- Treatment should be customized according to the patient's characteristics and tumor-related factors.
- Radiotherapy and systemic therapy are reserved for locally advanced disease and metastatic. For patients with advanced disease, standard treatment options include hedgehog inhibitors (e.g., vismodegib or sonidegib) and immunotherapy.

Epidemiology and Pathogenesis

Among non-melanoma skin tumors, which account for 95% of skin cancer cases, basal cell carcinoma (BCC) is the most common. Although the notification of BCC cases is not precise, it is estimated that they correspond to

B. M. Awni · R. R. Munhoz (✉)
Oncology Center, Hospital Sírio-Libanês, São Paulo, Brazil

S. M. R. Ferrer · A. S. Molina · M. F. Lissae · M. Sahade · C. M. Z. Abdalla
Hospital Sírio-Libanês, São Paulo, Brazil

C. M. Z. Abdalla et al. (eds.), *Oncodermatology*,
https://doi.org/10.1007/978-3-031-29277-4_14

more than 80% of skin cancer cases in general. Its global incidence is progressively increasing, affecting about one million new patients yearly. BCC is a slow-growing keratinocyte neoplasm from the follicular or interfollicular basal layer [1, 2].

BCC's global incidence is increasing as a result from population aging, chronic exposure to sunlight, climatic changes, and individual and social conditions [3]. In the United States, two million cases were reported between 1998 and 2012, which allows a projection of ten million new cases of BCC per year worldwide [2, 4]. The overall incidence ratio BCC:SCC is 4:1, but recently decreased to 2:1 because of the increasing incidence of SCC [5]. The incidence is higher in middle-aged and elderly individuals and the men/women ratio is 2:1 [1, 6]. In addition, consecutive BCCs are expected, with almost 29% of patients with a first BCC developing at least one more lesion throughout their lives [6].

BCCs characteristically develop in sun-exposed areas of the head and neck region. This anatomical predisposition highlights ultraviolet radiation (UVR) as an important environmental risk factor. Other risk factors are Fitzpatrick skin types I and II (lifetime risk for BCC is 30%), childhood sunburns, family history of skin cancer, use of tanning beds, chronic immunosuppression (e.g., twice the risk for HIV and 5–10 times greater in organ transplant patients), photosensitizing drugs (e.g., tetracyclines, calcium channel blockers, beta-blockers, or thiazide diuretics), and prior exposure to ionizing radiation and carcinogenic chemicals, especially arsenic [1].

Although most BCCs occur sporadically, some cases may develop in the context of germline mutations associated with hereditary syndromes, the foremost being Gorlin–Goltz syndrome (GGS) and, less frequently, Bazex syndrome and xeroderma pigmentosum [7]. GGS, also known as basal cell nevus syndrome, is a rare autosomal dominant inherited disease characterized by the development of BCCs from a young age and keratocystic odontogenic tumors, dyskeratotic palmar, and plantar pits. The syndrome's molecular pathogenesis results from defects in signaling in the hedgehog pathway, resulting in constitutive pathway activity and tumor cell proliferation. Therapeutic agents targeting the hedgehog pathway play a significant role in BCC's treatment [8].

BCC's molecular basis involves an interplay of somatic mutations, commonly induced by exposure to UV radiation and inherited genetic susceptibility, among them tumor suppressor genes and proto-oncogenes, including key components of the hedgehog pathway, the tumor suppressor TP53, and members of the RAS family of proto-oncogenes. The main pathway of BCC carcinogenesis is aberrant hedgehog signaling. Most BCCs carry inactivating mutations in PTCH1 (90%) and activating mutations in the SMO gene (10%), resulting in constitutive activation of the hedgehog pathway and subsequent cell proliferation and tumor growth. Advances in molecular sequencing technology have allowed the discovery of several mutations potentially involved in BCC carcinogenesis, including mutations in MYCN, PPP6C, STK19, LATS1, ERBB2, PIK23C, NRAS, K-RAS, and H-RAS, as well as loss of function PTPN14, RB1, and FBXW7 [9–11].

Clinical Presentation and Histopathology

BCCs are usually indolent and slow-growing tumors. Despite its high prevalence, metastases are extremely rare, with incidence rates ranging from 0.0028 to 0.55% [2]. Most BCCs predominantly affect the head and neck, consistent with the etiological role of UV exposure. Additional primary sites include the trunk and extremities and, rarely, non-hair-bearing areas [12].

There is no consensus on the classification of BCCs [13]; however, many consider histopathological aspects strictly for the clinical denomination. BCC has a variety of clinicopathologic forms, all with specific characteristics, and treatment options may vary according to the type of BCC. There are several variants described, but below are the main ones [4, 12].

The histopathological subtypes of BCC are classified according to the risk of tumor recurrence, with low-risk nodular, superficial, pigmented, and infundibulocystic (BCC with adnexal differentiation) and fibroepithelial. Those with a higher risk of recurrence and local destruction are basal, sclerosing/morphoic, infiltrating squamous carcinomas with sarcomatoid and micronodular differentiation [12].

Nodular Type

It is the most prevalent subtype representing 60–80% of all BCCs [14]. The classical clinical presentation is a shiny, pearly, smooth papule/nodule with prominent, dilated, and arborizing telangiectasias, often with erosions or ulcerations [4, 14]. Bleeding with minor trauma is frequent. Nodular BCCs are predominant on the head and neck, notably the cheeks, nasolabial folds, forehead, and eyelids. The differential diagnosis includes molluscum contagiosum, sebaceous hyperplasia, amelanotic melanoma, intradermal melanocytic nevus, Merkel cell carcinoma, fibrous papule of the nose, trichoepithelioma, and other adnexal neoplasms. For an ulcerated lesion, the differential diagnosis includes squamous cell carcinomas and keratoacanthomas (Fig. 14.1). Microscopically, it appears as large nests of basaloid cells in the dermis and peripheral palisade, in addition to surrounding mucinous tumor stroma (Figs. 14.2 and 14.3) [11].

Superficial Type

The superficial variety is responsible for approximately 20% of all BCCs, and the location is primarily on the trunk and limbs. This tumor often presents as a well-defined, erythematous, scaly, or slightly shiny macular lesion. Hypopigmented and atrophic areas are the result of spontaneous regression foci. It tends to occur in younger patients (mean age at diagnosis 57 years), and the differential diagnosis

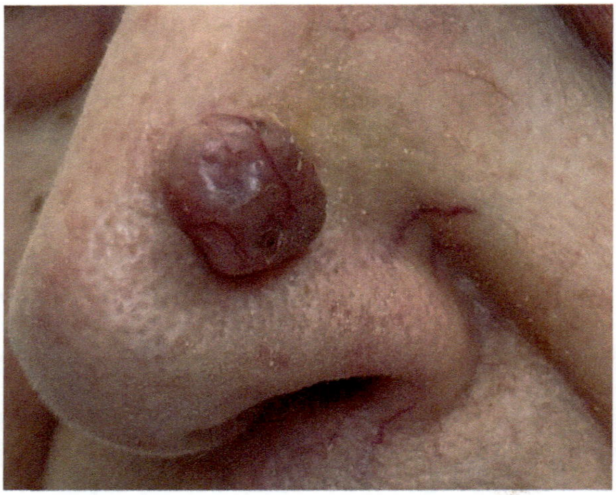

Fig. 14.1 Nodular BCC (Courtesy of Cristina Abdalla, MD)

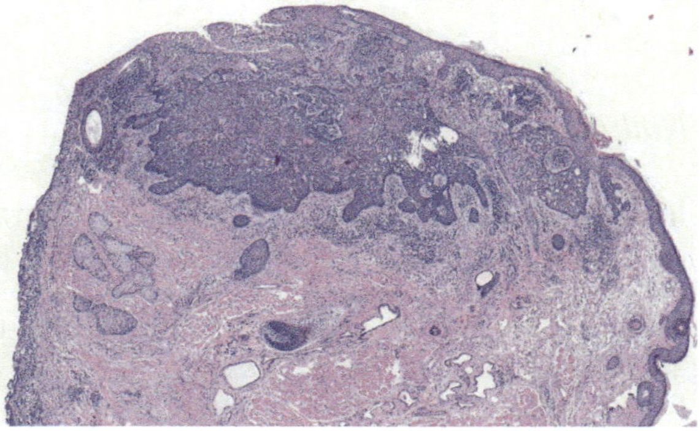

Fig. 14.2 Histopathology of nodular BCC (Courtesy of Melissa Fugimori, MD)

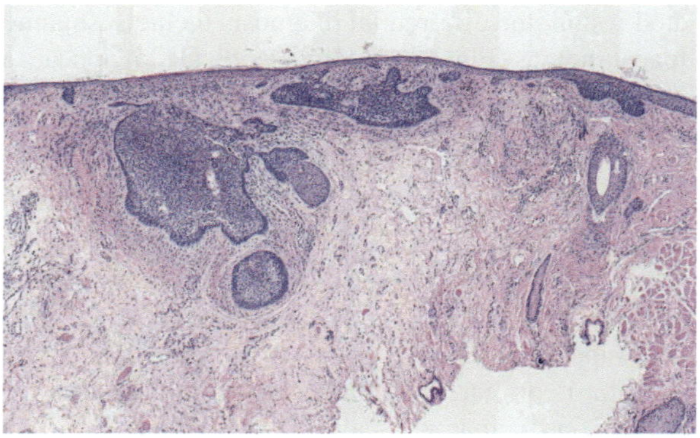

Fig. 14.3 Histopathology of nodular and superficial BCC (Courtesy of Melissa Fugimori, MD)

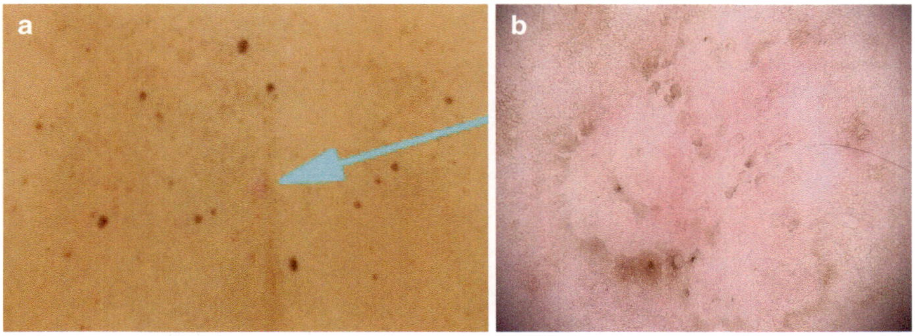

Fig. 14.4 Superficial BCC: (**a**) clinical picture (delicate pink macule), (**b**) dermoscopy of superficial BCC (Courtesy of Cristina Abdalla, MD)

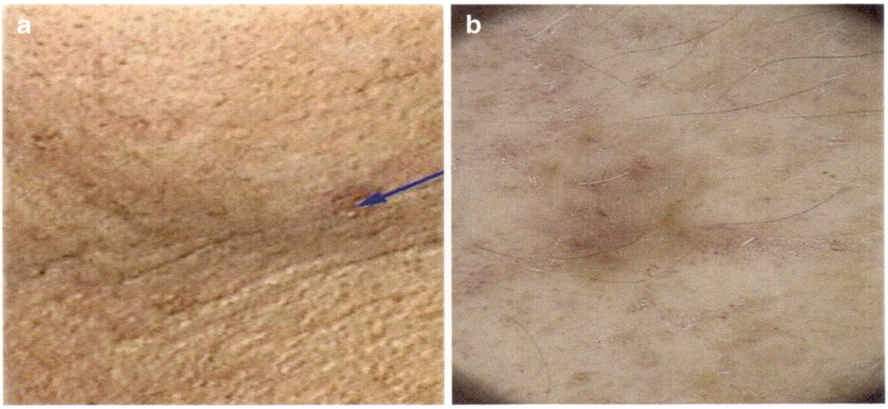

Fig. 14.5 Superficial BCC: (**a**) Clinical picture, (**b**) dermoscopy (Courtesy of Cristina Abdalla, MD)

includes psoriasis, nummular dermatitis, lichenoid keratosis, actinic keratosis, Bowen's disease, and early amelanotic melanoma. It is widespread in organ transplant patients [1, 12, 14] (Figs. 14.4 and 14.5). Histologically, it is characterized by foci of malignant, basaloid, palisaded tumors that adhere to the substrate of the epidermis and are usually restricted to the papillary dermis (Fig. 14.6) [11].

Morpheaform (Sclerosing, Desmoplastic) Type

This variant accounts for 5–10% of cases, is commonly seen on the face and neck, and tends to be invasive with the potential for extensive local destruction. Its designation is attributed to the clinical similarity with localized scleroderma: pink-to-ivory-white, shiny, smooth, scar-like, indurated plaques or depressions with

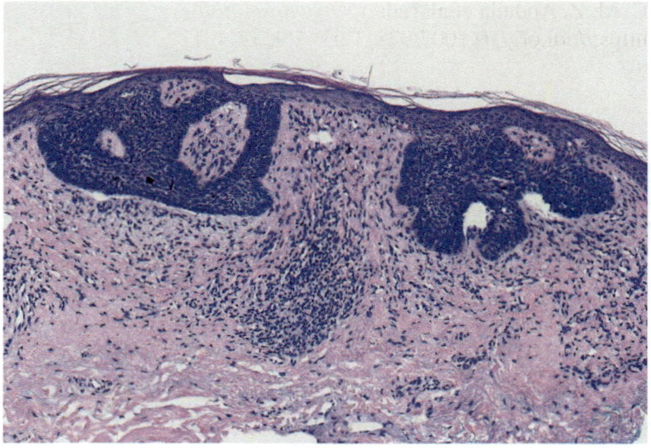

Fig. 14.6 Histopathology of superficial BCC (Courtesy of Melissa Fugimori, MD)

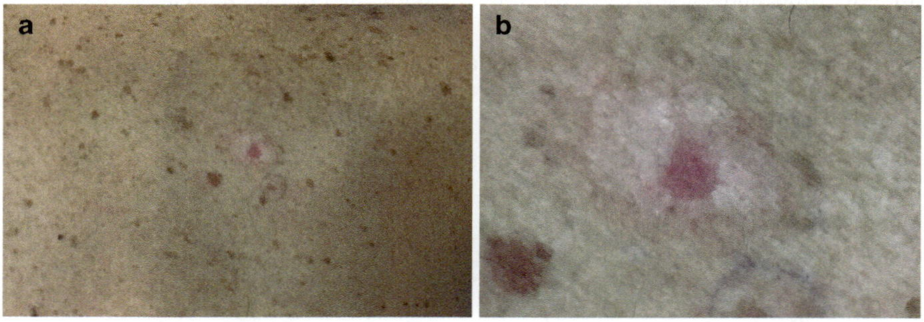

Fig. 14.7 Morpheaform BCC: (**a**) clinical picture, (**b**) higher magnification (Courtesy of Cristina Abdalla, MD)

ill-defined borders. Atrophy, telangiectasias, erosions, or small crusts may develop. The differential diagnosis includes localized scleroderma, a scar, dermatofibrosarcoma protuberans, Merkel cell carcinoma, amelanotic melanoma, microcystic adnexal carcinoma, and other adnexal neoplasms (Fig. 14.7) [12]. In morpheaform/infiltrative BCCs, there are thin, elongated filaments of basaloid tumor cells that penetrate the surrounding sclerotic collagen, which may appear sclerotic [11].

Fibroepithelial Type

This rare variant, also known as fibroepithelioma of Pinkus, mainly involves the trunk and appears mostly as a pink or flesh-colored sessile plaque or pedunculated papule or nodule. The differential diagnosis includes acrochordon or seborrheic keratosis (Fig. 14.8) [4, 13, 14]. Histologically, they exhibit fine filaments of basaloid keratinocytes in a reticular pattern and prominent loose stroma. The tumor cell proliferation index is high [11].

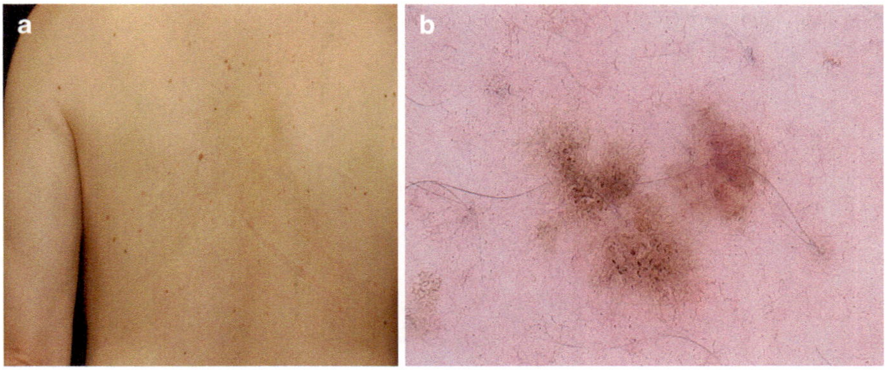

Fig. 14.8 Pinkus fibroepithelioma (**a**) clinical picture, (**b**) dermoscopy (Courtesy of Cristina Abdalla, MD)

Infiltrative Type

Infiltrative-type BCCs are often found together in the nodular and morphoic/sclerosing forms. They appear as opaque pink plaques that are thick, hardened, depressed, or flat, and there may be ulcerations, erosions, crusts, and papules on the surface. In histopathology, it is a subtype composed mainly of thin tumor nests that infiltrate deeply, with angled edges and with an irregular and permeable invasion pattern at the tumor edge [11].

Pigmented BCCs

It is a nodular or superficial BCC variant, more common in Asians and Africans. It features pigmented owing to basal cells that produce melanin, leading to clinically brown discoloration (Figs. 14.9, 14.10 and 14.11) [12]. Microscopically, an increased number of dendritic melanocytes is seen within tumor nests, found within basaloid cells or macrophages (Figs. 14.12 and 14.13) [11].

Basosquamous Carcinoma

It is a subtype characterized by tumors characteristic of nodular or superficial BCC and squamous cell carcinoma (SCC). Tumor nests are composed of basaloid cells, which intermingle with atypical squamous cells with eosinophilic cytoplasm (Fig. 14.14) [11].

Fig. 14.9 Pigmented BCC (Courtesy of Beatrice Abdalla, MD)

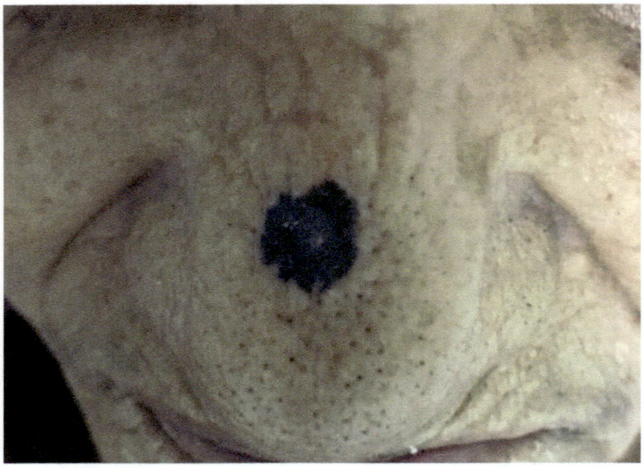

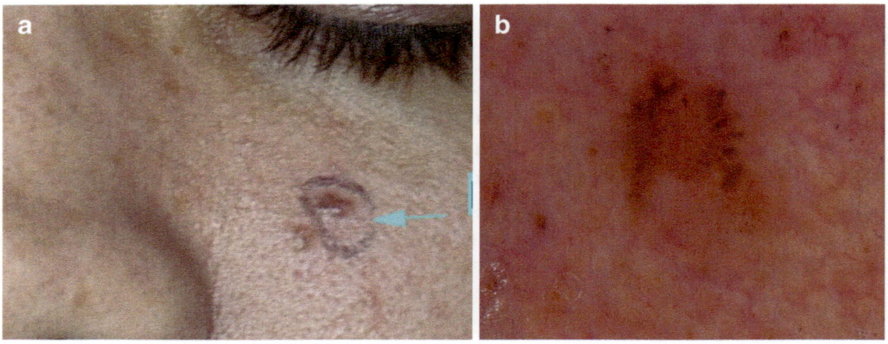

Fig. 14.10 Pigmented nodular BCC (**a**) clinical picture, (**b**) dermoscopy (Courtesy of Cristina Abdalla, MD)

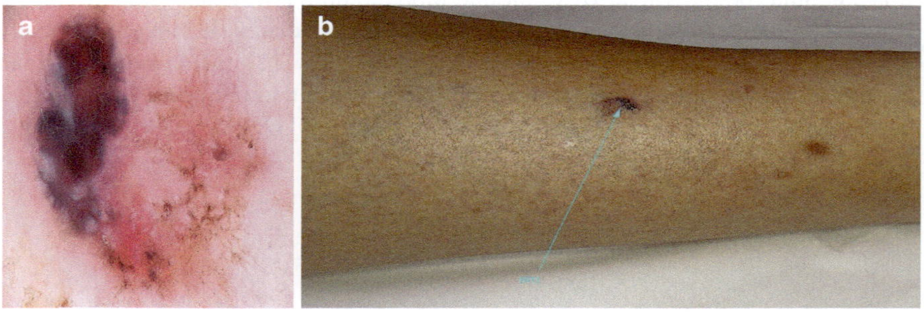

Fig. 14.11 Pigmented superficial and nodular BCC on the leg (**a**) clinical picture, (**b**) dermoscopy (Courtesy of Cristina Abdalla, MD)

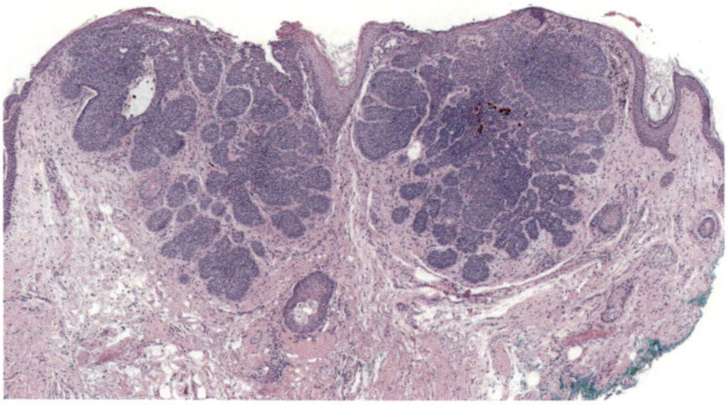

Fig. 14.12 Histopathology of pigmented BCC (Courtesy of Melissa Fugimori, MD)

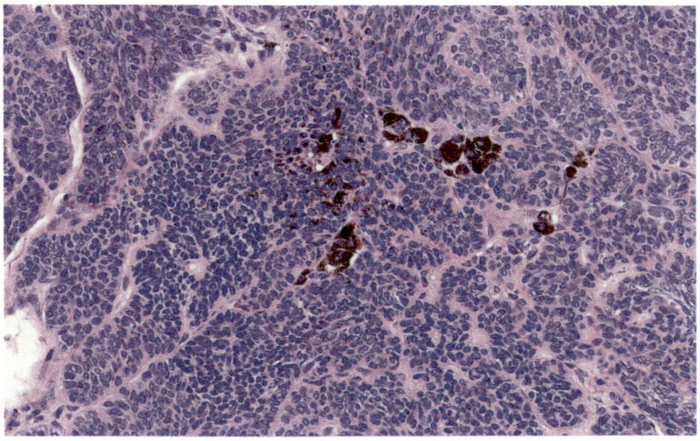

Fig. 14.13 Histopathology of pigmented BCC (Courtesy of Melissa Fugimori, MD)

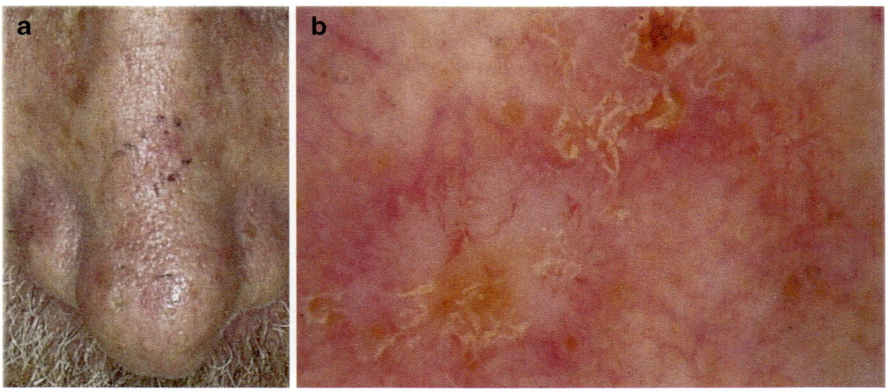

Fig. 14.14 Basosquamous cell carcinoma (**a**) clinical picture, (**b**) dermoscopy (Courtesy of Cristina Abdalla, MD)

Diagnosis

BCCs can have a wide variety of clinical presentations and are usually lesions that progressively enlarge over time, do not heal, and may bleed or ulcerate. In more detail, these lesions present as pearly, flesh-colored, or pink papules or plaques with overlying ulceration or telangiectatic vessels [4].

Dermoscopy improves the accuracy in diagnosing BCC, allowing the differentiation of the different clinical-pathological subtypes and ruling out differential diagnoses such as neoplastic and inflammatory diseases [14].

Obtaining a skin biopsy is the gold standard for diagnosing and guiding appropriate management based on histopathologic characteristics. Excisional, incisional, or punch biopsies are the preferred biopsy methods. Superficial shaving biopsies require careful interpretation because they can underestimate tumor depth [4, 14].

Novel noninvasive devices, such as confocal reflectance microscopy (RCM), optical coherence tomography (OCT), high-resolution ultrasonography, and confocal laser scanning microscopy, are tools of important sensitivity and specificity that can help in the diagnostic accuracy of BCCs [4].

Risk Stratification for BCC

BCC risk stratification based on risk factors for recurrence is of great importance for defining the therapeutic plan (Table 14.1). Collection of a detailed clinical history, including chronology, characteristics of the lesion and physical examination, questioning about medications in use and use of immunosuppressants, and biopsy of the suspicious lesion allow classifying BCCs at high and low risk of recurrence and, in this way, guide the most appropriate treatment [5, 11].

Table 14.1 Risk stratification in BCC

Risk	Low risk	High risk
Primary site and size	Trunk and extremities, <20 mm	Trunk and extremities, >20 mm Cheekbone, forehead, scalp, neck, and pretibial (any size)
Border	Well defined	Poorly defined
Primary vs. recurrent	Primary	Recurrent
Immunosuppression	No	Yes
Previous radiotherapy area	No	Yes
Histological subtype	Nodular and superficial	Aggressive patterns
Perineural invasion	No	Yes

Treatment of BCC

Surgical Treatments

Surgical excision with adequate margins remains the treatment of choice in most BCCs. However, treatment should be customized according to the patient's characteristics and factors related to the tumor, in addition to aiming at satisfactory aesthetic and functional results. An option for patients who are not candidates for surgery is exclusive radiotherapy [14, 15].

The definition of the surgical method is based on risk stratification through the analysis of clinical and pathological characteristics. Curettage and electrodesiccation (C&E), standard excision with a wide margin (4–5 mm) followed by postoperative pathological evaluation of the margins, Mohs micrographic surgery (MMS), and peripheral and deep en face margin assessment (PDEMA) are the surgical methods more common [14, 15].

Curettage and Electrodesiccation (C&E) It is a fast and cost-effective method, mainly for superficial lesions. The overall 5-year recurrence rates range from 1.2 to 40%, with high-risk tumors with higher recurrence rates. The major disadvantage is the lack of margin control. C&E should not be used to treat BCC in areas with terminal hair growth (scalp, pubic and axillary regions, or beard area) due to the risk of a tumor extending down follicular structures. If the subcutaneous layer is reached during C&E, surgical excision should be performed. This technique is considered less effective and selected for low-risk BCC [16].

Standard Excision with Postoperative Margin Assessment It is generally recommended as first-line therapy for BCC at low risk of recurrence. The clinical margins indicated that for well-circumscribed BCC lesions smaller than 2 cm in diameter, excision with 4-mm clinical margins should result in complete removal in more than 95% of cases. This technique has been reported to achieve 5-year recurrence rates of 0.8–17.4% for BCC, with lower recurrence rates associated with low-risk tumors and higher recurrence rates associated with high-risk tumors. The indication for this approach is also suitable for re-excision of low-risk primary BCC if positive margins are obtained after an initial excision [14, 15].

Surgery with Perioperative Frozen Sections for the Examination of the Entire Margins

Mohs Micrographic Surgery (MMS) The tumor is removed within a thin layer, less than 1 mm in thickness (called a stage), usually with a thin rim of normal-appearing skin around the lesion. This saucer-shaped tissue specimen is marked and frozen-sectioned so that the entirety of the undersurface and outer edges of the tumor are examined microscopically to minimize sampling error. The tissue is microscopically mapped and the slides are read by the Mohs surgeon so that, if any tumor focus persists, the posterior excision can be directed only to these areas, sparing the normal tissue. The 5-year recurrence rate for BCC treated with Mohs micrographic surgery was 1%, compared with 7.5% after cryosurgery, 7.7% after desiccation and curettage, 8.7% after radiotherapy, and 10.1% after surgical excision. The disadvantages of MMS include special training for MMS being required, the number of surgeons capable of performing MMS remaining low, and the technique not being available in every center. It can be very time-consuming and expensive, and the reconstruction may be deferred if the Mohs surgeon is not comfortable with more involved reconstructive procedures [5].

Peripheral and Deep En Face Margin Assessment (PDEMA) The tumor is removed with a 1-mm margin and divided into small circumferential units for a standard frozen section. These units are then labeled according to their cancer orientation. These marked units represent the entire circumference of the tumor and its peripheral deep margin slices or sections, representing the outermost surgical margin. A laboratory technician processes the samples using standard frozen section staining and mounting techniques. The pathologist and surgeon examined the frozen slides. If suspicious sites or evidence of tumor is seen on the slide, different tissue is excised from just that positive margin area. This procedure is repeated until the area is free of tumors. Reconstruction is performed immediately in all patients. PDEMA can be achieved by any surgeon offering frozen pathology services. The surgeon-directed en face technique eliminates the inadequacies of incomplete tumor assessment associated with standard frozen section techniques. It provides an equally effective, faster, and more available option for MMS. Recurrence rates are similar, around 1–3%, compared to MMS [5].

Nonsurgical Treatments

In patients with superficial BCC, topical therapies such as topical imiquimod, 5-fluorouracil (5-FU), photodynamic therapy, or cryotherapy may be considered. The cure rates are lower (approximately 10%) and should be reserved for nonsurgical candidates or cases of low-risk BCC. Recurrent BCC following treatment with topical therapies or PDT is considered a high-risk tumor and should be referred for conventional re-excision or MMS/PDEMA [5].

Cryotherapy (Cryosurgery) Application of liquid nitrogen to freeze the BCC lesion and destroy the tumor and a margin of surrounding normal tissue. At least three freeze-thaw cycles with liquid nitrogen (−196 °C, freezing duration of 40–60 s) with tissue temperature of −50 °C are required to destroy basal cell carcinoma. Techniques and liquid nitrogen delivery methods are variable, and protocols differ, including the number of freeze-thaw cycles. In prospective trials, cryotherapy has been shown to result in recurrence rates ranging from 5 to 39%. A limitation of cryotherapy is poorer cosmetic outcomes compared with other treatment options, as demonstrated by prospective randomized trials [5].

Imiquimod 5% Cream Approved by the US Food and Drug Administration for the treatment of non-facial superficial BCC. Imiquimod is applied 3–7 times per week, and the dosage is increased as tolerated to once or twice daily to maintain mild-to-moderate skin irritation. Studies have shown 73–82% cure rates when used once daily for 6–12 weeks. Smaller studies have shown similar responses for nodular BCC. Because of the concern of patient adherence to the more prolonged treatment, side effects, lower cure rate, and the availability of more effective therapies, imiquimod is recommended for treatment of non-superficial BCCs only in those patients who are poor surgical candidates or who have limited life expectancy [5, 17].

Photodynamic Therapy (PDT) with Photosensitizing Agents Including Methyl Aminolevulinate (MAL) and 5-Aminolevulinic Acid (ALA) Although PDT has been approved in Europe and other countries for the treatment of superficial and thin nodular BCC when other available therapies are not acceptable, US FDA approval has not been granted. PDT cure rates are 50% for superficial BCC versus an 83% cure rate for nodular BCC [18]. Currently, some cancer centers use PDT for premalignant or superficial low-risk lesions on any location on the body, although response rates may be higher on the face and scalp [5, 19].

5-Fluorouracil (5-FU) Although approved topical treatment for superficial BCC, it is commonly used in premalignant actinic keratosis (AK) and Bowen's disease. Clinical experience indicates 5-FU should be restricted to superficial BCCs in non-critical locations. It is applied twice daily for 4–6 weeks. Some patients may experience inflammatory reactions in 2–3 weeks [5, 20].

Nicotinamide Oral nicotinamide (vitamin B3) is safe, has protective effects against UV damage, and reduces 20% new BCC in 12-month follow-up [5, 21].

Radiotherapy Primary radiotherapy is a therapeutic option for treating high-risk BCC in patients with unresectable tumors or in cases where surgery is not recommended. With advances in RT techniques and the possibility of conformal radiation, excellent oncologic and aesthetic results can be achieved, with long-term disease control rates comparable to those obtained with surgical resection in select situations. Radiotherapy with adjuvant intent can also be discussed if there is a perineural invasion or positive margins without conditions for a salvage surgical procedure [22].

Treatment of Advanced/Metastatic BCC

Despite the high incidence, only a limited proportion of patients with BCC will ultimately demand systemic therapies due to recurrent/unresectable lesions or, even less frequently, due to distant metastases. Historically, standard cytotoxic chemotherapies have resulted in anecdotal and transient responses and have no established indication in treating advanced BCC.

Following the description of germline mutations of PTCH1 gene involved in the development of multiple and early-onset BCCs associated with the Gorlin–Goltz syndrome, the central role of the HH pathway was also characterized in sporadic BCCs. Indeed, somatic mutations in the PTCH1 or SMO have been described as key molecular drivers in most BCCs, resulting in aberrant HH pathway signaling [10]. Cyclopamine, a steroidal alkaloid, has been shown to result in teratogenic effects and midline deformities in developing embryos due to the blockade of HH signaling. These observations prompted the development of selective HH pathway inhibitors. Following promising results in a phase I study [23], vismodegib (GDC-0449), an orally administered small molecule, was investigated in a prospective, nonrandomized study. Among 33 patients with metastatic BCC and 63 with locally advanced BCC, vismodegib resulted in objective response rates of 30% and 43%, respectively, with a median duration of response of almost 8 months [24]. A subsequent open-label safety study including more than 1200 patients with advanced BCC confirmed the pronounced activity of vismodegib, with objective responses occurring in 68.5% and 36.9% of the patients with locally advanced and metastatic BCCs, respectively [25]. Sonidegib, a distinct HH inhibitor, has been approved for clinical use based upon the results of a pivotal phase II study that demonstrated response rates of approximately 40% and a significant improvement in disease-related symptoms [26]. Although approved for patients with advanced BCC, preliminary evidences also suggest a potential role of HH inhibitors in the neoadjuvant setting, as the potential for downstaging and less morbid surgeries has been demonstrated in a proof-of-concept study [27].

Despite the clinical activity, the prolonged use of HH inhibitors is often limited by adverse events that include dysgeusia, weight loss, myalgias, muscle spasms, and alopecia, and intermittent regimens of HH inhibitors have been investigated and are frequently used in clinical practice.

More recently, immunotherapy has emerged as a new systemic treatment option for patients who have progressed to or are intolerant of HH inhibitors and is currently approved for clinical use. A pivotal phase II study demonstrated clinically significant antitumor activity and an acceptable safety profile of the anti-PD-1 agent cemiplimab. In one of the study cohorts that included patients with locally advanced disease who were refractory or intolerant to HH inhibitors, cemiplimab resulted in an objective response rate of 31% and a median progression-free survival of 19 months, with a median time to response of 4.3 months; median duration of response had not been reached [28]. Among patients with documented metastases that were investigated in a distinct cohort of the same phase II trial, the objective response rate was 21.4%, and the median progression-free survival was 8.3 months [29].

More research and trials using immunotherapy in advanced BCC are ongoing.

Prognosis and Follow-Up

The prognosis for most patients with BCC is excellent and considerably improved through early diagnosis and appropriate management. However, delays in diagnosis and treatment can result in local destruction due to the aggressive biological behavior of the tumor, invading the skin, cartilage, and even bone. In addition, approximately 15% of BCC patients will develop a second-primary BCC within 1 year and up to 35% within 5 years [30, 31].

Follow-up of patients with BCC is necessary to detect local recurrences and new skin cancers, including non-melanoma and melanoma. Complete skin examination and biopsy are mandatory in suspected recurrences. The recommendation is a biannual reassessment during the initial 5 years posttreatment and annually thereafter [5].

References

1. Kim DP, Kus KJB, Ruiz E. Basal cell carcinoma review. Hematol Oncol Clin N Am. 2019;33(1):13–24.
2. Lewin JM, Carucci JA. Advances in the management of basal cell carcinoma. F1000Prime Rep. 2015;7. https://facultyopinions.com/prime/reports/m/7/53/.
3. Castanheira A, Boaventura P, Vieira F, Soares P, Mota A, Lopes JM. Clinicopathological features of head and neck cutaneous basal cell carcinoma observed at the Centro Hospitalar de Trás-os-Montes e Alto Douro ENT Department. Porto Biomed J. 2022;7(5):e190.
4. Niculet E, Craescu M, Rebegea L, Bobeica C, Nastase F, Lupasteanu G, et al. Basal cell carcinoma: comprehensive clinical and histopathological aspects, novel imaging tools and therapeutic approaches. Exp Ther Med. 2021;23(1):60.
5. Bichakjian CK, Olencki T, Aasi SZ, Alam M, Andersen JS, Berg D, et al. Basal cell skin cancer, version 1.2016, NCCN clinical practice guidelines in oncology. J Natl Compr Cancer Netw. 2016;14(5):574–97.
6. Asgari MM, Moffet HH, Ray GT, Quesenberry CP. Trends in basal cell carcinoma incidence and identification of high-risk subgroups, 1998–2012. JAMA Dermatol. 2015;151(9):976.
7. Parren LJMT, Frank J. Hereditary tumour syndromes featuring basal cell carcinomas: hereditary tumour syndromes. Br J Dermatol. 2011;165(1):30–4.
8. Lo ML. Nevoid basal cell carcinoma syndrome (Gorlin syndrome). Orphanet J Rare Dis. 2008;3(1):32.
9. Kilgour JM, Jia JL, Sarin KY. Review of the molecular genetics of basal cell carcinoma; inherited susceptibility, somatic mutations, and targeted therapeutics. Cancers. 2021;13(15):3870.
10. Epstein EH. Basal cell carcinomas: attack of the hedgehog. Nat Rev Cancer. 2008;8(10):743–54.
11. Naik PP, Desai MB. Basal cell carcinoma: a narrative review on contemporary diagnosis and management. Oncol Ther. 2022;10(2):317–35.
12. Marzuka AG, Book SE. Basal cell carcinoma: pathogenesis, epidemiology, clinical features, diagnosis, histopathology, and management. Yale J Biol Med. 2015;88(2):167–79.
13. Cives M, Mannavola F, Lospalluti L, Sergi MC, Cazzato G, Filoni E, et al. Non-melanoma skin cancers: biological and clinical features. IJMS. 2020;21(15):5394.

14. Cameron MC, Lee E, Hibler BP, Giordano CN, Barker CA, Mori S, et al. Basal cell carcinoma: contemporary approaches to diagnosis, treatment, and prevention. J Am Acad Dermatol. 2019;80(2):321–39.
15. Peris K, Fargnoli MC, Garbe C, Kaufmann R, Bastholt L, Seguin NB, et al. Diagnosis and treatment of basal cell carcinoma: European consensus-based interdisciplinary guidelines. Eur J Cancer. 2019;118:10–34.
16. Thissen MR, Neumann MH, Schouten LJ. A systematic review of treatment modalities for primary basal cell carcinomas. Arch Dermatol. 1999;135(10):1177–83.
17. Bath-Hextall F, Ozolins M, Armstrong SJ, Colver GB, Perkins W, Miller PSJ, et al. Surgical excision versus imiquimod 5% cream for nodular and superficial basal-cell carcinoma (SINS): a multicentre, non-inferiority, randomised controlled trial. Lancet Oncol. 2014;15(1):96–105.
18. Kuijpers DI, Thissen MR, Thissen CA, Neumann MH. Similar effectiveness of methyl aminolevulinate and 5-aminolevulinate in topical photodynamic therapy for nodular basal cell carcinoma. J Drugs Dermatol. 2006;5(7):642–5.
19. Arits AHMM, Mosterd K, Essers BA, Spoorenberg E, Sommer A, De Rooij MJM, et al. Photodynamic therapy versus topical imiquimod versus topical fluorouracil for treatment of superficial basal-cell carcinoma: a single blind, non-inferiority, randomised controlled trial. Lancet Oncol. 2013;14(7):647–54.
20. Love WE, Bernhard JD, Bordeaux JS. Topical imiquimod or fluorouracil therapy for basal and squamous cell carcinoma: a systematic review. Arch Dermatol. 2009;145(12):1431–8.
21. Chen AC, Martin AJ, Choy B, Fernández-Peñas P, Dalziell RA, McKenzie CA, et al. A phase 3 randomized trial of nicotinamide for skin-cancer chemoprevention. N Engl J Med. 2015;373(17):1618–26.
22. Likhacheva A, Awan M, Barker CA, Bhatnagar A, Bradfield L, Brady MS, et al. Definitive and postoperative radiation therapy for basal and squamous cell cancers of the skin: executive summary of an American Society for Radiation Oncology clinical practice guideline. Pract Radiat Oncol. 2020;10(1):8–20.
23. Von Hoff DD, LoRusso PM, Rudin CM, Reddy JC, Yauch RL, Tibes R, et al. Inhibition of the hedgehog pathway in advanced basal-cell carcinoma. N Engl J Med. 2009;361(12):1164–72.
24. Sekulic A, Migden MR, Oro AE, Dirix L, Lewis KD, Hainsworth JD, et al. Efficacy and safety of vismodegib in advanced basal-cell carcinoma. N Engl J Med. 2012;366(23):2171–9.
25. Basset-Séguin N, Hauschild A, Kunstfeld R, Grob J, Dréno B, Mortier L, et al. Vismodegib in patients with advanced basal cell carcinoma: primary analysis of STEVIE, an international, open-label trial. Eur J Cancer. 2017;86:334–48.
26. Migden MR, Guminski A, Gutzmer R, Dirix L, Lewis KD, Combemale P, et al. Treatment with two different doses of sonidegib in patients with locally advanced or metastatic basal cell carcinoma (BOLT): a multicentre, randomised, double-blind phase 2 trial. Lancet Oncol. 2015;16(6):716–28.
27. Bertrand N, Guerreschi P, Basset-Seguin N, Saiag P, Dupuy A, Dalac-Rat S, et al. Vismodegib in neoadjuvant treatment of locally advanced basal cell carcinoma: first results of a multicenter, open-label, phase 2 trial (VISMONEO study). EClinicalMedicine. 2021;35:100844.
28. Stratigos AJ, Sekulic A, Peris K, Bechter O, Prey S, Kaatz M, et al. Cemiplimab in locally advanced basal cell carcinoma after hedgehog inhibitor therapy: an open-label, multi-centre, single-arm, phase 2 trial. Lancet Oncol. 2021;22(6):848–57.
29. Lewis K, Peris K, Sekulic A, Stratigos A, Dunn L, Eroglu Z, et al. Interim analysis of phase 2 results for cemiplimab in patients with metastatic basal cell carcinoma (mBCC) who progressed or are intolerant to hedgehog inhibitors (HHIs). J Immunother Cancer. 2020;8(10):1136.
30. Wysong A, Aasi SZ, Tang JY. Update on metastatic basal cell carcinoma: a summary of published cases from 1981 through 2011. JAMA Dermatol. 2013;149(5):615–6.
31. Weinstock MA, Bogaars HA, Ashley M, Litle V, Bilodeau E, Kimmel S. Nonmelanoma skin cancer mortality. A population-based study. Arch Dermatol. 1991;127(8):1194–7.

Chapter 15
Benign Melanocytic Lesions

Maria Fernanda Vianna Hunziker and Ana Maria Fagundes Sortino

> **Key Points**
> - In melanocytic hyperplasias there is an increase of pigmentation and melanocytes in the basal layer, without nest formation.
> - Melanocytic nevi are benign neoplasms of melanocytes, characterized by the presence of nests within the epidermis and/or dermis.
> - World Health Organization (WHO) classification of melanocytic tumors recognizes the existence of benign tumors that may be related to melanomas as potential precursors or as simulants.

Benign Melanocytic Hyperplasias

Lentigines are benign pigmented macules that result from increased activity of epidermal melanocytes. There are two major types of lentigines: lentigo simplex (simple lentigo) and solar lentigo [1].

Lentigo Simplex

(Synonyms: simple lentigo, melanotic macule, and lentiginosis)

M. F. V. Hunziker (✉) · A. M. F. Sortino
Hospital Sírio-Libanês, São Paulo, SP, Brazil

C. M. Z. Abdalla et al. (eds.), *Oncodermatology*,
https://doi.org/10.1007/978-3-031-29277-4_15

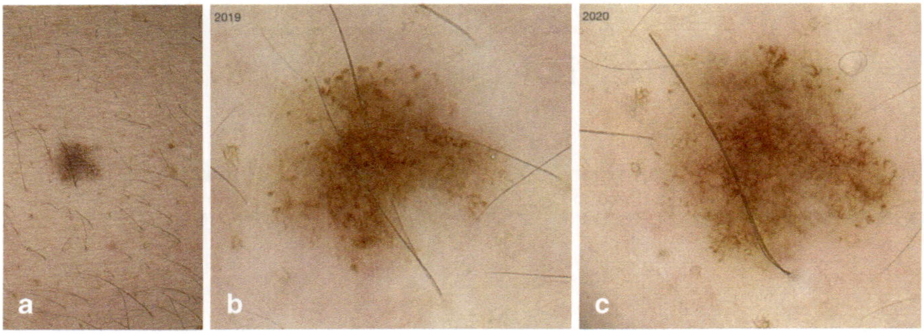

Fig. 15.1 Enlarging lesion on the arm of a 51-year-old male patient with moderately sun-damaged skin. (**a**) Clinical close-up image, (**b**) baseline dermoscopy in 2019, and (**c**) 1-year follow-up dermoscopy in 2020. The lesion was biopsied and diagnosed as a *lentigo*. Both dermoscopy images are polarized with 20 × magnification. (*Courtesy of Ana Maria Sortino MD, MSc*)

Lentigo simplex appears mostly in childhood as sharply circumscribed, round-to-oval, uniformly brown or brownish-black macules that are usually <5 mm in diameter. They can develop in both sun-protected and sun-exposed areas and may occur alone, in focal clusters (agminated), or have a generalized distribution (Fig. 15.1). Lentigo simplex may be present on the skin, conjunctivae, and mucous membranes (mucosal melanotic macule) [1].

Lentigines may occur as an isolated phenomenon or in association with a number of inherited disorders, including LEOPARD syndrome (lentigines, electrocardiographic conduction abnormalities, ocular hypertelorism, pulmonary valve stenosis, abnormalities of the genitalia, growth retardation, and sensorial deafness), Peutz–Jeghers syndrome, Laugier–Hunziker syndrome (idiopathic mucocutaneous pigmentation), and LAMB syndrome (lentigines, atrial myxoma, mucocutaneous myxomas, and blue nevi) [2].

Solar Lentigo

Solar lentigines are sharply circumscribed, uniformly pigmented macules that are located predominantly on the sun-exposed areas of the skin. They are induced by ultraviolet sun exposure and predominantly develop in older individuals. Children with xeroderma pigmentosum develop solar lentigines during the first years of life due to increased sun sensitivity [1, 2]. Dermoscopic features of solar lentigo include moth-eaten border, homogeneous light brown pigmentation, delicate pigmented network, fingerprint-like areas, and pseudonetwork in lesions located on the face and scalp (Fig. 15.2). Histologically, they present bulblike elongation of the rete ridges, basal layer hyperpigmentation, and increased number of melanocytes. Solar elastosis is usually seen in the dermis [3].

The "ink spot" lentigo is distinguished clinically by its dark color and markedly irregular outline. Its reticulated pattern resembles a spot of ink (Fig. 15.2c–d).

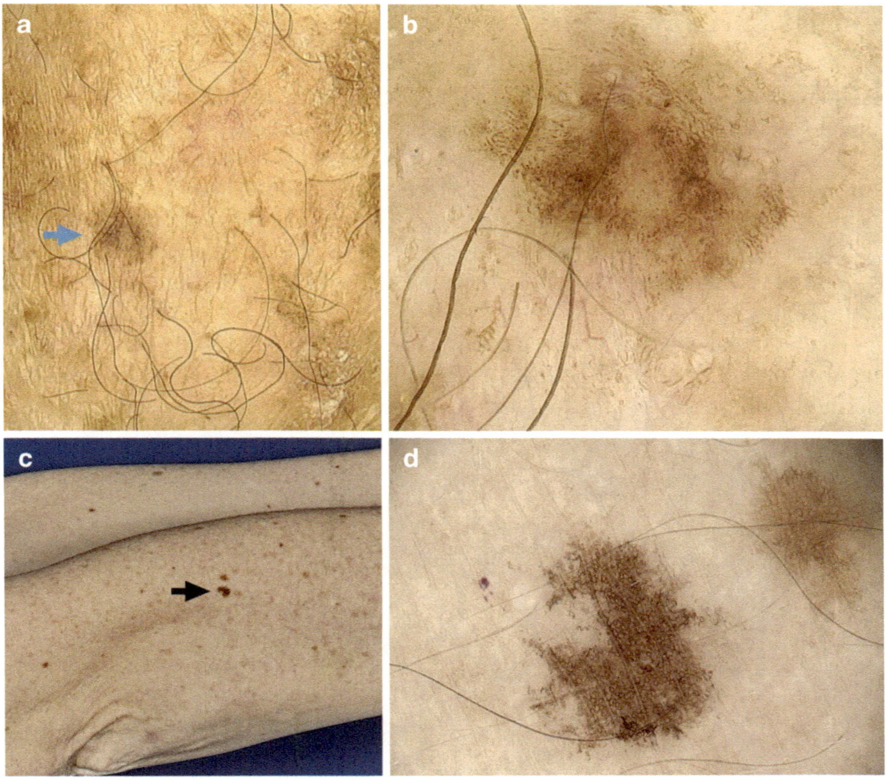

Fig. 15.2 *Upper images*: new pigmented lesion on the leg of an 88-year-old male patient with severely sun-damaged skin and personal history of multiple melanomas. The lesion was biopsied with a final diagnosis of *solar lentigo*. (**a**) Clinical close-up image, blue arrow; (**b**) dermoscopy shows delicate pigmented network, fingerprint-like focal areas, and diffuse light and dark brown small globules. *Lower images*: stable lesion on a 49-year-old female. (**c**) Clinical image, black arrow; (**d**) dermoscopy shows delicate brownish-black pigmented network. Both dermoscopy images are polarized with 20 × magnification. (*Courtesy of Ana Maria Sortino MD, MSc*)

Histology shows a lentiginous hyperplasia of the epidermis, hyperpigmentation of the basal layer, and minimal increase in the number of melanocytes [4].

Nevi

Melanocytic nevi represent benign proliferations of a type of melanocyte known as a "nevus cell." Nevus cells cluster as nests within the lower epidermis and/or dermis, while ordinary melanocytes are present in the basal layer of the epidermis. Acquired and congenital nevi will be discussed in the following sections [5].

Common Acquired Nevi

Acquired nevi can be classified as common or atypical, and there are several additional variants, including halo nevi, blue nevi, and Spitz nevi.

Nevi are more prevalent among those with fair skin, sun sensitivity, and freckling, and their development is influenced by age, sex, and sun exposure [6]. Heredity is also a factor related to nevi development. Germline polymorphisms that impact the number, morphology, and dermoscopic features of nevi have been identified in several genes, including interferon regulatory factor 4 (*IRF4*) and telomerase reverse transcriptase (*TERT*) [6].

Acquired melanocytic nevi begin to appear after 6 months of life and increase in number during childhood and adolescence. Considerable nevus turnover occurs during the first years of life, and many new nevi will appear, grow, and eventually enter senescence [7] (Fig. 15.3).

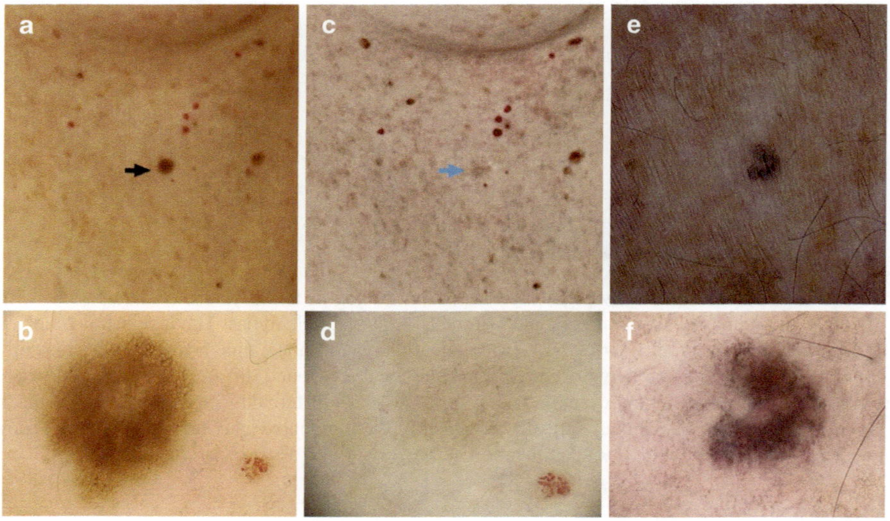

Fig. 15.3 Regressing lesions. Female patient in her 40 s, without personal history of skin cancer. (**a**) Close-up baseline clinical image of melanocytic nevus (black arrow). (**b**) Dermoscopy shows a central hypopigmented area with focal small brown globules surrounded by a brown pigmented network. (**c**) After 2-year close-up clinical image of a faded lesion (blue arrow). (**d**) Dermoscopy shows a structureless center with diffuse light-gray granules and remains of a delicate tan network. Complete excision was performed, and the pathology report was of a *lentigo simplex with histological regression*. Male patient in his 60 s, personal history of unknown primary metastatic melanoma. On total body clinical exam, a brownish-gray slightly palpable lesion was found. (**e**) Close-up clinical image of a nevus surrounded by vitiligo-like lesions. (**f**) Dermoscopy shows an asymmetric lesion, with a structureless center, diffuse dark-gray and bluish granules. Complete excision was performed, and the pathology report was of a *compound nevus, with extensive regression areas and abundant melanophages at the papillary dermis*. Both dermoscopy images are polarized with 20 × magnification. (*Courtesy of Ana Maria Sortino MD, MSc*)

Acquired nevi can be classified as junctional, compound, or intradermal nevus, according to the location of the nests of melanocytes: (1) in the dermal–epidermal junction, (2) in the dermal–epidermal junction and dermis, and (3) in the dermis, respectively (Fig. 15.4).

Common nevi have a variety of clinical appearances, but usually they are symmetric, round, or oval and have a homogeneous surface. They can be heavily or lightly pigmented, but most frequently they are brown or light brown in color (Fig. 15.4). Usually they are present in sun-exposed areas. Less frequently, they occur in palms, soles, nail matrix, and scalp. Acral nevi that involve the nail matrix can present as longitudinal melanonychia that is a tan, brown, or black streak caused by melanin deposition in the nail plate. Longitudinal melanonychia in multiple nails can frequently be observed in individuals with darker skin due to increased melanin production by normal nail matrix melanocytes. Melanonychia that develops in children is usually benign. However, pigmented streaks that develop in adults must be carefully evaluated. Dark, irregular, wide (≥4 mm) bands that become darker or wider over time may warrant biopsy to exclude melanoma. Also, the association with nail dystrophy and/or the extension of the pigmentation beyond the nail fold are signs of concern.

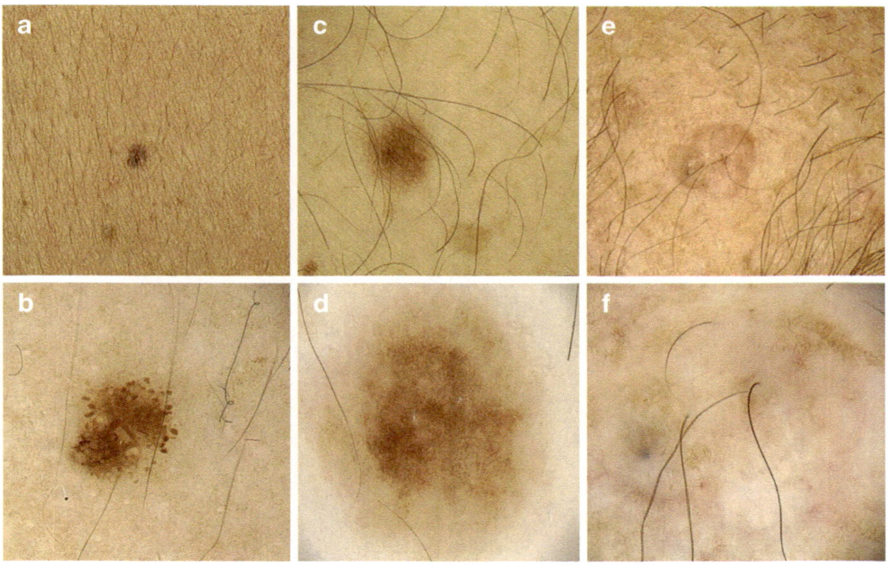

Fig. 15.4 Common acquired melanocytic nevi. (**a**) Close-up clinical image of a junctional nevus, (**b**) dermoscopy of a junctional nevus with a central thick network and peripheral globules. (**c**) Close-up clinical image of a compound nevus, (**d**) dermoscopy of a compound nevus with a central darker network and symmetrical tan structureless area at the periphery. (**e**) Close-up clinical image of a dermal nevus, (**f**) dermoscopy of a dermal nevus with structureless pinkish-white center, fragmented network areas and focal bluish-gray globule. All dermoscopy images are polarized with 20 × magnification. (*Courtesy of Ana Maria Sortino MD, MSc*)

Dermoscopic morphological patterns of acquired nevi include globular, globular-reticular, globular-homogeneous, reticular, reticular-homogeneous, and homogeneous. The pigment distribution can be uniform, central hyper- or hypopigmentation (Fig. 15.4), peripheral hypopigmentation, and multifocal hyper- or hypopigmentation. It has been suggested that most individuals harbor a predominant dermoscopic pattern in the melanocytic lesions [8]. Moreover, significant dermoscopic differences are site- and age-related. Acquired melanocytic lesions in children most often reveal a globular pattern, especially those located on the head, neck, and upper trunk. A reticular pattern is more often observed in acquired nevi on the extremities, as well as nevi that develop later in life [9].

Most acquired nevi remain benign throughout life. However, total body nevi count and the presence of dysplastic nevus are important risk factors for melanoma [6]. These patients should be followed with periodic total body skin examination and, in some cases, with body mapping and digital dermoscopy. Also, they should be counseled about sun-protection measures.

Sometimes it is hard to distinguish a benign and an early malignant melanocytic lesion with clinical and dermoscopic examinations, and a biopsy may be necessary (Fig. 15.5). When a melanocytic lesion is removed, whatever the reason, even when it looks banal on the bedside examination, the specimen should always be sent for histologic examination [5].

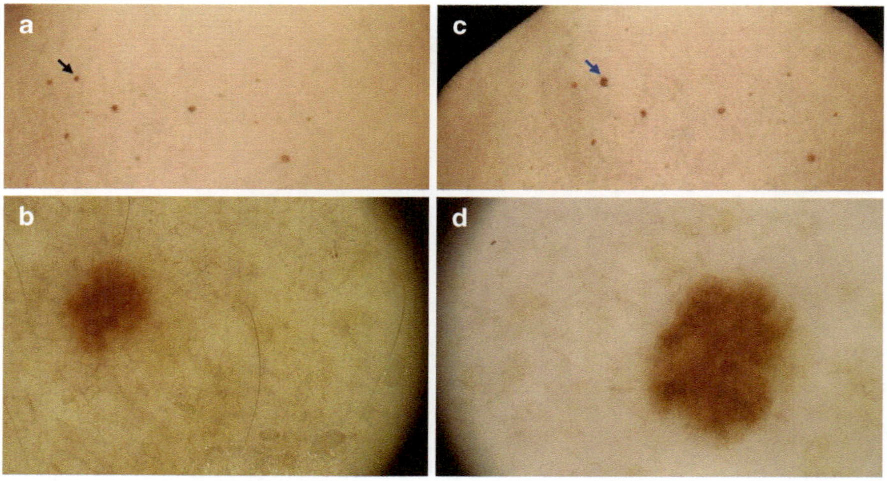

Fig. 15.5 Male patient in his 40 s, with moderately sun-damaged skin and growth of an acquired melanocytic nevus over a 2-year digital monitoring. (**a**) Close-up baseline clinical image in 2014, (**b**) baseline dermoscopy showing a small brown lesion with irregular hyperpigmented areas. (**c**) Close-up follow-up clinical image in 2016; (**d**) follow-up dermoscopy with increased irregular hyperpigmented areas and atypical pigment network. The lesion was biopsied and diagnosed as *low-grade dysplastic compound nevus* (mild atypia). Both dermoscopy images are polarized with 20 × magnification. (*Courtesy of Ana Maria Sortino MD, MSc*)

Dysplastic Melanocytic Lesions

Clark et al. described the atypical or dysplastic nevus as having clinical and pathologic features found in individuals of families predisposed to melanomas [10]. The WHO Working Group defines dysplastic nevus as a clinically atypical, histopathologically benign junctional or compound melanocytic tumor, >4 mm in breadth on fixed sections (>5 mm clinically), with architectural disorder plus cytological atypia [11].

Clinically, dysplastic nevi often measure at least 5 mm in diameter and characteristically have irregular, indistinct borders and variable pigmentation. Lesions can be a mixture of tan to brown or lightly colored, with a pink-red pigmentation. They are often slightly raised and frequently present a macular component that corresponds to the junctional component of a compound lesion.

The histological features of dysplastic nevi are intraepidermal lentiginous melanocytic hyperplasia with cytological and architectural atypia and dermal stromal response. One of the recommendations of the 1992 National Health Consensus Conference was the inclusion of a statement describing the presence and degree of cytologic atypia (none, mild, moderate, and severe) in the pathology report [12]. The morphologic variation of nevi, both clinically and histologically, and also from a genomic perspective, makes them potential simulants that need to be distinguished from melanoma.

The 2018 World Health Organization (WHO) classification of melanocytic tumors recognizes the existence of benign tumors that may be related to melanomas as potential precursors or as simulants. This classification encompasses nine melanoma pathways according to a progression model in which morphologically intermediate melanocytic tumors are considered as simulators or precursors to melanoma. These intermediate lesions can be subclassified into (a) a "classical" subgroup (superficial/thin compound: dysplastic nevus), which is placed within the morphologic and molecular progression spectrum of classical melanoma subtypes (superficial spreading and, possibly, nodular), and (b) a "nonclassical" subgroup (thick compound/dermal: "melanocytomas") whose genetic pathways diverge from classical melanoma subtypes [13].

It is important to recognize that although common and dysplastic nevi are benign tumors, they can be related to melanoma as simulators or precursors. Most nevi are, however, stable and more likely to regress than progress to melanoma [13]. Atypical/dysplastic nevi are phenotypic markers of increased risk of melanoma development, especially when in patients with other risk factors, like high nevi count and family or personal history of melanoma [14] (Fig. 15.6).

The combination of whole body examination, manual dermoscopy using the comparative approach [15], total body photographs, sequential digital dermoscopy of suspicious lesions without clear-cut melanoma features, and lifelong follow-up is recommendable in patients with atypical nevi (Fig. 15.7). Also, these patients should receive education on self-examination and sun protection. Routine ophthalmologic examination should be recommended, due to the increased prevalence of ocular melanocytic nevi and the risk of ocular melanoma.

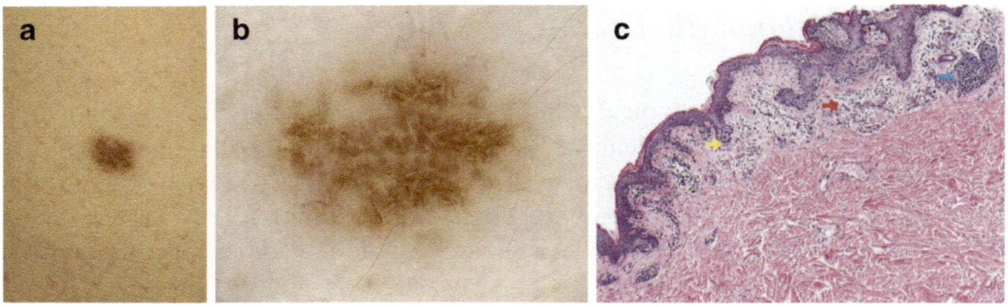

Fig. 15.6 *Low-grade dysplastic compound nevus* (moderate atypia) on the trunk of a 29-year-old male patient with more than 200 nevi. (**a**) Close-up clinical image; (**b**) polarized dermoscopy (20 ×) showing a central negative network and tan structureless peripheral areas; (**c**) histology (HE 45 ×) shows a junctional component extending laterally beyond intradermal nests, predominantly arranged in junctional nests along the basal layer of the acanthotic epidermis and with elongated ridges (yellow arrow). Nevus cells increased in size with visible nucleoli. Intradermal nests with preserved vertical maturation (blue arrow). Fibroplasia in the papillary dermis (red arrow). Perivascular lymphocytic infiltrate and melanophages in the superficial dermis. (*Courtesy of Ana Maria Sortino MD, MSc. and Ebe Christie de Oliveira MD*)

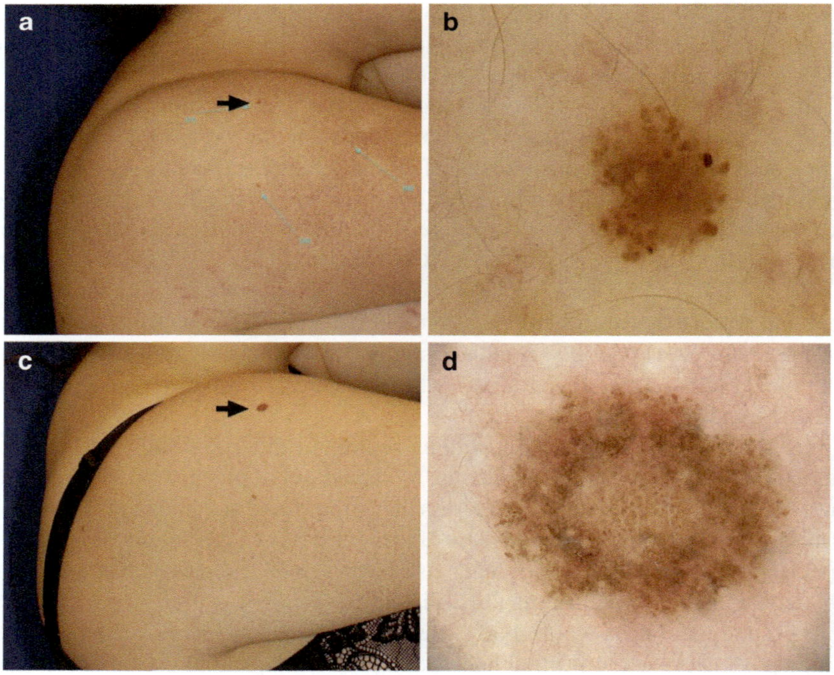

Fig. 15.7 Changes of a suspicious melanocytic nevi in a teenage girl over a 5-year period. (**a**) Clinical baseline image at age 13; (**b**) dermoscopy shows central structureless brown and peripheral irregular globules with different colors and sizes. (**c**) Clinical image showing accentuated enlargement after 5 years; (**d**) dermoscopy with a central negative network surrounded by fragmented atypical network and irregular dots and globules at the periphery. The lesion was completely excised with a histological diagnosis of a *compound dysplastic nevus*. All dermoscopy images are polarized with 20 × magnification. (*Courtesy of Ana Maria Sortino MD, MSc*)

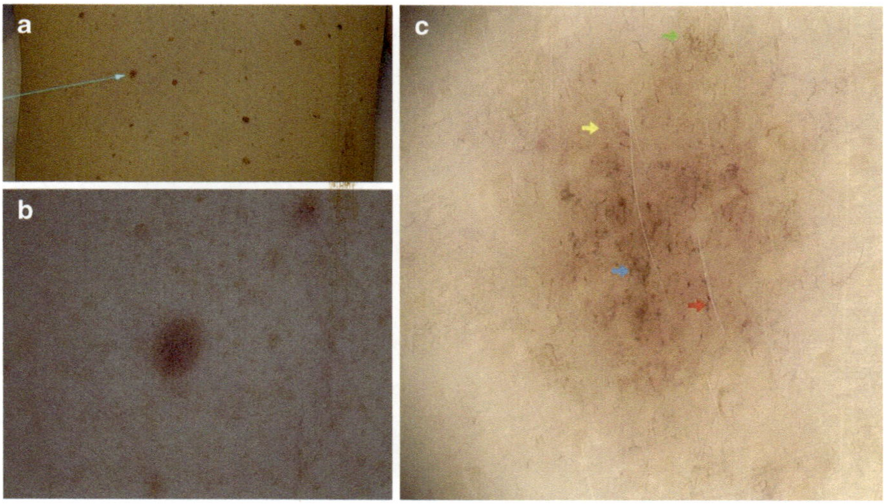

Fig. 15.8 Female patient in her 30 s, with atypical mole syndrome (AMS) and severe photodamage for her age. (**a**) Clinical overview image illustrating the impressive number of nevi on the back and the suspicious nevus (teal arrow). (**b**) Clinical close-up image of a brownish-red symmetrical suspicious nevus (diameter >6 mm). (**c**) Polarized dermoscopy (20 ×) allows the visualization of dotted vessels (red arrow), gray dots and granules (blue arrow), irregular brown and tan globules (yellow arrow), and atypical delicate pigment network. The excision disclosed a *high-grade dysplastic compound nevus* (severe atypia). (*Courtesy of Ana Maria Sortino MD, MSc*)

Lesions that are suspicious for melanoma on the bedside examination should be excised. Partial or superficial biopsies are discouraged to avoid sampling error and to reduce the risk of nevus recurrence. In atypical nevi with moderate to severe atypia and positive biopsy margins re-excision to exclude melanoma is recommended; [14, 16] severely dysplastic melanocytic lesions may merit re-excision with 5-mm margin [16] (Fig. 15.8).

Halo Nevi

(Synonym: Sutton's nevi)

Halo nevi are moles that develop a border of depigmentation resembling a halo. It occurs in approximately 1% of the population, usually before adulthood [17]. The halo phenomenon is thought to involve destruction of melanocytes by CD8+ cytotoxic T lymphocytes and has been associated with vitiligo and rare spontaneous regression of melanocytic lesions [18]. The halo phenomenon typically involves acquired melanocytic nevi, but may also be seen with congenital nevi, blue nevi, Spitz nevi, and melanoma.

The halo nevi correlate with the nevus regression and ultimately complete disappearance of the nevus, with a remaining depigmented macule. Eventually,

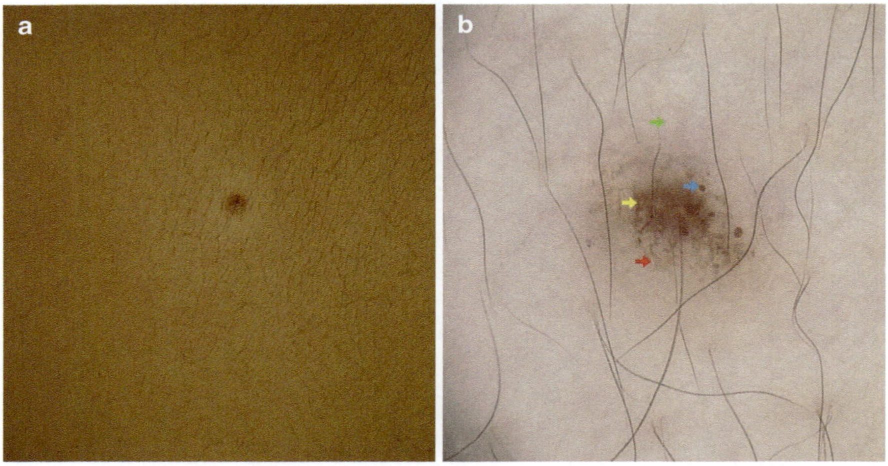

Fig. 15.9 Halo nevi on the back of a 13-year-old female patient. (**a**) Close-up clinical image showing a halo phenomenon around a symmetrical brown nevus. (**b**) Polarized dermoscopy (20 ×) showed asymmetrical multicomponent pattern, with irregular globules (blue arrow) and dots (yellow arrow), atypical pigment network, and peripheral hypopigmentation (green arrow). The lesion was excised, and the final diagnosis was a *dermal nevus*. (*Courtesy of Ana Maria Sortino MD, MSc*)

repigmentation occurs. The time period of this process is variable, but it may take years [17] (Fig. 15.9).

Blue Nevi and Dermal Melanocytes

Blue nevi are present in approximately 1–2% in Caucasians and 3–5% in Asians [19]. They are generally acquired, but less commonly may be congenital. Common blue nevi are deeply pigmented small lesions, usually less than 1 cm in diameter. Cellular blue nevi have a similar color but are often larger plaques or nodules (Fig. 15.10). Histologically, blue nevi present deeply pigmented spindle or epithelioid melanocytes in the dermis [2].

Related lesions include the hamartomatous dermal melanocytosis: (1) Mongolian spot, on the sacrum area; (2) nevi of Ota, on the face; and (3) nevi of Ito, on the arms or trunk [20].

Spitz Nevi

(Synonyms: spindle and epithelioid cell nevus)

A Spitz nevus is a melanocytic neoplasm of epithelioid and/or spindle cells that usually appears in childhood. These lesions are by nature benign, but their clinical,

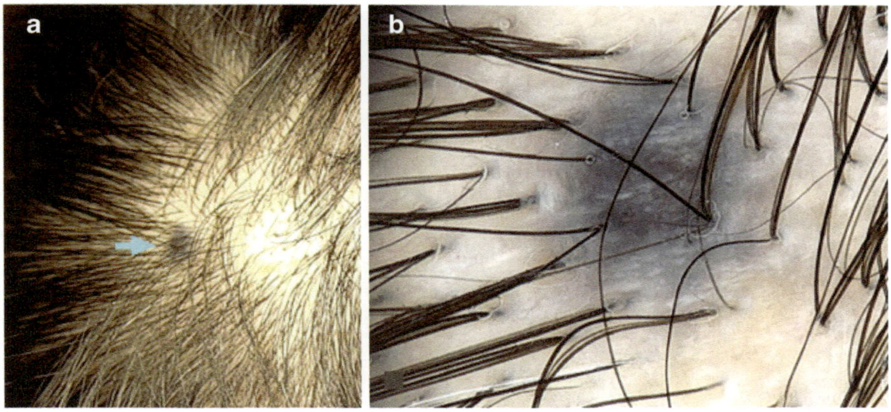

Fig. 15.10 Lesion on the scalp of a 49-year-old female patient with androgenic alopecia. It was unknown to the patient and found on whole-body skin examination. (**a**) Close-up clinical image showing ill-defined bluish lesion. (**b**) Polarized dermoscopy (30 ×) showed a brownish-blue center, a grayish-blue periphery, with irregular shiny white lines diffusely distributed. The lesion was excised, and the final diagnosis was *blue nevus*. (*Courtesy of Ana Maria Sortino MD, MSc*)

dermoscopic, and even histopathologic features sometimes overlap with those of melanoma.

Clinically, they usually present as pink, tan, red-brown dome-shaped papule or nodule, most commonly on the face or lower extremities of children and young individuals [21]. In 1975, Reed et al. [22] described a benign pigmented melanocytic lesion, thereafter named Reed nevus, that is currently regarded as the pigmented counterpart of Spitz nevus (Fig. 15.11).

Nonpigmented Spitz nevus commonly show on dermoscopy dotted vessels, monomorphic and uniformly distributed throughout the lesion [23] (Fig. 15.12). Another frequent additional feature of nonpigmented Spitz nevus is reticular depigmentation (negative network) that may present either as a whitish grid surrounding the vessels or as shiny white structures, orthogonally or in parallel to each other. Pigmented variants usually display the starburst pattern, consisting of a central area of homogeneous black-blue pigmentation and symmetrically distributed peripheral streaks or pseudopods (Fig. 15.11). Additional patterns have been described: globular, homogeneous, reticular (inverse white and superficial black network), and multicomponent pattern [24, 25].

Due to controversies involving clinical recognition, histopathologic criteria, and biological behavior for spitzoid lesions, recently the International Dermoscopy Society proposed a management guideline for theses lesions, according to clinical and dermoscopic features. Overall dermoscopic symmetry should be assessed, and lesions displaying spitzoid features (starburst, dotted vessels, reticular depigmentation) asymmetrically distributed should be excised to rule out melanoma. Dermoscopically symmetric flat spitzoid lesions should be managed according to the age of the patient. In patients older than 12 years old, these lesions should be managed with caution, because there is a considerable probability of malignancy.

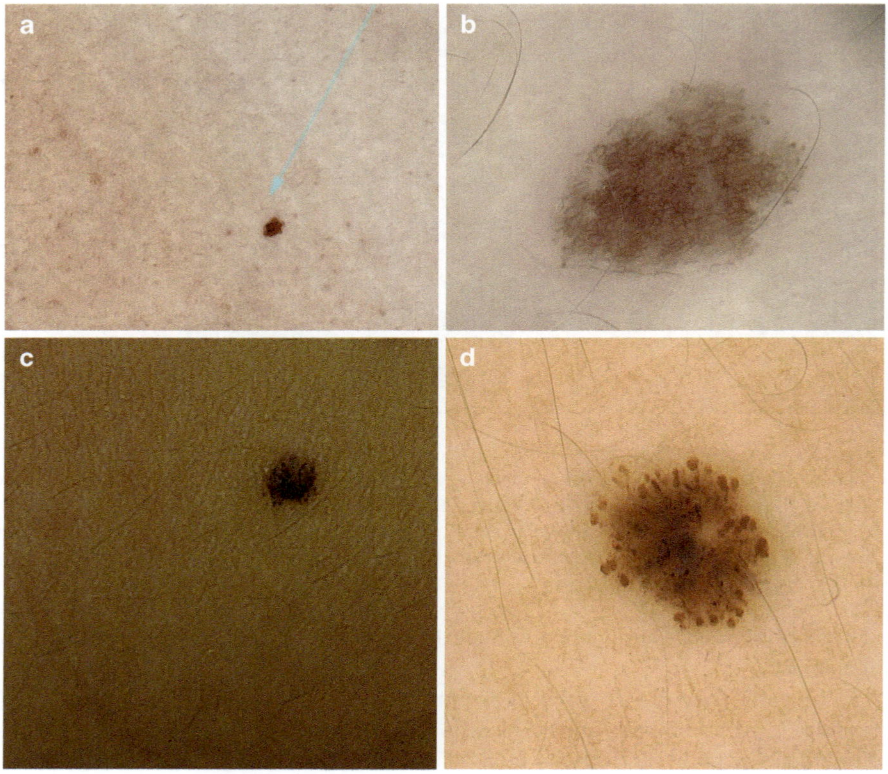

Fig. 15.11 *Upper images*: isolated pigmented lesion on the right gluteus of a 42-year-old female. (**a**) Close-up of the lesion (teal arrow); (**b**) polarized dermoscopy (30 ×) reveals an atypical pigment network with focal peripheral streaks and pseudopods. The lesion was biopsied with a final diagnosis of *Reed nevus*. *Lower images*: growing lesion on the abdomen of a 20-year-old female patient. (**a**) Close-up clinical image; (**b**) polarized dermoscopy (20 ×) showing central brownish-black clods, irregular hyperpigmentation, and teared peripheral globules. The lesion was biopsied with a final diagnosis of *junctional pigmented Spitz nevus*. (Courtesy of Ana Maria Sortino MD, MSc)

The recommendation is excision to rule out melanoma (Fig. 15.13). In patients younger than 12 years, Spitz nevus can be followed up until stabilization. Dermoscopically symmetric spitzoid nodules should be excised or closely monitored, irrespective of the age, to rule out atypical Spitz tumors [26].

Congenital Nevi

Congenital melanocytic nevi (CMN) are hamartomas of the neuroectoderm caused by genetic post-zygotic mosaicism for *NRAS* mutations in 80% of cases [27, 28]. They are classically present at birth or shortly thereafter (*tardive nevi*) [29, 30] and

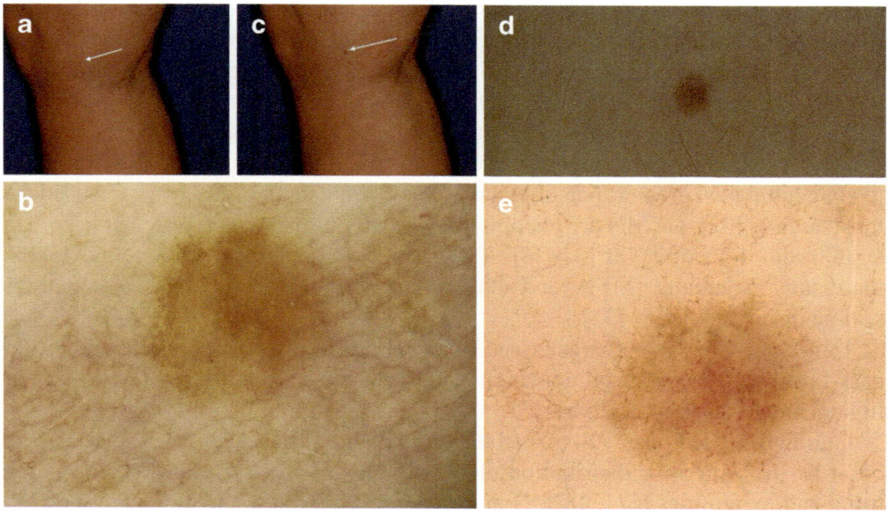

Fig. 15.12 Small pink lesion on the medial knee of a 43-year-old female patient with personal history of basal cell carcinoma and family history of multiple melanomas. (**a**) Baseline total body image; (**b**) polarized dermoscopy (20 ×) showing a central pigment network, structureless tan areas around the center, focal peripheral globules, and negative network. (**c**) One-year follow-up total body image, showing marked change. (**d**) Close-up clinical image; (**e**) polarized dermoscopy (20 ×) reveals gain of dotted vessels, structureless hyperpigmented areas, and negative network. The lesion was excised, and the final diagnosis was *Spitz nevus*. (*Courtesy of Ana Maria Sortino MD, MSc*)

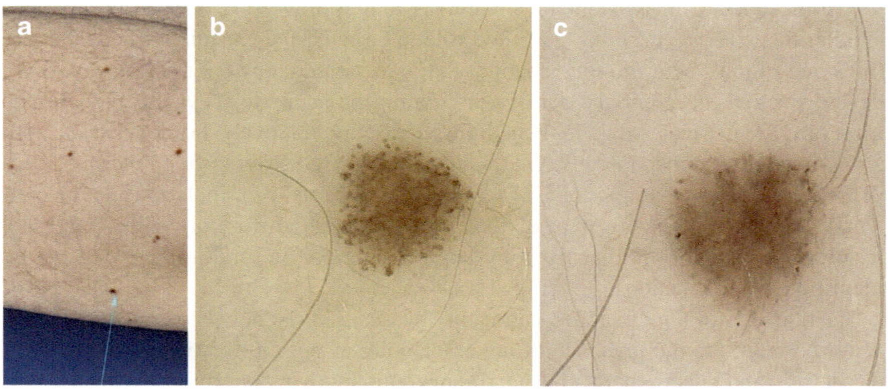

Fig. 15.13 New pigmented lesion on a 34-year-old female patient with personal history of melanoma. (**a**) Close-up clinical image (teal arrow). (**b**) Baseline dermoscopy showing central enlarged pigment network and peripheral teared globules. (**c**) Follow-up dermoscopy reveals growth, loss of globules, structureless brown, and remains of the network forming angulated lines (polygons). All dermoscopy images are polarized with 20 × magnification. The lesion was completely excised with a histological diagnosis of a *junctional pigmented Spitz nevus with pagetoid spread*. The case was discussed on a tumor board and re-excision with 5-mm margins was performed. (*Courtesy of Ana Maria Sortino MD, MSc*)

occur in approximately 1% of newborns. The current classification is based on the maximum diameter that the nevus is predicted to attain during adulthood [29, 31]. Small congenital nevi are less than 1.5 cm in the largest diameter, medium sized are those between 1.5 and 19 cm, and large congenital nevi are greater than or equal to 20 cm. Nomenclature regarding classification of large and giant congenital melanocytic nevi (GCMN) has been inconsistent [32]. We will use the term GCMN to refer to congenital nevi greater than or equal to 20 cm in diameter, as it has been used for most authors [32]. GCMN are uncommon with an estimated incidence between 1 in 20.000 and 1 in 500.000 [31–33]. They can be associated with satellite CMN, malignant melanoma (MM), and neurocutaneous melanosis. These associations will be discussed below [34].

Clinically, CMN are characterized by a smooth to mamillated surface, light- to dark-brown color, and well-demarcated borders. Over time, they may darken or lighten and acquire coarse hairs [32, 35].

Garment-related terms, like "bathing trunk" and "vest-like," have been used to describe the pattern of distribution of GCMN. The most common location is the trunk and extremities [31]. GCMN are commonly associated with benign melanocytic growths within the substance of the lesion, named "proliferative nodules." These nodules can be clinically and pathologically misdiagnosed as MM. Satellite CMN can be frequently observed in patients with GCMN. They correspond to smaller CMN that may be present at birth or months to years later [32]. In addition, mucosal nevi (31%) [36] and plexiform overgrowth (6%) [32] have been described in association with GCMN. Also, nevi extensively involving the extremities can affect growth and cause hypotrophy of the affected limb, due to substitution of fat tissue by nevus cells [36].

Dermoscopy can assist in the diagnosis and follow-up of CMN, particularly smaller ones. However, it has a limited role in large CMN, especially those that are thick and rugous. Morphologic changes that may be indicative of malignancy might develop below the papillary dermis and cannot be accurately evaluated with dermoscopy [35]. Most small and medium CMN are relatively homogeneous both clinically and dermoscopically. On the other hand, GCMN are often heterogeneous [37]. Dermoscopic features of CMN, irrespective of its size, include reticular network, globules that may form a cobblestone pattern, and diffuse pigmentation. Also, terminal hairs, perifollicular hypo-hyperpigmentation, and milia-like cysts can be identified in these lesions [38] (Fig. 15.14).

Distinct histologic features can help the distinction between congenital and acquired nevi: (1) the presence of nevomelanocytes within the lower two thirds of the dermis and subcutaneous tissue; (2) nevomelanocytes intermingled with collagen bundles in the reticular dermis as single cells; (3) nevomelanocytes around hair follicles, sebaceous glands, eccrine apparatus, vessel walls, and nerves; (4) a perivascular and perifollicular distribution of nevomelanocytes; and (5) arrector pili that may be enlarged, distorted, and infiltrated by nevomelanocytes. All these features are more pronounced in GCMN [29]. These findings, however, are not absolutely specific of congenital nevi. Many pathologists use the term "congenital nevi pattern" to describe histologic features of congenital melanocytic nevi when the history of the congenital nature of the lesion is unreliable [29].

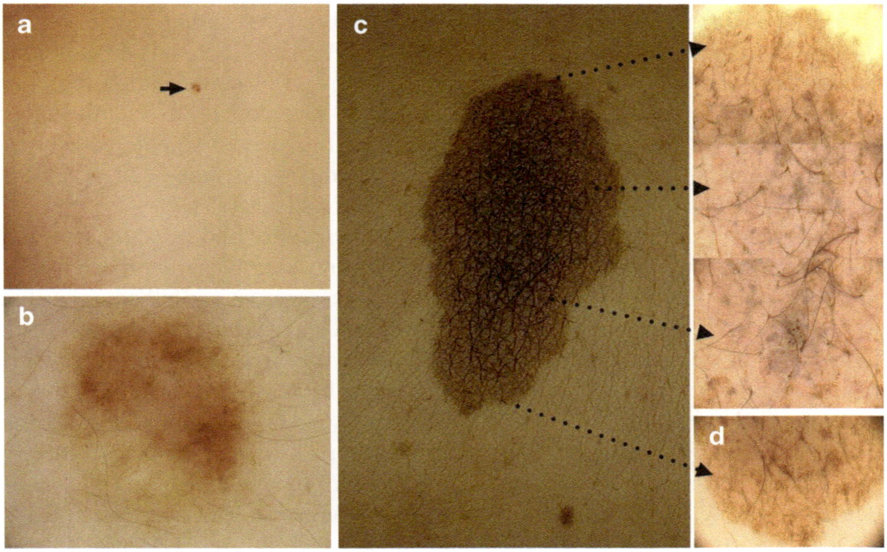

Fig. 15.14 (**a**) Clinical image of an isolated and suspicious melanocytic nevus on the back of a 12-year-old girl. (**b**) Polarized dermoscopy (20 ×) shows focal and irregular hyperpigmented areas, dotted vessels, and tan eccentric area. (**c**) Close-up clinical image of a nevus on the back of a 46-year-old female patient, present since childhood. The patient had a melanoma on the leg and chose to excise the large back lesion. (**d**) Collage of polarized dermoscopy (20 ×), from four different areas of the lesion, showing homogeneity of structures, mainly brown and bluish-gray clods, and peripheral enlarged pigment network. Both excisions revealed a *congenital-type compound melanocytic nevus*. (*Courtesy of Ana Maria Sortino MD, MSc*)

Because CMN, particularly GCMN, can be aesthetically displeasing, some patients experience a phycological burden and social difficulties. In addition, CMN may increase the risk of cutaneous melanoma, leptomeningeal melanoma, neurocutaneous melanocytosis (NCM), central nervous system (CNS) malformations, and, rarely, other tumors, like rhabdomyosarcoma and liposarcoma [34]. NCM is a benign or malignant, diffuse or localized, melanocytic proliferation in the leptomeninges and/or brain parenchyma associated with multiple CMN or GCMN. The presence of satellite lesions seems to be associated with an elevated risk of NCM [27]. Most patients are asymptomatic. When symptoms are present, they usually appear before the age of 2, though delayed presentation has been reported. Magnetic resonance imaging is usually the image modality of choice.

Patients with CMN can develop cutaneous or extracutaneous melanoma. The risk of MM in patients with CMN likely increases with the size of nevus and the number of satellite lesions [32, 39]. The overall absolute risk for all types of CMN taken together is low, of the order of 1–2%; however the incidence actually varies with the severity of the congenital phenotype [28]. Lifetime melanoma risk associated with GCMN is estimated to be between 1 and 15% [32, 39]. Melanomas associated with smaller CMN tend to appear after puberty and most likely originate at the dermo-epidermal junction (DEJ) and at the peripheral edge of the CMN. On the contrary, melanomas associated with large/GCMN develop earlier in life and frequently have their origin below the DEJ [37, 39]. Primary CNS melanoma in individuals with multiple CMN can either present as a solid tumor within the brain parenchyma or more commonly as leptomeningeal melanoma [28]. Nonmelanotic malignancies, including rhabdomyosarcoma, undifferentiated spindle cell tumor, neuroblastoma, melanoblastoma, myoblastic sarcoma, and malignant peripheral nerve sheath tumor, have been described in GCMN patients [39].

Management of CNM should consider size, symptoms, and psychological factors of each patient. Patients should be offered a multidisciplinary approach including pediatrician, dermatologist, neurologist, plastic surgeon, and others according to each case [40]. Early surgical resection may be beneficial in patients with CMN larger than 10 cm, although routine surgery has not been demonstrated to reduce risk of malignancy or CNS involvement [32, 39]. Moreover, regarding GCMN or multiple CMN, the complications of an extensive surgery ought to balance against the benefits [32, 39]. Management of CMN with single or combination laser therapy may show good results in short-term clearance of pigmentation, yet a high incidence of scaring, repigmentation, and complications have been reported. To date there is very-low-quality evidence for the efficacy and safety of CMN laser treatments in the long term [40]. Regular clinical and imaging follow-ups to assess spontaneous lightening or any proliferative changes in the CMN are advisable. Also, particularly for children with multiple CMN or GCMN, it is important to access neurological development closely. Early routine magnetic resonance imaging (MRI) to access CNS involvement is debatable in the literature. One must consider that imaging does not predict which patients will become symptomatic nor identify those who might benefit from a proven therapy. In addition, MRI often requires general anesthesia for young children, and its adverse effects for this age group have to be considered individually [32].

Nevus Spilus

(Synonyms: speckled lentiginous nevi, zosteriform lentiginous nevi)

Nevus spilus occurs in approximately 1–2% of the population and is present either at birth or in the first years of life. Clinically, it presents with a macular background with scattered superimposed more darkly pigmented macules or papules. Lesions are more commonly found on the trunk and extremities, although any site may be affected (Fig. 15.15) [41].

Nevus spilus has been associated with some abnormalities of vascular, central nervous system, and connective tissue origin. They can be associated with phacomatosis spilorosea and phacomatosis pigmentokeratotica [2]. Phacomatosis spilorosea is a rare syndrome characterized by the combination of a large macular nevus spilus and nevus roseus (a telangiectatic nevus of pale-pink color) in a segmental distribution [42]. Phacomatosis pigmentokeratotica (PPK) is a distinctive epidermal nevus syndrome first described in 1996, characterized by the presence of multiple

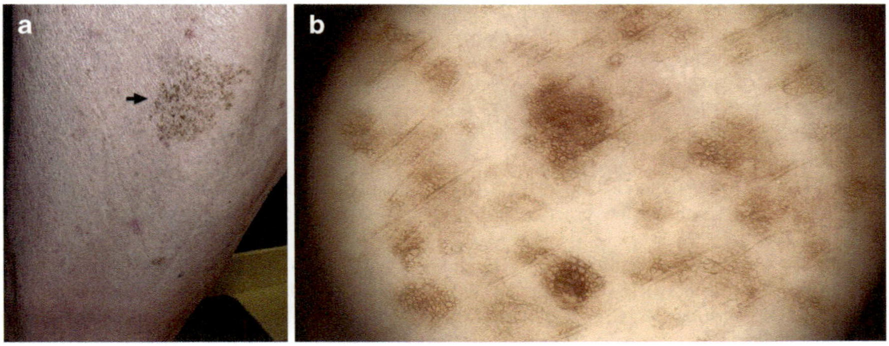

Fig. 15.15 Nevus spilus on the posterior tight of a 90-year-old male patient. The lesion has been present since early childhood and stable throughout life. (**a**) Close-up clinical image. (**b**) Polarized dermoscopy (20 ×) showing fragmented pigment network. (*Courtesy of Ana Maria Sortino MD, MSc*)

organoid nevi with sebaceous differentiation, a speckled lentiginous nevus, and skeletal and neurologic abnormalities. Cases without extracutaneous manifestations have been reported [43].

Rare cases of melanoma arise in nevus spilus. A changing lesion with irregular-shaped areas and variegated pigmentation should prompt a biopsy [41].

References

1. Schaffer J, Bolognia J, Hunt R. Benign pigmented skin lesions other than melanocytic nevi (moles). 2021. https://www.uptodate.com.
2. Kang S, Amagai M, Bruckner AL, Enk AH, Margolis DJ, McMichael AJ, Orringer JS, editors. Fitzpatrick's dermatology, 9e. New York: McGraw Hill; 2019.
3. Braun R. Solar lentigines. Dermoscopedia. 2019. https://dermoscopedia.org/w/index.php?title=Solar_lentigines&oldid=16362. Accessed 30 Jan 2022.
4. Bolognia JL. Reticulated black solar lentigo ('ink spot' lentigo). Arch Dermatol. 1992;128(7):934–40.
5. Hunt R, Schaffer JV, Bolognia JL. Acquired melanocytic nevi (moles). 2021. http://www.uptodate.com.
6. Orlow I, Satagopan JM, Berwick M, Enriquez HL, White KA, Cheung K, Dusza SW, Oliveria SA, Marchetti MA, Scope A, Marghoob AA, Halpern AC. Genetic factors associated with naevus count and dermoscopic patterns: preliminary results from the study of nevi in children (SONIC). Br J Dermatol. 2015;172(4):1081–9. https://doi.org/10.1111/bjd.13467.
7. Scope A, Marchetti MA, Marghoob AA, Dusza SW, Geller AC, Satagopan JM, Weinstock MA, Berwick M, Halpern AC. The study of nevi in children: principles learned and implications for melanoma diagnosis. J Am Acad Dermatol. 2016;75(4):813–23. https://doi.org/10.1016/j.jaad.2016.03.027.
8. Zalaudek I, Grinschgl S, Argenziano G, Marghoob AA, Blum A, Richtig E, Wolf IH, Fink-Puches R, Kerl H, Soyer HP, Hofmann-Wellenhof R. Age-related prevalence of dermoscopy patterns in acquired melanocytic naevi. Br J Dermatol. 2006;154(2):299–304. https://doi.org/10.1111/j.1365-2133.2005.06973.x.

9. Fonseca M, Marchetti MA, Chung E, Dusza SW, Burnett ME, Marghoob AA, Geller AC, Bishop M, Scope A, Halpern AC. Cross-sectional analysis of the dermoscopic patterns and structures of melanocytic naevi on the back and legs of adolescents. Br J Dermatol. 2015;173(6):1486–93. https://doi.org/10.1111/bjd.14035.
10. Clark WH Jr, Reimer RR, Greene M, Ainsworth AM, Mastrangelo MJ. Origin of familial malignant melanomas from heritable melanocytic lesions. 'The B-K mole syndrome'. Arch Dermatol. 1978;114(5):732–8.
11. Ferrara G, Argenziano G. The WHO 2018 classification of cutaneous melanocytic neoplasms: suggestions from routine practice. Front Oncol. 2021;11:675296. https://doi.org/10.3389/fonc.2021.675296.
12. NIH Consensus Conference. Diagnosis and treatment of early melanoma. JAMA. 1992;268(10):1314–9. https://doi.org/10.1001/jama.1992.03490100112037.
13. Elder DE, Bastian BC, Cree IA, Massi D, Scolyer RA. The 2018 World Health Organization classification of cutaneous, mucosal, and uveal melanoma: detailed analysis of 9 distinct subtypes defined by their evolutionary pathway. Arch Pathol Lab Med. 2020;144(4):500–22. https://doi.org/10.5858/arpa.2019-0561-RA.
14. Duffy K, Grossman D. The dysplastic nevus: from historical perspective to management in the modern era: part II. Molecular aspects and clinical management. J Am Acad Dermatol. 2012;67(1):19.e1–32. https://doi.org/10.1016/j.jaad.2012.03.013.
15. Argenziano G, Catricalà C, Ardigo M, Buccini P, De Simone P, Eibenschutz L, Ferrari A, Mariani G, Silipo V, Zalaudek I. Dermoscopy of patients with multiple nevi: improved management recommendations using a comparative diagnostic approach. Arch Dermatol. 2011;147(1):46–9. https://doi.org/10.1001/archdermatol.2010.389.
16. Wall N, De'Ambrosis B, Muir J. The management of dysplastic naevi: a survey of Australian dermatologists. Australas J Dermatol. 2017;58(4):304–7. https://doi.org/10.1111/ajd.12720.
17. Aouthmany M, Weinstein M, Zirwas MJ, Brodell RT. The natural history of halo nevi: a retrospective case series. J Am Acad Dermatol. 2012;67(4):582–6. https://doi.org/10.1016/j.jaad.2011.11.937.
18. Mundinger GS. Images in clinical medicine. Halo phenomenon. N Engl J Med. 2014;370(3):262. https://doi.org/10.1056/NEJMicm1306230.
19. Joseph M, Susana P. Blue nevi. Dermoscopedia. 2019. https://dermoscopedia.org/w/index.php?title=Blue_nevi&oldid=16844.
20. Ferrara G, Soyer HP, Malvehy J, Piccolo D, Puig S, Sopena J, Zalaudek I, Argenziano G. The many faces of blue nevus: a clinicopathologic study. J Cutan Pathol. 2007;34(7):543–51. https://doi.org/10.1111/j.1600-0560.2006.00650.x.
21. Ferrara G, Gianotti R, Cavicchini S, Salviato T, Zalaudek I, Argenziano G. Spitz nevus, Spitz tumor, and spitzoid melanoma: a comprehensive clinicopathologic overview. Dermatol Clin. 2013;31(4):589–98. https://doi.org/10.1016/j.det.2013.06.012.
22. Reed RJ, Ichinose H, Clark WH Jr, Mihm MC Jr. Common and uncommon melanocytic nevi and borderline melanomas. Semin Oncol. 1975;2(2):119–47.
23. Gaetanoli TR, Argenziano G. Spitz/Reed nevi. Dermoscopedia. 2019. https://dermoscopedia.org/Spitz_/_Reed_nevi.
24. Pedrosa AF, Lopes JM, Azevedo F, Mota A. Spitz/Reed nevi: a review of clinical-dermatoscopic and histological correlation. Dermatol Pract Concept. 2016;6(2):37–41. https://doi.org/10.5826/dpc.0602a07.
25. Argenziano G, Soyer HP, Ferrara G, Piccolo D, Hofmann-Wellenhof R, Peris K, Staibano S, Chimenti S. Superficial black network: an additional dermoscopic clue for the diagnosis of pigmented spindle and/or epithelioid cell nevus. Dermatology (Basel, Switzerland). 2001;203(4):333–5. https://doi.org/10.1159/000051784.
26. Lallas A, Apalla Z, Ioannides D, Lazaridou E, Kyrgidis A, Broganelli P, Alfano R, Zalaudek I, Argenziano G, International Dermoscopy Society. Update on dermoscopy of Spitz/Reed naevi and management guidelines by the International Dermoscopy Society. Br J Dermatol. 2017;177(3):645–55. https://doi.org/10.1111/bjd.15339.

27. Farabi B, Akay BN, Goldust M, Wollina U, Atak MF, Rao B. Congenital melanocytic naevi: an up-to-date overview. Australas J Dermatol. 2021;62(2):e178–91. https://doi.org/10.1111/ajd.13535.
28. Kinsler VA, O'Hare P, Bulstrode N, Calonje JE, Chong WK, Hargrave D, Jacques T, Lomas D, Sebire NJ, Slater O. Melanoma in congenital melanocytic naevi. Br J Dermatol. 2017;176(5):1131–43. https://doi.org/10.1111/bjd.15301.
29. Tannous ZS, Mihm MC Jr, Sober AJ, Duncan LM. Congenital melanocytic nevi: clinical and histopathologic features, risk of melanoma, and clinical management. J Am Acad Dermatol. 2005;52(2):197–203. https://doi.org/10.1016/j.jaad.2004.07.020.
30. Rhodes AR, Albert LS, Weinstock MA. Congenital nevomelanocytic nevi: proportionate area expansion during infancy and early childhood. J Am Acad Dermatol. 1996;34(1):51–62. https://doi.org/10.1016/s0190-9622(96)90834-8.
31. Martins da Silva VP, Marghoob A, Pigem R, Carrera C, Aguilera P, Puig-Butillé JA, Puig S, Malvehy J. Patterns of distribution of giant congenital melanocytic nevi (GCMN): the 6B rule. J Am Acad Dermatol. 2017;76(4):689–94. https://doi.org/10.1016/j.jaad.2016.05.042.
32. Alikhan A, Ibrahimi OA, Eisen DB. Congenital melanocytic nevi: where are we now? Part I. Clinical presentation, epidemiology, pathogenesis, histology, malignant transformation, and neurocutaneous melanosis. J Am Acad Dermatol. 2012;67(4):495.e1–514. https://doi.org/10.1016/j.jaad.2012.06.023.
33. Warner PM, Yakuboff KP, Kagan RJ, Boyce S, Warden GD. An 18-year experience in the management of congenital nevomelanocytic nevi. Ann Plast Surg. 2008;60(3):283–7. https://doi.org/10.1097/SAP.0b013e318095a784.
34. Kinsler VA, Chong WK, Aylett SE, Atherton DJ. Complications of congenital melanocytic naevi in children: analysis of 16 years' experience and clinical practice. Br J Dermatol. 2008;159(4):907–14. https://doi.org/10.1111/j.1365-2133.2008.08775.x.
35. Haliasos EC, Kerner M, Jaimes N, Zalaudek I, Malvehy J, Hofmann-Wellenhof R, Braun RP, Marghoob AA. Dermoscopy for the pediatric dermatologist part III: dermoscopy of melanocytic lesions. Pediatr Dermatol. 2013;30(3):281–93. https://doi.org/10.1111/pde.12041.
36. Ruiz-Maldonado R, Tamayo L, Laterza AM, Durán C. Giant pigmented nevi: clinical, histopathologic, and therapeutic considerations. J Pediatr. 1992;120(6):906–11. https://doi.org/10.1016/s0022-3476(05)81958-4.
37. Marghoob A. Congenital nevi. Dermoscopedia. 2019. https://dermoscopedia.org/w/index.php?title=Congenital_nevi&oldid=16533.
38. Seidenari S, Pellacani G. Surface microscopy features of congenital nevi. Clin Dermatol. 2002;20(3):263–7. https://doi.org/10.1016/s0738-081x(02)00223-7.
39. Eggen C, Lommerts JE, van Zuuren EJ, Limpens J, Pasmans S, Wolkerstorfer A. Laser treatment of congenital melanocytic naevi: a systematic review. Br J Dermatol. 2018;178(2):369–83. https://doi.org/10.1111/bjd.1609440.
40. Kim JY, Jeon JH, Choi TH, Kim BJ. Risk of malignant transformation arising from giant congenital melanocytic nevi: a 20-year single-center study. Dermatol Surg. 2022;48(2):171–5. https://doi.org/10.1097/DSS.0000000000003341.
41. Vaidya DC, Schwartz RA, Janniger CK. Nevus spilus. Cutis. 2007;80(6):465–8.
42. Fink C, Happle R, Enk A, Haenssle HA. Phacomatosis spilorosea: visual diagnosis and associated pathologies of a rare entity. J Eur Acad Dermatol Venereol. 2016;30(10):e69–70. https://doi.org/10.1111/jdv.13312.
43. Chantorn R, Shwayder T. Phacomatosis pigmentokeratotica: a further case without extracutaneous anomalies and review of the condition. Pediatr Dermatol. 2011;28(6):715–9. https://doi.org/10.1111/j.1525-1470.2011.01655.x.

Chapter 16
Malignant Melanocytic Tumors: Melanoma

Carlos Barcauí, Eduardo Bertolli, Juan Manuel Piñeiro-Maceira, Melissa Fugimori Lissae, Priscila Muniz Gonçalves de Moraes, and Rodrigo Ramella Munhoz

Key Points

- Cutaneous melanoma (CM) is the seventeenth most prevalent cancer worldwide according to the International Agency for Research on Cancer (IARC).
- There are four main types of CM: superficial spreading, nodular, lentigo maligna, and acral.
- Diagnosis is based on clinical examination, dermoscopy, and in selected cases confocal microscopy.

C. Barcauí
School of Medical Sciences, State University of Rio de Janeiro, Rio de Janeiro, Brazil

E. Bertolli
Cutaneous Oncology and Sarcoma Group, Hospital Sírio-Libanês, São Paulo, Brazil

Skin Cancer Department, AC Camargo Cancer Center, São Paulo, Brazil

Melanoma and Sarcoma Group, Beneficência Portuguesa de São Paulos, São Paulo, Brazil

J. M. Piñeiro-Maceira
Dermoscopy and Confocal Microscopy Section, Pedro Ernesto University Hospital-UERJ, Rio de Janeiro, Brazil

M. F. Lissae
Department of Pathology, Hospital Sírio-Libanês, São Paulo, Brazil

P. M. G. de Moraes
Oncology Center, Hospital Sírio-Libanês, São Paulo, Brazil

R. R. Munhoz (✉)
Cutaneous Oncology and Sarcoma Group, Hospital Sírio-Libanês, São Paulo, Brazil

Oncology Center, Hospital Sírio-Libanês, São Paulo, Brazil

C. M. Z. Abdalla et al. (eds.), *Oncodermatology*,
https://doi.org/10.1007/978-3-031-29277-4_16

- Excisional biopsy for histopathology remains the gold standard for accurate melanoma diagnosis.
- The prognosis is related by variables that include tumor thickness, ulceration, melanoma subtype, anatomical site, presence of nodal involvement, satellitosis/microsatellitosis, or in-transit or distant metastases.
- Surgery is the mainstay of treatment for CM, with wide local excision (WLE) associated with sentinel node biopsy (SNB) when indicated.
- Radiotherapy and systemic therapy are reserved for advanced stages or as adjuvant treatments in select scenarios.

Epidemiology and Biology of Melanoma

Cutaneous melanoma is the seventeenth most prevalent cancer worldwide according to the International Agency for Research on Cancer (IARC), with 324,635 cases estimated in 2020. The estimated global incidence rates are 3.8 new cases/100,000 men/year and 3.0 new cases/100,000 women/year [1, 2], with a significant variation across distinct geographic regions and ethnic groups. The highest incidence of CM is observed in Australia and New Zealand (41.6/100,000 men/year; 30.5/100,000 women/year), followed by Western Europe, North America, and Northern Europe. The lowest incidences are observed in South-Central Asia and Western Africa, which can be explained by epidemiological/demographic factors, but also potentially by underreporting and registry biases [3]. CM can have an aggressive behavior due to its potential to spread regionally and to distant sites through the lymphatic and hematogenous circulation. The absolute number of deaths expected in 2020 was 57,043, with a global mortality rate of 0.56 deaths/100,000 inhabitants (Boxes 16.1 and 16.2).

Risk Factors and Predisposing Conditions

Several risk factors are thought to be significant in the development of cutaneous melanoma, encompassing individual characteristics, environmental/acquired factors, and hereditary syndromes (Table 16.1).

The phototype, determined by skin color, eyes, and hair, is strongly associated with the risk of melanocytic tumors, with increased incidence among individuals with fair skin, blue or green eyes, and blond or red hair. Particularly for melanoma, additional factors include the presence of more than 50 common melanocytic nevi or more than 5 atypical nevi or personal history of other subtypes of skin cancers. Patients who have already had a melanoma are also more likely to develop a second-primary cutaneous malignancy. The relative risk is increased by a tenfold, but this risk decreases over time. Second-primary melanomas occur more frequently within

Table 16.1 Key risk factors for cutaneous melanoma

Risk factor	Considerations
Ultraviolet radiation/sun exposure	Intermittent and intense exposure, especially in childhood, adolescence, and early adulthood
Phenotype	Fair skin, blond or red hair, blue or green eyes
Melanocytic nevus	Multiple, dysplastic nevus
Immunosuppression	Organ-transplanted patients, chronic use of immunosuppressants
Personal history of neoplasms	Other skin tumors, hematologic neoplasms
Hereditary syndromes	
CDKN2A mutation	Younger age Multiple primary tumors Association with pancreatic cancer
BAP1 mutation	Cutaneous and uveal melanoma Association with mesothelioma
CDK4 mutation	Melanocytic nevus, melanoma Association with pancreatic cancer
MITF mutation	Dark hair, fair skin, and non-blue eyes Association with renal cell carcinoma
MC1R mutation	Red hair, freckles, fair skin Sensitivity to UV radiation
BRCA2 mutation	Association with breast, ovarian, and pancreatic cancer
Others—POT1, ACD, TERF2IP	Rare cause of hereditary melanoma Association with breast, ovarian, uterus, thyroid, colon, lung, kidney, prostate, and esophageal cancers

the first 2 years after the primary tumor, which probably reflects a higher level of surveillance in these patients. The chances of developing a second-primary tumor are greater in patients with atypical nevus syndrome and/or a family history of melanoma [4, 5]. Patients with history of non-melanoma skin cancer and actinic keratosis also have a relative risk of approximately 4.0, which is directly related to the patient's degree of exposure to ultraviolet rays.

Although the presence of multiple melanocytic nevi is considered a risk factor for melanoma, most (70%) of melanomas arise de novo, originating from healthy skin. Approximately 30% of melanomas are associated with melanocytic nevi regardless of whether they are atypical or common. Atypical nevi are, therefore, risk markers and not precursor lesions of melanoma [6].

Damage to the DNA induced by ultraviolet radiation, particularly through sunlight exposure, represents the most frequent acquired/environmental risk factor. History of intense and intermittent sun exposure, episodes of sunburn especially during childhood and adolescence, and presence of ephelides and solar lentigines can significantly contribute to an increased risk. As an example, the presence of signs of actinic damage, which is a subjective way of evaluating previous sun exposure, and history of sunburn are related to a relative risk of 2.0 [5].

Immunosuppression is also related to CM and is associated with a higher probability of developing a new lesion, in addition to an increased risk of relapse following the initial diagnosis. Overall survival is worse in these patients, and they are at increased risk of dying from metastatic melanoma. Previous hematologic malignancies, particularly chronic lymphocytic leukemia, also result in an increased risk of melanoma and an increased risk of dying from metastatic melanoma [7].

A family history of melanoma is also a risk factor and can be explained by non-pathogenic, inherited characteristics (e.g., phototype) and environmental/behavioral factors, in addition to hereditary syndromes. Regardless of the cause, a family history of melanoma in a first-degree relative confers a relative risk of 1.7. Hereditary syndromes, defined by the presence of pathogenic germline mutations in the DNA or genetic polymorphisms, contribute to a relatively small percentage of CM. In the context of a hereditary predisposition, mutations affecting the CDKN2A gene and, less frequently, CDK4 contribute to the majority of cases and define the familial atypical multiple mole melanoma (FAMMM) syndrome or dysplastic nevus syndrome. Additional mutations affecting different genes, including BAP1, MITF, MC1R, and BRCA2, contribute to a smaller percentage of cases (Table 16.1) [5].

Currently, according to the Melanoma Genetics Consortium, genetic counseling is indicated in the following situations:

- Family history of invasive cutaneous melanoma or pancreatic cancer (three members affected on one side of the family).
- Three or more invasive primary cutaneous melanomas, including the first starting before 45 years of age.
- One or more intradermal melanocytic tumors with BAP-1 mutation and family history of mesothelioma, meningioma, and/or uveal melanoma.
- Two or more intradermal melanocytic tumors with BAP-1 mutation.

Further details on the updated recommendations on indications for genetic research in families with melanoma can be found at www.genomel.org. As with any laboratory test, the pros and cons of this research must be evaluated and, mainly, its impact on the management of these patients.

Biology of Melanoma

Melanoma can originate de novo or from precursor lesions, such as melanocytic nevi or melanoma in situ, and its development is related to the accumulation of genetic alterations that result in uncontrolled cell proliferation, as well as acquisition of immune evasion mechanisms. Of note, CM can also be found in association with distinct precursor lesions. Most melanomas exhibit aberrant activation of the RAS/RAF/MEK/ERK signaling cascade, known as the mitogen-activated protein kinase (MAPK) pathway, responsible for cell cycle regulation and apoptosis inhibition. Additional signaling pathways potentially affected in CM include PI3K, SWI/SNF, telomerase, p53, and RB. Pathogenic mutations present in CM affect key genes involved in cell proliferation, replication, and survival (BRAF, NRAS, NF1, KIT, TERT), transcription active ion (ARID2, ARID1A), resistance to apoptosis (PTEN, TP53), and cell cycle control (CDKN2A) [8].

The level of sun exposure associated with cutaneous melanoma leads to clinical, anatomopathological, and molecular differences. Chronically sun-damaged (CSD) melanomas usually arise from anatomical sites with high levels of sun exposure (e.g., head and neck, truck), have a higher number of non-synonymous somatic mutations (mutational burden), and are characterized by mutations in NRAS, neurofibromin 1 (NF1), KIT, and BRAF non-V600E genes. Non-CSD melanomas typically affect individuals at younger ages and are usually associated with preexisting nevi, tend to have a lower mutation burden, and harbor BRAF V600E mutations in approximately 60% of the cases [8].

Specific subtypes of melanoma also display a distinct biology, natural history, and molecular characteristics; in contrast to the previously described distribution of BRAF mutations present in cutaneous melanoma, acral melanomas are enriched for NRAS (15%) and KIT (15%) mutations, with only 15% of the patients presenting with a BRAF mutation; similarly, mutations affecting the BRAF, NRAS, and KIT genes occur in 5%, 15%, and 30% of mucosal melanoma; uveal melanoma is an entirely distinct entity in terms of clinical presentation, molecular aspects, and clinical course, as is characterized by the presence of aberrations affecting GNAQ (25–30%), GNA11 (32–55%), and BAP1 (30%) genes.

Clinical Variants of Melanoma

There are four main types of CM: superficial spreading, nodular, lentigo maligna, and acral. All originate in the epidermis where the melanocytes are located and have a radial intraepithelial followed by a vertical growth phase. The time of these phases varies according to the histopathological type. Melanoma is considered invasive when it invades through the basal membrane into the dermis. The occurrence of metastases is directly related to the tumor thickness, the presence of ulceration, and mitotic count, defined by the number of mitoses/mm^2 found in the dermis (invasive component). All clinical presentations may, in their evolution, present hypo-/amelanotic and/or ulcerate areas.

A new classification based on the correlation between genetic alterations observed in different types of melanomas has gained relevance in the literature: melanomas associated with chronic UV-induced damage, melanomas not associated with chronic UV-induced damage, and acral melanomas:

- **Superficial Spreading Melanoma**: This subtype represents approximately 70% of melanomas and is more frequent in patients between 40 and 60 years old. Historically, it has been described on the trunk of men and on the legs of women, but can occur on any area of the body in both genders. The classic clinical presentation of this type of neoplasm is a macule, which evolves into an asymptomatic, blackened, asymmetric plaque (“A”), with irregular borders (“B”), varied color (+ 3 colors) (“C”), and diameter above 6 mm (“D”). The ABCD rule was created then, in the 1980s, by a group from the University of New York. The main complaint is the change/growth of a “mole” reported by the patient or one of their relatives, adding the “E” for evolution to the ABCD (Figs. 16.1a–c and 16.2a–c).

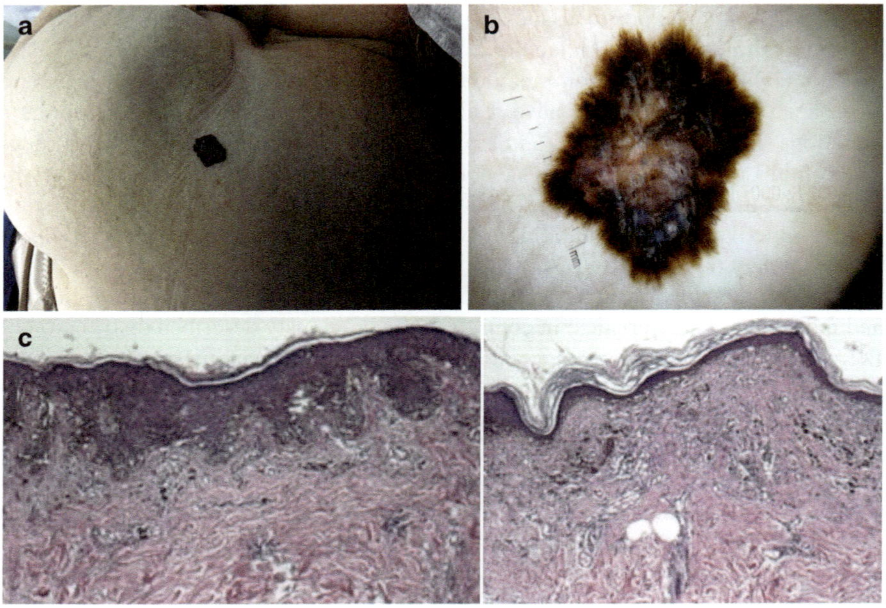

Fig. 16.1 (**a**) Superficially spreading melanoma on the scapular region of a 55-year-old woman. Black plaque with irregular borders. The "ugly duck" sings among this patient's nevi. Courtesy of Dr. Carlos Barcaui. (**b**) Dermoscopy of superficial spreading melanoma showing a multicomponent pattern with an irregular pigmented network, irregular black blotches, white cicatricial areas, peppering, and shiny white streaks. Courtesy of Dr. Carlos Barcaui. (**c**) Histopathology of superficial spreading melanoma (Clark II, Breslow 0.5 mm). Note the proliferation of melanoma cells occupying the epidermis, with fusion of interpapillary cones (left, H&E 100 ×), and invading the dermis. in which an area of fibrosis with an inflammatory reaction containing melanophages is observed, corresponding to a phenomenon of partial regression of the lesion (right, H&E 40 ×). (Courtesy of Dr. Carlos Barcaui)

The radial growth phase of superficial spreading melanoma has an asymmetrical proliferation of atypical melanocytes, singly and in clusters throughout all levels of the epithelium (buckshot scatter). Invasive component is characterized by solid masses or may have a fascicular arrangement, consisting of epithelioid cells, nevus cell-like, or even spindle-shaped cells without maturation during their descent into the dermis. The epithelioid cells have abundant cytoplasm, often showing fine or dusty melanin pigmentation, and contain pleomorphic vesicular nuclei with prominent eosinophilic nucleoli; scattered mitotic figures including atypical forms may be evident. Actinic damage is often little visible. Desmoplasia and/or neurotropism are uncommon [9–11].

- **Nodular Melanoma**: This subtype is the second most common in fair-skinned individuals, representing 15–30% of melanomas, and is the most frequent in those aged over 60 years. Unlike other types, its incidence is not increasing. It affects men more frequently than women. Nodular melanomas arise more frequently in the trunk, upper extremities, and head and neck. It presents, clinically, as a papule that develops into a brown, black, or pink nodule. It is the form that

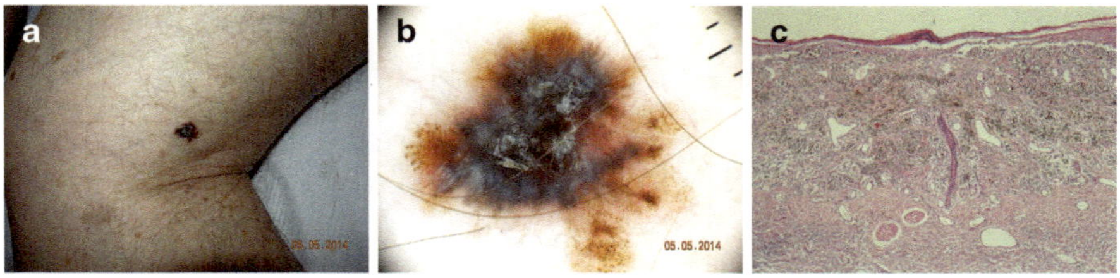

Fig. 16.2 (**a**) Superficially spreading melanoma on the popliteal region of a 63-year-old male patient. Courtesy of Dr. Carlos Barcaui. (**b**) Dermoscopy of the superficial spreading melanoma multicomponent pattern. Asymmetrical lesion of light brown, dark brown, black, red, and bluish gray coloration, showing peripheral streaks, an irregular network, amorphous areas, a blue-white veil, and shiny white streaks. Courtesy of Dr. Carlos Barcaui. (**c**) Histopathology of superficial spreading melanoma (Clark IV, Breslow 0.78 mm) showing extensive dermal involvement and involvement of the epithelium of a sweat duct in the central portion of the photo. (H&E 40 ×). (Courtesy of Dr. Carlos Barcauí)

displays the fastest vertical growth phase and is therefore often diagnosed belatedly (Fig. 16.3a, b).

- **Lentigo Maligna**: Corresponds to 10–15% of melanomas and is more frequent in individuals over 70 years with intense photodamage. It preferentially affects the head and neck region, mainly the nose and malar region. It has a prolonged radial growth phase, remaining intraepithelial (in situ) for a long period before progressing to the invasive vertical phase, which occurs in approximately 5% of cases. Clinically, it presents as a blackish brownish macula, with irregular edges that progress to a plaque and, eventually, to a nodule (invasive phase) (Fig. 16.4a, b).

  Lentigo maligna melanoma (LMM) exhibits an epidermal component of atypical melanocytes, singly and in nests, located along the dermoepidermal junction, and epidermal thinning and loss of rete ridges. Invasive component is characterized by spindle or epithelioid melanocytes. There are variable cytological atypia, mitotic figures, considerable nuclear pleomorphism, and tumor giant cells. There are moderate to severe solar elastosis, macrophages with pigment, and lymphocytes at the upper dermis usually [10, 12, 13].
- **Acral Lentiginous Melanoma**: It represents approximately 5% of melanomas. However, due to the low occurrence of melanomas related to sun exposure in blacks and Asians, it represents 70 and 45% of melanomas in these ethnic groups, respectively. It occurs in the palmoplantar region, fingers, and the nail apparatus. Involvement of the feet is three times more frequent than that of the hands, where the involvement of the nail apparatus prevails and, rarely, of the palmar region. It is more frequent in individuals over 60 years of age and affects both men and women, with a slight predominance in females (1.8:1.0). Palmoplantar lesions present as an irregularly shaped macule, with color ranging from brown to black, evolving into a plaque or nodule which may ulcerate. Its diagnosis is often late, with more advanced Median Breslow Thickness Index, which results in a poor prognosis [13]. It can also present in the hypo-/amelanotic form, making its diagnosis even more difficult. It may also be confused with plantar warts, traumatic ulcers, or pyogenic granuloma. The role of repeated trauma in the etiology of

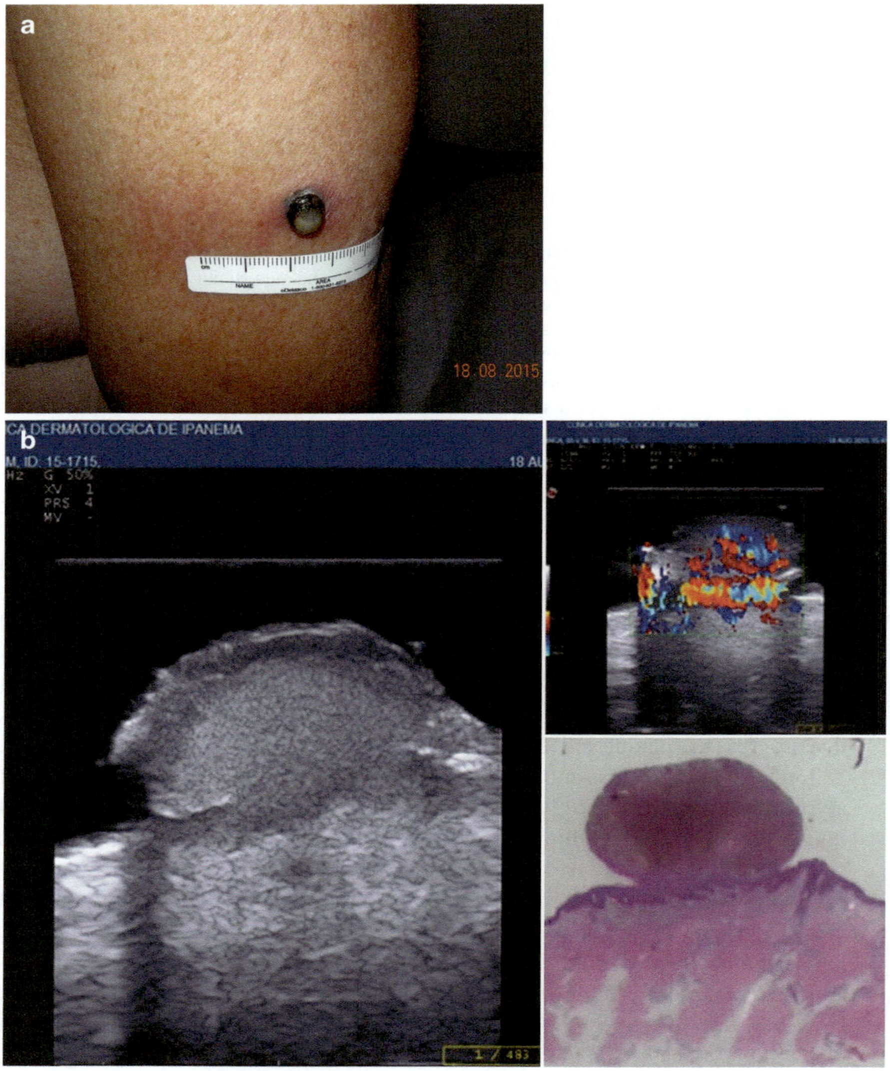

Fig. 16.3 (**a**) Nodular melanoma on the left arm of a 65-year-old male patient. Lesion covered by a pustule. The smaller image shows pigment leakage in the periphery of the lesion. Courtesy of Dr. Carlos Barcaui. (**b**) High-frequency ultrasound (22 MHz) of nodular melanoma showing positive intra- and perilesional Doppler mapping. Perfect correlation of the ultrasound image with the small increase in histopathology in H&E. Breslow nodular melanoma, 3.7 mm; 2 mitoses/mm^2. (Courtesy of Dr. Carlos Barcaui)

melanoma in the palmoplantar regions is controversial. From a molecular biological perspective, it is characterized by having a large number of genetic abnormalities and KIT mutations (Figs. 16.5a–c and 16.6).

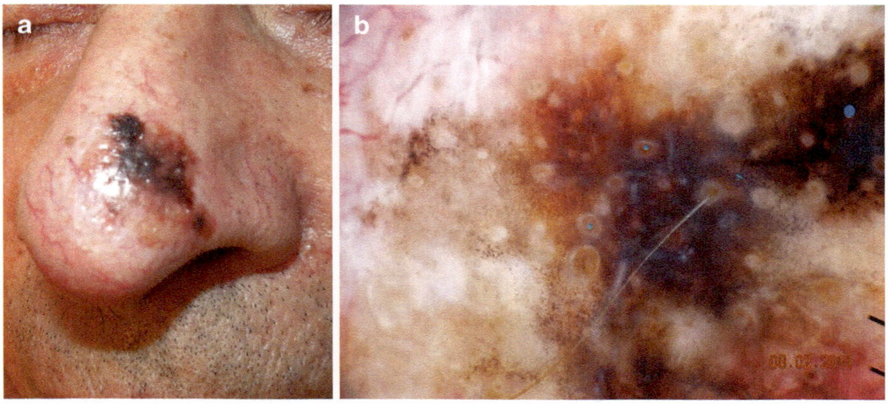

Fig. 16.4 (**a**) Lentigo maligna. Extensive lesion, with a long-lasting radial growth phase, without invading the dermis. Courtesy of Dr. Carlos Barcaui. (**b**) Dermoscopy of Lentigo Maligna—note the light brown, dark brown, black, red, and bluish-gray colors. From a structural point of view, multiple bluish gray dots (>) can be seen forming an annular-granular pattern, asymmetrically pigmented follicular openings (*), amorphous areas (blue circle), and shiny white streaks. (Courtesy of Dr. Carlos Barcaui)

Melanoma of the nail apparatus accounts for 0.3–1.4% of melanomas. The most affected portion is the nail matrix, where most melanocytes in the nail apparatus are located, but it can also occur in the subungual bed and the epithelium adjacent to the lamina. It often presents as an irregular band of blackish-brown pigmentation—melanonychia, usually greater than 3 mm. It may eventually affect the proximal nail fold—Hutchinson's sign. In its later phase, it can cause dystrophy and destruction of the nail apparatus. The English eponym ABCDEF was created to highlight the most frequent clinical findings of nail melanoma: A, age, African Americans; B, brown to black bands; C, change in the nail band; D, dominant digit; E, extension (Hutchinson's sign); and F, family or personal history of melanoma (Figs. 16.7a–e and 16.8).

Acral lentiginous melanomas have a radial growth phase characterized by irregular epidermal hyperplasia and scattered, basally located, atypical melanocytes, with some nesting. The atypical melanocytes have nuclear pleomorphism and hyperchromatism and may be round with a clear halo or heavily pigmented dendritic processes. The invasive component may have epithelioid or spindle cells; mitotic activity; desmoplastic stromal response; osteosarcomatous change in the stroma; presence of giant, nevoid, and clear cells; neural differentiation; and perineural infiltration. A heavy bandlike chronic inflammatory cell infiltrate is frequently present [10, 11, 14].

- **Atypical Melanoma Variants**: Less common forms of melanoma can be found both in the skin and in the mucosal membranes. In general, these special types of melanoma have an atypical clinical presentation or are located in peculiar anatomical sites, which causes a delay in diagnosis and, consequently, a worsening of the prognosis. Atypical variants include desmoplastic melanoma (Fig. 16.9a–g), amelanotic melanoma (Fig. 16.10a–c), mucosal melanoma, min-

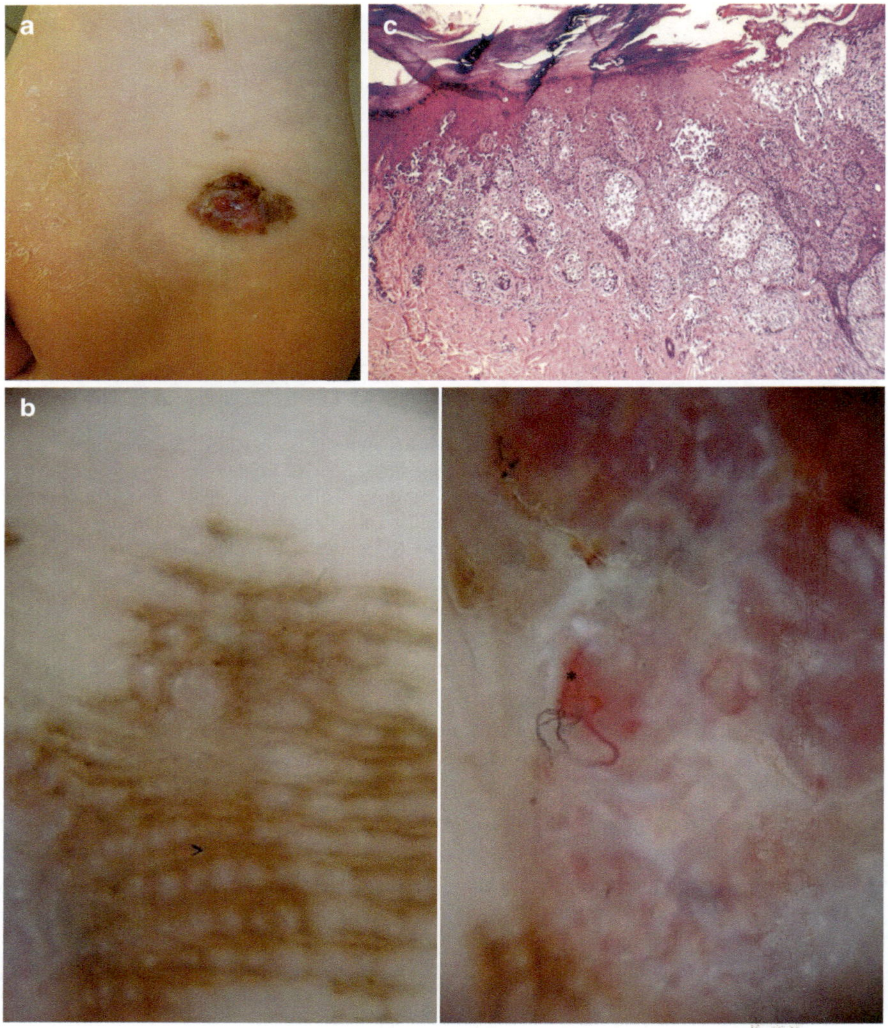

Fig. 16.5 (**a**) Melanoma in the plantar region associated with congenital melanocytic nevus in a 53-year-old Caucasian patient. Courtesy of Dr. Carlos Barcaui. (**b**) Dermoscopy of acral melanoma. On the left, a pattern of parallel sulci with a double line is observed (>), suggestive of benignity and probably related to the congenital nevus present before the melanoma. On the right, we highlight the vascular pattern showing irregular linear vessels (*) in the hypomelanotic component of the tumor. Courtesy of Dr. Carlos Barcaui. (**c**) Histopathology of ulcerated melanoma of the plantar region (Clark IV, Breslow 8 mm). There is an extensive invasion of the dermis by masses of tumor cells, as well as a pagetoid rise in the epidermis. (Courtesy of Dr. Carlos Barcaui)

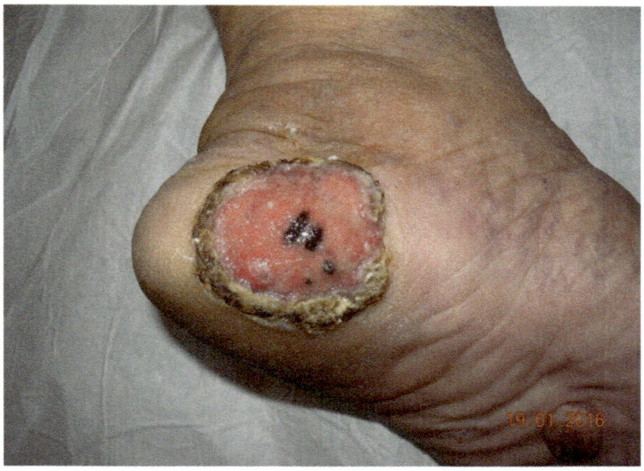

Fig. 16.6 Hypo/amelanotic melanoma in the plantar region. The lesion was treated for more than 1 year as a stasis ulcer due to the poorly pigmented appearance of the lesion. (Courtesy of Dr. Carlos Barcaui)

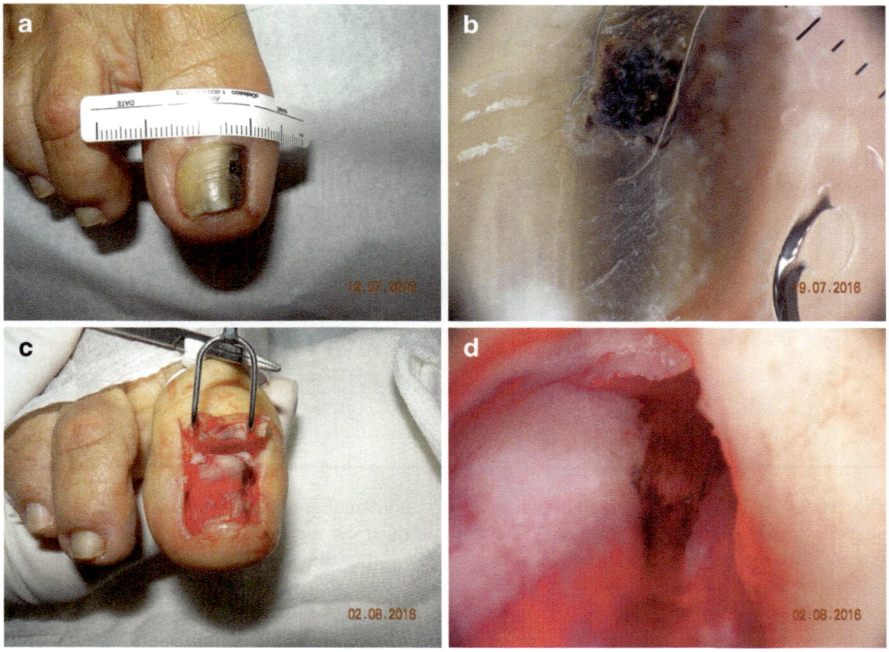

Fig. 16.7 (**a**) Melanonychia, approximately 3 mm thick, and fracture of the nail plate. Melanoma in situ. Courtesy of Dr. Carlos Barcaui. (**b**) Dermoscopy of the nail plate showing melanic and hematic pigment being extruded through the nail plate. Courtesy of Dr. Carlos Barcaui. (**c**) After nail plate ablation and proximal fold folding, a pigmented lesion affecting the nail matrix and bed is observed. Courtesy of Dr. Carlos Barcaui. (**d**) Perioperative dermoscopy of the nail matrix shows melanin pigment distributed in irregular lines and forming streaks. Courtesy of Dr. Carlos Barcaui. (**e**) Histopathology of melanoma in situ. Note the occupation of the entire thickness of the subungual epithelium by atypical melanocytes, without involvement of the subungual connective tissue (H&E 100 ×). (Courtesy of Dr. Carlos Barcaui)

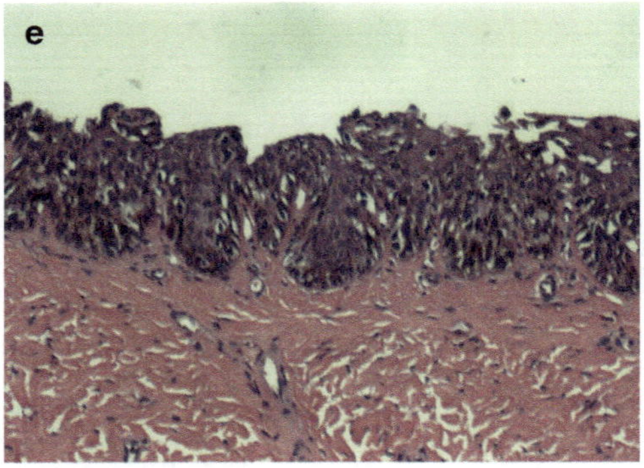

Fig. 16.7 (continued)

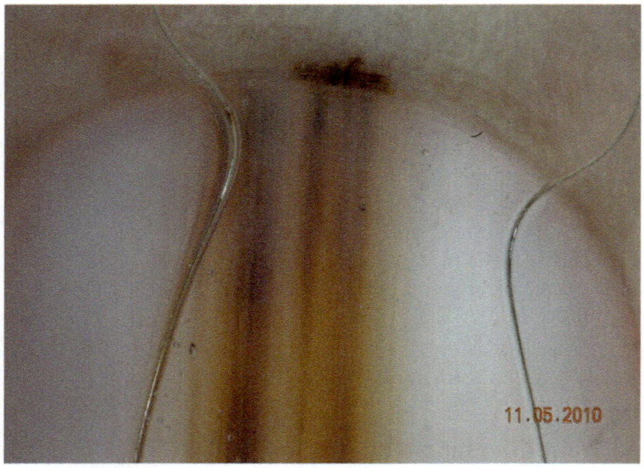

Fig. 16.8 Dermoscopy of subungual melanoma shows irregularly sized bands of light and dark brown pigment and pigment leakage in the proximal nail fold—Hutchinson's sign. (Courtesy of Dr. Carlos Barcaui)

Fig. 16.9 (**a**) Desmoplastic melanoma associated with malignant lentigo. Lesion in a keloid-shaped, poorly delimited plaque with irregular pigment on the surface, in a 76-year-old male patient with extensive photodamage. Courtesy of Dr. Carlos Barcaui. (**b**) Dermoscopy of desmoplastic melanoma associated with malignant lentigo. Note the irregular pigmented network (>), erythema, and shiny white streaks (*). Courtesy of Dr. Carlos Barcaui. (**c**) High-frequency ultrasound (22 MHz) of desmoplastic melanoma associated with malignant lentigo showing an irregularly shaped, non-circumscribed hypoechoic image, affecting the dermis to the subcutaneous tissue. Courtesy of Dr. Carlos Barcaui. (**d**) Desmoplastic melanoma associated with malignant lentigo. Excisional biopsy of the lesion. Courtesy of Dr. Carlos Barcaui. (**e**) The histopathology of desmoplastic melanoma associated with malignant lentigo showed a malignant neoplasm of spindle cells affecting the entire length of the dermis. In the higher magnification detail, the fusiform aspect of the cells can be seen. Courtesy of Dr. Carlos Barcaui. (**f**) Immunohistochemistry of desmoplastic melanoma associated with malignant lentigo positive S100 in the dermal component of the tumor and in Langerhans cells in the epidermis. Courtesy of Dr. Carlos Barcaui. (**g**) Immunohistochemistry of desmoplastic melanoma associated with malignant lentigo positive for Melan A showing atypical melanocytes in confluent distribution in the hyperplasia epidermis in the right half of the photo. (Courtesy of Dr. Carlos Barcaui)

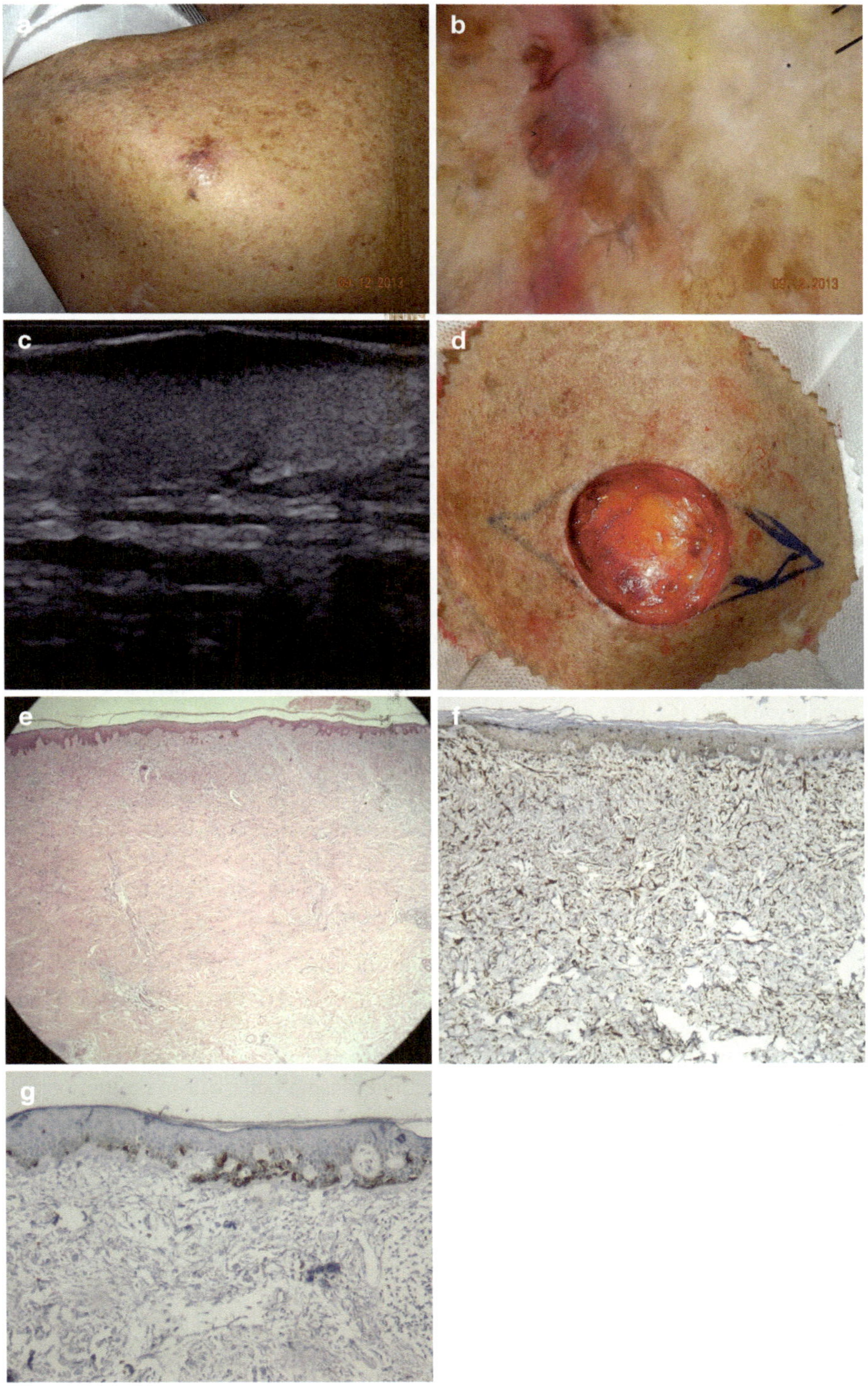
a
b
c
d
e
f
g
09.12.2013

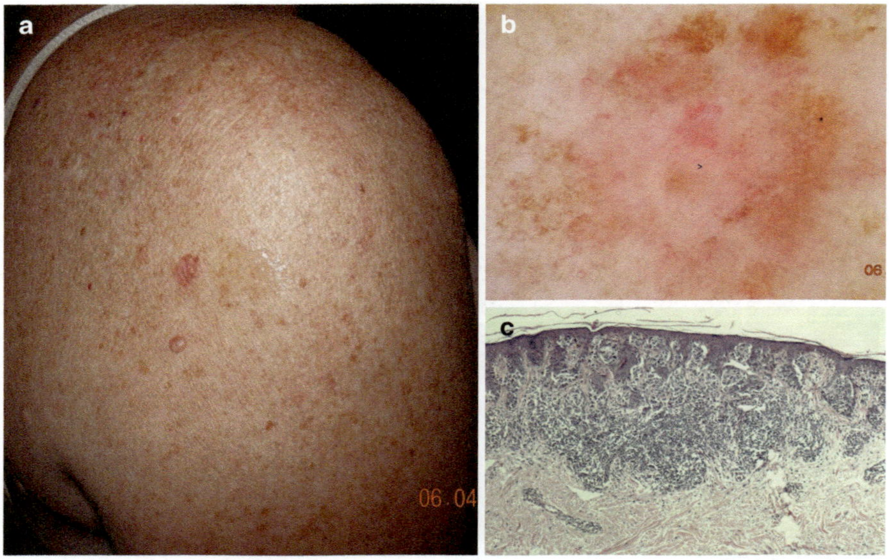

Fig. 16.10 (**a**) Amelanotic melanoma associated with a melanocytic nevus, a pinkish lesion in a 56-year-old female patient with a previous family history of melanoma. Courtesy of Dr. Carlos Barcaui. (**b**) Dermoscopy of amelanotic melanoma associated with melanocytic nevus showing punctiform vessels (>), erythema, and pigmented network remnants in the periphery (*). Courtesy of Dr. Carlos Barcaui. (**c**) Amelanotic melanoma (Clark II Breslow 0.55 mm) associated with melanocytic nevus. (Courtesy of Dr. Carlos Barcaui)

imal deviation melanoma (nevus), malignant blue nevus, and primary dermal melanoma (Fig. 16.11a–c). Other less frequent histopathological variants that have an aberrant antigenic profile during the vertical growth phase are spitzoid melanoma, verrucous melanoma, ballooning cell melanoma, signet-ring cell melanoma, myxoid melanoma, and polypoid melanoma.

– **Desmoplastic Melanoma**: Desmoplastic/spindle-cell melanomas are composed of strands of spindle-shaped cells surrounded by mature collagen and are subdivided into entirely desmoplastic lesion and desmoplastic melanoma mixed with conventional melanoma. Multinucleate cells, neural transformation, neurotropism, and lymphocytes and plasma cells within the tumor may be seen. Heterotopic bone and cartilage and sweat duct proliferation can be found. Aggressive variants of osteogenic desmoplastic melanoma have been reported. A component of lentigo maligna in the epidermis overlying or toward one edge of the lesion can be found. The tumor cells are positive for vimentin in all cases and for S100 protein and neuron-specific enolase. Desmoplastic neurotropic melanoma is considered a variant (Fig. 16.9a–g) [10, 15, 16].

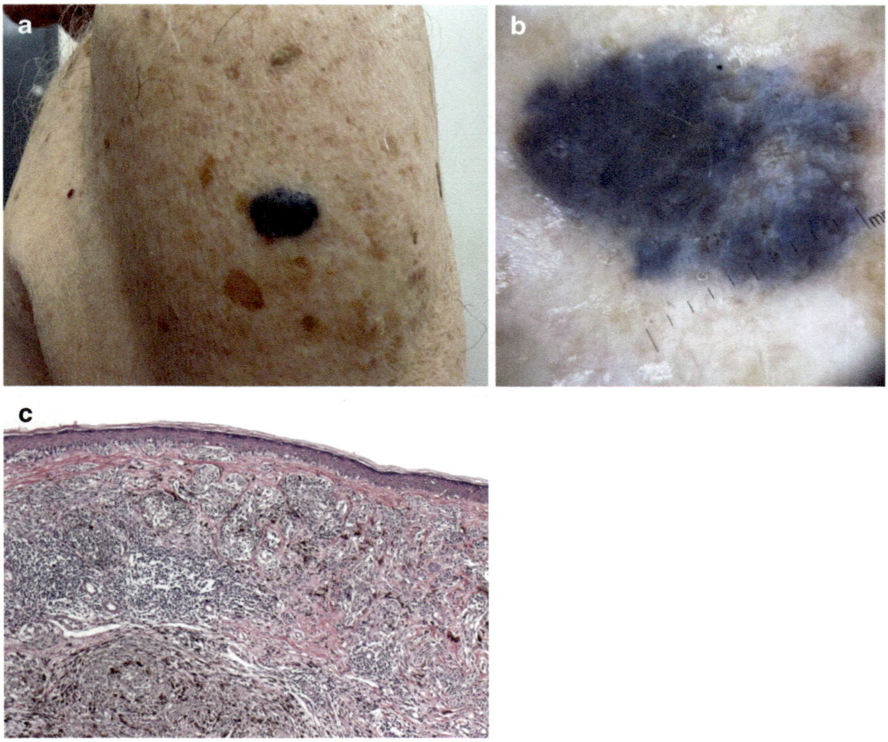

Fig. 16.11 (**a**) Primary dermal melanona, melanophage-rich variant, Clark IV, Breslow 3.3 mm, 1 mitosis/mm^2. Lesions on a blackened plaque with a bluish hue. Courtesy of Dr. Carlos Barcaui. (**b**) Dermoscopy of primary dermal melanona, melanophage-rich variant, Clark IV, Breslow 3.3 mm, 1 mitosis/mm^2—diffuse homogeneous pattern, differential diagnosis with blue nevus. Courtesy of Dr. Carlos Barcaui. (**c**) Histopathology—melanophage-rich melanoma (Clark IV, Breslow 3.3 mm, mitotic index 1/mm^2)—extensive occupation of the dermis by atypical melanocytic cell masses, focus of lymphocytic inflammation, and numerous melanophages. There is a small neoplastic component in the portion. Lower epidermis (H&E 40 ×). (Courtesy of Dr. Carlos Barcaui)

– **Spitz Melanoma**: Spitz melanomas (malignant Spitz tumor) histologically exhibit large epithelioid melanocytes resembling those found in Spitz nevi and can be of any size (usually >1 cm). Epidermal component is characterized by asymmetry, poor circumscription, consumption of the epidermis, ulceration, and enlarged, irregular, and confluent nests. The dermal component consists of asymmetric, nodular, or sheet-like clusters of melanocytes, reduction of maturation, melanin deeply located, lymphocyte infiltrates, and necrosis. Cytologically, there are nuclear enlargement and pleomorphism, nuclear membranes irregularity, hyperchromatism, and eosinophilic nucleoli. High mitotic

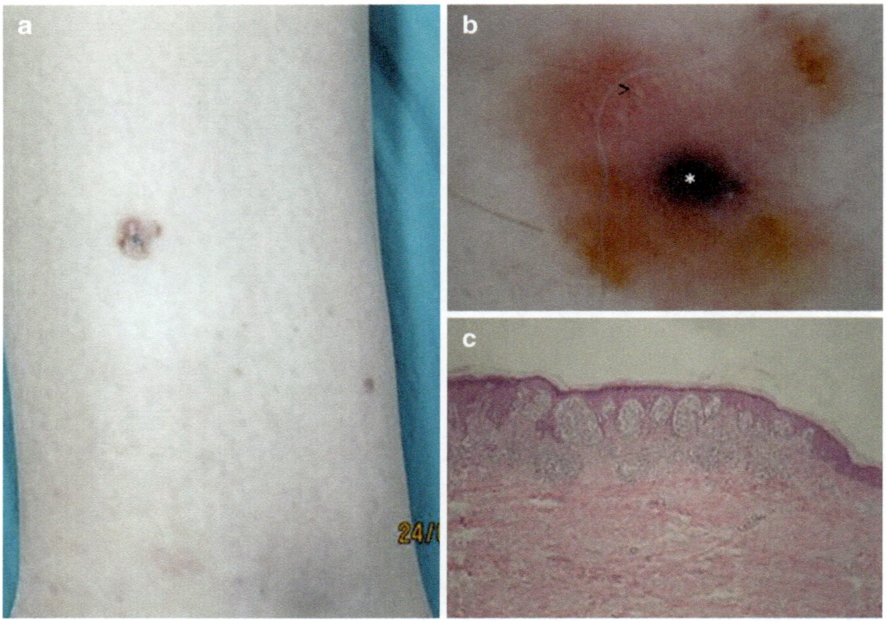

Fig. 16.12 Spitzoid melanoma (Clark II, Breslow 0.35 mm). (**a**) Pinkish poorly delimited plaque with a darker center. (**b**) Dermoscopy—punctate vascular pattern (>), an irregular network in the periphery, and central blackened amorphous area (*). (**c**) Histopathology—acanthotic epidermis containing nests of atypical cells, large and elongated, at the dermoepidermal junction, extending to the papillary dermis; presence of lymphohistiocytic inflammation under the neoplasm (H&E 40 ×). (Courtesy of Dr. Carlos Barcaui)

activity, atypical forms, and deep mitosis suggest melanoma. Spitz melanoma has not only the morphologic features of Spitz tumors but also has their genetic hallmarks (spectrum of MAPK activating alterations) and has a better prognosis than other types of cutaneous melanomas (Fig. 16.12a–c) [17, 18].

Diagnosis

Dermatologic Assessment

Most melanomas are initially noted by the patient or by one of his family members or friends, who report the appearance or change of a "mole" [19]. The dermatological physical examination of the entire body surface is the first step in order not to miss the diagnosis of a melanoma, particularly in individuals at higher risk. In these patients, the guidance for monthly skin self-examination should be emphasized. It is very important that the total skin examination is standardized and systematically performed allowing for an appropriate assessment of areas encompassing the feet, buttocks, scalp, and genital region. During the examination, even if at first glance there is one lesion that stands out from the others, the so-called "ugly duckling" sign, all lesions must be examined, as synchronous melanomas may occur.

The sensitivity for diagnosing melanoma through the dermatologist's naked eye is approximately 70%. The addition of dermoscopy techniques increases the diagnostic sensitivity to 90% in the hands of trained physicians [20].

For pigmented suspicious lesions on nail apparatus, dermoscopy is a powerful semiologic tool and can be performed on the lamina, matrix/bed, proximal periungual tissue, and the distal edge of the lamina. Basically, on the nail plate, the melanoma appears as a band with irregular blackish-brown lines. On the free edge of the nail, dermoscopy makes it possible to assess whether the pigment is in the lower or upper part of the nail, which indicates the location of the lesion in the distal or proximal matrix, respectively. In the proximal nail fold, with a dermatoscope, the presence of pigment (micro-Hutchinson's sign) can be seen before it becomes clinically apparent (Hutchinson's sign) (Fig. 16.5). Nail bed/matrix dermoscopy, originally described in Brazil, is an invasive test performed after the removal of the nail plate, with noncontact polarized light dermoscopy. The homogeneous pattern indicates benignity and the irregular one, melanoma. Its main contribution is the better observation and delimitation of the lesion [21, 22].

Digital dermoscopy consists of capturing and storing digital dermoscopy images. Image acquisition can be performed using any equipment that has a digital camera coupled to a dermatoscope (e.g., a camera, smartphone, tablet, or videodermatoscope). The storage of images allows the creation of a database that can be used to compare the evolution of the lesion over time, for teledermoscopy and, more recently, for artificial intelligence using convolutional neural networks (CNN) (Figs. 16.13 and 16.14).

Total body mapping comprises the photographic documentation of the entire body surface (total body photograph) followed by digital dermoscopy of the selected lesions. This two-step method, when applied to high-risk patients, allows for early detection of melanoma and reduces the number of unnecessary biopsies of benign

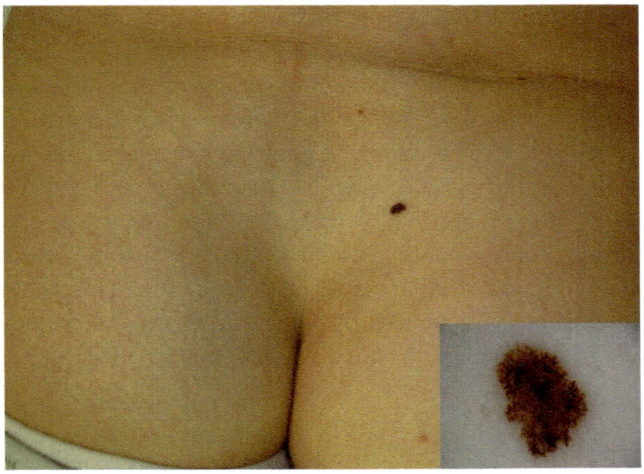

Fig. 16.13 The importance of the total body examination. In situ melanoma was detected in a patient whose reason for consultation was acne on the buttock. In detail, dermoscopy shows an enlarged pigmented network. (Courtesy of Dr. Carlos Barcaui)

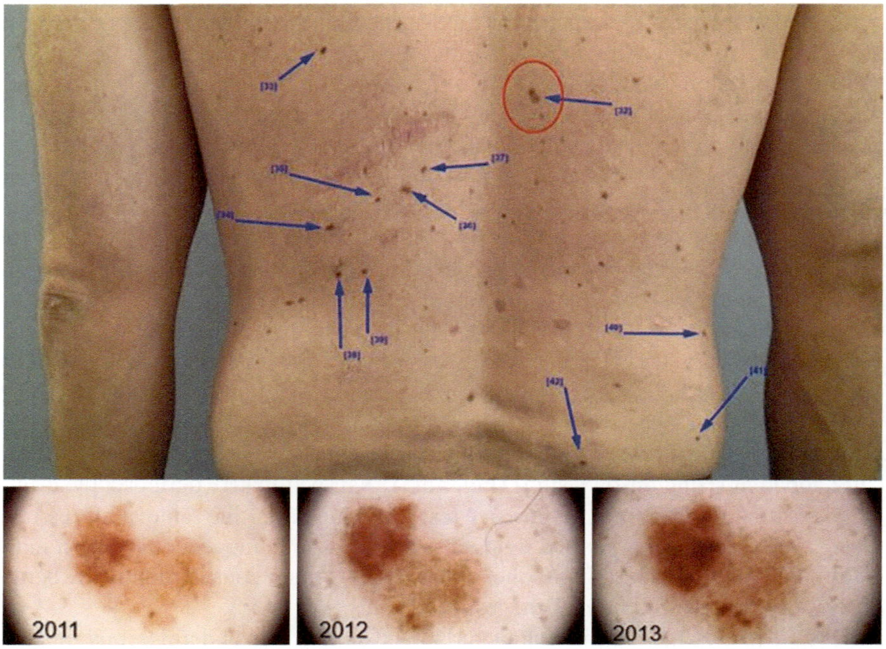

Fig. 16.14 Total body mapping. Dermoscopic follow-up allowed the diagnosis of this melanoma in situ (a slow grower) after 3 years of follow-up due to changes observed in the pigmented network. (Courtesy of Dr. Carlos Barcaui)

lesions. Depending on the follow-up period, greater are the chances of an early diagnosis of melanoma [22]. More recently, three-dimensional total body mapping equipment is being used in some centers in the USA and Australia. This equipment works with 96 simultaneous cameras that build an image of a patient's avatar with high resolution. One of the advantages of this device is the speed in obtaining images.

Confocal laser reflectance microscopy is a method in which near-histological level images are obtained from the reflection of diode laser beams (830 nm) on cell structures, which have different refractive indices. It is an in vivo, noninvasive test that allows observation of the entire surface of the lesion in horizontal sections (the same orientation as dermoscopy and different from histopathology, which is generally performed in vertical sections). Its disadvantages are the high cost of the equipment, the long learning curve, and the fact that images are viewed in grayscale. Its main applications in the diagnosis of melanoma are doubtful lesions in dermoscopy (mainly in children and patients resistant to biopsy), lesions located on the face (mainly lentigo maligna) both for diagnosis and delimitation of surgical margins, and hypo- or achromic lesions. When used by experienced physicians, its sensitivity and specificity for diagnosing melanoma are 86–100% and 72–91%, respectively [23, 24] (Fig. 16.15).

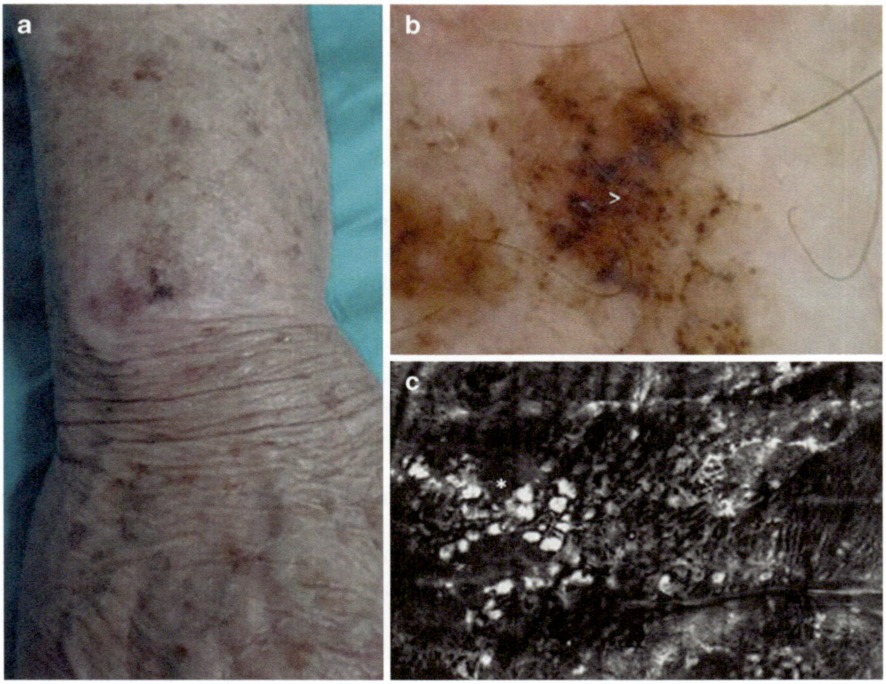

Fig. 16.15 Lentigo maligna melanoma (Clark II Breslow 0.26 mm). (**a**) Clinical—macular lesion on the forearm of a 73-year-old female patient. (**b**) Dermoscopy—global globular pattern (more frequent in childhood), note irregular dots and globules (>). (**c**) Confocal laser microscopy (Vivascope 1500) note the architectural disarrangement and cell polymorphism (*). The clearest and most irregular cells are atypical melanocytes. (Courtesy of Dr. Carlos Barcaui)

Ultrasonography is a noninvasive, nonradioactive diagnostic imaging method based on the reflection of sound waves through tissue. The recent development of high-frequency (HFUS >18 MHz) and high-resolution transducers enabled a better assessment of skin structures. In cutaneous melanocytic neoplasms, the method allows delimiting the lesion margin by the difference in refraction between the tumoral area, which is hypoechoic, and the perilesional region, which is hyperechoic. Thus, in melanoma, the HFUS is used to establish tumor thickness, margins, and vascularization. The evaluation with HFUS for the detection of melanoma metastases in regional lymph nodes has greater sensitivity and specificity when compared to clinical examination, which may be relevant due to the use of drugs for treating metastatic melanomas. On ultrasound, metastatic lymph nodes are round, with sharp edges and a hypoechoic or echolucent center (necrosis), whereas in reactional lymphadenopathies they present an elliptical aspect with a hyperechoic center and central vascularization [24].

Biopsy Techniques and Recommendations

In the presence of a suspicious lesion, an excisional biopsy should be performed with 1–3 mm margins, including the entire skin up to the subcutaneous tissue. The entire tumor must be represented, to avoid underestimating the Breslow thickness and additional risk variables. For limbs lesions, the biopsy should rather be performed vertically (along the path of the lymphatic vessels), even though this is not the direction of the tension lines of the skin, in order not to impair any future sentinel lymph node biopsy. The procedure must be performed according to oncologic principles, with particular attention not to transect the tumor during the anesthetic procedure. Primary closure or healing by second intention is preferable. Flaps or grafts should be avoided upfront (Fig. 16.16a, b). Exceptionally and in selected scenarios, an incisional biopsy can be performed in the case of extensive lesions, with a low index of suspicion or located in peculiar sites, such as the face, palmoplantar region, pinna, or genital region. It does not affect the patient's prognosis, but it can lead to an underestimation of the tumor depth and additional risk variables (Fig. 16.17).

Superficial shave biopsies are discouraged for suspected melanomas. Saucerization, or deep scalloped shaving biopsy, which can reach as far as the reticular dermis including the entire lesion, is acceptable when used in select situations according to the guidelines of the American Academy of Dermatology (AAD) and the National Comprehensive Cancer Network (NCCN). Dermoscopy-guided biopsy is helpful, particularly in cases of melanoma of the nail apparatus with involvement of the nail bed and/or matrix.

The correct specimen identification, clinical information, and proper sample handling are important for diagnosing. The specimen should be placed in a 10% buffered formalin solution. The use of unbuffered formalin may hinder future research on mutations such as BRAF, for example, which may impact on the use of systemic therapy.

It is important to highlight that a proper communication between surgeon/dermatologist and pathologist is extremely valuable and determinant in challenging cases and patients' outcome. Differential diagnoses include melanocytic nevus, atypical mole (dysplastic nevus), Spitz nevus, and cafe-au-lait spots. Dysplastic nevus (Clark nevus) is a premalignant lesion, with was described with five histological criteria: lentiginous melanocytic hyperplasia, melanocytic nuclear atypia, lamellar fibroplasia, concentric eosinophilic fibroplasia, and patchy lymphocytic infiltrates [25]. Spitz nevus is characterized by nuclear cytoplasmic ratio less than 4:1, single prominent nucleoli, inconspicuous nucleoli, corrugation of nuclear envelope, and flattening of adjacent nuclei [26].

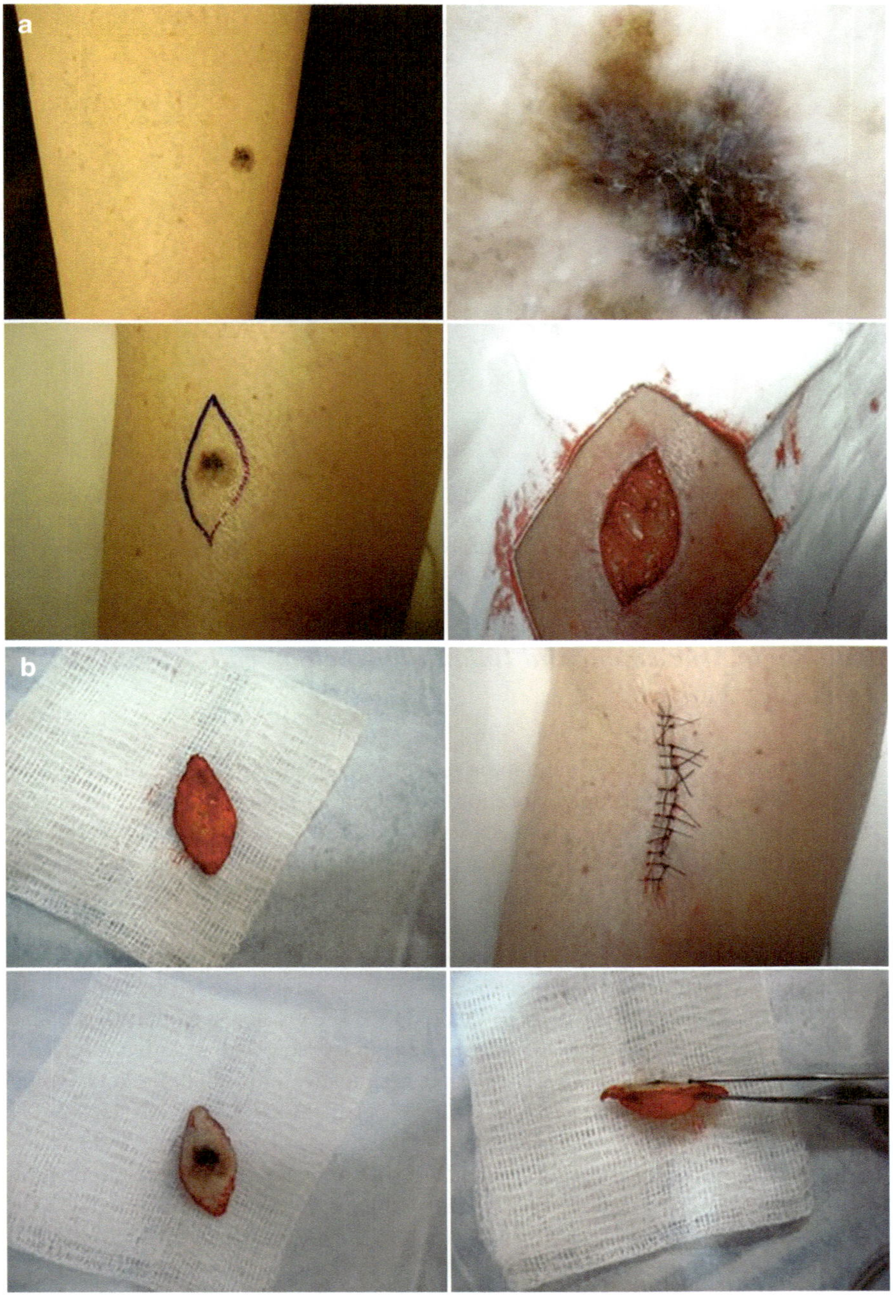

Fig. 16.16 (**a**) A suspicious pigmented lesion on the leg of a 42-year-old female patient. Excision was performed in the vertical direction in order not to prejudice future enlargement and possible sentinel lymph node research. 1–3 mm along the side margins of the fatty tissue. Courtesy of Dr. Carlos Barcaui. (**b**) The entire lesion was excised, and primary closure was performed as advisable. (Courtesy of Dr. Carlos Barcaui)

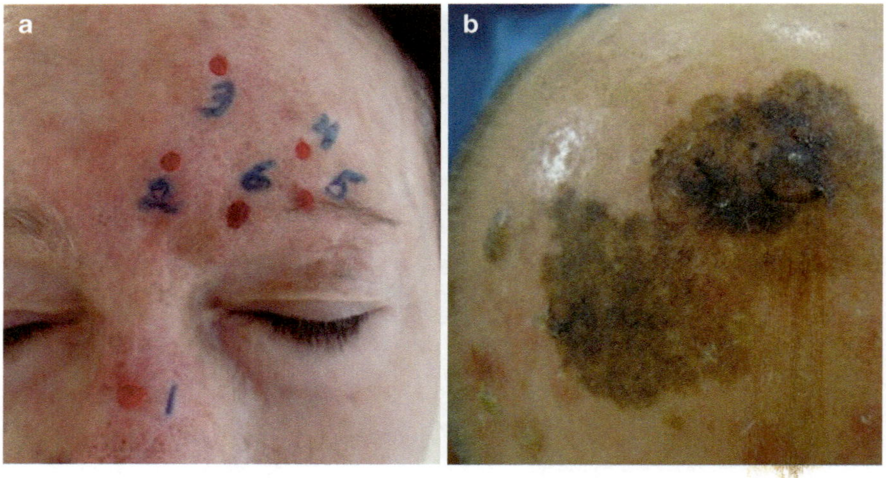

Fig. 16.17 A punch biopsy is acceptable in the case of extensive lesions located on the face. The procedure does not change the prognosis and must be guided by dermoscopy. (**a**) There is an extensive hypomelanotic malignant lentigo melanoma, occupying almost the left hemiface of the patient. (**b**) Extensive lentigo maligna melanoma on the scalp. (Courtesy of Dr. Carlos Barcaui)

Pathologic Assessment and Immunohistochemical/ Molecular Markers

The histological features of melanoma range from epithelioid to spindled cells and include different cytoplasmic morphologies, such as clear cell, rhabdoid, signet-ring shape, ballooning, and plasmacytoid appearance. Architectural patterns vary widely, including nests, trabeculae, sheets, whorls, rosettes, nodules, and papillary formations. The differential diagnoses include lymphomas, poorly differentiated carcinomas, neuroendocrine tumors, sarcomas, and germ cell tumors. Immunohistochemical staining can be used to confirm the diagnosis and to differentiate melanoma from other tumors, and established markers are S100 (sensitivity of 97–100%; however specificity is limited), HMB45 (greater specificity), melan-A (specificity of 95–100%), and vimentin (sensitivity 96%—if negative, is used to rule out melanoma) [27]. Prognostic and diagnostic molecular markers include GNAQ/GNA11, CDKN2A, BAP1, SF3B1, EIF1AX, VDR, MC1R, MITF, and HAPLN1.

In addition, molecular markers associated with potential therapeutic implications in CM include BRAF mutations, typically affecting codons V600E and V600K, NRAS, KIT, and NTRK gene fusions, which occur in less than 1% of CM [28].

The pathology report may provide the essential data elements for complete reporting of malignant tumors and ideal patient care. In the cases of melanoma in situ, the description of the tumor site, histologic type, ulceration, tumor regression, and margin status are required. Elements for reporting invasive melanoma include histologic type, maximum tumor thickness in millimeters (Breslow), macroscopic satellite nodule, ulceration, anatomic level (Clark), mitotic rate, microsatellite, lymphovascular invasion, neurotropism, tumor-infiltrating lymphocytes (TILs), regression of the tumor, and margin status for invasive and for in situ melanoma. If nodes are present in the specimen, the total number of lymph nodes with tumor, number of sentinel lymph nodes compromised by tumor, nodal site with tumor (subcapsular and/or intramedullary), size of largest nodal metastatic deposit, extranodal extension, matted nodes, total number of lymph nodes examined (sentinel and non-sentinel), and the number of sentinel nodes examined must be reported. The presence of distant metastasis and additional findings should be reported if applicable [29].

Risk Stratification and Staging

The prognosis for patients with CM is influenced by variables that include the tumor thickness (Breslow index), presence of ulceration, mitotic rate, presence of lymphovascular or perineural invasion, neurotropism, density and distribution of tumor-infiltrating lymphocytes (TILs), regression, melanoma subtype (e.g., desmoplastic melanoma is less frequently associated with nodal metastasis and has a more favorable prognosis, as well as patient characteristics such as age, gender, and anatomical site of the tumor), presence of regional disease (nodal involvement, satellitosis/microsatellitosis, or in-transit metastases), and presence of distant metastases. Advanced age is a poor prognostic factor, and it is known that elderly patients tend to have more advanced tumors, with a higher mitotic rate, lesions that are more commonly ulcerated, and a higher incidence of primary in the head and neck. CM developing in females is potentially marked by more favorable outcomes, although this observation remains controversial, and may be explained not only by biological aspects but also factors such as diagnosis at earlier stages and higher compliance with skin examinations. In non-metastatic patients, nodal involvement and superior anatomical location (compared to the lower extremity) lead to worse clinical outcome. The presence of discontinuous, non-nodal melanoma deposits, defined as satellites, microsatellites, or in-transit metastases, is also of poor prognostic value. The site of metastasis has an important correlation with survival: patients with metastasis in the skin, subcutaneous tissue, and lymph nodes have a better evolution, with a progressively worse prognosis for those with pulmonary, non-pulmonary visceral, and central nervous system (CNS) involvement, respectively.

The most commonly used CM staging tool is based upon the description of T (tumor) N (nodal) M (metastasis) categories, according to eighth Edition of the American Joint Committee on Cancer staging system (Table 16.2) [30].

The indication for additional evaluation, including imaging evaluation, for clinical staging purposes varies according to variables of the primary tumor, findings on physical examination, and symptoms described by the patient, which should be always appropriately investigated. There are no prospective studies that defined a

Table 16.2 AJCC eighth Ed TNM classification and staging groups—melanoma

T[a]	N	M
T1—≤1.0 mm a—Non-ulcerated and <0.8 mm b—<0.8 ulcerated or 0.8–1.0 mm	**N0—No signs of LN involvement or S/MS/ITM**	**M0—No signs of distant metastases**
T2—>1.0–2.0 mm a—Non-ulcerated b—Ulcerated	**N1—1 positive LN or presence of S/MS/ITM and negative LN** a—Sentinel b—Clinical c—S/MS/MT com LN negative	**M1—Presence of distant metastases** a—Skin/SC/LN/soft parts b—Lungs c—Extrapulmonary visceral sites d—CNS 0—Normal LDH 1—Elevated LDH
T3—>2.0–4.0 mm a—Non-ulcerated b—Ulcerated	**N2–2–3 positive LN or 1 positive LN and S/MS/ITM** a—Sentinel b—Clinical c—S/MS/IM and positive LN	
T4—> 4.0 mm a—Non-ulcerated b—Ulcerated	**N3—4 or more positive LN or 2 LN or more and S/MS/ITM** a—Sentinel b—Clinical c—S/MS/ITM and positive LN	

Staging group	T	N	M
0	Tis	N0	M0
IA	T1a	N0	M0
IB	T1b	N0	M0
	T2a	N0	M0
IIA	T2b	N0	M0
	T3a	N0	M0
IIB	T3b	N0	M0
	T4a	N0	M0
IIC	T4b	N0	M0
IIIA	T1a–T2a	N1a or N2a	M0
IIIB	T0	N1b or N1c	M0
	T1a–T2a	N1b–N2b	M0
	T2b–T3a	N1a–N2b	M0
IIIC	T0	N2b/N2c/N3b/N3c	M0
	T1a–T3a	N2c/N3	M0
	T3b–T4a	N1–N3	M0
	T4b	N1a–N2c	M0
IIID	T4b	N3	M0
IV	Any	Any	M1

[a] *Tx* primary non-evaluable, *T0* no evidence of primary tumor, *Tis* melanoma in situ, *LN* lymph node, *S* satellitosis, *MS* microsatellitosis, *ITM* in-transit metastases, *SC* subcutaneous, *CNS* central nervous system

Table 16.3 Imaging recommended for clinical stages

Clinical stage	Exams indicated for staging
In situ, clinical stages I, IIA	Routine imaging tests are not recommended
Clinical stage IIIA	Consider thoracic and abdomen CT (include neck CT in primary head and neck tumors) PET-TC is not routinely recommended
Clinical stages IIB, IIC, IIIB, IIIC, and IIID	Thoracic and abdomen CT (include neck CT in primary head and neck tumors) Consider PET/CT if "bulky" or multifocal nodal involvement Consider central nervous system RM
Clinical stage IV	Thoracic and abdomen CT (include neck CT in primary head and neck tumors) Consider PET/CT in oligometastatic patients who are candidates for surgical resection Central nervous system RM Laboratory tests including lactic dehydrogenase (DHL)

pattern of evaluations for staging and stating strategies may vary. The choice of imaging test for diagnosing and follow-up depends on the risk of systemic disease and may include ultrasonographic evaluations, computed topographies (CT), magnetic resonance imaging (MRI), or more advanced techniques [31, 32]. For any clinical stage, physical examination, with a detailed evaluation of the skin for suspicious lesions and regional nodal basins, is mandatory. In low-risk melanomas (e.g., melanoma in situ, stage I), no additional investigations are required. Current indications are summarized in Table 16.3. The role of positron emission tomography (PET/CT) in melanoma is not universal; however, a PET/CT should be considered especially for patients at very high-risk regional disease (bulky or multifocal nodal involvement) or in the setting of oligometastatic disease [33]. A central nervous system (CNS) MRI may be considered in CS III and is mandatory in CS IV due to high risk of CNS involvement. Serum lactic dehydrogenase (DHL) values play an independent prognostic role and should be incorporated for those with stage IV disease.

If regional or distant metastatic disease is suspected, a confirmatory biopsy should be pursued, if not contraindicated.

Treatment of Localized Disease

In the absence of nodal or distant metastases, surgery is the main treatment for CM. Patients should undergo wide local excision (WLE) associated with sentinel node biopsy (SNB) when indicated.

Table 16.4 Surgical margins—localized disease

Breslow thickness	Local surgical excision margins
In situ	0.5 cm
<1.0 mm	1.0 cm
1–2.0 mm	1–2 cm
>2.0 mm	2 cm

Surgical margins for WLE should be performed according to Breslow thickness (Table 16.4). Reconstruction following WLE may be challenging according to the extension of the resection as well as the primary site, with particularly challenging scenarios represented by melanomas arising in the head and neck and the extremities. The involvement of surgeons trained in reconstructive surgery in oncologic patients may lead to better aesthetic and functional outcomes [34].

Sentinel node biopsy (SNB) currently represents a staging tool for CM and should be offered for T2a patients and above (Breslow thickness >1.0 mm) without evidence of clinical nodal disease. For T1b patients (Breslow 0.8–1.0 mm or Breslow <1.0 mm with ulceration), the current recommendation is to discuss with patients about pros and cons of the procedure. SNB technique for CM is well established since 1992 and comprises the identification of sentinel nodes with preoperative lymphoscintigraphy, followed by surgical removal and pathologic assessment of excised nodes [35].

If SNB is negative (no signs of melanoma in the sentinel node), no additional surgical procedures are indicated [36]. For patients with a positive SNB, which defines a locoregional disease, further management must be discussed. The results of two large, multicenter, prospective studies suggest that there is no additional survival benefit from complete lymph node dissection (CLND) in these patients undergoing adequate surveillance, and surgery can be considered in case of nodal relapse [37–39]. Nevertheless, in certain scenarios, especially if appropriate imaging follow-up is not available, CLND can still be considered [40].

Systemic therapies following initial surgical approach with curative intent, or adjuvant treatments, are currently approved for patients with nodal involvement and/or non-nodal regional disease (satellitosis/microsatellitosis/in-transit metastases) and can also be considered for individuals with oligometastatic disease undergoing complete surgical resection. More recently, a randomized studies also demonstrated a significant improvement in recurrence-free survival and distant-metastases free survival with immunotherapy for patients with high-risk, stage II disease—these results, however, have not been fully incorporated into clinical practice yet, mainly due to the lack of an improvement in overall survival and concerns about potential toxicities [41].

Despite the decades of controversies, interferon (either conventional or in its pegylated form) no longer corresponds to a standard adjuvant treatment for melanoma patients, as different pivotal trials confirmed the benefits in terms of RFS resulting from either single-agent anti-PD-1 monoclonal antibodies—nivolumab or pembrolizumab—or dabrafenib/trametinib for those harboring a BRAF V600E or V600K mutation [42].

The first study to confirm the success in the adjuvant setting of therapies initially approved for those with advanced disease was the EORTC 18071 study [43]. In this phase III randomized trial, patients with stage IIIA–C disease according to the seventh Edition of the AJCC staging system, and at least 1 mm of melanoma in the lymph node if stage IIIA, were randomized to ipilimumab for up to 3 years versus placebo. The study's primary endpoint demonstrated a significant reduction in the risk of relapse with ipilimumab. Nevertheless, the incorporation of ipilimumab in the adjuvant setting was limited due to safety concerns and promising results with anti-PD-1 agents and BRAF/MEK inhibitors. It is important to highlight, however, that this was the sole randomized trial to demonstrate a significant overall survival benefit among contemporary practice-changing studies—in a recent update, ipilimumab was associated an absolute overall survival (OS) improvement of 8.7% at 7 years, when compared to placebo (HR 0.73; $p = 0.002$) [44]. Four subsequent randomized trials defined nivolumab, pembrolizumab, or dabrafenib/trametinib as the current standard of care options for the adjuvant treatment of patients with locoregional melanoma. In the ChekMate-238 study, patients with stage IIIB/C or oligometastatic stage IV disease (according to the seventh Edition of the AJCC staging system) were randomized to nivolumab or ipilimumab for up to 12 months [45]. The efficacy of adjuvant pembrolizumab was investigated in KEYNOTE-054 [46] and Intergoup/SWOG 1404 [47] phase III studies, having placebo or high-dose interferon/ipilimumab as comparator arms, respectively. For patients with BRAF V600E or V600K-mutant melanoma, the combination of dabrafenib and trametinib for up to 12 months was compared to placebo in the COMBI-AD study [48]. Across all four randomized trials, the experimental arms containing nivolumab or pembrolizumab, or dabrafenib/trametinib, resulted in statistically significant improvements in RFS, leading to regulatory approvals worldwide and a rapid incorporation into clinical practice. However, mature OS data are still pending.

Therefore, 1 year of adjuvant nivolumab or pembrolizumab should be considered for patients with stage III (and selected stage IV) melanoma following complete surgical resection; for those diagnosed with a BRAF-mutant melanoma, 1 year of dabrafenib/trametinib can also be regarded as a standard treatment option, with an apparent similar impact in terms of RFS, albeit with a distinct toxicity profile (Fig. 16.5). As of today, there are no randomized trials directly comparing immunotherapy and targeted therapy in the adjuvant setting, and a balanced and shared decision should be pursued following a careful discussion encompassing potential adverse events, contraindications, drug interactions, and patients' expectations [49]. Of note, the preclusion of a CLND following a positive SLB should not affect decisions regarding adjuvant systemic therapies. Also, despite the lack of definitive studies addressing the optimal approach for patients with clinical non-nodal regional disease (satellitosis/in-transit metastases), upfront surgery followed by adjuvant treatment remains the main treatment in those scenarios and justified by the high risk of relapse associated with these presentations. For patients who are not suitable for surgery, topical treatments (e.g., imiquimod, diphencyprone) and intralesional therapies should also be considered, according to clinical status and possibility of access.

For patients with clinical nodal disease, either at initial presentation or during follow-up, lymphadenectomy is still the standard of care. However, mounting data and proof-of-concept studies provided preliminary evidence to support a potential transition toward neoadjuvant approaches for those with clinical/macroscopic nodal

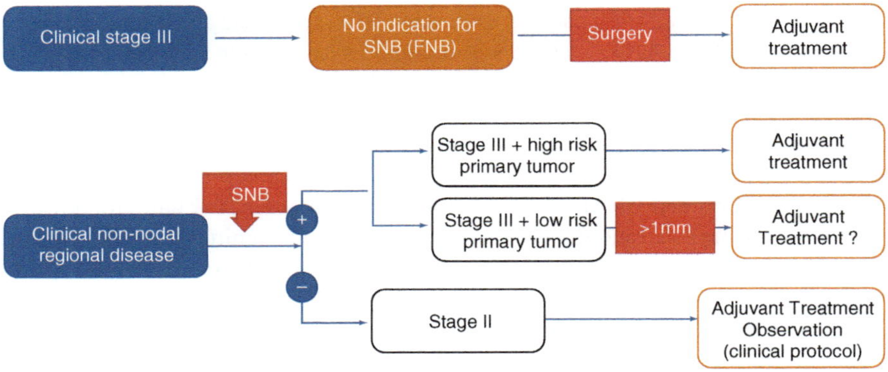

Fig. 16.18 Treatment algorithms for patients with locoregional melanoma. *SNB* sentinel node biopsy, *FNB* fine needle biopsy. (Courtesy of Dr. Rodrigo Ramella Munhoz)

involvement of non-nodal regional disease in the near future. Across different studies investigating immunotherapy (particularly the combination of ipilimumab and nivolumab) or targeted therapy, neoadjuvant treatments resulted in remarkably high pathologic complete response rates and promising RFS curves [49]. Nevertheless, definitive, randomized studies establishing the optimal neoadjuvant regimen are still warranted, despite the optimistic projections for the near future.

Although individuals with high-risk stage II melanoma (stage IIB/IIC) have outcomes similar to patients with stage IIIA or event stage IIIB disease based on the eighth Edition of the AJCC staging system, these patients were excluded from the previously discussed clinical trials and, currently, are not candidates for adjuvant anti-PD-1 or BRAF/MEK inhibitors. Nevertheless, randomized trials comparing either nivolumab or pembrolizumab are currently ongoing (NCT04309409, NCT03405155, NCT03553836), some of which already incorporating gene-expression panels as tools for optimized patient selection. In a recent presentation, pembrolizumab resulted in a statistically significant improvement in RFS for patients with stage IIB/IIC melanoma when compared to placebo, but mature results are still pending [41]. Naturally, long-term follow-up of these studies is eagerly awaited, and a careful consideration of potential risks and chronic adverse events will be critical when considering the extension of the indication of adjuvant treatments for patients with stage II disease. Figure 16.18 summarizes the suggested treatment algorithm for localized disease.

Treatment of Advanced Melanoma

Despite the high curability that can be achieved in patients presenting with localized disease, with early diagnosis resulting in 5-year survival rates above 90%, melanoma is generally perceived as an aggressive neoplasm and associated with significant risks of relapse and metastases. For those not amenable to treatment with curative intent, paradigm-changing advances have been accomplished and translated into clinical practice over the last decade, resulting in a significant transformation in the prognosis of patients with advanced disease, for whom historically, survival rates at 5 years rarely exceeded 10–15% [50].

Even though surgery (metastasectomy) and radiotherapy should be considered among the available options for the management of advanced disease in select situations, systemic therapy is the main treatment for most patients. Traditional cytotoxic chemotherapies, considered customary indications for patients with advanced melanoma for decades and incorporated as control arm in distinct clinical trials, include dacarbazine, vinblastine, cisplatin/carboplatin, and taxanes, either used in combination or in monotherapy. In addition to response rates that range from 10 to 25% and usually present short-lived benefits, these agents resulted in an arguable, if existent, impact on survival and often limiting toxicities. Nonselective forms of immunotherapy, including high-dose interleukin-2 (IL-2) or biochemotherapy, had their widespread use hampered by the complexity of this treatment and need for highly specialized centers, unfavorable safety profile, and objective (albeit durable and potentially curative) responses limited to a small proportion of individuals. The incorporation of both immune-checkpoint blockers against CTLA-4 and PD-1 and targeted therapy aiming at BRAF mutations yielded significant improvements in response and survival and now correspond to the standard of care, with 34% to more than 50% of the patients diagnosed with advanced melanoma alive at 5 years [50].

Activating mutations of the BRAF gene, which are found in approximately 40–60% of patients with metastatic melanoma, result in constitutive activation of the growth-promoting MAPK pathway [51]. Targeting the aberrantly activated MAPK pathway was confirmed as an efficacious approach for the treatment of advanced disease. Initially approved for clinical use in monotherapy, the selective BRAF inhibitors vemurafenib and dabrafenib resulted in response rates of approximately 50% in the BRM-3 and BEAK-3 randomized studies, with significant improvements in PFS and/or OS when compared to standard cytotoxic chemotherapy regimens [52, 53]. Nevertheless, secondary resistance to single-agent BRAF inhibitors was almost universal, and the possibility of prolonged disease control remained limited; in this setting combined BRAF/MEK inhibition emerged as an efficacious alternative to enhance the benefits from MAPK pathway inhibition [54]. Indeed, the superiority of combined approaches in comparison to single-agent BRAF inhibition has been confirmed in at least four pivotal, randomized trials. The combination of dabrafenib plus trametinib was compared to single-agent dabrafenib or vemurafenib in the COMBI-d and COMBI-v trials, respectively [55, 56]. Both studies have consistently shown increased response rates, with objective responses occurring in 68% of the cases (including 19% of complete responses), and gains in PFS and OS favoring the use of the combination, resulting in 5-year survival rate of 34% [57]. In the coBRIM trial, the combination of vemurafenib and cobimetinib was compared to single-agent vemurafenib in BRAF-mutant melanoma patients. Combined blockade resulted in prolonged PFS and OS (median PFS 12.3 vs 7.2 months; $p < 0.0001$/median OS 22.3 vs 17.4 months, HR 0.70; 95% CI 0.55–0.90;

$p = 0.005$) and a higher objective response rate (70% vs 50%) [56]. More recently, a third combination of BRAF/MEK inhibitors, encorafenib and binimetinib, also demonstrated superior outcomes in comparison to single-agent vemurafenib, with a median OS of more than 33 months [58]. Of note, the most frequent toxicities associated with combined BRAF/MEK inhibition may vary according to the regimen or combination. As an example, photosensitivity and rash tend to occur more frequently with vemurafenib/cobimetinib, whereas pyrexia is a typical adverse event associated with dabrafenib/trametinib.

Additional driver mutations can be relevant in the setting of advanced disease, including KIT mutations and NRAS mutations [51]. Nevertheless, the clinical outcomes and success of targeting these mutations have been limited. As an example, mutations affecting the NRAS gene, an upstream effector of the MAP and PI3K pathways, occur in approximately 20% of the cases. Despite the strong rationale, only a modest improvement in PFS was demonstrated in a randomized study that compared binimetinib to dacarbazine in patients with NRAS-mutant melanoma (median PFS 2.8 vs 1.5 months; HR 0.62; 95%; $p < 0.001$), with no significant difference in OS [59]. Similarly, the use of imatinib for patients with c-KIT mutations, enriched in acral and mucosal melanomas, was demonstrated in rapid, although usually transient, responses [60, 61].

In addition to targeted therapy, the use of immunotherapy in the form of monoclonal antibodies targeting immune coreceptors associated with the modulation of immune synapse, or checkpoints, is regarded as one of the major breakthroughs in oncology in recent years, resulting in the possibility of sustained responses and prolonged survival. In 2011, the first agent of this class was approved for the treatment of advanced melanoma. Ipilimumab, an anti-CTLA-4 monoclonal antibody, resulted in survival gains in both first- and second-line settings, with response rates of 10–15% and approximately 21% of the patients alive beyond 3 years [62, 63]. Despite the practice-changing impact of CTLA-4 blockade, even more persuasive results developed from the anti-PD1 agents pembrolizumab and nivolumab, leading to multiple regulatory approvals since 2014. In phase I studies, pembrolizumab and nivolumab resulted in ORR of approximately 30%, with median OS of 16–23 months [64, 65]. Subsequent randomized studies confirmed the efficacy of these anti-PD-1 agents, initially after progression on ipilimumab and/or BRAF inhibitors. In KEYNOTE 002, a randomized phase II trial, patients with ipilimumab-refractory disease were randomly assigned to two regimens of pembrolizumab or chemotherapy. Pembrolizumab resulted in statistically significant improvement in the 6-month progression-free rate, the primary endpoint of the study, as well as in ORR [66]. Similarly, nivolumab superiority over investigator's choice of chemotherapy following failure to ipilimumab was demonstrated in the CheckMate 037 study, with objective responses occurring in 31.7% of the patients treated with nivolumab vs 10.6% with chemotherapy, in addition to a more favorable toxicity profile [67]. In immunotherapy-naïve patients and also in the first-line setting, both pembrolizumab and nivolumab showed superiority in terms of efficacy and tolerability when compared to ipilimumab. In the phase III KEYNOTE-006 study, pembrolizumab demonstrated a significant improvement in ORR, PFS, and OS in comparison to ipilimumab, with a 2-year survival rate for pembrolizumab of 55% vs 43% (HR 0.68; $p = 0.0008$) [68]. Nivolumab also resulted in superior outcomes when compared to chemotherapy in treatment-naïve, BRAF wild-type patients in the CheckMate 066 study, with a 5-year OS rate of 39% with nivolumab versus 17% with dacarbazine [69].

More recently, the combination of ipilimumab and nivolumab was also incorporated into clinical practice. In the pivotal CheckMate 067 study, which comprised three treatment arms (ipilimumab and nivolumab, single-agent nivolumab, and single-agent ipilimumab), both nivolumab-containing regimens resulted in improvement in OS, PFS, and ORR versus ipilimumab [70]. In a recent update, 49% of the patients treated with the combination and 42% of those who received single-agent nivolumab were alive at 6.5 years [71]. Despite the higher ORR and prolonged PFS in the exploratory direct comparison of ipilimumab and nivolumab versus single-agent nivolumab, there was no statistically significant improvement in OS; it is also important to note that combined CLTA-4 and PD-1 blockade was associated with a significant and clinically relevant increase in the risk of immune-related adverse events. The subsequent CheckMate 511 randomized trial suggested a more favorable toxicity profile with an alternative regimen with a reduced dose of ipilimumab, with comparable outcomes [72].

Contemporary studies also confirmed the activity of ipilimumab/nivolumab and dabrafenib/trametinib in individuals with central nervous system (CNS) metastases, with intracranial response rates exceeding 50% and the possibility of prolonged disease control in selected patients [73–75]. Nevertheless, CNS involvement defines a challenging subgroup of patients, for whom the therapeutic approach must be tailored in a multidisciplinary form, contemplating variables that include the number, size, and anatomical location of CNS lesions, symptoms, use of steroids, and possibility of local approaches (surgery, stereotactic body radiation therapy, etc.).

Additional treatment options have also been investigated in prospective studies, however with less meaningful results and limited incorporations. As an example, the triplet combination of vemurafenib/cobimetinib/atezolizumab (an anti-PD-L1 agent) resulted in modest PFS gains and increased toxicity when compared to vemurafenib/cobimetinib, with no improvement in ORR or OS [76]. Also, preliminary results of a randomized study comparing a novel combination of nivolumab and relatlimab, an anti-*lymphocyte-activation gene 3* (LAG-3) monoclonal antibody, suggesting a PFS improvement have been recently presented, but mature data are awaited [77]. Another promising approach already approved for clinical use yet with limited applicability is the intralesional oncolytic attenuated herpesvirus talimogene laherparepvec (T-VEC). In a phase III trial with patients with stage IIIB–IV melanoma amenable to direct tumor injection, T-VEC produced an improved durable response rate compared to intratumoral GM-CSF alone (16.3% vs 2.1%; odds ratio 8.9; $p < 0.001$) [78].

In summary, remarkable advances in the past 10 years with both immunotherapy and molecular-driven approaches have significantly prolonged the life expectancy and improved the quality of life of patients with advanced melanoma (Table 16.5). According to contemporary algorithms, first-line treatment options encompass the

Table 16.5 Summary of pivotal clinical trials and contemporary treatment options for patients with advanced melanoma

Study	Author/year	Phase	*N*	Intervention	ORR (%)	mPFS (months)	Survival data
Immune-checkpoint blockade							
KEYNOTE 001	Ribas (2016)	1	655	Pembrolizumab	33	5.2	mOS 23 months
KEYNOTE 002	Ribas (2015)	3	540	Pembrolizumab 2 mg/kg × pembrolizumab 10 mg/kg vs CT	38 × 46 × 8	4.2 × 5.6 × 2.6	NR
KEYNOTE 006	Robert (2015)	3	834	Pembrolizumab q 14 days × pembrolizumab q 21 days × ipilimumab	33.7 × 32.9 × 11.9	5.5 × 4.1 × 2.8	2 years OS 55% × 55% × 43%
–	Topalian (2014)	1	107	Nivolumab	31	3.7	mOS 16.8 months
CheckMate 037	Weber (2015)	3	405	Nivolumab versus CT	32 × 5	4.7 × 4.2	NR
CheckMate 066	Robert (2015)	3	418	Nivolumab vs dacarbazine	40 × 13.9	5.1 × 2.2	NR × 10.8 months
CheckMate 069	Postow (2015)	2	142	Ipilimumab/nivolumab vs ipilimumab	61 × 11	NR × 4.4	NR
CheckMate 067	Larkin (2015)	3	945	Ipilimumab/nivolumab vs nivolumab vs ipilimumab	57.6 × 43.7 × 19	11.5 × 6.9 × 2.9	NR
CheckMate 511	Lebbe (2019)	3b/4	360	Ipilimumabe1/nivolumabe3 vs ipilimumabe3/ nivolumabe1	45.6 × 50.6	9.9 × 8.9	NR
Relativity-047	Lipson (2021)	3	714	Relatlimab/nivolumab vs nivolumab	NA	10.1 × 4.6	NA

MAPK pathway blockade							
coBRIM	Ascierto (2016)	3	495	Vemurafenib + cobimetinib × vemurafenib	70 × 50	12.3 × 7.2	mOS 22.3 months × 17.4 months
COMBI-v	Robert (2015)	3	704	Dabrafenib + trametinib vs vemurafenib	64 × 51	11.4 × 7.3	mOS 25.6 months × 18.3 months
COMBI-d	Long (2015)	3	423	Dabrafenib + trametinib vs dabrafenib	69 × 53	11.0 × 8.8	mOS 25.1 months × 18.7 months
COLUMBUS	Dummer (2018)	3	577	Encorafenib + binimetinib vs encorafenib or vemurafenib	64 × 52 × 41	14.9 × 9.6 × 7.3	33.6 × 23.5 × 16.9
TRILOGY IMspire150	Gutzmer (2020)	3	514	Vemurafenib + cobimetinib + atezolizumab vs vemurafenib + cobimetinib	66.3 × 65	15.1 × 10.6	NR
Other							
OPTiM	Andtbacka (2019)	3	436	T-VEC vs GM-CSF	31.5 × 6.4	NE	23.3 × 18.9

NA not available, *T-VEC* intratumoral talimogene laherparepvec, *GM-CSF* granulocyte-macrophage colony-stimulating factor, *NE* not evaluable anti-BRAF/MEK combinations vemurafenib/cobimetinib, dabrafenib/trametinib, and encorafenib/binimetinib for BRAF-mutant melanoma patients, with preliminary evidence also suggesting a potential role for the triplet combination of vemurafenib/cobimetinib/atezolizumab. Also, immunotherapies with nivolumab, pembrolizumab, ipilimumab/nivolumab, single-agent ipilimumab, or T-VEC are also standard treatment options for both BRAF-mutant and BRAF "wild-type" melanoma patients. Importantly, the optimal first-line treatment for patients with advanced melanoma harboring a BRAF mutation remains to be determined, and treatment decision relies on variables that include potential contraindications, comorbidities, toxicity profiles of distinct options, presence of symptoms, disease volume, etc.; in this setting, mature results and results of ongoing studies looking at the best sequencing and potential combinations of BRAF/MEK inhibition and immune-checkpoint blockade are necessary. Also, the incorporation of predictive and prognostic biomarkers remains of utmost importance to allow for a better patient selection in a setting of escalating costs associated with cancer care and often limiting toxicities, and a better characterization of resistance mechanisms to either immunotherapy or targeted therapy is also mandatory for a rational development of future treatment strategies and compounds.

Follow-Up and Surveillance

The optimal follow-up strategy for patients with melanoma remains debatable and is influenced by clinicopathologic risk factors, clinical staging, and initial treatment. The primary objective is to identify potentially curable recurrence, second-primary skin cancer, and diagnosis of a metastatic disease with a low tumor burden. Patients should be carefully educated regarding self-assessment measures and behavioral strategies, including the use of approaches aiming at reducing exposure to UV radiation [79].

Regardless of stage and additional risk factors, patients diagnosed with melanoma should undergo a careful dermatologic surveillance. Current recommendations suggest a dermatologic physical examination (including dermatoscopy) every 6 months in the first 5 years and then annually, or more frequently, if clinically indicated. Ancillary techniques, including digital dermoscopy and total body mapping, can also be considered. The risk of a second-primary cutaneous malignancy should be contemplated [79, 80].

For patients with low-risk disease (melanoma in situ, stages I–IIA), there is no clear role for follow-up imaging on follow-up, and a careful physical and dermatologic examination is indicated. For those presenting with high-risk stage II or locoregional disease, a higher risk for recurrence justifies the consideration for additional imaging techniques that typically include ultrasonography or computed tomography or magnetic resonance imaging, performed every 3–6 months during the initial years and then less frequently; of note, PET/CT should not be routinely indicated for these patients as a follow-up strategy. It is important to highlight that patients with a positive SLDB not undergoing a CLND should be carefully monitored for local and nodal recurrences, particularly with ultrasonography of the regional nodal basin. Patients at a higher risk for recurrence (high-risk stage III or resected stage IV) should be followed closely, with more frequent imaging and clinical assessment [79, 80].

Box 16.1 General Considerations—Mucosal Melanoma

Epidemiology

Primary mucosal melanomas represent approximately 1.4% of all melanomas and arise from melanocytes located in mucosal membranes lining respiratory, gastrointestinal, and urogenital tract. The incidence is higher in females, due to the numbers of cases found in the female genital tract, and increases with age. There is no association between mucosal melanomas and nevus count or familial predisposition to melanomas [28, 81–84].

Etiopathogenesis

Unlike the cutaneous melanomas, mucosal melanomas have no apparent association with ultraviolet (UV) radiation exposure. Trauma has been suggested as a possible cause [83, 84]. Because of their rareness, no modifiable risk factor has yet been identified, and there are no well-established protocols for staging and treatment of mucosal melanomas [31, 81–84].

Clinical Presentation

Clinical presentation depends on the location of advanced tumors, although some patients already have distant metastatic disease [31]. In the head and neck region, it usually presents recurrent epistaxis, nasal obstruction, loss of smell, proptosis, limited ocular movement, and headaches [85]. Vulvovaginal mucosal melanomas present with pruritus, vaginal bleeding or discharge, dyspareunia, or a mass, and anorectal mucosal melanoma generally presents with bleeding, pain, a mass, tenesmus, or change in bowel habit [82].

Histopathology

The mucosal lentiginous and nodular patterns are the most common, with epithelioid and/or spindled melanocytes with variable pigmentation, ovoid nuclei, and prominent nucleoli. The epidermis usually presents a lentiginous growth with single cells and small nests. Ulceration and vascular invasion can be found in advanced lesions. The tumor cells usually express melan-A (MART1), HMB45 antigen, SOX10, and MITF [83, 84].

Treatment

Due to the difficulties with diagnosis, the anatomical location, and the infrequency, there have been no large randomized controlled trials to evaluate for the best treatment approach. Mucosal melanoma is a disease with a very poor prognosis, and most patients will develop incurable metastatic disease, irrespective of surgical excision. The 5-year survival rate is 25%. Mutations involving KIT and NRAS are frequent, and mutations in the BRAF gene occur in less than 5% of the cases [82–84].

For patients with localized disease, complete surgical resection of mucosal melanoma with negative pathological margins should be pursued, and adjuvant radiation therapy or systemic agents should be discussed, despite the lack of definitive data. Systemic treatment is indicated for unresectable or metastatic disease and may include immunotherapy, particularly with combined regimens (e.g., ipilimumab and nivolumab), targeted therapy, and chemotherapy.

Box 16.2 General Considerations—Uveal Melanoma

Epidemiology

Uveal melanoma (UM) is the most common primary intraocular malignant tumor in adults and arises from melanocytes located in the iris, ciliary body, or choroid, representing 3–5% of all melanomas. The median age of diagnosis is approximately 62 years. There is no sex predilection [85–87].

Risk Factors

The risk factors include fair skin, light eye color, inability to tan, ocular or oculodermal melanocytosis, age, gender, choroidal nevi, and germline *BAP1* mutations [86–88].

Clinical Presentation

Choroidal melanoma can present as dome-shaped or mushroom-like mass, retinal detachment, vitreous hemorrhage, and macular edema. Ciliary body melanoma can exhibit as nodular mass with extraocular extension, shallowing of the anterior chamber, lens changes, and decreased or increased intraocular pressure. Visual symptoms resulting from tumor growth or local complications correspond to the most frequent clinical presentation [86, 89–91].

Diagnosis

UM can be diagnosed through funduscopic examination by an experienced clinician, by using ultrasonography, fluorescein angiography, indocyanine green angiography, and enhanced depth imaging optical coherence tomography. Although a biopsy is not mandatory, a fine-needle aspiration biopsy can be considered [87–89].

Histopathology

UM may have spindle cells and/or epithelioid cells, prominent nucleoli and intranuclear pseudoinclusions, mitotic figures, necrotic foci, scattered lymphocytic infiltrates, and pigment-laden macrophages. Tumor cells variably express melanocytic markers and may show nuclear BAP1 protein loss [85, 90] (Fig. 16.19a–d).

Treatment

For patients with localized disease, options include resection, radiotherapy, enucleation, or orbital exenteration [87, 89]. Prognostic factors for a worse outcome included tumor size, location, diffuse growth pattern, extraocular extension, histologic features such as cell type, increased mitotic activity, tumor-infiltrating macrophages and lymphocytes, expression of human leukocyte antigen and insulin-like growth factor receptor-1, types of extravascular matrix patterns, loss of nuclear BAP1 expression, metastasis, and recurrence. Furthermore, cytogenetic abnormalities are prognostic and include chromosome 3 loss and chromosome 8q gain, lack of chromosome 6p gain, the class 2 gene expression profile, and BAP1 mutation [85, 90, 91]. Common sites of metastases include the liver (89%), lungs (29%), and bones (17%) [91]. Advanced UM remains a challenging disease, as BRAF mutations are absent and immune-checkpoint blockade results in low response rates. More recently, tebentafusp, a bi-specific T-cell-engaging protein, was the first agent to result in a survival improvement in advanced UM.

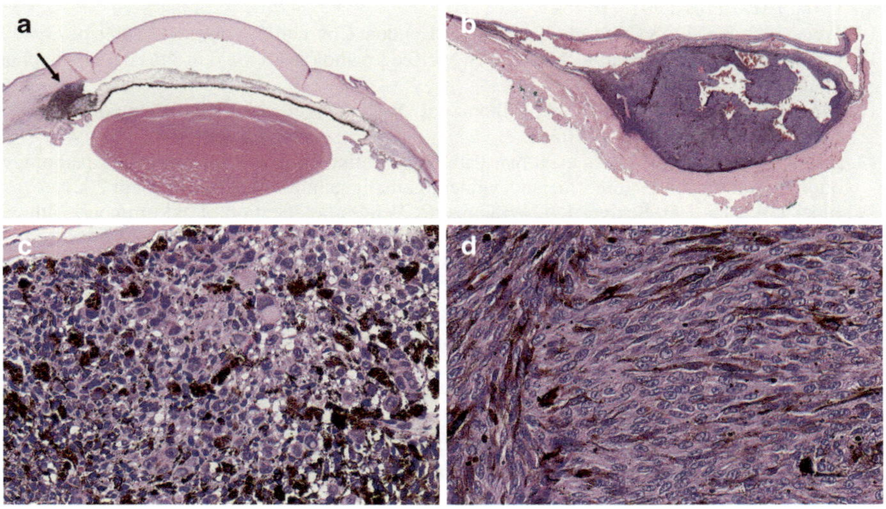

Fig. 16.19 (**a**) Histopathology of ciliary body melanoma (arrow) (hematoxylin and eosin). Iris melanoma, 11.2 ×. Courtesy of Dr. Melissa Fugimori Lissae. (**b**) Histopathology of choroidal melanoma (hematoxylin and eosin). Choroidal melanoma, 14.5 ×. Courtesy of Dr. Melissa Fugimori Lissae. (**c**) Histopathology of uveal melanoma. Epithelioid cells, 400 ×. High magnification showing epithelioid cell type, pigmented, with large polygonal cells, atypical nuclei, prominent nucleoli, and sometimes intranuclear pseudoinclusions (hematoxylin and eosin). Courtesy of Dr. Melissa Fugimori Lissae. (**d**) Histopathology of uveal melanoma. Spindle cells, 400 ×. High magnification showing spindle cell type, pigmented, with large oval nuclei and distinct nucleoli (hematoxylin and eosin). (Courtesy of Dr. Melissa Fugimori Lissae)

References

1. International Agency for Research on Cancer. Melanoma of skin ASR. Global Cancer Observatory 2019;1–2.
2. International Agency for Research on Cancer. Non-melanoma skin cancer fact sheet. World Health Organ. 2020;419:2–3.
3. IARC. World cancer report 2020. Cancer Control 2020;199.
4. Doubrovsky A, Menzies SW. Enhanced survival in patients with multiple primary melanomas. Arch Dermatol. 2003;139(8):1013–8.
5. Gandini S, Sera F, Cattaruzza MS, Pasquini P, Zanetti R, Masini C, et al. Meta-analysis of risk factors for cutaneous melanoma: III. Family history, actinic damage and phenotypic factors. Eur J Cancer. 2005;41(14):2040–59.
6. Pampena R, Kyrgidis A, Lallas A, Moscarella E, Argenziano G, Longo C. A meta-analysis of nevus-associated melanoma: prevalence and practical implications. J Am Acad Dermatol. 2017;77(5):938.
7. Kubica AW, Brewer JD. Melanoma in immunosuppressed patients. Mayo Clin Proc. 2012;87(10):991–1103.
8. Shain AH, Bastian BC. From melanocytes to melanomas. Nat Rev Cancer. 2016;16:345–58.
9. Elder DE, Massi D, Scolyer RA, Willemze R. WHO classification of skin tumours. 4th ed. Lyon: IARC Press; 2018. p. 76–7.
10. Weedon D. Weedon's skin pathology. 3rd ed. London: Churchill Livingstone; 2009. p. 739–42.
11. Calonje JE, Brenn T, Lazar AJ, McKee PH. McKee's pathology of the skin. 4th ed. Philadelphia: Saunders; 2011. p. 1226–9.
12. Elder DE, Massi D, Scolyer RA, Willemze R. WHO classification of skin tumours. 4th ed. Lyon: IARC Press; 2018. p. 102–4.
13. Hale CS. Lentigo maligna melanoma. PathologyOutlinescom. 2013. https://www.pathologyoutlines.com/topic/skintumormelanocyticlentigomaligna.html. Accessed 14 Sept 2021.
14. Elder DE, Massi D, Scolyer RA, Willemze R. WHO classification of skin tumours. 4th ed. Lyon: IARC Press; 2018. p. 116–8.
15. Elder DE, Massi D, Scolyer RA, Willemze R. WHO classification of skin tumours. 4th ed. Lyon: IARC Press; 2018. p. 105–7.
16. Albahra S, Hosler GA. Desmoplastic melanoma. PathologyOutlines.com. 2021. https://www.pathologyoutlines.com/topic/skintumormelanocyticdesmoplasticmelanoma.html. Accessed 14 Sept 2021.
17. Elder DE, Massi D, Scolyer RA, Willemze R. WHO classification of skin tumours. 4th ed. Lyon: IARC Press; 2018. p. 108–10.
18. Raghavan SS, Peternel S, Mully TW, North JP, Pincus LB, LeBoit PE, et al. Spitz melanoma is a distinct subset of spitzoid melanoma. Mod Pathol. 2020;33:1122–34.
19. Sharon CE, Sinnamon AJ, Ming ME, Chu EY, Fraker DL, Karakousis GC. Association of marital status with T stage at presentation and management of early-stage melanoma. JAMA Dermatol. 2018;154(5):574–80.
20. Vestergaard ME, Macaskill P, Holt PE, Menzies SW. Dermoscopy compared with naked eye examination for the diagnosis of primary melanoma: a meta-analysis of studies performed in a clinical setting. Br J Dermatol. 2008;159(3):669–76.
21. Hirata SH, Yamada S, Almeida FA, Enokihara MY, Rosa IP, Enokihara MM, et al. Dermoscopic examination of the nail bed and matrix. Int J Dermatol. 2006;45(1):28–30.
22. Hirata SH, Yamada S, Almeida FA, Tomomori-Yamashita J, Enokihara MY, Paschoal FM, et al. Dermoscopy of the nail bed and matrix to assess melanonychia striata. J Am Acad Dermatol. 2005;53(5):884–6.
23. Farnetani F, Scope A, Braun RP, Gonzalez S, Guitera P, Malvehy J, et al. Skin cancer diagnosis with reflectance confocal microscopy: reproducibility of feature recognition and accuracy of diagnosis. JAMA Dermatol. 2015;151(10):1075.

24. Waldman RA, Grant-Kels JM, Curiel CN, Curtis J, Rodríguez SG, Hu S, et al. Consensus recommendations for the use of non-invasive melanoma detection techniques based on results of an international DELPHI process. J Am Acad Dermatol. 2019;85(3):745–9.
25. Clark WH, Elder ED, Guerry D 4th, Epstein MN, Greene MH, Horn MV. A study of tumor progression: the precursor lesions of superficial spreading and nodular melanoma. Hum Pathol. 1984;15(12):1147–65.
26. Valdebran M, Elbendary A, Arudra SKC, Torres KM, Elattar I, Elston DM. Nuclear and cytoplasmic features in the diagnosis of banal nevi, Spitz nevi, and melanoma. J Am Acad Dermatol. 2016;75(5):1032–7.
27. Ohsie SJ, Sarantopoulos GP, Cochran AJ, Binder SW. Immunohistochemical characteristics of melanoma. J Cutan Pathol. 2008;35:433–44.
28. Yang K, Oak ASW, Slominski RM, Brozyna AA, Slominski AT. Current molecular markers of melanoma and treatment targets. Int J Mol Sci. 2020;21(10):3535.
29. Scolyer RA, Rawson RV, Gershenwald JE, Ferguson PM, Prieto VG. Melanoma pathology reporting and staging. Mod Pathol. 2019;33:15–24.
30. American Joint Committee on Cancer. AJCC cancer staging manual. 8th ed. Chicago: Springer; 2018. p. 245–54.
31. Grupo Brasileiro de Melanoma. Recomendação para o Tratamento do Melanoma Cutâneo. 2019. p. 32–34.
32. National Comprehensive Cancer Network (NCCN). NCCN Clinical Practice Guidelines in Oncology. Melanoma. Version 2.2021. Fort Washington (PA): National Comprehensive Cancer Network; 2021. https://www.nccn.org/professionals/physician_gls/pdf/cutaneous_melanoma.pdf.
33. Acland KM, O'Doherty MJ, Russell-Jones R. The value of positron emission tomography scanning in the detection of subclinical metastatic melanoma. J Am Acad Dermatol. 2000;42(4):606–11.
34. Campagnari M, Jafelicci AS, Carneiro HA, Brechtbuhl ER, Bertolli E, Duprat Neto JP. Dermal substitutes use in reconstructive surgery for skin tumors: a single-center experience. Int J Surg Oncol. 2017;2017:1–8.
35. Morton DL, Wen DR, Wong JH, Economou JS, Cagle LA, Storm FK, et al. Technical details of intraoperative lymphatic mapping for early stage melanoma. Arch Surg. 1992;127(4):392–9.
36. Bertolli E, de Macedo MP, Calsavara VF, Pinto CAL, Duprat Neto JP. A nomogram to identify high-risk melanoma patients with a negative sentinel lymph node biopsy. J Am Acad Dermatol. 2019;80(3):722–6.
37. Leiter U, Stadler R, Mauch C, Hohenberger W, Brockmeyer N, Berking C, et al. Complete lymph node dissection versus no dissection in patients with sentinel lymph node biopsy positive melanoma (DeCOG-SLT): a multicentre, randomised, phase 3 trial. Lancet Oncol. 2016;17(6):757–67.
38. Leiter U, Stadler R, Mauch C, Hohenberger W, Brockmeyer N, Berking C, et al. Final analysis of DeCOG-SLT trial: no survival benefit for complete lymph node dissection in patients with melanoma with positive sentinel node. J Clin Oncol. 2019;37(32):3000–8.
39. Faries MB, Thompson JF, Cochran AJ, Andtbacka RH, Mozillo N, Zager JS, et al. Completion dissection or observation for sentinel-node metastasis in melanoma. N Engl J Med. 2017;376(23):2211–22.
40. Hui JYC, Burke E, Broman KK, Marmor S, Jensen E, Tutlle TM, et al. Surgeon decision-making for management of positive sentinel lymph nodes in the post-multicenter selective lymphadenectomy trial II era: a survey study. J Surg Oncol. 2021;123(2):646–53.
41. Luke JJ, Ascierto PA, Carlino MS, Gershenwald JE, Grob JJ, Hauschild A, et al. KEYNOTE-716: phase III study of adjuvant pembrolizumab versus placebo in resected high-risk stage II melanoma. Future Oncol. 2020;16(3):4429–38.
42. Luke JJ, Flaherty KT, Ribas A, Lon GV. Targeted agents and immunotherapies: optimizing outcomes in melanoma. Nat Rev Clin Oncol. 2017;14:463–82.

43. Eggermont AMM, Chiarion-Sileni V, Grob JJ, Dummer R, Wolchok JD, Schmidt H, et al. Prolonged survival in stage III melanoma with Ipilimumab adjuvant therapy. N Engl J Med. 2016;375:1845–55.
44. Eggermont AMM, Chiarion-Sileni V, Grob JJ, Dummer R, Wolchok JD, Schmidt H, et al. Adjuvant ipilimumab versus placebo after complete resection of stage III melanoma: long-term follow-up results of the European Organisation for Research and Treatment of Cancer 18071 double-blind phase 3 randomised trial. Eur J Cancer. 2019;119:1–10.
45. Weber J, Mandala M, Del Vecchio M, Gogas HJ, Arance AM, Cowey L, et al. Adjuvant nivolumab versus ipilimumab in resected stage III or IV melanoma. N Engl J Med. 2017;377:1824–35.
46. Eggermont AMM, Blank CU, Mandala M, Long GV, Atkinson V, Dalle S, et al. Adjuvant pembrolizumab versus placebo in resected stage III melanoma. N Engl J Med. 2018;378:1789–801.
47. Grossman KF, Othus M, Patel SP, Tarhini AA, Sondak VK, Petrella TM, et al. Final analysis of overall survival (OS) and relapse-free-survival (RFS) in the intergroup S1404 phase III randomized trial comparing either high-dose interferon (HDI) or ipilimumab to pembrolizumab in patients with high-risk resected melanoma. J Clin Oncol. 2021;39(suppl 15):abstract 9501.
48. Dummer R, Hauschild A, Santinami M, Atkinson V, Mandala M, Kirkwood JM, et al. Five-year analysis of adjuvant dabrafenib plus trametinib in stage III melanoma. N Engl J Med. 2020;383:1139–48.
49. Menzies AM, Amaria RN, Rozeman EA, Huang AC, Tetzlaff MT, Van de Wiel BA, et al. Pathological response and survival with neoadjuvant therapy in melanoma: a pooled analysis from the International Neoadjuvant Melanoma Consortium (INMC). Nat Med. 2021;27(2):301–9.
50. Curti BD, Faries MB. Recent advances in the treatment of melanoma. N Engl J Med. 2021;348:2229–40.
51. The Cancer Genome Atlas Network. Genomic classification of cutaneous melanoma. Cell. 2015;161(7):1681–96.
52. McArthur GA, Chapman PB, Robert C, Larkin J, Haanen JB, Dummer R, et al. Safety and efficacy of vemurafenib in BRAF (V600E) and BRAF (V600F) mutation-positive melanoma (BRIM-3): extended follow-up of a phase 3, randomized, open-label study. Lancet Oncol. 2014;15:323–32.
53. Hauschild A, Grob JJ, Demidov LV, Jouary T, Gutzmer R, Millward M, et al. Dabrafenib in BRAF-mutated metastatic melanoma: a multicentre, open-label, phase 3 randomised controlled trial. Lancet. 2012;380(9839):358–65.
54. Rizos H, Menzies AM, Pupo GM, Carlino MS, Fung C, Hyman J, et al. BRAF inhibitor resistance mechanisms in metastatic melanoma: spectrum and clinical impact. Clin Cancer Res. 2014;20(7):1965–77.
55. Robert C, Karaszewska B, Schachter J, Rutkowski P, Mackiewicz A, Stroiakovski D, et al. Improved overall survival in melanoma with combined dabrafenib and trametinib. N Engl J Med. 2015;372:30–9.
56. Ascierto PA, McArthur GA, Dréno B, Atkinson V, Liszkay G, Di Giacomo AM, et al. Cobimetinib combined with vemurafenib in advanced BRAFV600-mutant melanoma (coBRIM): updated efficacy results from a randomised, double-blind, phase 3 trial. Lancet Oncol. 2016;17(9):1248–60.
57. Robert C, Grob JJ, Stroyakovskiy D, Karaszewska B, Hauschild A, Levchenko E, et al. Five-year outcomes with dabrafenib plus trametinib in metastatic melanoma. N Engl J Med. 2019;381:626–36.
58. Dummer R, Flaherty K, Robert C, Arance AM, Groot JW, Garbe C, et al. Five-year overall survival (OS) in COLUMBUS: a randomized phase 3 trial of encorafenib plus binimetinib versus vemurafenib or encorafenib in patients (pts) with BRAF V600-mutant melanoma. J Clin Oncol. 2021;39(15_suppl):abstract 9507.
59. Dummer R, Schadendorf D, Ascierto PA, Arance A, Dutriax C, Di Giacomo AM, et al. Binimetinib versus dacarbazine in patients with advanced NRAS-mutant melanoma (NEMO): a multicentre, open-label, randomised, phase 3 trial. Lancet Oncol. 2017;18(4):435–45.

60. Kim KB, Eton O, Davis DW, Frazier ML, McConkey DJ, Diwan AH, et al. Phase II trial of imatinib mesylate in patients with metastatic melanoma. Br J Cancer. 2008;99(5):734–40.
61. Guo J, Si L, Kong Y, Flaherty KT, Xu X, Zhu Y, et al. Phase II, open-label, single-arm trial of imatinib mesylate in patients with metastatic melanoma harboring c-KIT mutation or amplification. J Clin Oncol. 2011;29(21):2904–9.
62. Hodi FS, O'Day SJ, McDermott DF, Weber RW, Sosman JA, Haanen JB, et al. Improved survival with ipilimumab in patients with metastatic melanoma. N Engl J Med. 2010;363:711–23.
63. Schadendorf D, Hodi FS, Robert C, Weber IS, Margolin K, Hamid O, et al. Pooled analysis of long-term survival data from phase II and phase III trials of Ipilimumab in unresectable or metastatic melanoma. J Clin Oncol. 2015;33:1889–94.
64. Ribas A, Hamid O, Daud A, Hodi FS, Wolchok JD, Kefford R, et al. Association of pembrolizumab with tumor response and survival among patients with advanced melanoma. JAMA. 2016;315(15):1600–9.
65. Topalian SL, Hodi FS, Brahmer JR, Gettinger SN, Smith DC, McDermott DF, et al. Five-year survival and correlates among patients with advanced melanoma, renal cell carcinoma, or non-small cell lung cancer treated with nivolumab. JAMA Oncol. 2019;5(10):411–1420.
66. Ribas A, Puzanov I, Dummer R, Scadendorf D, Hamid O, Robert C, et al. Pembrolizumab versus investigator-choice chemotherapy for ipilimumab-refractory melanoma (KEYNOTE-002): a randomised, controlled, phase 2 trial. Lancet Oncol. 2015;16(8):908–18.
67. Larkin J, Minor D, D'Angelo S, Neyns B, Smylie M, Miller WH Jr, et al. Overall survival in patients with advanced melanoma who received nivolumab versus investigator's choice chemotherapy in CheckMate 037: a randomized, controlled, open-label phase III trial. J Clin Oncol. 2018;36(4):383–90.
68. Schachter J, Ribas A, Long GV, Arance A, Grob JJ, Mortier L, et al. Pembrolizumab versus ipilimumab for advanced melanoma: final overall survival results of a multicentre, randomised, open-label phase 3 study (KEYNOTE-006). Lancet. 2017;390(10105):1853–62.
69. Robert C, Long GV, Brady B, Dutriaux C, Di Giacomo AM, Mortier L, et al. Five-year outcomes with nivolumab in patients with wild-type BRAF advanced melanoma. J Clin Oncol. 2020;38(33):3937–46.
70. Larkin J, Chiarion-Sileni V, Gonzalez R, Grob JJ, Rutkowski P, Lao CD, et al. Five-year survival with combined nivolumab and ipilimumab in advanced melanoma. N Engl J Med. 2019;381:1535–46.
71. Wolchok JD, Chiarion-Sileni V, Gonzalez R, Grob JJ, Rutkowski P, Lao CD, et al. CheckMate 067: 6.5-year outcomes in patients (pts) with advanced melanoma. J Clin Oncol. 2021;39(15_suppl):abstract 9506.
72. Lebbé C, Meyer N, Ortier L, Marquez-Rodas I, Robert C, Rutkowski P, et al. Evaluation of two dosing regimens for nivolumab in combination with ipilimumab in patients with advanced melanoma: results from the phase IIIb/IV CheckMate 511 trial. J Clin Oncol. 2019;37(11):867–75.
73. Long GV, Atkinson V, Lo S, Guminski AD, Sandhu SK, Brown MP, et al. Five-year overall survival from the anti-PD1 brain collaboration (ABC study): randomized phase 2 study of nivolumab (nivo) or nivo+ipilimumab (ipi) in patients (pts) with melanoma brain metastases (mets). J Clin Oncol. 2021;39(15_suppl):abstract 9508.
74. Tawbi HA, Forsyth PAJ, Hodi FS, Lao CD, Moschos SJ, Hamid O, et al. Efficacy and safety of the combination of nivolumab (NIVO) plus ipilimumab (IPI) in patients with symptomatic melanoma brain metastases (CheckMate 204). J Clin Oncol. 2019;37(15_suppl):abstract 9501.
75. Davies MA, Saiag P, Robert C, Grob JJ, Flaherty KY, Arance A, et al. Dabrafenib plus trametinib in patients with BRAFV600-mutant melanoma brain metastases (COMBI-MB): a multicentre, multicohort, open-label, phase 2 trial. Lancet Oncol. 2017;18(7):863–73.
76. Gutzmer R, Stroyakovskiy D, Gogas H, Robert C, Lewis K, Protsensko S, et al. Atezolizumab, vemurafenib, and cobimetinib as first-line treatment for unresectable advanced BRAFV600 mutation-positive melanoma (IMspire150): primary analysis of the randomised, double-blind, placebo-controlled, phase 3 trial. Lancet. 2020;395(10240):1835–44.
77. Lipson EJ, Tawbi HA, Schadendorf D, Ascierto PA, Matamala L, Gutiérrez EC, et al. Relatlimab (RELA) plus nivolumab (NIVO) versus NIVO in first-line advanced melanoma:

primary phase III results from RELATIVITY-047 (CA224-047). J Clin Oncol. 2021;39(15_ suppl):abstract 9503.
78. Andtbacka RH, Kaufman HL, Collichio F, Amatruda T, Senzer N, Chesney J, et al. Talimogene laherparepvec improves durable response rate in patients with advanced melanoma. J Clin Oncol. 2015;33(25):2780–8.
79. Damude S, Hoekstra-Weebers JEHM, Francken AB, Meulen ST, Bastiaannet E, Hoekstra HJ. The MELFO-study: prospective, randomized, clinical trial for the evaluation of a stage-adjusted reduced follow-up schedule in cutaneous melanoma patients-results after 1 year. Ann Surg Oncol. 2016;23(9):2762–71.
80. Krüger U, Kretschmer L, Thoms KM, Padeken M, Bertsch HP, Schön MP, et al. Lymph node ultrasound during melanoma follow-up significantly improves metastasis detection compared with clinical examination alone. Melanoma Res. 2011;21(5):457–63.
81. Mihajlovic M, Vlajkovic S, Jovanovic P, Stefanovic V. Primary mucosal melanomas: a comprehensive review. Int J Clin Exp Pathol. 2012;5(8):739–53.
82. Tyrrell H, Payne M. Combatting mucosal melanoma: recent advances and future perspectives. Melanoma Manag. 2018;5(3):MMT11.
83. Pietro VG, Dehner LP, Pfeifer JD, Wick MR. Genital and mucosal melanocytic tumors: mucosal melanomas. 4th ed. Lyon: IARC Press; 2018. p. 121–2.
84. Amim MB, Edge S, Greene F, Byrd DR, Brookland RK, Washington MK, et al. Principles of cancer staging: AJCC cancer staging manual. 8th ed. New York: Springer; 2017. p. 3–30.
85. Coupland S, Folberg R, Kivel T, Pietro VG. Ocular melanocytic tumors: uveal melanoma. 4th ed. Lyon: IARC Press; 2018. p. 137–8.
86. Krantz BA, Dave N, Komatsubara KM, Marr BP, Carvajal RD. Uveal melanoma: epidemiology, etiology, and treatment of primary disease. Clin Ophthalmol. 2017;11:279–89.
87. Kaliki S, Shields CL. Uveal melanoma: relatively rare but deadly cancer. Eye (Lond). 2017;31(2):241–57.
88. Singh M, Durairaj P, Yeung J. Uveal melanoma: a review of the literature. Oncol Ther. 2018;6(1):87–104.
89. Grisanti S, Tura A. Uveal melanoma. In: Noncutaneous melanoma. Brisbane: Exon Publications; 2018. p. 1–188. https://doi.org/1 0.15586/codon.noncutaneousmelanoma.2018.chl.
90. Tretter EM, Schoenfield LR. Melanoma-uvea. PathologyOutlines.com. 2018. https://www.pathologyoutlines.com/topic/eyeuveamelanoma.html. Accessed 13 Sept 2021.
91. Tarlan B, Kıratlı H. Uveal melanoma: current trends in diagnosis and management. Turk J Ophthalmol. 2016;46(3):123–37.

Chapter 17
Appendageal Tumors

Francisco Aparecido Belfort, Laryssa Gonçalves de Gouvea Faiçal, Luiz Guilherme Cernaglia Aureliano De Lima, and André Luis de Freitas Perina

Introduction

Skin appendage tumors are a group of neoplasms that either differentiate toward or arise from the pilosebaceous apparatus, apocrine glands, or eccrine glands. Mostly with a nonspecific clinical presentation as subcutaneous nodules, papules, plaques, or tumors without peculiar morphological or dermoscopic aspects, they often end up not being included in the differential diagnosis of biopsied lesions and are setting as a histopathological finding [1, 2]. There is a great variety of cells that takes part of the structure of the pilosebaceous apparatus (divided into hair follicle, adjacent sebaceous gland, and, in some body sites, apocrine gland) and the eccrine glands, with their deeper secretory portion and excretory portion, which is more superficial. The ductal portion (excretory) of the eccrine and apocrine glands are identical considering the morphological point of view, only being possible to distinguish them according to the anatomical area or if the duct is identified penetrating the hair follicle; however, in some cases, the apocrine duct can also arise directly into the epidermis [3]. This similarity between the glands, just as the variety of cells that form the skin appendages, makes great difficulty and heterogeneity in classifying these tumors, since they can be predominantly of hair lineage, sebaceous, eccrine, apocrine (or indistinguishable between eccrine and apocrine), or even a mixture of these distinct lineages. In addition, it is postulated that some (if not all) may originate from pluripotent cells that undergo differentiation into one or more of these

F. A. Belfort (✉) · L. G. C. A. De Lima
NOCS - Hospital Sírio-Libanês, São Paulo, Brazil

L. G. de Gouvea Faiçal
AMO Clinic, Salvador, Bahia, Brazil

A. L. de Freitas Perina
NOCS - Hospital Sírio-Libanês, São Paulo, São Paulo, Brazil

C. M. Z. Abdalla et al. (eds.), *Oncodermatology*,
https://doi.org/10.1007/978-3-031-29277-4_17

lineages in variable proportions [4, 5]. The majority of these types of tumors are benign or have indolent behavior, but there are extremely aggressive subtypes, with a potential for metastasis or high rates of local recurrence, and some with unpredictable behavior. The last ones mentioned are classified as atypical cutaneous adnexal tumors or tumors of uncertain malignant potential [6]. Beyond the possibility of having lesions with considerable aggressiveness, some types of adnexal tumors may be markers of genetic syndromes associated with internal malignancies; therefore, their correct recognition helps in the follow-up and management of these high-risk patients. Another subject to be considered is the similarity that some adnexal tumors have with cutaneous metastasis from other neoplasms, such as breast and salivary gland tumors [7]. To complete the challenge, the rarity of some of these tumors makes difficult their recognition by the pathologist and the existence of guidelines for their correct management [4]. For the dermatologist, some benign tumors are easily recognized clinically, such as syringoma, but most of malignant adnexal tumors have a resemblance or are indistinguishable from other more common tumors; basal cell carcinoma is the most important differential diagnosis, because they often present arboriform telangiectasias in dermoscopy, and it is also not uncommon the polymorphic or atypical vascular pattern [2]. Because of the great challenge that is the correct diagnosis and classification of adnexal tumors, a practical approach becomes fundamental for the correct management of these neoplasms. In this sense, the focus should be given to the following questions: The tumor resembles which type of adnexal structure? Is the tumor benign or malignant? Is it a primary cutaneous adnexal tumor or a cutaneous metastasis of an internal neoplasm? Is it possible that this lesion represents the cutaneous expression of some systemic syndrome?

The correct answer to these questions will guide clinical management and prognosis. Histopathological examination remains the gold standard in the diagnosis of cutaneous adnexal tumors, in addition to complete clinical information, associated with immunohistochemistry and molecular analysis [1].

Epidemiology, Risk Factors, and Genetic Determinants

As in other parts of the world, statistics about cutaneous malignancies are based on only two categories: melanoma and non-melanoma. The last category covers neoplasms of the skin appendages, but the largest part of the group is represented by basal cell and squamous cell carcinomas, which are by far the most predominant. The age-adjusted incidence in the United States is estimated to be 5.1 cases/million/year and in Europe 2.1–5.3 cases/million/year. Despite being considered rare, the incidence of adnexal tumors has been increasing significantly in recent years, a fact related to the increased life expectancy of the population and improvement in detection of these tumors [6–8]. In general, they are more frequent in males and Caucasians and between the fourth and sixth decades of life. As for the preferential location, the sebaceous and follicular tumors are more commonly diagnosed in the head and neck region, where there is the highest concentration of these skin appendages; the eccrine neoplasms can originate in any body site, but predominate in the palmoplantar regions, while the apocrine ones predominate in the armpits, anogenital regions, and eyelids [3]. As for the most prevalent subtypes and lineages, according to the French database [8], in a sample of 2177 cases from 2014 to 2018, we have that 88% of adnexal tumors are distributed between sudoriferous tumors (50%) and follicular tumors (38%). Among the sweat tumors, porocarcinoma (23%), microcystic adnexal carcinoma (10%), and hidradenocarcinoma (9%) predominate. Extramammary Paget disease, classified as site-specific, accounts for 20% of this sample. Among the tumors of follicular origin, the most prevalent is trichoblastic carcinoma (80%), followed by proliferating trichilemmal tumor (13%), with the remaining 7% shared among the other subtypes [8]. Although ultraviolet radiation and immunosuppression are considered triggering factors, little is known about the etiology and pathogenesis of adnexal tumors. Specific genetic alterations are imputed as the cause of some of them, mainly in the setting of hereditary syndromes (most with alterations in tumor suppressor genes) [9–12]. Presence of multiple tumors, particularly in head and neck region, raises the suspicion of a syndromic patient. It's extremely important that physicians know how to recognize and correctly manage these patients, since they can have internal and cutaneous malignancies. In Table 17.1 we will describe the main cutaneous adnexal tumors related to hereditary syndromes and their main characteristics [2, 9–11, 13].

Initial Assessment

Recognizing an adnexal tumor is essential to distinguish it from different tumors of the skin such as basal cell, squamous cell, Merkel cell carcinomas, and metastasis, with so variable conducts and evolutions. As previously mentioned, adnexal tumors can occur as single or multiple lesions like nonspecific papules, nodules, or plaques rarely diagnosed without the aid of histopathological investigation. Features such as asymmetry, irregular borders, varied colors, erosion, and ulceration may suggest malignancy in lesions that have been evolving for some time. Dermatoscopy is a very useful tool in the diagnosis of other skin neoplasms with well-defined dermatoscopic findings, but in appendageal tumors scenario rarely can distinguish them from other tumors. In general, tumors of follicular origin are those that most mimic basal cell carcinoma, even in histology; besides the linear arboriform vessels encountered, blue-gray dots or globules are often found too. The presence of "white structures" may be a clue in favor of adnexal tumors of follicular lineage, but not specific. Yellowish structures with blurred arboriform vessels, on the other hand, are patterns that indicate sebaceous lineage. Sudoriferous gland tumors have a great dermatoscopic variability and can mimic basal cell carcinomas, squamous cell carcinomas, and melanoma. The finding of polymorphic or atypical vessels is also common in malignant adnexal tumors, but this doesn't distinguish them from malignant tumors of more frequent lineages [12, 14].

Table 17.1 Main characteristics of the cutaneous adnexal tumors related to hereditary syndromes

Appendageal tumor	Clinical aspects	Dermoscopy	Syndrome	Molecular findings	Malignancies and other findings
Fibrofolliculomas/ trichodiscomas	White to skin-colored papules; smooth; head, neck, upper trunk	F: well-demarcated areas/ globules of whitish coloration with a central yellowish-brown spot, may present a prominent vascular component. Fibrofolliculomas with central open comedo is a diagnostic clue to Birt–Hogg–Dube´ syndrome T: whitish globular structures, blue-gray nests, and blurred linear vessels	Birt–Hogg–Dubé syndrome Consider in young adult with five fibrofolliculomas, with at least one histologically confirmed and FLCN mutation detected	FLCN mutations (folliculin protein) Autosomal dominant	Renal tumors/multiple pulmonary cysts with spontaneous pneumothorax risk Acrochordons
Trichilemmomas	Skin-colored papules or verrucous growths—head	Radial linear vessels (and occasionally hairpin) with distal thickening adopting a triangular form in the periphery of the lesion (red iris-like structure), with white shiny areas surrounding them, a whitish keratin mass/central hyperkeratotic crust	Cowden syndrome/ PTEN hamartoma tumor syndrome	Heterozygous germline mutation in the PTEN gene on chromosome 10q23 Autosomal dominant	Breast, thyroid, and endometrial carcinoma Check for other facial papules, oral papillomatosis, acral keratoses, sclerotic fibromas, lipomas, skin tags, macrocephaly, hamartomatous polyps of the gastrointestinal tract

Appendageal tumor	Clinical aspects	Dermoscopy	Syndrome	Molecular findings	Malignancies and other findings
Trichoepitheliomas Spiradenomas Cylindromas	T: skin-colored to pink papules/central face S: solitary, intradermal, round oval, and blue or pink C: smooth, dome-shaped, hairless, reddish-brown papules or nodules on the head and neck (but also the trunk and extremities)	T: small, thin, infocus arborizing vessels, shiny white areas/background and milialike cyst C: a homogeneous pink or pink, orange area with arborizing telangiectasias. In some of them, blue ovoid nests or blue globules can be seen	Brooke–Spiegler syndrome Multiple familial trichoepitheliomas MFT1 Familial cylindromatosis	Germline mutations in the cylindromatosis (CYLD) gene on chromosome 16q12 Autosomal dominant	Salivary and parotid gland tumors Spiradenoma may transform into spiradenocarcinoma Cylindroma may transform into cylindrocarcinoma Trichoepithelioma may transform into *basal cell carcinoma*

(continued)

Table 17.1 (continued)

Appendageal tumor	Clinical aspects	Dermoscopy	Syndrome	Molecular findings	Malignancies and other findings
Sebaceous adenomas Sebaceomas Sebaceous carcinoma	Yellow to yellow-red nodules, head and neck, but also trunk and extremities	S: adenoma/sebaceoma: (two patterns) central crater with crown vessels embracing an opaque structureless ovoid white-yellow center, blood crusts or without a central crater with branching but unfocussed arborizing vessels over a white to yellow background and few, loosely arranged, yellow comedolike globules S. Carcinoma: polymorphous atypical vessels, homogeneous yellowish background and ulceration	Muir–Torre syndrome Consider in anyone under 50 years with a solitary sebaceous adenoma, multiple sebaceous tumors, or a sebaceous tumor not on the head and neck	Immunohistochemistry for MLH-1, MSH-2, and MSH-6 and subsequent microsatellite instability analysis Autosomal dominant	Colorectal, genitourinary tract, *breast cancer*, *lymphoma*, *leukemia* (rarely), salivary gland tumors, lower and upper respiratory tract tumors, and *chondrosarcoma* Check for keratoacanthomas; desmoid tumors, pilomatricomas
Hidrocistomas	Translucent to blue; eyelids	Central homogeneous area, translucent to opaque skin-colored (31.8%), yellowish (31.8%), blue (22.7%), or less frequently pinkish-blue or gray and also vascular structures (81.8%), usually arborizing vessels, and whitish structures (22.7%)	Schöpf–Schulz–Passarge syndrome	Homozygous mutation in the WNT10A gene on chromosome 2q35 Autosomal recessive	Basal cell carcinoma, porocarcinoma and squamous cell carcinoma The neoplastic risk in SSPS is controversial Check for palmoplantar keratoderma, eccrine syringofibroadenomas, hypotrichosis, hypodontia, nail dystrophy, facial telangiectatic erythema

Appropriate management for skin lesions with a suspicious clinical appearance begins with a biopsy, preferably excisional, which is not always possible. When requesting the pathological examination, one should always provide as much information as possible, such as type of biopsy (punch, incisional, or excisional), the anatomical site of the lesion, size, time of evolution, gender, age, family history, any previous treatments, and differential diagnoses (and here, remembering adnexal tumors is fundamental). Evaluation by a pathologist with expertise in cutaneous adnexal tumors is of utmost importance to a correct diagnosis and to provide prognostic factors such as risk of relapse due to local infiltration, risk of lymph node dissemination, or distant metastasis. Therefore, every clinical or surgical approach will be based on the histological report, hence the need for absolute trust in it. The pathologist needs to examine the lesion thoroughly in order to identify the different biological behavior (malignant or benign), mainly based on peripheral growth pattern, so the analysis of the relationship with the adjacent tissues is very important. Using morphological basis and similarity with the normal tissues, the pathologist can evaluate if the tumor has a glandular, follicular, or sebaceous differentiation. For example, apocrine differentiation is characterized by the presence of secretion by decapitation and accumulation of supranuclear zymogen granules PAS-positive and diastase-resistant. However, it's very common the coexistence of eccrine and apocrine differentiation and superposition of morphologic and immunohistochemical factors that turn more difficult the definition of these kinds of lesions. Other factor that makes the differential diagnosis more difficult, is the plasticity of this group of neoplasms, represented by capacity of unicystic growth pattern, hyperpigmentation by melanocytic colonization, epidermal perforating aspect, and divergent differentiation, particularly for other cutaneous adnexal lineages. The histopathological criteria for malignancy are poor delimitation, asymmetry, infiltrative growing, deep extension, desmoplastic reaction, lymphoid reaction, necrosis, embolization, cytologic pleomorphism, and stromal epithelium clefts; these criteria have great variability and different relevance in the dependence of histologic subtype. Just one or two of these criteria, in an isolated manner, could be insufficient for malignant definition. Despite the great controversy and variety of classifications, the most accepted and used by pathologists is that of skin tumors by the World Health Organization—WHO [6]—updated in 2018, which we will mention in Table 17.2.

Some adnexal tumors are clinically indistinguishable from metastasis from other neoplasms, in particular breast, colon, salivary glands, and others in smaller numbers (Fig. 17.1a, b).

However, the microscopy evaluation can distinguish the great majority of them, except breast and salivary gland ones, that can have very similar histological counterparts and need essentially a clinical approach to distinguish primary and cutaneous metastasis.

Table 17.2 Classification of malignant and benign adnexal cutaneous tumors adapted from the World Health Organization—WHO (fourth Ed)

Malignant tumors with apocrine and eccrine differentiation Adnexal adenocarcinoma NOS Microcystic adnexal carcinoma Porocarcinoma Porocarcinoma in situ Malignant neoplasms arising from spiradenoma, cylindroma, or spiradenocylindroma Malignant mixed tumor Hidradenocarcinoma Mucinous carcinoma Endocrine mucin-producing sweat gland carcinoma Digital papillary adenocarcinoma Adenoid cystic carcinoma Apocrine carcinoma Squamous eccrine ductal carcinoma Syringocystadenocarcinoma papilliferum Secretory carcinoma Cribriform carcinoma Signet-ring cell/histiocytoid carcinoma	*Benign tumors with apocrine and eccrine differentiation* Hidrocystoma/cystadenoma Syringoma Poroma Syringofibroadenoma Hidradenoma Spiradenoma Cylindroma Tubular adenoma Syringocystadenoma papilliferum Mixed tumor Myoepithelioma
Malignant tumors with follicular differentiation Pilomatrical carcinoma Proliferating trichilemmal tumors Trichoblastic carcinoma/carcinosarcoma Trichilemmal carcinoma	*Benign tumors with follicular differentiation* Trichoblastoma Pilomatricoma Trichilemmoma Trichofolliculoma Pilar sheath acanthoma Tumor of the follicular infundibulum Melanocytic matricoma Spindle cell predominant trichodiscoma
Malignant tumors with sebaceous differentiation Sebaceous carcinoma	*Benign tumors with sebaceous differentiation* Sebaceous adenoma Sebaceoma
Site-specific tumors Mammary Paget disease Extramammary Paget disease Adenocarcinoma of anogenital mammary-like glands Hidradenoma papilliferum Fibroadenoma of anogenital mammary-like glands Phyllodes tumor of anogenital mammary-like glands	

From a clinical point of view, consider that approximately 5% of cancer patients may develop cutaneous metastasis but less than 1% of them will have cutaneous metastasis as the first manifestation [15, 16]. In this context, it is of utmost importance to mention in the request for pathological examination the presence of another malignancy, provided it is known. Distinction clinical data between primary adnexal tumors and metastasis from other carcinomas can be summarized as shown in Table 17.3.

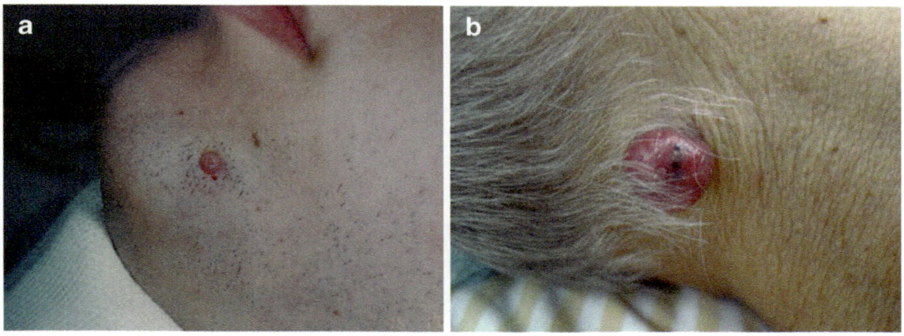

Fig. 17.1 (**a**) Relapsed hidradenoma in the cheek of young man. (**b**) Metastasis of adenocarcinoma of the colon in the posterior aspect of the neck

Table 17.3 Differential diagnosis between primary adnexal tumors and metastasis from other carcinomas

	Adnexal tumors	Metastasis
Occurrence	0.5%	2.5%
Average age	4th to 6th decades	70 years old
Male/female	1.5/1	1/2
Local	CP (70%) face > scalp	Male: CP > thorax > abdomen Female: thorax/abdomen
Number of lesions	Single	Multiple
Duration	>6 months	<6 months
Morphology	Nodule	Nodule > keratotic Inflammatory aspect
Survival rate	5 years: 96%	Median: 2–36 months

Management of Local and Advanced Disease

After the biopsy, preferably excisional, has been performed, careful analysis by dermatopathologist will provide the details for the suitable management. Clinical and image staging should be done, depending on the severity of each case.

The differential diagnosis between benign and malignant is the first step. We will exemplify with a dorsal tumor as shown in Fig. 17.2a, b.

In Fig. 17.2a we see a sebaceous adenoma, confirmed as a benign lesion, that was treated by a simple excision with minimum margins; in Fig. 17.2b, a sebaceous carcinoma that received wide margins, after the appropriate oncological staging.

The pathologist has more difficulty when faced with the so-called "adnexal tumors of undetermined malignant potential (ATUMP)." This concept applies to those tumors in which the limit for malignancy is not settle, remaining the doubt between two types, as exemplified by the subtypes below [8]:

- Atypical hidradenoma/hidradenocarcinoma.
- Atypical poroma/porocarcinoma.
- Atypical mixed tumor/malignant mixed tumor.

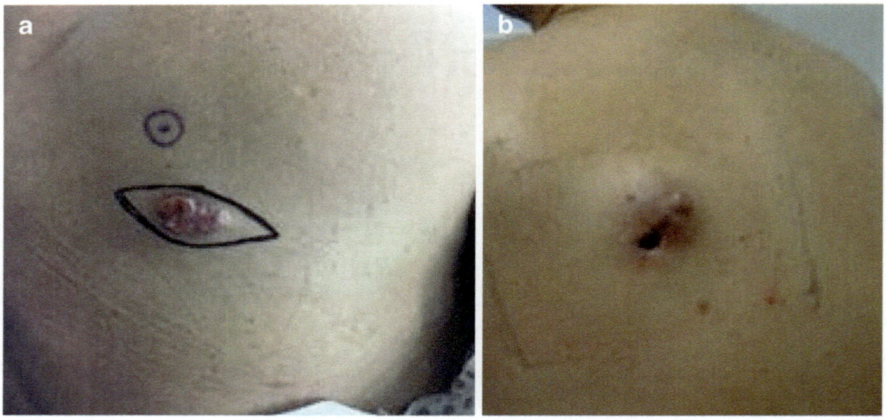

Fig. 17.2 (**a**) Sebaceous adenoma—back localization. (**b**) Sebaceous carcinoma—back localization

- Atypical myoepithelioma/malignant myoepithelioma.
- Atypical sebaceoma or adenoma/sebaceous carcinoma.

Although immunohistochemistry and molecular profiling resources contribute to a better definition, there are still lesions that the guidance given by pathologists is "make a complete excision and follow-up."

As commented in the introduction, there is a need to seek a consensus for the most appropriate therapeutic management, as several questions remain, such as:

- In surgical treatment, which margins are adequate?
- When to use micrographic surgery?
- Is sentinel lymph node biopsy useful?
- Which one and when to perform image examinations?
- How to do follow-up and for how long to keep it?
- How to treat metastatic disease?
- Is there a place for immunotherapy or targeted drugs?

The main limiting factors are related to the numerous subtypes, with heterogeneous behavior and little existing literature about it, preventing evidence-based decisions.

Given the data above, as most lesions will have their final diagnosis after the histological report, the initial treatment varies a little. Never remove any lesion and not refer for histological examination. Always provide all possible data in the request for pathological examination, as mentioned above.

In a global way, the management of these different types of adnexal tumors is the same, with small details in some specific subtypes.

Benign lesions, which usually present as uncharacteristic papules or nodules, similar in appearance to normal skin, usually between 1 and 2 cm in size, asymptomatic and slow growing, are treated by a *simple excision* with margins around of 0.5 cm, as shown in Figs. 17.3a–c and 17.4a, b.

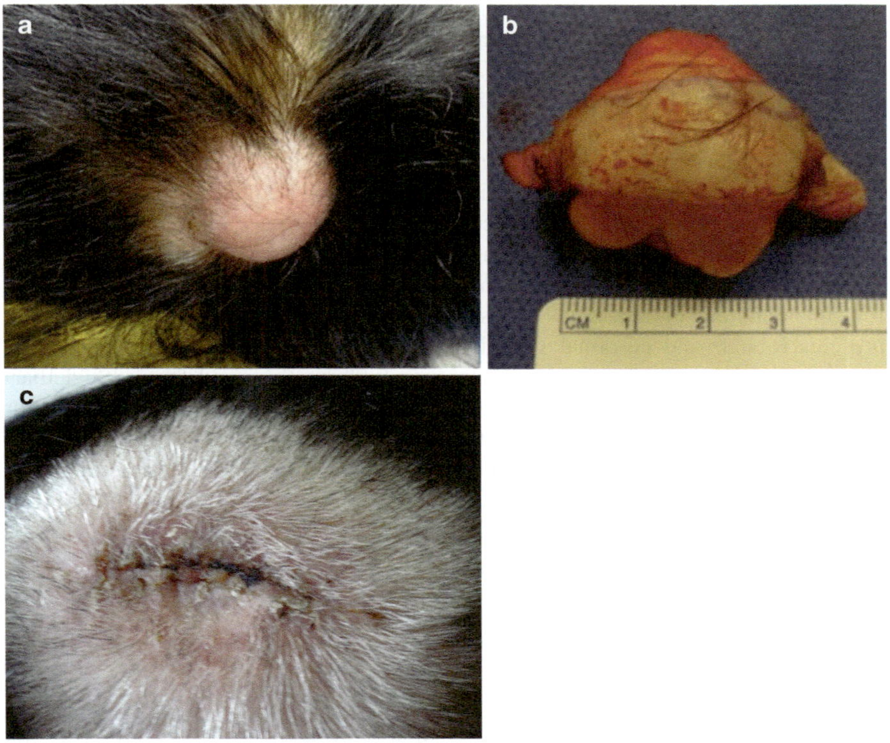

Fig. 17.3 (**a**) Syringocystadenoma papilliferum of the scalp. (**b**) Surgical piece of (**a**). (**c**) Recent scare of the patient of (**a**)

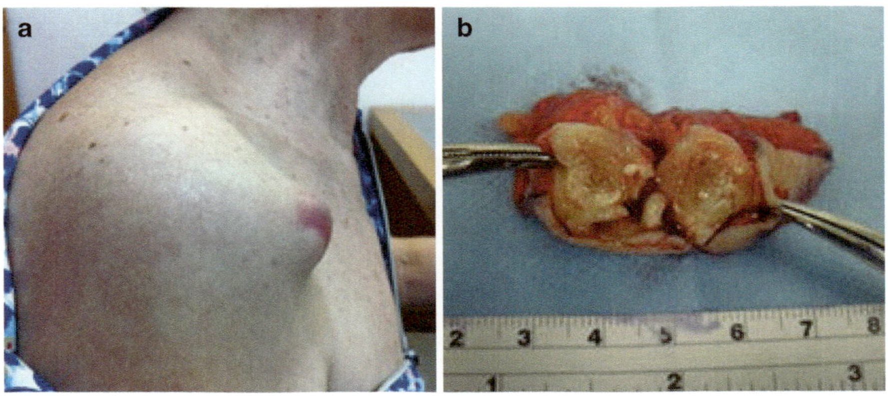

Fig. 17.4 (**a**) Trichilemmal cyst of the right shoulder of a woman. (**b**) Trichilemmal cyst—surgical piece of the patient of (**a**)

In syndromic patients with multiple benign tumors, other forms of therapy can be used, such as removal by electrocautery or electro-resection, laser therapy, and saucerization.

Malignant lesions have similar clinical appearance to benign ones, but a fast growing, often ulcerated.

Starting the topic of malignant tumors therapy by those with eccrine/apocrine lineage, it's necessary to make a description of the most frequent or aggressive ones.

Eccrine Porocarcinoma: usually occurs in the sixth decade of life, most common in the head and neck and torso, as a nodule or plaque or verrucous papule, asymptomatic, usually ulcerated, with a high relapse rate (20%) and a significant capacity for cutaneous and lymph node metastases (20%). At histological examination, it presents lobular and cordonal growths arising from the epidermis composed of small cells with vesicular core and scanty cytoplasm (basaloid features), demarcated from close epidermal keratinocytes. Neoplastic cells near sites of dermal invasion may have a higher degree of cytological pleomorphism. It should be differentiated from simple hidroacanthoma, extramammary Paget and squamous cell in situ in its intraepidermal phase, as well as metastatic carcinoma when in the invasive phase [17]. An example of this kind of tumor is presented in Fig. 17.5a–d.

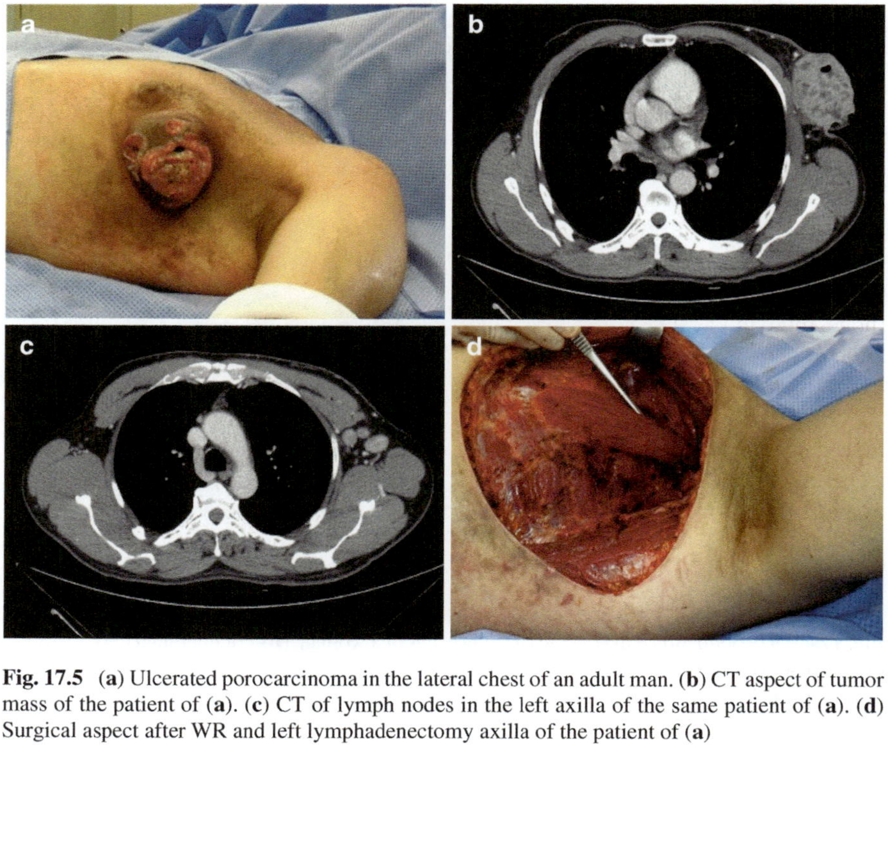

Fig. 17.5 (**a**) Ulcerated porocarcinoma in the lateral chest of an adult man. (**b**) CT aspect of tumor mass of the patient of (**a**). (**c**) CT of lymph nodes in the left axilla of the same patient of (**a**). (**d**) Surgical aspect after WR and left lymphadenectomy axilla of the patient of (**a**)

Eccrine Ductal Adenocarcinoma: predominantly in adult females, on the chest wall. It presents as a slow-growing plaque, up to 5 cm, and the differential diagnosis with metastasis from breast carcinoma is necessary, as it has an infiltrative and ductular growth pattern [17].

Another tumor from eccrine/apocrine origin is *microcystic adnexal carcinoma* [17]. It presents as a plaque or nodule, with gradual enlargement, slightly colored, beige or yellowish. It rarely produces metastasis. The differential diagnosis is with syringoma, desmoplastic trichoepithelioma, sclerodermiform basal cell carcinoma, and papillary eccrine adenocarcinoma. Histology shows small keratinocytes cysts, occasionally associated with lumens of small basaloid cells more superficially. Medially basaloid strands predominate, which decrease in size as they deepen into the dermis, until they remain as only two or three cells, presenting a general aspect of a deeply infiltrative lesion without cytological pleomorphism, and perineural invasion is common, which justifies the frequent recurrences, such as the case in Fig. 17.6a, b.

Mucinous Carcinoma: clinically presents as a single, painless, slow-growing, soft consistency nodule. Common on the eyelids in females. The epithelial cells have monomorphic round nuclei, admixed with abundant slightly basophilic mucin, interspersed with fibrovascular septa. Most significant differential diagnosis is with metastatic breast and gastrointestinal tract tumors. It has indolent behavior with low metastatic potential.

Apocrine Carcinoma: also known as apocrine adenocarcinoma, it predominates in the armpit, fifth to sixth decades, without predilection for sex or race. Size around 2 cm, painless, relatively slow growth until it was noticed by the patient. Distinguishing it from a breast tumor is primordial. Indication for SN research is debatable [18]. They usually present as intradermal lesions with cells with finely granular eosinophilic cytoplasm, showing tubular, tubulopapillary, or solid patterns, often with lymphovascular invasion.

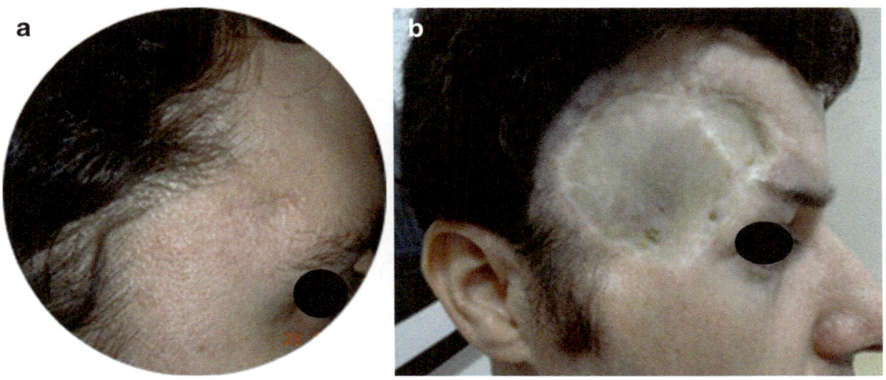

Fig. 17.6 (**a**) Young man with third recurrence aspect of microcystic adnexal carcinoma of right temporal region (Sept 2007). (**b**) The same patient after 12 years and three more resections, the last one in 2009

Among the tumors with *follicular differentiation*, we are going to mention the *pilomatrical carcinoma* [6] (malignant pilomatricoma, matrical carcinoma, matrix carcinoma, and pilomatrix carcinoma are synonyms) whose benign counterpart is the calcified epithelioma of Malherbe. It occurs after the age of 50 years, present as a single, often ulcerated nodule, predominant on the face. Histologic examination shows dermal lobules, with keratin and ghost cells, filaments, and serpiginous strands of basaloid cells with nuclear pleomorphism and numerous mitosis. Presence of infiltrative pattern and mass necrosis are common findings. Basal cell carcinoma with matrix distinction is the most common differential diagnosis.

Surgical treatment of these types of tumors is the gold standard, always after confirmed by biopsy and histological analysis.

The primary tumor must be submitted to wide and three-dimensional margins, with 1.0–2.0 cm distance beyond the tumor [7].

Always Try the Simplest Reconstruction. In the case of Fig. 17.7a–d, the flap slippage and suturing were adequate, but we used skin grafting to repair a relapsed eccrine carcinoma of the scalp of Fig. 17.8a–c, also with good evolution, allowing the repair to be done after proper examination of the resection margins.

Depending on the professional experience and in areas where tissue preservation is imperative, surgery with microscopically controlled margins (Mohs or similar) has gained a lot of space [7, 17].

The use of sentinel lymph node research can be indicated in specific cases, but there is not enough literature for its inclusion in the therapeutic routine [7, 18, 19]. Classic lymphadenectomy is indicated in cases of clinically compromised lymph nodes.

For the treatment of malignant tumors with sebaceous differentiation, the surgical strategy does not change. Remember that we have components from pilosebaceous apparatus, with tumors starting from the sebaceous unit (duct or gland) and those starting from the apocrine gland.

Among these starting from apocrine glands, *sebaceous carcinoma* [17] can occur anywhere but is predominant on the eyelids, with an average age of 62 years. It presents as a painless nodule on the eyelid border or conjunctiva (Fig. 17.9a–d). Differential diagnosis should include squamous cell carcinoma, basal cell carcinoma, Paget disease, melanoma, and metastasis. Always remember to look for signs of Muir–Torre syndrome [20].

Among the *"site"-specific tumors*, we find those predominating in mammary region and anal genital region tissue, including extramammary Paget disease, adenocarcinoma of anogenital mammary-like glands, hidradenoma papilliferum, fibroadenoma of anogenital mammary-like glands, and phyllodes tumor of anogenital mammary-like glands.

Extramammary Paget can be a primary cutaneous adenocarcinoma or be a secondary involvement of a gastrointestinal or urinary tract tumor. When primary, its cell of origin is an epidermal extension of an adenocarcinoma originated from apocrine or eccrine glands, or it may originate from stem cells or even from Toker cells. Its clinical appearance takes the form of well-demarcated eczematous plaques, predominantly in the anal genital region. Its differential diagnosis is with squamous

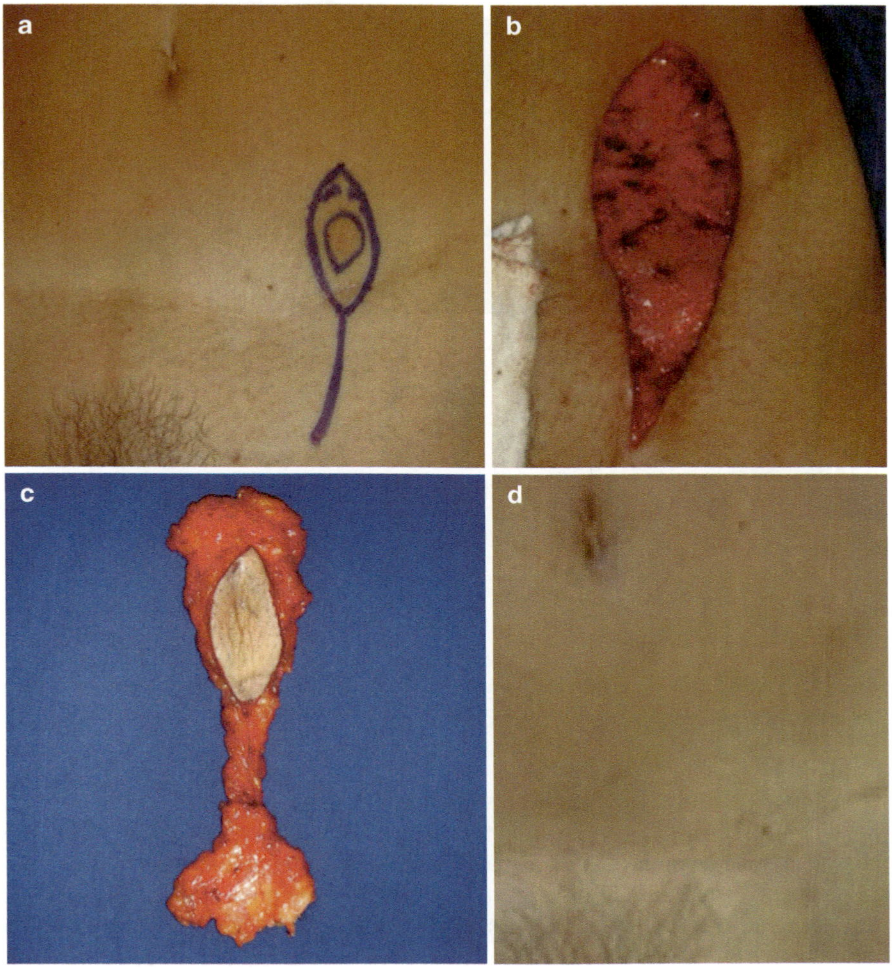

Fig. 17.7 (**a**) Eccrine carcinoma of the abdominal wall of an adult woman (clinical aspect—Aug 2005). (**b**) Surgical aspect after resection of the patient of (**a**). (**c**) Surgical piece of the patient of (**a**). (**d**) Clinical aspect of the patient of (**a**), 16 years later

cell carcinoma and amelanotic melanoma. Preferential surgical treatment of the primary lesion is wide excision with 1.0 cm margins. Surgery with microscopically controlled margins has been progressively more used. Associating sentinel lymph node research is still a controversial issue. An example of a patient with extramammary Paget is shown in Fig. 17.10a–d.

The absence of a standard practice related to surgical management (margins and indication of sentinel lymph node research) also happens regarding systemic treatment and radiotherapy. Under these aspects, the lack of randomized studies remains.

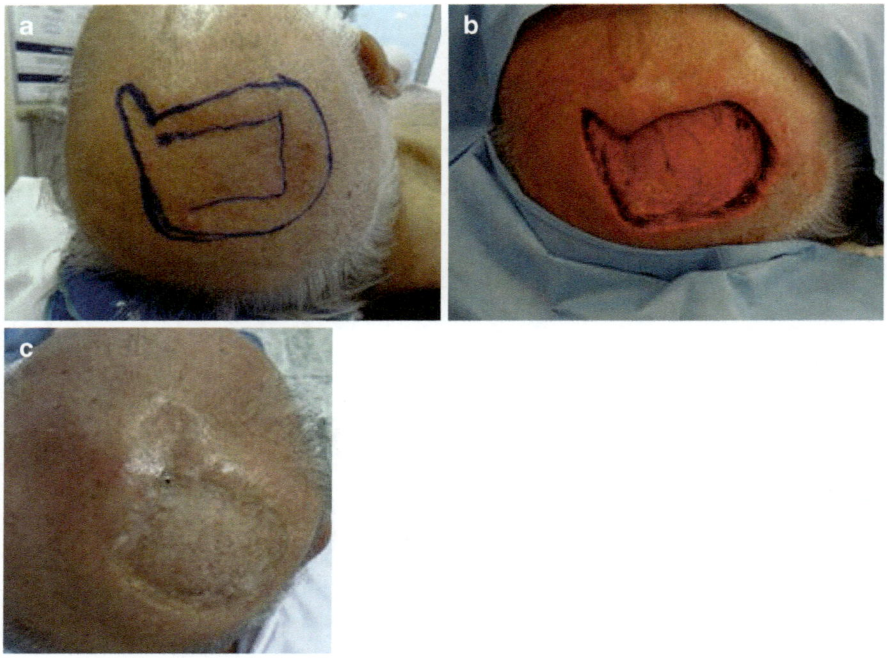

Fig. 17.8 (**a**) Recurrent eccrine carcinoma of the scalp with margins delineated in a 70-year-old man. (**b**) Surgical aspect after resection of the patient of (**a**). (**c**) Same patient of (**a**) after 2 years

Adjuvant radiotherapy has been supported by some authors in search of better local control results. The indication for this type of treatment is based on high-risk characteristics as tumors greater than 5 cm, angiolymphatic and perineural invasion, positive margins, high-grade tumors, multifocal presentation, lymph node involvement, and local relapse. These high-risk criteria are similar of that used for other, better-known non-melanoma skin tumors, such as squamous cell carcinoma [21, 22].

Adjuvant systemic treatment is not usually indicated.

In the metastatic setting, systemic treatment with platinum-based chemotherapy is commonly reported. Specific situations may bring rationale from other therapies such as anti-PDL1 immunotherapy in sebaceous carcinomas with microsatellite instability (Muir–Torre syndrome) and anti-estrogen hormone therapy in sudoriferous carcinomas with hormone receptors positive by immunohistochemistry [23–25].

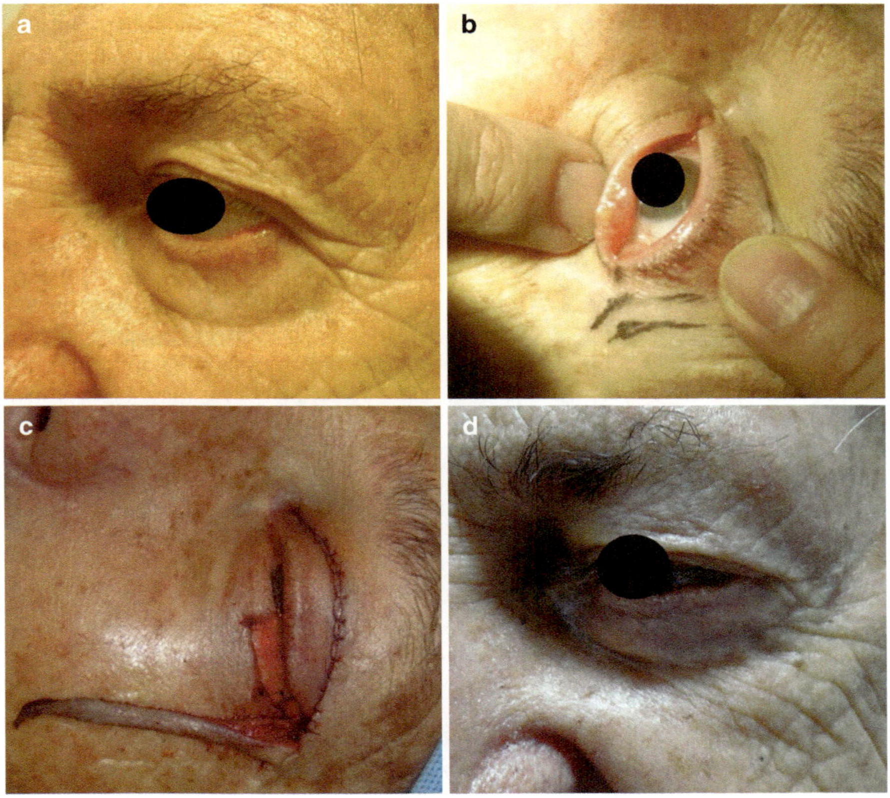

Fig. 17.9 (**a**) Sebaceous carcinoma of the left lower eyelid (2006). (**b**) Mucosal aspect of the same lesion of the patient of (**a**). (**c**) Surgical bed and the upper eyelid flap of the patient of (**a**) (courtesy of pro. Max Pereira). (**d**) Evolution after 5 years of patient of (**a**)

Follow-Up and Prognostic

The monitoring of patients with malignant adnexal tumors should be quarterly in the first year (always complete physical examination, chest X-ray, and ultrasound of the drainage areas every 6 months), biannually in the second until the fifth year, and annually thereafter, provided there is no manifestation of any relapse. More specific exams, such as tomography or nuclear magnetic resonance or even positron emission tomography (PET-CT), should be ordered in specific cases, based on the evolution of each patient.

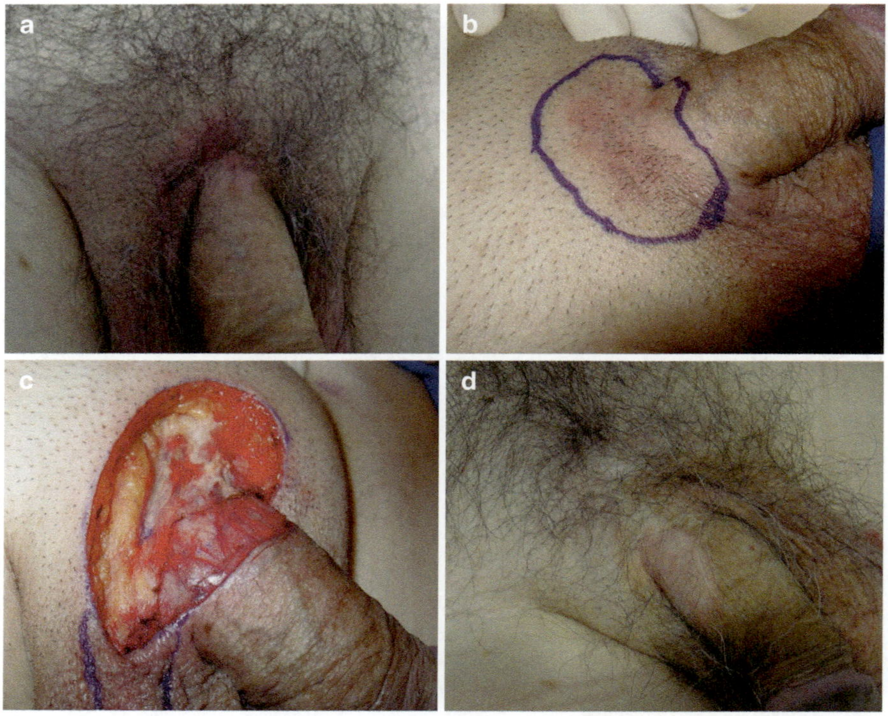

Fig. 17.10 (**a**) Extramammary Paget disease—pubic and inguinal region (2004) of a 65-year-old man. (**b**) Presurgical aspect the patient of (**a**). (**c**) Surgical aspect after immediate resection of the patient of (**a**). (**d**) Clinical aspect after 6 years of surgical resection of the patient of (**a**)

References

1. Danialan R, Mutyambizi K, Aung P, Prieto VG, Ivan D. Challenges in the diagnosis of cutaneous adnexal tumours. J Clin Pathol. 2015;68(12):992–1002. https://doi.org/10.1136/jclinpath-2015-203228.
2. Zaballos P, Gómez-Martín I, Martin JM, Bañuls J. Dermoscopy of adnexal tumors. Dermatol Clin. 2018;36(4):397–412. https://doi.org/10.1016/j.det.2018.05.007.
3. Mackie RM, Calonje E. Tumours of the skin appendages. In: Burns T, Breathnach S, Cox N, Griffiths C, editors. Rook's textbook of dermatology, vol. 2. 7th ed. London: Blackwell; 2004. p. 37.1–37.34. https://doi.org/10.1002/9780470750520.ch37.
4. Alsaad KO, Obaidat NA, Ghazarian D. Skin adnexal neoplasms—part 1: an approach to tumours of the pilosebaceous unit. J Clin Pathol. 2007;60(2):129–44. https://doi.org/10.1136/jcp.2006.040337.
5. Obaidat NA, Alsaad KO, Ghazarian D. Skin adnexal neoplasms—part 2: an approach to tumours of cutaneous sweat glands. J Clin Pathol. 2007;60(2):145–59. https://doi.org/10.1136/jcp.2006.041608.
6. Massi D, Cree IA, Elder DE, Kazakov DV, Scolyer RA. Appendageal tumours. In: Elder DE, Massi D, Scolyer RA, Willenze R, editors. WHO classification of skin tumours. 4th ed. Lyon: International Agency for Research on Cancer; 2018. p. 154–222.

7. Prieto-Granada C, Castner N, Chen A, Li J, Yue B, Wong JY, Iyengar S, Sondak VK, Zager JS, Messina JL. Behavior of cutaneous adnexal malignancies: a single institution experience. Pathol Oncol Res. 2020;26(1):239–44. https://doi.org/10.1007/s12253-018-0427-3.
8. Battistella M. Adnexal tumours: facing clinic-pathological challenges. In: Paper presented at the 15th EADO CONGRESS, Paris, France, 25 April 2019.
9. Mccalmont TH, Pincus LB. Adnexal neoplasms. In: Bolognia JL, Schaffer JV, Cerroni L, editors. Dermatology. 4th ed. Amsterdam: Elsevier; 2018. p. 1930–52.
10. Mester J, Eng C. Estimate of de novo mutation frequency in probands with PTEN hamartoma tumor syndrome. Genet Med. 2012;14(9):819–22. https://doi.org/10.1038/gim.2012.51.
11. Menko FH, van Steensel MA, Giraud S, Friis-Hansen L, Richard S, Ungari S, Nordenskjöld M, Hansen TV, Solly J, Maher ER, European BHD Consortium. Birt–Hogg–Dubé syndrome: diagnosis and management. Lancet Oncol. 2009;10(12):1199–206. https://doi.org/10.1016/S1470-2045(09)70188-3.
12. Papageorgiou V, Apalla Z, Sotiriou E, Papageorgiou C, Lazaridou E, Vakirlis S, Ioannides D, Lallas A. The limitations of dermoscopy: false-positive and false-negative tumours. J Eur Acad Dermatol Venereol. 2018;32(6):879–88. https://doi.org/10.1111/jdv.14782.
13. Kazakov DV. Brooke–Spiegler syndrome and phenotypic variants: an update. Head Neck Pathol. 2016;10(2):125–30. https://doi.org/10.1007/s12105-016-0705-x.
14. Lallas A, Moscarella E, Argenziano G, Longo C, Apalla Z, Ferrara G, Piana S, Rosato S, Zalaudek I. Dermoscopy of uncommon skin tumours. Australas J Dermatol. 2014;55(1):53–62. https://doi.org/10.1111/ajd.12074.
15. Messina JL. Adnexal primary or metastatic carcinoma? Paper presented at the HemOnctoday melanoma and cutaneous malignancies. New York, NY, 18 March 2016.
16. Schwartz RA. Cutaneous metastatic disease. J Am Acad Dermatol. 1995;33(2 Pt 1):161–82. https://doi.org/10.1016/0190-9622(95)90231-7.
17. North JP, McCalmont TH, Ruben BS. Cutaneous adnexal tumours. In: Robinson JK, Corona R, editors. UpToDate pathways®. Waltham: Wolters Kluwer; 2021.
18. Sekine C, Kawase K, Yoshida K. Sentinel lymph node biopsy of primary apocrine sweat gland carcinoma of the axilla: a case report and review of the literature. Int J Surg Case Rep. 2020;77:122–5. https://doi.org/10.1016/j.ijscr.2020.10.067.
19. Goyal A, Marghitu T, Goyal N, Rubin N, Patel K, Goyal K, O'Leary D, Bohjanen K, Maher I. Surgical management and lymph-node biopsy of rare malignant cutaneous adnexal carcinomas: a population-based analysis of 7591 patients. Arch Dermatol Res. 2020;313(8):623–32. https://doi.org/10.1007/s00403-020-02143-5.
20. Ponti G, Ponz de Leon M. Muir–Torre syndrome. Lancet Oncol. 2005;6(12):980–7. https://doi.org/10.1016/S1470-2045(05)70465-4.
21. Wang LS, Handorf EA, Wu H, Liu JC, Perlis CS, Galloway TJ. Surgery and adjuvant radiation for high-risk skin adnexal carcinoma of the head and neck. Am J Clin Oncol. 2017;40(4):429–32. https://doi.org/10.1097/COC.0000000000000178.
22. Chamberlain RS, Huber K, White JC, Travaglino-Parda R. Apocrine gland carcinoma of the axilla: review of the literature and recommendations for treatment. Am J Clin Oncol. 1999;22(2):131–5. https://doi.org/10.1097/00000421-199904000-00005.
23. Domingo-Musibay E, Murugan P, Giubellino A, Sharma S, Steinberger D, Yuan J, Hunt MA, Lou E, Miller JS. Near complete response to Pembrolizumab in microsatellite-stable metastatic sebaceous carcinoma. J Immunother Cancer. 2018;6(1):58. https://doi.org/10.1186/s40425-018-0357-3.
24. Robson A, Lazar AJ, Ben Nagi J, Hanby A, Grayson W, Feinmesser M, Granter SR, Seed P, Warneke CL, McKee PH, Calonje E. Primary cutaneous apocrine carcinoma: a clinicopathologic analysis of 24 cases. Am J Surg Pathol. 2008;32(5):682–90. https://doi.org/10.1097/PAS.0b013e3181590ba4.
25. Seong MK, Kim EK, Han K, Seol H, Kim HA, Noh WC. Primary apocrine sweat gland carcinomas of the axilla: a report of two cases and a review of the literature. World J Surg Oncol. 2015;13:59. https://doi.org/10.1186/s12957-015-0473-1.

Chapter 18
Merkel Cell Carcinoma

Andreia Cristina de Melo, Mariana Petaccia de Macedo, and Frederico José Ribeiro Teixeira Junior Teixeira

Key Points

- Merkel cell carcinoma (MCC) is one of the most aggressive poorly differentiated malignant neuroendocrine neoplasms.
- There are two genomic groups: one related to the integration of Merkel cell polyomavirus (MCPyV) and the other one of DNA damage secondary to ultraviolet (UV) light.
- Clinically presents as a solitary, rapidly growing, non-tender, red or violet nodule in an immunocompromised individual or in a sun-exposed skin of an elderly, fair-skinned patient.
- The diagnosis of MCC may be challenging for the pathologist.
- Surgery is often the first-line treatment for localized MCC. Adjuvant radiotherapy (RT) to the primary tumor site is often recommended or as an alternative option.
- Immunotherapy using checkpoint inhibitors is the favored starting treatment approach for advanced or metastatic MCC.

A. C. de Melo (✉)
Division of Clinical Research and Technological Development, Brazilian National Cancer Institute, INCA, Rio de Janeiro, Brazil
e-mail: andreia.melo@inca.gov.br

M. P. de Macedo
Laboratory of Pathology, Hospital Sírio-Libanês, São Paulo, Brazil

F. J. R. T. J. Teixeira
Surgical Oncology, General Surgery Service, Hospital das Clínicas, Faculdade de Medicina da Universidade de São Paulo, São Paulo, Brazil

C. M. Z. Abdalla et al. (eds.), *Oncodermatology*,
https://doi.org/10.1007/978-3-031-29277-4_18

Epidemiology

Since the first description of Merkel cell carcinoma (MCC) in 1972, the understanding of the biology and the management of patients has advanced substantially [1]. MCCs are most frequently found in the dermis but can arise from intraepidermal to subcutaneous layers [2]. Currently, no consensus has been reached regarding the most likely candidate for the MCC cell of origin.

The incidence of MCC in the USA, some European countries, and Australia increased substantially after 2000; the reason is unclear but might be related to an aging population and improvements in diagnostic recognition [3, 4]. Australia currently has the highest reported incidence of MCC (up to 1.6 cases per 100,000 person-years) [5].

MCC arises almost exclusively in those of advanced age and 90% of patients are >50 years of age. The median age of presentation falls within the late seventh decade, but incidence continues to increase even as patients reach 80 or even 90 years of age [6]. MCC also has a higher incidence among immunosuppressed populations [7].

Risk Factors

Merkel cell carcinoma (MCC) is a poorly differentiated malignant neuroendocrine neoplasm and one of the most aggressive skin cancers. Synonyms for this neoplasm include trabecular carcinoma, Toker tumor, or primary neuroendocrine carcinoma of the skin [8–11]. Although similarities such as neuroendocrine nature point toward the Merkel cell as a potential cell of origin of MCC, some inconsistencies are evident. MCC is more commonly found as a dermal lesion, and its distribution is more common in sun-exposed area in counterpoint to the epidermis location of Merkel cell and its density normally being found in locations such as the hand and feet. No definitive proven cell of origin for MCC is established [12].

MCC may be divided into two well-described genomic groups: one related to the integration of Merkel cell polyomavirus (MCPyV) and the other one of DNA damage secondary to ultraviolet (UV) light. This distinction may represent the pathways of MCC formation. Approximately 80% of MCC are related to MCPyV infection, a virus described in 2008 that belongs to the family *Polyomaviridae* of double-stranded DNA viruses [9, 11, 13–15]. The mechanism of neoplastic transformation associated with the MCPyV includes two of its encoded proteins known as large T antigen (LT-ag) and small T antigen (ST-ag) and requires the integration of the viral genome into the host genome and truncation of the LT-ag [9].

The mutational findings differ among virus-positive MCC (VP-MCC) and virus-negative MCC (VN-MCC) groups. VP-MCC shows a lower mutation burden, while VN-MCC usually shows more mutations, an UV-associated signature, and recurrent mutations in tumor suppressor genes like *TP53* and *RB1* [9, 11, 14, 16, 17].

Risk factors for MCC development are reminiscent of the possible mechanisms distinguishing VP- and VN-MCC. Immunosuppression and old age are associated with a higher frequency of MCC and also white ethnicity. Global incidences of MCC are coincident with UV indices, and distribution of the lesions into the most common affected sites shows preferentially affection of sun-exposed areas. Immunosuppression may include HIV patients, solid organ transplantation, and those with immunosuppressive therapies such as in lymphoma treatment. To date, there is no proven germline predisposition syndrome associated with an increased incidence of MCC [9, 18].

Diagnosis: Dermatologic Assessment

MCC typically presents as a solitary, rapidly growing, non-tender, red or violet nodule in an immunocompromised individual or in a sun-exposed skin of an elderly, fair-skinned patient. However, up to 19% are present on the buttock or other minimally sun-exposed areas. The head and neck are the most common anatomic sites of the primary lesion followed by the lower limbs and upper extremities.

The clinical features are nonspecific, which often lead to confusion with a benign lesion. A cyst or acneiform lesion is the single most common presumptive diagnosis. Delay in diagnosis could allow disease progression, and early clinician recognition of this disease may improve survival rates [19]. Furthermore, up to 15% of patients with MCC will present with a tumor-positive lymph node without an unknown primary cutaneous tumor [20, 21].

The five most common clinical features are used to create an acronym AEIOU: asymptomatic/lack of tenderness, expanding rapidly (≤3 months), immunosuppression, older than age 50, and location on a UV-exposed site. Heath M et al. in a cohort of 195 patients described the first systematic analysis of the clinical features of MCC, 89% of patients met three or more criteria, 52% met four or more criteria, and 7% met all five criteria [6]. During the dermatological assessment, other clinical features, such as overlying scale and nearby actinic keratoses, solar lentigines, and telangiectasia, are common.

Diagnosis: Biopsy and Pathology

These tumors are often (>45%) indeterminate to clinically benign and unsuspected at the time of biopsy. Knowledge of MCC as a diagnostic possibility in solitary cutaneous growths and attention to the clinical description of a nodular lesion should encourage the surgeon to perform a deeper or excisional biopsy [22].

MCC is currently classified in the fourth edition of the WHO classification of skin tumors under the keratinocytic/epidermal tumors, different from the previous edition, where it was listed under neural tumors [8].

The diagnosis of MCC may be challenging for the pathologist. MCC usually presents in the microscope as a highly cellular dermal lesion and may be characterized either as a well-circumscribed nodule or infiltrative lesion, composed of poorly differentiated uniform round cells with scarce cytoplasm. Cells are usually small to intermediate in size and may also be arranged in a trabecular architecture. The nuclear detail shows neuroendocrine features such as salt and pepper chromatin. Mitoses are very common and necrosis may be found. Additional findings include hyperchromasia, nuclei molding, and crush artifact commonly seen in neuroendocrine neoplasms. Rarely it may also show epidermotropic growth [8–10].

The majority of MCC rise as a single lesion, but the association to other neoplasms such as basal cell carcinoma, adnexal tumors, and especially squamous cell carcinoma is well described and usually not associated with MCPyV infection [23].

A wide range of other neoplasms comprises the histological differential diagnosis of MCC, including but not limited to the following: lymphoma, poorly differentiated carcinomas, metastatic neuroendocrine neoplasms, melanoma, neuroblastoma, Ewing sarcoma, and basal cell carcinoma. Immunohistochemical studies are very helpful and almost mandatory in diagnosing MCC, especially when in the metastatic scenario. Classically MCC shows positivity for epithelial markers such as CAM5.2, AE1/AE3, cytokeratin 20 (CK20), 34BE12, and EMA and also for neuroendocrine markers such as chromogranin, synaptophysin, and CD56. TTF-1 positivity is a useful marker for confirming a small cell neuroendocrine carcinoma metastatic from the lung. CK20 is a very helpful marker in MCC revealing a very characteristic paranuclear dot representing the keratin filaments grouped around the nuclei (Fig. 18.1). Despite a wide range of useful IHC markers, still many MCC remains diagnosed solely as a high-grade neuroendocrine carcinoma when in the metastatic scenario [8, 9, 11, 18, 24, 25].

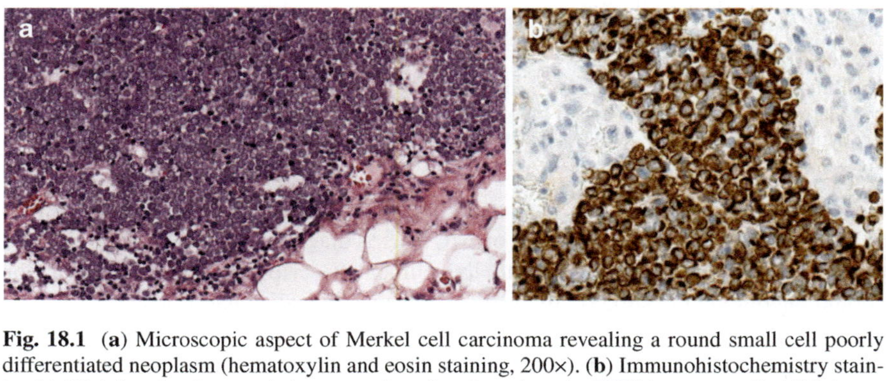

Fig. 18.1 (**a**) Microscopic aspect of Merkel cell carcinoma revealing a round small cell poorly differentiated neoplasm (hematoxylin and eosin staining, 200×). (**b**) Immunohistochemistry staining highlighting the characteristic paranuclear dot of cytokeratin CK20 in tumor cells (400×)

Risk Stratification and Staging

MCC is currently staged following the AJCC eighth edition. The pTNM pathology staging is based on findings from the primary tumor and the lymph nodes metastatic status. Primary tumor staging is based on the tumor clinical diameter and also the degree of infiltration into the skin layers and adjacent structures. Lymph node staging is based on the detection or not of metastatic cells in the lymph node parenchyma and further divided into those detected clinically, radiologically, or only by histopathology. Lymph node staging is also influenced by the presence or not of in-transit metastasis [26].

Other histopathological parameters are relevant for prognosis, including depth of tumor infiltration, tumor growth pattern, mitotic count, intratumoral lymphocytes, presence of secondary malignancy, and the other variables common to most other malignant tumors such as perineural and vascular invasion. These variables show a correlation to poor prognosis [8].

Tumor depth of infiltration is measured from the granular layer to the deepest infiltrative MCC neoplastic cell, and the greater the depth is correlated to a worst tumor behavior. MCC may present as either a nodular or an infiltrative lesion. The nodular pattern is of a well-delineated, circumscribed, solid, or polypoid lesion. The infiltrative pattern is characterized by isolated cells infiltrating the collagen, with trabecula or strands of cells, and correlated to poorer prognosis in MCC (Fig. 18.2).

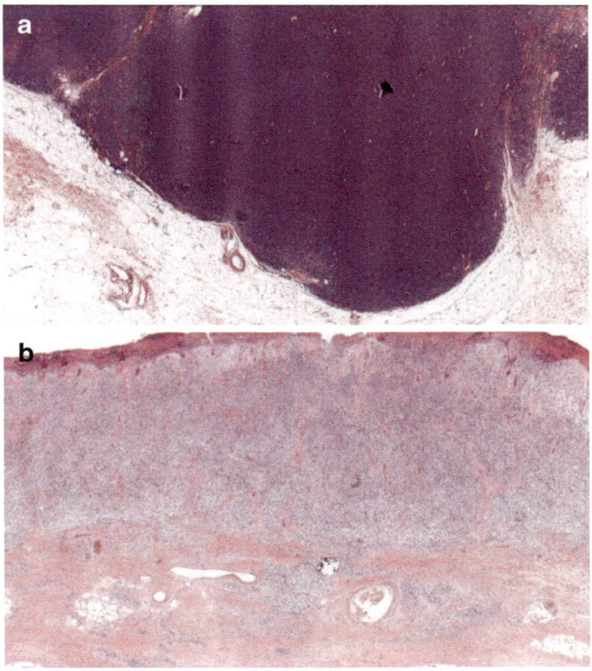

Fig. 18.2 Microscopic findings (hematoxylin and eosin) of the growth patterns observed in Merkel cell carcinoma. (**a**) Nodular growth pattern characterized by a well-delineated circumscribed lesion (200×), in contrast to infiltrative pattern in (**b**) highlighting a poorly delineated infiltrative lesion (100×)

The mitotic index correlates with tumor size and prognosis and should be reported as a number of mitoses per square millimeters (mm^2) [9, 10, 18, 25, 27, 28].

The lymph node status is a very important predictor of survival and risk of metastasis in MCC, and it should be completely represented in macroscopy for microscopic representation. For negative cases analyzed by hematoxylin and eosin (H&E), multiple new levels of H&E staining and IHC should be performed to allow small microscopic disease [26].

Treatment of Localized Disease

Surgery

Surgery is often the first-line treatment for localized MCC, as complete excision significantly improves overall survival [29]. Local treatment of MCC often includes wide excision of the primary site, which can lead to significant morbidity and delayed wound healing. Surgical excision with 1–2 cm margins is typically recommended. However, the effect of surgical margin size on local recurrence or survival remains controversial.

For patients without clinically detectable metastatic disease, sentinel lymph node biopsy (SLN) sampling is recommended because the presence of occult regional lymph nodal involvement (16–38%) is one of the most important prognostic factors [28, 30–32].

Because of this high incidence of occult nodal disease, SLN biopsy has become the standard of care in patients without clinically apparent lymphadenopathy and is recommended by the National Comprehensive Cancer Network (NCCN) [18, 19].

In a recent systematic review and meta-analysis, the SLN status was a strong predictor of overall survival (OS) and disease-free survival (DFS) in MCC patients. SLN biopsy predicted better OS and DFS as compared to the nodal observation in cN0 MCC patients. Pathologically negative SLN patients had significantly better OS and DFS as compared to SLN-positive patients. SLN-positive patients may suffer MCC-related death and recurrence 4.42 and 2.58 times more frequently per unit time than SLN-negative patients [33].

Recently, the Mayo Clinic experience of 150 patients who underwent SLN biopsy was published. Occult nodal metastasis is common in MCC (26%). Patients with positive SLN had almost twice the incidence of regional and distant recurrences. No clinical or pathological factors could identify a population at sufficiently low enough risk for occult nodal metastasis to safely omit SLN biopsy. Therefore, SLN biopsy should be recommended for all patients with primary MCC and no clinical evidence of lymphadenopathy [34].

Adjuvant Radiotherapy

MCC has long been known to be highly radiosensitive [35]. Adjuvant radiotherapy (RT) to the primary tumor site is often recommended as few retrospective studies have shown improvement in DFS with the addition of radiation treatment to the primary site [36]. However, the morbidity risks associated with RT can be avoided with a low local recurrence rate in a subset of patients (such as those with tumors <2 cm in size without other adverse prognostic features) [37].

In a study of 179 Canadian patients, among those who had a narrow excision (<1 cm), adjuvant RT was associated with a lower local recurrence rate (25% vs. 5%, $p = 0.03$). For patients who had more than 1 cm margins, local recurrence was 7% regardless of whether the patient received adjuvant RT or not [38].

In another recent study including 188 MCC patients without clinical nodal involvement, surgical margins of more than 1 cm were associated with a lower local recurrence rate among patients who underwent surgery alone. However, for patients who received adjuvant RT, local control was excellent (1% local recurrence) regardless of surgical margin size even for patients who had microscopically positive margins [39].

For large primary MCCs, if surgical resection is not feasible, definitive RT can be considered as an alternative option. In such cases, the in-field disease control rate for definitive RT (60–66 Gy) is about 70–80% [40].

The decision on management following SLN biopsy is more challenging. The NCCN guidelines for use of adjuvant radiation in the case of a negative SLN are broad, leaving the option of observation versus adjuvant radiation in "high-risk" patients (e.g., profound immunosuppression or inaccurate SLN mapping) [18]. While the use of adjuvant radiation may decrease the risk of locoregional recurrence in some patients with MCC, no benefit has been proven in this specific low-risk population [36]. Some groups of experts do not routinely recommend adjuvant radiation to the nodal basin in patients with a negative SLN [34].

When patients have positive sentinel lymph nodes, the question about how to manage them is more difficult. Most would agree that definitive treatment with either completion nodal dissection, radiation to the nodal field, or both should be performed. However, if multimodality therapy to the nodal basis is necessary stills an answered question. The NCCN recommends the management of clinically detectable or occult nodal disease using imaging investigations for distant metastases, followed by lymph node dissection and/or radiotherapy to the nodal basin [18].

For patients with clinical nodal involvement, pathologic confirmation of lymph node involvement is recommended before the completion of lymphadenectomy. In the setting of clinical evident lymph node disease, few authors have shown improvement in regional recurrence rates with the addition of adjuvant radiation [41–43].

Due to the low number of patients and heterogeneous use of adjuvant radiation, it is impossible to determine if there is any benefit to multimodality treatment to the positive nodal basin. One small prospective study with a mixed population of clinical and occult regional disease includes radiation alone, completion nodal dissection, or completion nodal dissection with adjuvant radiation as modalities of treatment. In this study Fang et al. described 50 patients with regional nodal disease, none of the patients with microscopic disease developed recurrence, and there was no statistically significant difference between recurrence rates, regardless of treatment modality, in the group with clinically palpable nodes [44]. In another study conducted by Jouary et al., patients without clinical evidence of nodal metastasis were randomized to either adjuvant radiation or observation. The group receiving adjuvant radiation did show a significant decrease in regional recurrence. However, the study was stopped early due to a drop in recruitment with increased use of SLN biopsy in MCC [45].

Adjuvant Chemotherapy or Chemoradiotherapy

The role of adjuvant chemotherapy (alone or in combination with radiotherapy) after surgery in MCC is controversial, and there are no prospective trials. A retrospective study evaluated 4815 patients diagnosed with MCC of the head and neck between 1998 and 2011. A total of 1995 patients received surgery alone, 2330 were treated with adjuvant radiotherapy, 393 received the combination of chemotherapy and radiotherapy after surgery, and 97 received adjuvant chemotherapy alone. Adjuvant chemoradiotherapy and radiotherapy alone provided a survival benefit compared with surgery with no additional treatment (HR 0.62, 95% CI 0.47–0.81, and HR 0.80, 95% CI 0.70–0.92, respectively), and the adjuvant chemotherapy alone was associated with lower overall survival (HR 1.74, 95% CI 1.10–2.75) [46].

Adjuvant and Neoadjuvant Immunotherapy

So far, there are limited data on the use of immunotherapy in the adjuvant setting for MCC, and its use is being evaluated in randomized trials. The use of neoadjuvant immunotherapy in the management of patients with MCC remains also under investigation.

The CheckMate 358 is a multicohort trial investigating nivolumab alone or in combination in virus-associated solid tumors. Considering the MCC cohort, 39 patients with resectable stage IIA to IV disease received nivolumab at 240 mg on days 1 and 15, with surgery planned on day 29. Tumor response was assessed radiographically and pathologically. Among the 39 patients, 3 (7.7%) did not undergo surgery (1 due to progression and 2 due to adverse events). Of the 36 patients who underwent surgery, 17 had pathologic complete response (47.2%), and among 33 evaluable cases for a radiographic response, a tumor reduction of more than 30% was observed in 18 cases (54.5%). With a median follow-up of 20.3 months, the median recurrence-free survival was not reached, and the 12- and 24-month rates were 77.5% and 68.5%, respectively. The recurrence-free survival rates for patients with or without pathologic complete response were 100% versus 59.6% and 88.9% versus 52.2% for 12- and 24-month (HR 0.12, 95% CI 0.01–0.93). No patient with a pathologic complete response had tumor relapse during observation [47].

Treatment of Advanced Disease

Immunotherapy using checkpoint inhibitors is the favored starting treatment approach for advanced or metastatic MCC as it induces greater responses and survival compared to historical chemotherapy results. Avelumab (anti-PD-L1) and pembrolizumab (anti-PD-1) have been approved by the Food and Drug Administration to treat patients with advanced or metastatic MCC, in the first or subsequent lines.

A total of 88 patients have received avelumab (10 mg/kg every 2 weeks) in the JAVELIN Merkel 200 study—part A. In this phase II trial, all participants had received prior chemotherapy, and 40% of the patients had received two or more lines of cytotoxic chemotherapy. A total of 29 objective responses (33%) were observed (complete responses in 11%) [48].With a median follow-up of 65.1 months (range, 60.8–74.1 months), the median overall survival was 12.6 months (95% CI 7.5–17.1 months); the 48- and 60-month overall survival rates were 30% (95% CI 20–40%) and 26% (95% CI 17–36%), respectively [49].

A real-world experience with avelumab in patients with metastatic MCC from an expanded access program was recently reported. Patients with progressive disease during or after chemotherapy were considered eligible for the program. A total of 494 patients received avelumab, and among 240 evaluable patients, the objective response rate was 46.7% (complete response in 22.9%), and the disease control rate was 71.2% [50].

In the JAVELIN Merkel 200 study, part B, 29 previously untreated patients were treated with avelumab [51], and in a preplanned analysis, the objective response rate was 62%, with a durable response of at least 6 months in 83% of responding patients.

In a phase II study, 50 untreated stage III unresectable or metastatic MCC patients received pembrolizumab (2 mg/kg every 3 weeks) for up to 2 years [52]. With a median follow-up of 31.8 months, the overall response rate was 58% (complete response 30%, partial response 28%). The median progression-free survival was 16.8 months (95%CI 4.6–43.4), and the 3-year progression-free survival was 39.1%. The median overall survival was not reached, and the 3-year overall survival was 59.4% for all patients and 89.5% for patients with complete or partial response [53].

In a phase I/II trial, 25 patients who were treatment-naïve or who had received 1 to 2 prior systemic therapies received nivolumab (anti-PD-1) (240 mg every 2 weeks) [54]. The overall response rate was 68% considering the 22 response-evaluable patients (71% in untreated participants and 63% of patients with 1 to 2 prior lines).

In the case of not responding or relapsing to immunotherapy or for the patients with contraindication to immunotherapy, chemotherapy still has a role; however, data are not based on prospective trials. The combination of etoposide and carboplatin is often the initial treatment option, and alternative schemas are cyclophosphamide in combination with vincristine and doxorubicin or weekly carboplatin. Despite a relatively high response rate, the impact on survival of systemic chemotherapy in metastatic MCC is poor [55].

MCC is a radiosensitive tumor, and radiotherapy can be prescribed as a palliative option for symptomatic areas in patients not responding to systemic therapies [56].

Follow-Up

Because of the high rate of recurrence, patients diagnosed with MCC must be closely followed. The NCCN guidelines recommend physical examination (including lymph nodes palpation) every 3–6 months for 3 years and then every 6–12 months thereafter, and routine imaging should be considered for high-risk patients [18].

References

1. Toker C. Trabecular carcinoma of the skin. Arch Dermatol. 1972;105(1):107–10.
2. Harms PW. Update on Merkel cell carcinoma. Clin Lab Med. 2017;37(3):485–501.
3. Paulson KG, Park SY, Vandeven NA, Lachance K, Thomas H, Chapuis AG, et al. Merkel cell carcinoma: current US incidence and projected increases based on changing demographics. J Am Acad Dermatol. 2018;78(3):457–463.e2.
4. Stang A, Becker JC, Nghiem P, Ferlay J. The association between geographic location and incidence of Merkel cell carcinoma in comparison to melanoma: an international assessment. Eur J Cancer. 2018;94:47–60.
5. Schadendorf D, Lebbé C, Zur Hausen A, Avril M-F, Hariharan S, Bharmal M, et al. Merkel cell carcinoma: epidemiology, prognosis, therapy and unmet medical needs. Eur J Cancer. 2017;71:53–69.
6. Heath M, Jaimes N, Lemos B, Mostaghimi A, Wang LC, Peñas PF, et al. Clinical characteristics of Merkel cell carcinoma at diagnosis in 195 patients: the AEIOU features. J Am Acad Dermatol. 2008;58(3):375–81.
7. Ma J, Brewer J. Merkel cell carcinoma in immunosuppressed patients. Cancers. 2014;6(3):1328–50.
8. Elder D, Massi D, Scoyler R, Willemze R. WHO classification of skin tumors. 4th ed. Lyon: IARC; 2018.
9. Harms PW, Harms KL, Moore PS, DeCaprio JA, Nghiem P, Wong MKK, et al. The biology and treatment of Merkel cell carcinoma: current understanding and research priorities. Nat Rev Clin Oncol. 2018;15(12):763–76.
10. Andea AA, Coit DG, Amin B, Busam KJ. Merkel cell carcinoma: histologic features and prognosis. Cancer. 2008;113(9):2549–58.
11. Tetzlaff MT, Harms PW. Danger is only skin deep: aggressive epidermal carcinomas. An overview of the diagnosis, demographics, molecular-genetics, staging, prognostic biomarkers, and therapeutic advances in Merkel cell carcinoma. Mod Pathol. 2020;33(Suppl 1):42–55.

12. Kervarrec T, Samimi M, Guyétant S, Sarma B, Chéret J, Blanchard E, et al. Histogenesis of Merkel cell carcinoma: a comprehensive review. Front Oncol. 2019;9:451.
13. Feng H, Shuda M, Chang Y, Moore PS. Clonal integration of a polyomavirus in human Merkel cell carcinoma. Science. 2008;319(5866):1096–100.
14. Harms PW, Collie AMB, Hovelson DH, Cani AK, Verhaegen ME, Patel RM, et al. Next generation sequencing of Cytokeratin 20-negative Merkel cell carcinoma reveals ultraviolet-signature mutations and recurrent TP53 and RB1 inactivation. Mod Pathol. 2016;29(3):240–8.
15. Goh G, Walradt T, Markarov V, Blom A, Riaz N, Doumani R, et al. Mutational landscape of MCPyV-positive and MCPyV-negative Merkel cell carcinomas with implications for immunotherapy. Oncotarget. 2016;7(3):3403–15.
16. Mauzo SH, Ferrarotto R, Bell D, Torres-Cabala CA, Tetzlaff MT, Prieto VG, et al. Molecular characteristics and potential therapeutic targets in Merkel cell carcinoma. J Clin Pathol. 2016;69(5):382–90.
17. Moshiri AS, Doumani R, Yelistratova L, Blom A, Lachance K, Shinohara MM, et al. Polyomavirus-negative Merkel cell Carcinoma: a more aggressive subtype based on analysis of 282 cases using multimodal tumor virus detection. J Invest Dermatol. 2017;137(4):819–27.
18. https://www.nccn.org/professionals/physician_gls/pdf/mcc.pdf.
19. Bichakjian CK, Lowe L, Lao CD, Sandler HM, Bradford CR, Johnson TM, et al. Merkel cell carcinoma: critical review with guidelines for multidisciplinary management. Cancer. 2007;110(1):1–12.
20. Becker JC, Stang A, DeCaprio JA, Cerroni L, Lebbé C, Veness M, et al. Merkel cell carcinoma. Nat Rev Dis Primer. 2017;3(1):17077.
21. Vandeven N, Lewis CW, Makarov V, Riaz N, Paulson KG, Hippe D, et al. Merkel cell carcinoma patients presenting without a primary lesion have elevated markers of immunity, higher tumor mutation burden, and improved survival. Clin Cancer Res. 2018;24(4):963–71.
22. Pulitzer M. Merkel cell carcinoma. Surg Pathol Clin. 2017;10(2):399–408.
23. Busam KJ, Jungbluth AA, Rekthman N, Coit D, Pulitzer M, Bini J, et al. Merkel cell polyomavirus expression in Merkel cell carcinomas and its absence in combined tumors and pulmonary neuroendocrine carcinomas. Am J Surg Pathol. 2009;33(9):1378–85.
24. Llombart B, Monteagudo C, López-Guerrero JA, Carda C, Jorda E, Sanmartín O, et al. Clinicopathological and immunohistochemical analysis of 20 cases of Merkel cell carcinoma in search of prognostic markers. Histopathology. 2005;46(6):622–34.
25. Skelton HG, Smith KJ, Hitchcock CL, McCarthy WF, Lupton GP, Graham JH. Merkel cell carcinoma: analysis of clinical, histologic, and immunohistologic features of 132 cases with relation to survival. J Am Acad Dermatol. 1997;37(5 Pt 1):734–9.
26. Trinidad CM, Torres-Cabala CA, Prieto VG, Aung PP. Update on eighth edition American Joint Committee on Cancer classification for Merkel cell carcinoma and histopathological parameters that determine prognosis. J Clin Pathol. 2019;72(5):337–40.
27. Mott RT, Smoller BR, Morgan MB. Merkel cell carcinoma: a clinicopathologic study with prognostic implications. J Cutan Pathol. 2004;31(3):217–23.
28. Smith FO, Yue B, Marzban SS, Walls BL, Carr M, Jackson RS, et al. Both tumor depth and diameter are predictive of sentinel lymph node status and survival in Merkel cell carcinoma. Cancer. 2015;121(18):3252–60.
29. Tai PT, Yu E, Tonita J, Gilchrist J. Merkel cell carcinoma of the skin. J Cutan Med Surg. 2000;4(4):186–95.
30. Prieto Muñoz I, Pardo Masferrer J, Olivera Vegas J, Medina Montalvo MS, Jover Díaz R, Pérez Casas AM. Merkel cell carcinoma from 2008 to 2012: reaching a new level of understanding. Cancer Treat Rev. 2013;39(5):421–9.
31. Smith VA, Camp ER, Lentsch EJ. Merkel cell carcinoma: identification of prognostic factors unique to tumors located in the head and neck based on analysis of SEER data. Laryngoscope. 2012;122(6):1283–90.
32. Lemos BD, Storer BE, Iyer JG, Phillips JL, Bichakjian CK, Fang LC, et al. Pathologic nodal evaluation improves prognostic accuracy in Merkel cell carcinoma: analysis of 5823 cases as the basis of the first consensus staging system. J Am Acad Dermatol. 2010;63(5):751–61.

33. Sadeghi R, Adinehpoor Z, Maleki M, Fallahi B, Giovanella L, Treglia G. Prognostic significance of sentinel lymph node mapping in Merkel cell carcinoma: systematic review and meta-analysis of prognostic studies. Biomed Res Int. 2014;2014:1–9.
34. Sims JR, Grotz TE, Pockaj BA, Joseph RW, Foote RL, Otley CC, et al. Sentinel lymph node biopsy in Merkel cell carcinoma: the Mayo Clinic experience of 150 patients. Surg Oncol. 2018;27(1):11–7.
35. Leonard JH, Ramsay JR, Kearsley JH, Birrell GW. Radiation sensitivity of Merkel cell carcinoma cell lines. Int J Radiat Oncol Biol Phys. 1995;32(5):1401–7.
36. Rush Z, Fields RC, Lee N, Brownell I. Radiation therapy in the management of Merkel cell carcinoma: current perspectives. Expert Rev Dermatol. 2011;6(4):395–404.
37. Frohm ML, Griffith KA, Harms KL, Hayman JA, Fullen DR, Nelson CC, et al. Recurrence and survival in patients with Merkel cell carcinoma undergoing surgery without adjuvant radiation therapy to the primary site. JAMA Dermatol. 2016;152(9):1001–7.
38. Harrington C, Kwan W. Radiotherapy and conservative surgery in the locoregional management of Merkel cell carcinoma: the British Columbia Cancer Agency experience. Ann Surg Oncol. 2016;23(2):573–8.
39. Tarabadkar ES, Fu T, Lachance K, Hippe DS, Pulliam T, Thomas H, et al. Narrow excision margins are appropriate for Merkel cell carcinoma when combined with adjuvant radiation: analysis of 188 cases of localized disease and proposed management algorithm. J Am Acad Dermatol. 2021;84(2):340–7.
40. Sundaresan P, Hruby G, Hamilton A, Hong A, Boyer M, Chatfield M, et al. Definitive radiotherapy or chemoradiotherapy in the treatment of Merkel cell carcinoma. Clin Oncol (R Coll Radiol). 2012;24(9):e131–6.
41. Lee J, Poon I, Balogh J, Tsao M, Barnes E. A review of radiotherapy for Merkel cell carcinoma of the head and neck. J Skin Cancer. 2012;2012:1–6.
42. Veness MJ. Merkel cell carcinoma: improved outcome with the addition of adjuvant therapy. J Clin Oncol. 2005;23(28):7235–6; author reply 7237–8.
43. Foote M, Harvey J, Porceddu S, Dickie G, Hewitt S, Colquist S, et al. Effect of radiotherapy dose and volume on relapse in Merkel cell cancer of the skin. Int J Radiat Oncol Biol Phys. 2010;77(3):677–84.
44. Fang LC, Lemos B, Douglas J, Iyer J, Nghiem P. Radiation monotherapy as regional treatment for lymph node-positive Merkel cell carcinoma. Cancer. 2010;116(7):1783–90.
45. Jouary T, Leyral C, Dreno B, Doussau A, Sassolas B, Beylot-Barry M, et al. Adjuvant prophylactic regional radiotherapy versus observation in stage I Merkel cell carcinoma: a multicentric prospective randomized study. Ann Oncol. 2012;23(4):1074–80.
46. Chen MM, Roman SA, Sosa JA, Judson BL. The role of adjuvant therapy in the management of head and neck Merkel cell carcinoma: an analysis of 4815 patients. JAMA Otolaryngol Head Neck Surg. 2015;141(2):137–41.
47. Topalian SL, Bhatia S, Amin A, Kudchadkar RR, Sharfman WH, Lebbé C, et al. Neoadjuvant nivolumab for patients with resectable Merkel cell carcinoma in the CheckMate 358 trial. J Clin Oncol. 2020;38(22):2476–87.
48. Kaufman HL, Russell JS, Hamid O, Bhatia S, Terheyden P, D'Angelo SP, et al. Updated efficacy of avelumab in patients with previously treated metastatic Merkel cell carcinoma after ≥1 year of follow-up: JAVELIN Merkel 200, a phase 2 clinical trial. J Immunother Cancer. 2018;6(1):7.
49. Nghiem P, Bhatia S, Brohl AS, Hamid O, Mehnert JM, Terheyden P, et al. Avelumab in patients with previously treated Merkel cell carcinoma (JAVELIN Merkel 200): updated overall survival data after more than five years of follow up. J Clin Oncol. 2021;39(15_Suppl):9517.
50. Walker JW, Lebbé C, Grignani G, Nathan P, Dirix L, Fenig E, et al. Efficacy and safety of avelumab treatment in patients with metastatic Merkel cell carcinoma: experience from a global expanded access program. J Immunother Cancer. 2020;8(1):e000313.

51. D'Angelo SP, Russell J, Lebbé C, Chmielowski B, Gambichler T, Grob J-J, et al. Efficacy and safety of first-line avelumab treatment in patients with stage IV metastatic Merkel cell carcinoma: a preplanned interim analysis of a clinical trial. JAMA Oncol. 2018;4(9):e180077.
52. Nghiem P, Bhatia S, Lipson EJ, Sharfman WH, Kudchadkar RR, Brohl AS, et al. Durable tumor regression and overall survival in patients with advanced Merkel cell carcinoma receiving pembrolizumab as first-line therapy. J Clin Oncol. 2019;37(9):693–702.
53. Nghiem P, Bhatia S, Lipson EJ, Sharfman WH, Kudchadkar RR, Brohl AS, et al. Three-year survival, correlates and salvage therapies in patients receiving first-line pembrolizumab for advanced Merkel cell carcinoma. J Immunother Cancer. 2021;9(4):e002478.
54. Topalian SL, Bhatia S, Hollebecque A, Awada A, Boer JPD, Kudchadkar RR, et al. Abstract CT074: Non-comparative, open-label, multiple cohort, phase 1/2 study to evaluate nivolumab (NIVO) in patients with virus-associated tumors (CheckMate 358): efficacy and safety in Merkel cell carcinoma (MCC). In: Clinical trials [Internet]. American Association for Cancer Research; 2017. p. CT074. http://cancerres.aacrjournals.org/lookup/doi/10.1158/1538-7445.AM2017-CT074.
55. Iyer JG, Blom A, Doumani R, Lewis C, Tarabadkar ES, Anderson A, et al. Response rates and durability of chemotherapy among 62 patients with metastatic Merkel cell carcinoma. Cancer Med. 2016;5(9):2294–301.
56. Iyer JG, Parvathaneni U, Gooley T, Miller NJ, Markowitz E, Blom A, et al. Single-fraction radiation therapy in patients with metastatic Merkel cell carcinoma. Cancer Med. 2015;4(8):1161–70.

Chapter 19
Cutaneous Malignancies of Mesenchymal Origin: Sarcomas

Alessandra Corte Real Salgues, Mauricio Fernando Ribeiro, Fabio de Oliveira Ferreira, Carlos Diego Holanda Lopes, Luiz Guilherme Cernaglia Aureliano de Lima, and Caio Lamounier

Key Points
- Cutaneous sarcomas are a heterogenous group of malignant mesenchymal neoplasms that originate at the dermis and subcutis.
- Dermatofibrosarcoma protuberans is the most common cutaneous sarcoma.
- Atypical fibroxanthoma is more common in elderlies and immunosuppressed patients in sun-exposed areas.
- Angiosarcomas are usually high-grade and occur primarily or associated with radiotherapy or chronic lymphedema (Stewart-Treves syndrome).
- Kaposi sarcoma is a vascular-derived malignancy classified as classic (sporadic), endemic, iatrogenic, AIDS-related, and MSM without HIV infection.

A. C. R. Salgues (✉) · C. D. H. Lopes
Oncology Center, Hospital Sírio-Libanês, São Paulo, São Paulo, Brazil

M. F. Ribeiro
Division of Medical Oncology and Hematology, Princess Margaret Cancer Center - University of Toronto, Toronto, Canada

F. de Oliveira Ferreira · L. G. C. A. de Lima
Oncology Center, Hospital Sírio-Libanês, São Paulo, São Paulo, Brazil

Instituto do Cancer do Estado de São Paulo, São Paulo, São Paulo, Brazil

C. Lamounier
Instituto do Cancer do Estado de São Paulo, São Paulo, São Paulo, Brazil

C. M. Z. Abdalla et al. (eds.), *Oncodermatology*,
https://doi.org/10.1007/978-3-031-29277-4_19

Dermatofibrosarcoma Protuberans

Epidemiology

First named as dermatofibrosarcoma protuberans (DFSP) by Hoffman in 1925, DFSP is a rare tumor, but one of the most common cutaneous sarcomas, with an overall incidence of 0.8–4.5 cases per million persons per year in the USA, accounting for 0.1% of all malignant tumors [1, 2].

Usually, DFSP is a low-grade sarcoma derived from dermal fibroblast characterized by indolent clinical course, with high local recurrence rates and infiltrative behavior, despite its low metastatic potential (less than 5% of cases) [3, 4]. Nevertheless, approximately 10–15% contain a high-grade sarcomatous component or can be prone to fibrosarcomatous transformation, increasing the risk of distant metastasis [1, 4].

The median age at diagnosis is between the third and fifth decades of life, with slightly higher incidence in Afro-Americans and conflicting data of gender predominance [1]. However, it has also been described in children and older adults, and giant cell fibroblastoma, an intermediate-grade soft tissue tumor of childhood, is considered a variant of DFSP, with similar genomic alterations [4].

More than 90% of the DFSP cases have a t(17;22) translocation that produces a platelet-derived growth factor beta (PDGFB)/collagen type 1A1 (COL1A1) fusion product, leading to the self-propagation of tumor cells, generating the rationale to use multikinase inhibitors to treat advanced disease [2].

Risk Factors

There is no specific risk factor for the development of DFSP, and it can arise in any part of skin, healthy or chronically damaged, being more common in the trunk (40–50%), followed by upper and lower extremity (30–40%), and less frequently in the head/neck (10–15%) and genitals [1, 3].

Diagnosis

Clinical findings of classic DFSP include a slowly-progressive painless cutaneous plaque, solitary or multiple, reddish-brown in color that, without treatment, usually progresses to ulcerated/bleeding nodules or masses [1, 5].

Less frequently, DFSP manifests as a pigmented variant called Bednar tumor, characterized by a pigmented cutaneous lesion with irregular surface [4].

Findings on dermoscopy include delicate pigmented network, vessels, structureless light brown areas, shiny white streaks, pink background coloration, and structureless hypo- or depigmented areas, being helpful to suspect DFSP (still unspecific), but definitive diagnosis depends on core or incisional biopsies [6].

Histologically, DFSP is characterized by a spindle-cell proliferation in a storiform or fascicular pattern, with low to moderate atypia, and mitotic rate that arises within the dermis and extends into subcutaneous, sometimes into muscle, fascia, and bone. DFSP has an infiltrative pattern as "honeycomb" or irregular fingerlike projections [1]. Occasionally, DFSP arises in the subcutaneous tissue, with limited dermis involvement [3]. Immunohistochemistry is usually CD34 positive and factor XIIIa negative, while in dermatofibromas, the main differential diagnosis, a converse staining pattern is found [1]. Higher mitotic rate, intense atypia, and necrosis suggest fibrosarcomatous transformation, which is frequently CD34 negative [2, 5].

Detection of *PDGFB/COL1A1* fusion using fluorescent in situ hybridization (FISH) or reverse transcription-polymerase chain reaction (RT-PCR) is not mandatory for diagnosis, but recommended in suspicious cases without immunohistochemical confirmation or in advanced cases before the multikinase inhibitor imatinib initiation [2]. The presence of *PDGFB/COL1A1* fusion is a predictive biomarker of response to treatment [7].

Staging

There is no standardized universal staging system for DFSP.

The Short German Guidelines for DFSP divided DFSP into three stages: stage I, localized tumor; stage II, lymph node metastasis; and stage III, distant spread. Both clinical and prognostic utilities for this classification are uncertain [8].

Other staging systems include the (1) American Joint Committee on Cancer (AJCC) staging system for soft tissue sarcoma, which analyzes tumor size, regional lymph node metastasis, distant metastasis, and definition of grade, dividing these tumors in four prognostic stage groups, and (2) the American Musculoskeletal Tumor Society (MSTS) staging system, which is based on histologic grade [9, 10].

Imaging studies for staging workup are not routinely indicated, unless there are signs and symptoms suggestive of metastatic disease, presence of adverse prognostic histologic patterns (like fibrosarcomatous transformation), or for recurrent tumors [11].

The NCCN suggests preoperative MRI for treatment planning, if extensive extracutaneous extension or recurrent tumor is suspected [11].

Treatment of Localized Disease

The optimal treatment for localized disease is surgical excision with negative margins. Status of surgical margins is the most important prognostic factor, with recurrence rates of roughly 50% for coincident margins and even higher ones for positive margins [1, 11].

The choice of surgical techniques depends on tumor size and localization, considering the achievement of negative margins, cosmetic and functional aspects. Treatment options include wide local excision (WLE) with 2–4 cm margins, Mohs micrographic surgery (MMS), and complete circumferential and peripheral deep margin assessment (CCPDMA) [1, 2].

There is no randomized controlled trial comparing those techniques, although retrospective analyses suggest lower recurrence rate (less than 1%) with MMS [12].

Given the infiltrative characteristic of DFSP, frequently invading surrounding tissue in the form of irregular fingerlike projections in a subclinical extension, it is recommended that WLE should be performed with 2–4-cm margins to investing the fascia, muscle, or pericranium, with mandatory histologic assessment to guarantee clear margins [1, 11]. Reconstruction involving skin grafting is often required, but it must be postponed until negative margins are confirmed [1].

For challenging areas, such as the head and neck, or areas where WLE is unfeasible, MMS or CCPDMA is preferred.

MMS involves tumor resection with immediate histological analysis of the resected tissue by frozen section examination using immunostaining for CD34, which allows for the achievement of negative margins with minimal amount of healthy tissue [11, 13].

Given the rarity of lymph node metastasis (less than 1%), sentinel lymph node biopsy is not routinely performed; however, lymphadenectomy is recommended if lymph node involvement is clinically apparent [14]. For positive margins, re-resection is recommended whenever possible, but adjuvant radiotherapy may be considered for cases that re-excision is not feasible due to the proximity to critical sites, and there is no data for adjuvant systemic treatment [1, 11].

Recurrence usually occurs within the first 3 years after surgery, and the treatment of choice is re-resection followed by radiotherapy, if not given prior to that [2].

For inoperable or locally advanced lesions, radiotherapy can be considered either as the primary modality or with neoadjuvant intent, as with the systemic treatment with imatinib [2].

Treatment of Advanced Disease

As noted previously, more than 90% of DFSP have the t(17;22) translocation that leads to *PDGFB/COL1A1* fusion, promoting hyperexpression of PDGFR-B receptor and progression of tumor cells [2].

Imatinib is an oral multikinase inhibitor that inhibits PDGFR-B receptor, leading to inhibition of DFSP cell growth. In a systemic review of DFSP treated with imatinib, objective response was described in 60.5% of the cases, with stable disease in 27.6%. Apparently, there are no differences between 400 and 800 mg daily of imatinib, and, although the presence of t(17;22) is considered a predictive biomarker of response to imatinib, shrinkage of tumors lacking this genomic alteration has been described [7].

Other tyrosine kinase inhibitors, such as sunitinib and sorafenib, have shown activity in DFSP, and conventional chemotherapy used to treat other soft-tissue sarcomas plays a very limited role in DFSP management [15, 16].

Follow-Up

Clinical follow-up every 6–12 months is indicated considering a high risk of local recurrence. Biopsies should be performed in any suspicious lesions [11, 17].

Atypical Fibroxanthoma

Epidemiology

Atypical fibroxanthoma (AFX) is a rare, low-grade, cutaneous neoplasm with uncertain epidemiologic aspects, first reported by Helwig in the early 1960s [18]. Historically, AFX was regarded as a superficial variant of malignant fibrous histiocytoma (MFH), and those terms had been used interchangeably [19]. Nowadays, these tumors have been recategorized in distinct subtypes of neoplasms, such as AFX and undifferentiated pleomorphic sarcoma (UPS).

AFX is more common in elderlies, with peak incidence in the seventh or eighth decade of life, and has a male predilection [20]. In younger patients, AFX has been reported with cancer predisposilion disorders, such as the Li-Fraumeni syndrome and xeroderma pigmentosum, and their incidence is also higher in immunosuppressed populations, with an estimated incidence of 78 per 100,000 transplant patients [22].

Most frequently, AFX occurs on chronically sun-exposed skin of the head and neck; although distant metastases have been reported, some authors have questioned its metastatic potential [22].

Risk Factors

Ultraviolet (UV) light exposure is a risk factor for the development of AFX, as most lesions typically occur on sun-exposed skin, and UV-induced mutational signature in dipyrimidines sites has been documented in these lesions [19]. Other risk factors described in the literature include radiation therapy and immunosuppression [20].

Diagnosis

Clinically, AFX manifests as a firm, solitary, erythematous, or skin-colored papule or nodule, with or without ulceration and bleeding, which may mimic a benign lesion or other types of skin cancers, such as basal cell carcinomas and amelanotic melanomas [22].

Findings of dermoscopy include red and white structureless areas with an atypical polymorphous vascular pattern and irregular linear vessels, being dermoscopically indistinguishable from basal cell carcinomas [23].

The accurate diagnosis requires a skin biopsy and immunohistochemical studies, though there are no specific immunohistochemical markers; AFX remains a diagnosis of exclusion [19].

Pathologic analysis usually shows atypical spindle or epithelioid cells limited to the dermis, with nuclear pleomorphism and atypical mitoses. Immunohistochemistry helps to differentiate AFX from other cutaneous neoplasms. Vimentin, smooth muscle actin, CD68, and CD10 are often positive, while S100 and cytokeratins are negative in AFX and positive in desmoplastic melanoma and spindle-cell cutaneous squamous cell carcinoma, respectively [18, 20].

Staging

Given the rarity of AFX, evidence-based recommendations regarding imaging and staging are lacking.

At the time of diagnosis, staging workup includes a full skin examination, with focus on tumor site and regional lymph nodes. Physical examination could be complemented by lymph node ultrasound; though no other imaging studies are routinely indicated without the presence of symptoms, they can be helpful for surgical planning in cases of suspected deep invasion of adjacent or critical anatomic structures [18, 20].

The role of sentinel lymph node biopsy in AFX is uncertain and it is not usually recommended [19].

Treatment of Localized Disease

The treatment of choice is complete surgical resection with margins of 1–2 cm or Mohs micrographic surgery, which is often preferred since most AFX tumors arise on head/neck skin, where anatomical issues and aesthetic considerations may pose challenges to standard wide excisions [18, 20, 21]. Although there are no head-to-head comparisons between these two modalities in randomized trials, recurrence rates are lower after complete removal with negative margins, regardless of the chosen surgical approach.

For either inoperable tumors or patients deemed inappropriate candidates for surgery, radiotherapy with dosages ranging from 60 to 65 Gy can be useful for disease control [18].

There is no clear role for adjuvant or neoadjuvant systemic treatment, given the lack of data, and adjuvant radiotherapy could be considered in cases of positive margins not suitable for an additional resection [19].

Treatment of Advanced Disease

Metastatic disease is rare and there is no standard treatment for these cases. Most common sites of metastasis are parotid gland, lymph nodes, and subcutaneous tissue, usually occurring within 12–14 months of the initial diagnosis [22].

Treatment options reported include metastasectomy or cytotoxic chemotherapy regimens employed in other subtypes of soft-tissue sarcomas (i.e. ifosfamide and doxorubicin) [22].

Follow-Up

These patients should be followed up with at least full skin examination and imaging (provided suspicious clinical findings are present) every 6 months [19], due to the risk of recurrence and metastatic disease.

Cutaneous Undifferentiated Pleomorphic Sarcoma

Epidemiology

Cutaneous undifferentiated pleomorphic sarcoma (cUPS) (also known as pleomorphic dermal sarcoma) is a tumor with similar clinical and histologic features to AFX, but presenting more frequently with adverse features, for instance, deep subcutaneous invasion, high histologic grade, tumor necrosis, lymphovascular and/or perineural invasion, conferring more aggressive behavior [20, 24].

As AFX, cUPS commonly occur in sun-exposed areas of elderly patients, at median age of 80 years and with marked male predilection [20, 25].

Local recurrence and metastasis are more frequent in cUPS than AFX, occurring in 30% and 20% of the patients, respectively [26].

Risk Factors

AFX and cUPS have similar molecular phenotypes, with the presence of UV-signature mutations in *TP53* and *TERT*, suggesting the role of UV light in tumorigenesis. Also, a higher risk has been reported in immunosuppressed patients [19].

Diagnosis

Clinical presentation consists on firm, ulcerated, red or amelanotic, fast-growing exophytic/nodular lesions arising in sun-exposed areas of the body, with a predilection for the head and neck. Bleeding is common [20, 25].

Dermatoscopically, cUPS is characterized by red and white structureless areas and enlarged and/or linear irregular vessels. These findings may be similar to poorly differentiated squamous cell carcinomas, amelanotic melanomas, and AFX. Definitive diagnosis requires a skin biopsy [27]. Histopathological features include pleomorphic epithelioid and atypical spindle cells, with extensive subcutaneous invasion, tumor necrosis, and abundant atypical mitoses. Immunohistochemical staining is important to rule out other differential diagnoses, being cUPS a diagnosis of exclusion [20, 28].

Staging

There is no specific staging system for cUPS.

As with other high-grade sarcomas, AJCC 8th edition staging system for soft-issue sarcomas is usually employed, which assesses tumor size (T), lymph node involvement (N), presence or absence of distant metastases (M), and histologic grade (G).

Even though the role of complementary imaging studies at the time of diagnosis is unclear, it should always be considered as cUPS is a high-grade sarcoma with metastatic potential, and the presence of distant metastasis can change the treatment intent. Also, sentinel lymph node biopsy might be of benefit for these patients [19, 25].

Treatment of Localized Disease

The treatment of choice for localized disease is surgical excision with wide margins. There is limited evidence regarding optimal margins and surgical technique, but histological assessment to ensure negative margins is highly important [19, 20]. In a retrospective study of 27 patients with cUPS, the mean surgical excision margin was 1.2 cm, and all patients experiencing recurrence had positive deep margin at first excision [29].

The effectiveness of primary or adjuvant radiotherapy in cUPS is unknown, with little evidence to support indication [19, 26].

Treatment of Advanced Disease

Conventional chemotherapy seems to be ineffective for the treatment of unresectable or metastatic cUPS, and there is no standard treatment for these patients [19].

Like other skin cancers, cUPS has a high tumor mutation burden, with typical UV-signature and elevated immune cell infiltration, a rationale for the use of immune checkpoint inhibitors (ICI); recent data have demonstrated clinical activity of ICI, such as pembrolizumab and nivolumab, in unresectable or metastatic cUPS (even with reports of complete response) [26].

Follow-Up

There is no consensus regarding the optimal follow-up for these patients. However, routine surveillance with follow-up every 6 months is recommended to assess for local or metastatic recurrence [19].

Cutaneous Leiomyosarcoma

Epidemiology

Cutaneous leiomyosarcomas (cLMS) comprise a rare subgroup of soft tissue sarcomas (STS), with an incidence rate of 0.2 cases per 100,000 persons per year. They account for nearly 5% of all STS, predominantly affecting individuals around the sixth decade of life. These neoplasms are subdivided into LMS of dermal origin (superficial LMS) and subcutaneous form. The former presumably originates from arrector pili muscles of the dermis, while the latter arises from smooth muscle of subcutaneous vessels [30, 31].

While dermal LMS tend to affect more often men and present indolent behavior with frequent local recurrences, rarely metastasizing, subcutaneous LMS do not display gender predilection and have unquestionable metastatic potential, mostly to the lungs. Aneiros-Fernandez and colleagues described dermal LMS rates of metastatic relapse and mortality after a median follow-up of 4.4 years as 4.2% and 3.3%, respectively. For subcutaneous LMS, rates are definitely more worrisome: 43.2% and 37.8%, respectively [32].

Risk Factors

Risk factors related to the development of cutaneous leiomyosarcoma are unknown, although there are reports of predisposing factors, such as precancerous lesions, like leiomyomas, and history of previous injury or local trauma [33].

Diagnosis

LMS usually manifest as intracutaneous or subcutaneous skin-colored/violaceous nodules on the lower extremities, head and neck, or chest of elderly individuals; due to unspecific clinical characteristics, cutaneous metastases or even more favorable conditions (such as epidermal cysts) are differential diagnosis [20, 30, 31].

There are few reports of dermoscopic findings of cLMS, which include an aspecific nonpigmented pattern with the presence of arborizing vessels and spread telangiectasias on a background of whitish area [34].

On histologic assessment, tumor cells are spindle-shaped, resembling smooth muscle cells with atypia, mitotic figures, and variable rate of nuclear pleomorphism; immunohistochemical staining for caldesmon, desmin, and smooth muscle actin helps to differentiate from other spindle-cell malignancies. Importantly, the depth of invasion in dermal LMS provides important prognostic information and must be disclosed in pathology reports [20, 30–32]. Tumor size >5 cm, deep location with fascia involvement, and high histological grade have all been correlated with decreased survival in dermal LMS [35].

Staging

As other cutaneous sarcomas, no guideline is available regarding staging and imaging workup. Due to the metastatic potential, especially for the subcutaneous form, complementary imaging studies should be considered, especially chest CT scan, since the lungs are the main site of metastasis. The AJCC 8th edition staging system for soft tissue sarcoma is generally used to prognosticate and guide therapeutic interventions.

Treatment of Localized Disease

Surgical resection with margins >1 cm is the most important treatment, providing curative perspectives. Though radioresistant, adjuvant radiation therapy can be discussed in selected cases, as for adjuvant chemotherapy in high-grade and deep invasive lesions. Note that this is an exceedingly rare subgroup of LMS, and recommendations regarding management are usually extrapolation from extrauterine LMS studies and case series [20, 30–32].

Treatment of Advanced Disease

General principles of systemic treatment applied for LMS from other sites are also applied for cutaneous LMS; cytotoxic regimens involving gemcitabine plus docetaxel, dacarbazine, and doxorubicin are oftentimes adopted to treat advanced disease [20, 30–32].

Follow-Up

Although consensus-based surveillance guidelines after treatment of cLMS are lacking, frequent follow-up, notably in the first years after treatment, should be considered.

Liposarcoma

Epidemiology

Superficial liposarcomas (SL) are an extremely rare subgroup of STS that arises in the dermis or subcutaneous tissue and usually occur in individuals between 50 and 70 years of age [20, 36].

Risk Factors

Given the rarity of SL, no risk factor has been associated with the development of these neoplasms.

Diagnosis

These neoplasms can arise in virtually every site of the body and usually present as painless lumps or masses, frequently confounded with lipomas or epidermal cysts.

They are usually subdivided according to histologic subtypes in atypical lipomatous tumor (well-differentiated—WDL), dedifferentiated (DDL), myxoid/round cell (MRCL), and pleomorphic (PL) [36, 37]. Biological behavior is usually associated with histologic subtypes (better outcomes for WDL), grade, depth of invasion—underlying fascia and muscle involvement—and size of the lesion.

Overall, despite having metastatic potential, superficial liposarcomas tend to present less frequently with distant metastases, with a better prognosis when compared with their deeper counterparts.

On H & E staining, these tumors display variable degree of adipocytic differentiation. WDL exhibit normal-appearing adipocytes admixed with atypical stromal cells and frequently contain cells with multivacuolated cytoplasm and atypical nucleus (lipoblasts). DDL exhibit a composite of well-differentiated areas and areas with marked different morphology, presumably related to dedifferentiation within the primary tumor [37]. Importantly, though rare, areas with epithelioid shape demand differential diagnosis with melanoma and carcinomas [38]. ML present a characteristic abundance of mucin areas, oftentimes being associated with round cells, where higher proportions are indicative of poor prognosis. Lastly, PL displays features of high-grade sarcomas, with atypical spindle cells, multivacuolated lipoblasts, necrosis, and several mitotic figures [37, 38]. Along with morphologic features, assessment of immunostaining for p16, CDK4, and MDM2 is useful in determining the diagnosis, especially in WDL/DDL lesions, where amplifications in 12q13–15 (involving *CDK4*, *MDM2*, *HMGA2*, *CPM*, etc.) are common events. For MRCL, *FUS-DDIT3* fusion is highly specific and related to t(12;16) (q13p11), occurring in 95% of the cases; in 5%, t(12;22)(q13q12) generates *EWSR1-DDIT3*. For PL, no characteristic molecular events have been reported to date [37].

Staging

As noted previously, no guideline is available regarding staging and imaging workup for cutaneous sarcomas as LS, with limited data available, and the AJCC 8th edition staging for soft tissue sarcoma is used as the staging system of choice.

Treatment of Localized Disease

Wide local excision with at least 1 cm margins is the standard of care. Adjuvant radiotherapy can be discussed based on the depth of invasion, histologic grade, and subtype, which are all important prognostic characteristics. The same rationale could be adopted for indicating adjuvant chemotherapy. As described by Winchester et al. [36] in a case series of 13 patients with primary superficial liposarcomas, histologic subtypes other than WDL presented with larger primary lesions (up to 25 cm), and the only 2 deaths occurred in patients with MRCL.

Treatment of Advanced Disease

Metastatic disease is usually managed with cytotoxic chemotherapy extrapolating data from liposarcomas of other primary sites. Importantly, since superficial liposarcomas are extremely rare malignancies, the best treatment approach should be ideally discussed in multidisciplinary sarcoma boards. It is worth underscoring that every single sarcoma patient should be referred to specialized sarcoma centers, owing to the rarity and sometimes unpredictable behavior of these entities [20, 36].

Follow-Up

Due to metastatic potential, frequent follow-up should be considered. There is no consensus regarding the standard follow-up approach for this specific subgroup of malignancies.

Angiosarcoma

Epidemiology

Angiosarcoma is a high-grade sarcoma derived from vascular endothelial cells arising in cutaneous, soft tissues or visceral sites. Cutaneous angiosarcoma (cAS) is divided into primary (that occurs sporadically) and secondary cAS, related to history of radiotherapy or chronic lymphedema (Stewart-Treves syndrome) [39].

cAS represents less than 1% of all cutaneous sarcomas, with an incidence of 0.5 cases per 1 million persons per year in the USA. However, it is the most aggressive of all cutaneous sarcomas, with high rates of local recurrence and tendency to metastasize despite optimal treatment [20, 40].

Primary cAS commonly affect sun-damaged skin of the head and neck in elderlies, while radiaction-associated angiosarcomas frequently affect patients treated with radiotherapy after breast-conserving surgeries (median latency interval of 7–8 years). Lymphoedema-associated angiosarcoma is mostly reported in the upper extremity of patients submitted to lymphadenectomy, with latency period of 10–15 years. In younger individuals, cAS is rare, usually related to radiotherapy and genetic predisposing syndromes, such as xeroderma pigmentosum, Aicardi syndrome, and congenital lymphoedema [39, 41, 42, 43].

Risk Factors

As noted above, radiotherapy is a risk factor for the development of cAS, as well as chronic exposure to UV radiation, since the majority of primary cAS occur in sun-damaged skin.

cAS has also been described as secondary to arteriovenous fistulas for hemodialysis, immunosuppression, and foreign material retention [39].

Diagnosis

Clinically, cAS manifests as a hematoma-like lesion, being frequently misdiagnosed with benign lesions. Margins are poorly defined and may present as an ulceration, nodule, or plaque. cAS is characterized by rapid progression and is associated with high rate of lymph node metastasis [20, 40, 41].

Dermatoscopy findings include pink-purple "steam-like" areas with a white or skin-colored central region, strengthening of the purple color at the periphery of the lesions in radiotherapy-associated cAS, and macules with color gradation from dark reddish to purplish polymorphous atypical vessel-like features in classic cAS [44].

Histologically, cAS varies from irregular, anastomosing ectatic vessels with large endothelial cells, nuclear atypia, and mitoses to solid aggregates of polygonal spindle cells, atypical nuclei, and mitoses, depending on the degree of differentiation. Immunohistochemical findings include positivity for CD31, CD34, and podoplanin, which are endothelial cell markers, and for nuclear transcription factors, such as FLI-1 and ERG [39].

Staging

Like CUPS, cAS is a high-grade sarcoma, and further imaging studies should be considered at the time of diagnosis, including chest CT and evaluation of lymph node involvement.

AJCC 8th edition for soft tissue sarcoma is used as the preferable staging system; however, some authors suggest subdividing cAS into two categories: low and high risk [39, 41, 44].

Treatment of Localized Disease

Standard of care for localized disease is surgical resection with negative margins. There is limited evidence regarding optimal margins, but achievement of at least 3-cm margins is recommended; margin of less than 1 cm are associated with inferior survival outcomes [39, 45]. Unfortunately, positive margins are frequest due to difficulties in achieving wide margins in certain areas of the body, especially in the head and neck due to proximity with key anatomical structures [41].

As other cutaneous sarcomas of the head and neck, Mohs surgery is a treatment option for these cases, although there is limited data for the utility of this technique in cAS, with only retrospective studies and cases reports [46, 47].

Adjuvant radiotherapy with a >50 Gy dose is often recommended to reduce the risk of local recurrence and also should be discussed for patients with radiation-associated tumors with a long interval since previous radiotherapy (especially in cases with positive margins) [41, 45]. Data for neoadjuvant chemotherapy are scarce, but the overall sensitivity of AS to anthracycline-based regimens and paclitaxel, with frequent responses observed in the clinical practice, should stimulate the debate in multidisciplinary rounds; adjuvant chemotherapy remains questionable [39].

Treatment of Advanced Disease

Cytotoxic chemotherapy with anthracyclines-based regimens and taxanes is considered the gold standard for treatment of metastatic cAS with some series demonstrating paclitaxel as the most commonly used treatment as a first-line therapy [39, 41, 45].

Bevacizumab, a vascular endothelial growth factor (VEGF) inhibitor, in monotherapy or in combination with paclitaxel, has been reported to be effective for the treatment of metastatic cAS, and recently, the use of immunotherapy with ipilimumab and nivolumab demonstrated an objective response rate of 25% in these patients [40, 48]. Florou et al (2019) reported clinical activity (partial response) in 5 out of 7 angiosarcoma patients (71%) treated with immunotherapy (i.e. pembrolizumab plus axitinib, ipilimumab plus nivolumab, or the anti-CTLA-4 AGEN-1884), with one heavily pretreated patient achieving durable remission [49].

Follow-Up

Posttreatment cancer surveillance guidelines are lacking. Frequent follow-up should be considered.

Kaposi Sarcoma (KS)

Epidemiology

First described in 1872 in elderly European men by Moritz Kaposi, KS is a vascular-derived malignancy arising in the context of chronic human herpesvirus-8 (also known as KS herpesvirus—KSHV) infection and immunocompromise. This a highly heterogenous group of diseases, subclassified according to their etiology and biological behavior as follows: classic (sporadic), endemic, iatrogenic, AIDS-related, and MSM without HIV infection [50].

KS incidence across the world tends to reflect KSHV seroprevalence which, for reasons not fully understood, can range from <10% in northern Europe and the USA to >90% in some populations of sub-Saharan Africa. Moreover, KS incidence is closely related to HIV seroprevalence (more commonly associated with HIV-1) and access to combination antiretroviral therapy (cART); KS age-standardized incidence rates per 100,000 persons may vary from <0.3 in most European countries (except for eastern and Mediterranean regions) and Canada to 4–22.0 in Africa [51].

Risk Factors

Recipients of solid-organ transplants are at a substantially higher risk of developing KS (iatrogenic KS), with roughly 200-fold when compared with the general population; importantly, AIDS-related immunosuppression can increase the risk for up to 20,000 times when compared with the general population, turning access to cART the most important factor to both reduce the incidence and to treat initial stages of AIDS-related KS [50–52].

Diagnosis

Sporadic (or classic) KS usually presents with violaceous skin-confined painless papules/macules in elderlies or middle-aged patients, usually on the limbs; prevalence is higher in Eastern Europe, Mediterranean, and Middle East regions. It usually follows an indolent course, rarely displaying visceral or gastrointestinal mucosal involvement. Likewise, MSM without HIV infection KS tends to present with skin-limited disease and indolent behavior, rarely displaying widespread involvement of the body. Iatrogenic KS is also manifested as a skin-localized disease in patients following solid-organ transplants; mucosal involvement can occur, and the risk of developing this condition is correlated to the degree of immunosuppression. Decreasing (or modifying) immunosuppressive medications is usually helpful in managing this condition.

Endemic KS can occur in both HIV-negative children and adults, being most prevalent in sub-Saharan Africa. Its biological behavior differs according to age, resembling sporadic KS in adults and displaying an aggressive course in children/young adults. The latter frequently presents lymphadenopathy, lymphedema, and visceral involvement including gastrointestinal and respiratory tract. With disease progression, skin lesions may become exophytic and ulcerated masses; visceral involvement can produce hemoptysis, dry cough, dyspnea, gastrointestinal obstruction, and bleeding, which should prompt broader investigation with CT scans, gastroscopy, and/or bronchoscopy, whenever present. AIDS-related (epidemic) KS is closely related to viral load and CD4+ T-lymphocyte counts; it is usually manifested by widespread skin involvement, lymphadenopathy (in 50% of the cases), lymphedema (20%), and visceral involvement (15%) [50, 53, 54]. Mucosal involvement is common in AIDS-related KS, occurring in roughly 20% of the cases; oral lesions can manifest as ulcerated and bleeding nodules, which could also lead to complications owing to secondary infections [50].

As usual, a proper pathologic assessment deserves clinical correlation, since microscopic features may vary according to the stage of tumor progression. Overall, KS microscopic features in hematoxylin and eosin (H & E) staining comprise vascular proliferation of the dermis with vessels lacking endothelial lining, red blood cell (RBC) extravasation, hemosiderin deposition, and inflammatory infiltrate, along with spindle cells frequently showing hyaline inclusions. Flat lesions tend to be especially challenging, since they can resemble inflammatory conditions or minor vascular diseases; they usually present with focal perivascular infiltrates of inflammatory cells, siderophages, and mild extravasation of RBC. The immunohistochemical (IHC) profile of KS suggests a mesenchymal/endothelial (either lymphatic or vascular) origin, staining positive for CD34, podoplanin, LYVE1, VEGFR3, and vimentin. In challenging cases, IHC staining for a KSHV protein (e.g., KSHV LANA) can be performed to confirm the diagnosis, if available, being considered positive when a distinct granular nuclear staining is present, irrespective of the proportion of spindle cells stained [50, 55].

Staging

There is no standardized AJCC TNM staging system for KS. AIDS-related KS is classified according to the modified AIDS Clinical Trials Group staging, which categorizes patients into two subgroups (good and poor risk) considering disease burden (T), immune system involvement (I), and systemic illness (S). Regarding disease burden, patients presenting with good risk (T0) are those who have disease confined to the skin, lymph nodes, and/or minimal oral disease; poor risk (T1) patients present tumor-associated edema, ulceration, extensive oral lesions, gastrointestinal, and/or other non-nodal visceral disease. Immune system involvement categorizes patients based on CD4+ cell counts as $\geq$150 μL (I0) or $<$150/μL (I1). Lastly, patients with Karnofsky performance status (KPS) $>$70 are considered good risk (S0), while those with KPS $<$70, B symptoms, or HIV-related illnesses are classified as poor risk (S1) [50, 56, 57].

Classic KS is classified based on the involvement and aspect of skin lesions. Stage I (macronodular) consists of small macules/papules confined to inferior limbs; stage II (infiltrative) is characterized by plaques restricted to lower extremities. When multiple angiomatous plaques and nodules (some of them ulcerated) are present and confined to the lower extremities, it is classified as stage III. When these lesions extend beyond lower extremities, we classify as stage IV [58].

Treatment

Providing symptomatic relief and improving quality of life are important goals of KS treatment. When opting for treatment initiation and deciding which modalities would best serve the patient, one should always consider disease-related symptoms, impaired functionality, comorbidities versus potential toxicities, as well as involved organs and pace of progression. Oftentimes, when feasible, reducing the degree of immunosuppression can be an effective treatment by itself; in early-stage T0 AIDS-related KS, introducing or modifying cART is usually the first-line approach, able to provide disease control especially when managing treatment-naïve patients. In iatrogenic KS patients, reducing the degree of immunosuppression (or changing immunosuppressors) can be a useful strategy, if not posing unacceptable risk of graft rejection [50].

Most prospective data assessing the employment of cytotoxic agents come from AIDS-related KS, being often extrapolated for other forms; in fact, treatment of other forms relies on retrospective studies and case series. Even though paclitaxel and liposomal anthracyclines yield response rates of roughly 58%, pegylated liposomal doxorubicin is the recommended frontline regimen for progressive AIDS-related KS or T1 disease, owing to its more favorable toxicity profile with regards to neurotoxicity and alopecia; paclitaxel is usually recommended for anthracycline-refractory KS or as first line when liposomal anthracyclines are deemed unaffordable. Other regimens, such as combination vincristine and bleomycin or single-agent etoposide, provide inferior 48-week progression-free survival (PFS) rates (44% and 20%, respectively, as opposed to 64% with paclitaxel), but are still often used as preferred choices in low-income settings [50, 59–61].

Novel agents including anti-PD1 antibodies are under investigation, showing intriguing results even in chemotherapy-refractory scenario [62, 63]. A recently published phase II trial assessing the use of ipilimumab plus nivolumab in patients with classic KS reported an impressive 87% response rate, with 8 out of 13 patients experiencing complete metabolic response on PET-CT after median follow-up period of two years, highlighting the potential of these new agents to change the management of this subgroup of diseases. In addition, based on the phase I/II 12-C-0047, the US FDA approved in 2020 pomalidomide as an alternative to HIV-negative KS patients and HIV-positive experiencing progression upon cART. Lastly, other treatment modalities, such as surgical resection, radiation therapy, and topical agents, are always welcome as part of the therapeutic arsenal to manage isolated symptomatic KS lesions [50, 64].

Follow-Up

Importantly, there are no data to support any specific follow-up workup or prophylaxis for KS; adequate cART for AIDS-related KS can be an effective way to reduce likelihood of developing the condition in this specific setting [50].

A resume of cutaneous malignancies of mesenchymal origin could be seen in Table 19.1.

Table 19.1 Summary of cutaneous malignancies of mesenchymal origin

	Epidemiology and risk factors	Diagnosis	Staging	Treatment of localized disease	Treatment of advanced disease
Dermatofibrosarcoma protuberans	• Most common cutaneous sarcoma, with an overall incidence of 0.8–4.5 cases per million persons per year • More common during the third to fifth decades of life in the trunk (40–50%), extremities (30–40%), and head and neck (10–15%) • 10–15% contain a high-grade component • 90% have a t(17;22) translocation • There are no specific risk factors	• Clinically: slowly progressive painless cutaneous plaque, solitary or multiple, colored/brownish red (if untreated, it progresses to ulcerated/bleeding nodules or masses, high local recurrence rate, and low metastatic potential) • Histologically: spindle-cell proliferation in a storiform or fascicular pattern, with low to moderate atypia and mitotic rate • Infiltrative pattern as "honeycomb" or irregular fingerlike projections • Usually, CD34 positive and factor XIIIa negative • PDGFB/COL1A1 fusion (FISH or RT-PCR) is recommended in suspicious cases without immunohistochemical confirmation	• No standardized staging system • Considered preoperative MRI if extensive extracutaneous extension or recurrent tumor is suspected	• Surgical excision with negative margins • Technical options: wide local excision with 2–4 cm margins, Mohs micrographic surgery, and complete circumferential and peripheral deep margin assessment (CCPDMA)	• Tyrosine kinase inhibitors

(continued)

Table 19.1 (continued)

	Epidemiology and risk factors	Diagnosis	Staging	Treatment of localized disease	Treatment of advanced disease
Atypical fibroxanthoma	• Low-grade cutaneous neoplasm with uncertain epidemiologic aspects due to recent reclassification • Risk factors: UV light exposure, radiotherapy, and immunosuppression	• Clinically: firm, solitary, erythematous, or skin-colored papule or nodule, with or without ulceration and bleeding, which may be similar to benign lesions or other types of skin cancer • Histologically: atypical spindle or epithelioid cells limited to the dermis, with nuclear pleomorphism and atypical mitoses with no specific immunohistochemical markers	• No standardized staging system • Staging workup: full skin examination, considered lymph node ultrasound, and imaging studies in cases with suspected deep invasion	• Complete surgical resection with margins of 1–2 cm or Mohs micrographic surgery	• There is no standard treatment • Treatment options include metastasectomy or cytotoxic chemotherapy
Cutaneous undifferentiated pleomorphic sarcoma	• Similar clinical and histologic features to AFX with adverse features as deep subcutaneous invasion, high histologic grade, tumor necrosis, lymphovascular and/or perineural invasion • Median age at diagnosis is 80 years • Local recurrence and metastasis are more frequent than AFX • Risk factors: UV light exposure and immunosuppression	• Clinically: firm, ulcerated, red, or amelanotic nodular lesion, fast growing, exophytic in sun-exposed areas, with a predilection for the head and neck region • Histologically: pleomorphic epithelioid cells and atypical spindle cells, with extensive subcutaneous invasion, tumor necrosis, and abundant atypical mitoses with no specific immunohistochemical markers	• There is no specific staging system • AJCC eighth edition staging for soft tissue sarcoma is usually employed • Complementary imaging studies at the time of diagnosis are unclear	• Surgical excision with wide margins • There is limited evidence regarding optimal margins and surgical technique, but histological assessment to accomplish negative margins is highly important	• There is no standard treatment • Immune checkpoint has demonstrated clinical activity

	Epidemiology and risk factors	Diagnosis	Staging	Treatment of localized disease	Treatment of advanced disease
Cutaneous leiomyosarcoma	• Rare subgroup with incidence rate of 0.2 cases per 100,000 persons per year • Median age at diagnosis 60 years • Risk factors are unknown • Reports of predisposing factors: precancerous lesions like leiomyomas and history of previous injury or local trauma	• Clinically: intracutaneous or subcutaneous skin-colored/violaceous nodules on the lower extremities, head and neck, or chest • Histologically: tumor cells are spindle-shaped, resembling smooth muscle cells with atypia, mitotic figures, and variable rate of nuclear pleomorphism; immunohistochemical staining for caldesmon, desmin, and smooth muscle actin helps to differentiate from other spindle-cell malignancies	• There is no specific staging system • Due to the metastatic potential, especially of subcutaneous form, complementary images studies should be considered • AJCC eighth edition staging for soft tissue sarcoma is generally used for staging these patients	• Surgical resection with margins >1 cm is the most important treatment	• Cytotoxic regimens involving gemcitabine plus docetaxel, ifosfamide, and doxorubicin are oftentimes adopted to treat advanced disease
Liposarcoma	• Extremely rare • Individuals between 50 and 70 years old • Risk factors: unknown	• Clinically: painless lumps or masses, frequently confounded with lipomas or epidermal cysts • Histologically: normal-appearing adipocytes admixed with atypical stromal cells, and frequently contain cells with multivacuolated cytoplasm and atypical nucleus (lipoblasts)	• There is no specific staging system • AJCC eighth edition staging for soft tissue sarcoma is usually employed	• Wide local excision with at least 1 cm margins is the standard of care	• Metastatic disease is usually managed with cytotoxic chemotherapy extrapolating data from liposarcomas of other primary sites

(continued)

Table 19.1 (continued)

	Epidemiology and risk factors	Diagnosis	Staging	Treatment of localized disease	Treatment of advanced disease
Angiosarcoma	• cAS represents less than 1% of all cutaneous sarcomas, with an incidence of 0.5 cases per 1 million persons per year • Elderly individuals • Risk factors: radiotherapy, UV light exposure	• Clinically: hematoma-like lesion, but may present with ulceration, nodule, or plaque • Histologically: cAS varies from irregular, anastomosing ectatic vessels with large endothelial cells, nuclear atypia, and mitoses to solid aggregates of polygonal spindle cells, atypical nuclei, and mitoses • Immunohistochemical findings include positivity for CD31, CD34, and podoplanin, which are endothelial cell markers, and for nuclear transcription factors, such as FLI-1 and ERG	• Further imaging studies should be considered at the time of diagnosis, including chest CT and evaluation of lymph node involvement • AJCC eighth edition for soft tissue sarcoma is used as the staging system; however some authors suggest subdividing cAS into two categories: low and high risk	• Standard of care for localized disease is surgical resection with negative margins	• Cytotoxic chemotherapy with anthracyclines-based regimens and taxanes is considered the gold standard for treatment of metastatic cAS

	Epidemiology and risk factors	Diagnosis	Staging	Treatment of localized disease	Treatment of advanced disease
Kaposi sarcoma (KS)	• KS is a vascular-derived malignancy arising in the context of chronic human herpesvirus-8 infection and immunocompromise • Incidence is closely related to HIV seroprevalence and access to combination antiretroviral therapy • Risk factors: immunosuppression, HIV infection	• Clinically violaceous skin-confined painless papules/macules in elderlies or middle-aged patients, usually on the limbs • Histologically: comprise vascular proliferation of the dermis with vessels lacking endothelial lining, red blood cell (RBC) extravasation, hemosiderin deposition, and inflammatory infiltrate, along with spindle cells frequently showing hyaline inclusions • Immunohistochemical findings include positivity for CD34, podoplanin, LYVE1, VEGFR3, and vimentin	• There is no specific staging system AIDS-related KS is classified according to the modified AIDS Clinical Trials Group staging, which categorizes patients into two subgroups (good and poor risk) considering disease burden (T), immune system involvement (I), and systemic illness (S)	• Providing symptomatic relief and improving quality of life are important goals of KS treatment • Surgery may be considered for single symptomatic lesion	• When feasible, reducing the degree of immunosuppression can be an effective treatment by itself • In early-stage (T0) AIDS-related KS, introducing or modifying cART is usually the first-line approach • Cytotoxic chemotherapy includes paclitaxel and liposomal anthracyclines

References

1. Reha J, Katz SC. Dermatofibrosarcoma protuberans. Surg Clin N Am. 2016;96(5):1031–46.
2. Hao X, Billings SD, Wu F, et al. Dermatofibrosarcoma protuberans: update on the diagnosis and treatment. J Clin Med. 2020;9(6):1752.
3. Thway K, Noujaim J, Joner RL, et al. Dermatofibrosarcoma protuberans: pathology, genetics, and potential therapeutic strategies. Ann Diagn Pathol. 2016;24:64–71.
4. Rutkowski P, Debiec-Rychter M. Current treatment options for dermatofibrosarcoma protuberans. Expert Rev Anticancer Ther. 2015;15(8):901–9.
5. Mujtaba B, Wang F, Taher A, et al. Dermatofibrosarcoma protuberans: pathological and imaging review. Curr Probl Diagn Radiol. 2020;50(2):236–40.
6. Bernard J, Poulalhon N, Argenziano G, et al. Dermoscopy of dermatofibrosarcoma protuberans: a study of 15 cases. Br J Dermatol. 2013;169(1):85–90.
7. Navarrete-Dechent C, Mori S, Barker CA, et al. Imatinib treatment for locally advanced or metastatic dermatofibrosarcoma protuberans. JAMA Dermatol. 2019;155(3):361–9.
8. Ugurel S, Kortmann RD, Mohr P, et al. Short German guidelines: dermatofibrosarcoma protuberans. J German Soc Dermatol. 2008;6(1):S17–8.
9. Yoon SS, Maki RG, Asare EA, et al. Soft tissue sarcoma of the trunk and extremities. In: Amin MB, editor. AJCC cancer staging manual. 8th ed. Chicago: AJCC; 2017. p. 507.
10. Enneking WF, Spanier SS, Goodman MA. Current concepts review. The surgical staging of musculoskeletal sarcoma. J Bone Joint Surg Am. 1980;62(6):1927.
11. National Comprehensive Cancer Network (NCCN). NCCN clinical practice guidelines in oncology. https://www.nccn.org/professionals/physician_gls Accessed 19 Aug 2021.
12. Wacker J, Khan-Durani B, Hartschuh W. Modified Mohs micrographic surgery in the therapy of dermatofibrosarcoma protuberans: analysis of 22 patients. Ann Surg Oncol. 2005;11(4):438.
13. DuBay D, Cimmino V, Lowe L, et al. Low recurrence rate after surgery for dermatofibrosarcoma protuberans. Cancer. 2004;100(5):1008–16.
14. Lal P, Sharma R, Mohan H, et al. Dermatofibrosarcoma protuberans metastasizing to lymph nodes: a case report and review of literature. J Surg Oncol. 1999;72(3):178–80.
15. Kamar FG, Kairouz VF, Sabri AN. Dermatofibrosarcoma protuberans (DFSP) successfully treated with sorafenib: case report. Clin Sarcoma Res. 2013;3(1):5.
16. Ong HS, Ji T, Wang LZ, et al. Dermatofibrosarcoma protuberans on the right neck with superior cava syndrome: case report and literature review. Int J Oral Maxillofac Surg. 2013;42(6):707.
17. Gan J, Feng L. Follow-up after treatment of dermatofibrosarcoma protuberans. Cancer. 2019;125(19):3467.
18. Ziemer M. Atypical fibroxanthoma. J Dtsch Dermatol Ges. 2012;10:537–48.
19. Soleymani T, Aasi SZ, Novoa R, et al. Atypical fibroxanthoma and pleomorphic dermal sarcoma updates on classification and management. Dermatol Clin. 2019;37:253–9.
20. Kohlmeyer J, Steimle-Grauer SA, Hein R. Cutaneous sarcomas. J Dtsch Dermatol Ges. 2017;15(6):630–48.
21. Phelan PS, Rosamna IS, Council ML. Atypical fibroxanthoma: the Washington University experience. Dermatol Surg. 2019;45(12):1450–8.
22. Kolb L, Schmieder GJ. Atypical fibroxanthoma. [Updated 2021 Sep 9]. In: StatPearls [Internet]. Treasure Island (FL): StatPearls Publishing; 2021. https://www.ncbi.nlm.nih.gov/books/NBK459342/.
23. Moscarella E, Piana S, Specchio F, et al. Dermoscopy features of atypical fibroxanthoma: a multicenter study of the International Dermoscopy Society. Astralas J Dermatol. 2018;59(4):309–14.
24. Cohen PR. Cutaneous undifferentiated pleomorphic sarcoma is a pleomorphic dermal sarcoma. Dermatol Online J. 2020;26(5):13030/qt1tx8b3hr.
25. Soleymani T, Hollmig AT. Conception and management of a poorly understood spectrum of dermatologic neoplasms: atypical fibroxanthoma, pleomorphic dermal sarcoma, and undifferentiated pleomorphic sarcoma. Curr Treat Options Oncol. 2017;18:50.

26. Klein S, Persa OD, Mauch C, et al. First report on two cases of pleomorphic dermal sarcoma successfully treated with immune checkpoint inhibitors. Oncoimmunology. 2019;8(12):e1665977. (6 pages)
27. Salerni G, Alonso C, Sanchez-Granel G, et al. Dermoscopic findings in an early malignant fibrous histiocytoma on the face. Dermatol Pract Concept. 2017;7(3):44–6.
28. Mentzel R. Sarcomas of the skin in the elderly. Clin Dermatol. 2011;29(1):80–90.
29. Lonie S, Yau B, Henderson M, et al. Management of pleomorphic dermal sarcoma. ANZ J Surg. 2020;90(11):2322–4.
30. Luke JJ, Keohan ML. Advances in the systemic treatment of cutaneous sarcomas. Semin Oncol. 2012;39(2):173–83. https://doi.org/10.1053/j.seminoncol.2012.01.004. PMID: 22484
31. Bhatt MD, Nambudiri VE. Cutaneous sarcomas. Hematol Oncol Clin North Am. 2019;33(1):87–101. https://doi.org/10.1016/j.hoc.2018.08.007. PMID: 30497679
32. Aneiros-Fernandez J, Antonio Retamero J, Husein-Elahmed H, Ovalle F, Aneiros-Cachaza J. Primary cutaneous and subcutaneous leiomyosarcomas: evolution and prognostic factors. Eur J Dermatol. 2016;26(1):9–12. https://doi.org/10.1684/ejd.2015.2681. PMID: 26678649
33. Queiros CS, Filipe P, de Almeida LS. Cutaneous leiomyosarcoma: a 20-year retrospective study and review of the literature. An Bras Dermatol. 2021;96(3):278–83.
34. De Giorgi V, Scarfi F, Silverti F, et al. Cutaneous leiomyosarcoma: a clinical, dermoscopic, pathologic case study. Exp Oncol. 2019;41(1):80–1.
35. Fauth CT, Bruecks AK, Temple W, Arlette JP, DiFrancesco LM. Superficial leiomyosarcoma: a clinicopathologic review and update. J Cutan Pathol. 2010;37(2):269–76.
36. Winchester DS, Gardner KH, Lehman JS, Otley CC. Superficial liposarcoma: a retrospective review of 13 cases. J Am Acad Dermatol. 2016;74(2):391–3.
37. Yang L, Chen S, Luo P, Yan W, Wang C. Liposarcoma: Advances in Cellular and Molecular Genetics Alterations and Corresponding Clinical Treatment. J Cancer. 2020;11(1):100–7. https://doi.org/10.7150/jca.36380. PMID: 31892977; PMCID: PMC6930414.
38. Chambers M, Badin DJ, Sriharan AA, Linos KD. Expanding the differential of cutaneous epithelioid tumors: a case of dedifferentiated liposarcoma with epithelioid features involving the skin, with review of the literature. J Cutan Pathol. 2020;47(6):554–60.
39. Shustef R, Kazlouskaya V, Prieto VG, et al. Cutaneous angiosarcoma: a current update. J Clin Pathol. 2017;70(11):917–25.
40. Ishida Y, Otsuka A, Kabashima K. Cutaneous angiosarcoma: update on biology and latest treatment. Curr Opin Oncol. 2018;30(2):107–12.
41. Dossett LA, Harrington M, Cruse W, et al. Cutaneous angiosarcoma, vol. 39. Curr Probl Cancer; 2015. p. 258.
42. D'Angelo S, Antonescu C, Kuk D, et al. High-risk features in radiation-associated breast angiosarcomas. Br J Cancer. 2013;109:2340–6. https://doi.org/10.1038/bjc.2013.590.
43. Kokkali S, Moreno JD, Klijanienko J, Theocharis S. Clinical and molecular insights of radiation-induced breast sarcomas: is there hope on the horizon for effective treatment of this aggressive disease? Int J Mol Sci. 2022;23(8):4125. https://doi.org/10.3390/ijms23084125. PMID: 35456944; PMCID: PMC9029574.
44. De Giorgi V, Grazzini M, Gori A, et al. Dermoscopy pattern of cutaneous angiosarcoma. Eur J Dermatol. 2010;21(1):107–9.
45. Fujisawa Y, Yoshino K, Fukimura T, et al. Cutaneous angiosarcoma: the possibility of new treatment options especially for patients with large primary tumor. Front Oncol. 2018;8:46.
46. Buehler D, Rice SR, Moody JS, et al. Angiosarcoma outcomes and prognostic factors: a 25-year single institute experience. Am J Clin Oncol. 2014;37(5):473–9.
47. Prodanovic E, Youker S, Hurley Y. Slow Mohs increasing histopathology identification of angiosarcoma. J Am Acad Dermatol. 2009;60(3):AB137.
48. Wagner MJ, Othus M, Patel SP, et al. Multicenter phase II trial (SWOG S1609, cohort 51) of ipilimumab and nivolumab in metastatic or unresectable angiosarcoma: a substudy of dual anti-CTLA-4 and anti-PD-1 blockade in rare tumors (DART). J Immunother Cancer. 2021;9(8):1–8.

49. Florou V, Rosenberg AE, Wieder E, et al. Angiosarcoma patients treated with immune checkpoint inhibitors: a case series of seven patients from a single institution. j. immunotherapy cancer. 2019;7:213. https://doi.org/10.1186/s40425-019-0689-7.
50. Cesarman E, Camania B, Keown SE, et al. Kaposi sarcoma. Nat Rev Dis Primers. 2019;5(1):9.
51. Mesri E, Cesarman E, Boshoft C. Kaposi's sarcoma and its associated herpesvirus. Nat Rev Cancer. 2010;10:707–19.
52. International Collaboration on HIV and Cancer. Highly active antiretroviral therapy and incidence of cancer in human immunodeficiency virus-infected adults. J Natl Cancer Inst. 2000;22:1823–30.
53. Bower M, Dalla Pria A, Coyle C, et al. Prospective stage-stratified approach to AIDS-related Kaposi's sarcoma. J Clin Oncol. 2014;32(5):409–14.
54. Atillasoy ES, Santoro A, Weinberg JM. Lymphoedema associated with Kaposi's sarcoma. J Eur Acad Dermatol Venereol. 2001;15(4):364–5. PMID: 11730058.
55. Schneider JW, Dittmer DP. Diagnosis and treatment of kaposi sarcoma. Am J Clin Dermatol. 2017;18(4):529–39. https://doi.org/10.1007/s40257-017-0270-4. PMID: 28324233; PMCID: PMC5509489.
56. Krown SE, Metroka C, Wernz JC. Kaposi's sarcoma in the acquired immune deficiency syndrome: a proposal for uniform evaluation response, and staging criteria. AIDS Clinical Trials Group Oncology Committee. J Clin Oncol. 1989;7(9):1201–7.
57. Krown SE, Testa MA, Huang J. AIDS-related Kaposi's sarcoma: prospective validation of the AIDS Clinical Trials Group Oncology Committee. J Clin Oncol. 1997;15(9):3085–92.
58. Brambilla L, Boneschi V, Taglioni M, Ferrucci S. Staging of classic Kaposi's sarcoma: a useful tool for therapeutic choices. Eur J Dermatol. 2003;13(1):83–6. PMID: 12609790.
59. Stewart S, Jablonowski H, Goebel FD, et al. Randomized comparative trial of pegylated liposomal doxorubicin versus bleomycin and vincristine in treatment of AIDS-related Kaposi's sarcoma. International Pegylated Liposomal Doxorubicin Study Group. J Clin Oncol. 1998;16(2):683–91.
60. Krown SE, Moser CB, MacPhail P, et al. Treatment of advanced AIDS-associated Kaposi sarcoma in resource-limited settings: a three-arm, open label, randomized, non-inferiority trial. Lancet. 2020;395(10231):1195–207.
61. Freeman EE, McMahon DE, Laker-Oketta M. Time to address disparities in the standard of care for Kaposi sarcoma. Lancet. 2020;395(10231):1169–70.
62. Galanina N, Goodman AM, Cohen PR, Frampton GM, Kurzrock R. Successful treatment of HIV-associated Kaposi sarcoma with immune checkpoint blockade. Cancer Immunol Res. 2018;6(10):1129–35.
63. Delyon J, Biard L, Renaud M, Resche-Rigon M, Le Goff J, Dalle S, Heidelberger V, Da Meda L, Toullec L, Carcelain G, Mourah S, Caillat-Zucman S, Allain V, Battistella M, Lebbe C. PD-1 blockade with pembrolizumab in classic or endemic Kaposi's sarcoma: a multicentre, single-arm, phase 2 study. Lancet Oncol. 2022;23(4):491–500. https://doi.org/10.1016/S1470-2045(22)00097-3. Epub 2022 Mar 10. PMID: 35279271.
64. Zer A, Icht O, Yosef L, Avram D, Jacobi O, Fenig E, Kurman N, Peretz I, Shamai S, Merimsky O, Ben-Ami E, Shapira Frommer R, Schwarzbach AE, Bernstine H, Weitzen R, Vornicova O, Bar-Sela G, Stemmer SM, Lotem M. Phase II single-arm study of nivolumab and ipilimumab (Nivo/Ipi) in previously treated classical Kaposi sarcoma (cKS). Ann Oncol. 2022;33(7):720–7. https://doi.org/10.1016/j.annonc.2022.03.012. Epub 2022 Mar 23. PMID: 35339649.

Chapter 20
Hematolymphoid Tumors

José Antonio Sanches, Denis Miyashiro, Jade Cury Martins, Juliana Pereira, and Cláudia Regina Cardin Mendes de Oliveira

Key Points

- Primary cutaneous lymphomas are the second most frequent extranodal non-Hodgkin lymphomas.
- Mycosis fungoides, a cutaneous T-cell lymphoma, represent approximately 50% of the primary cutaneous lymphomas. It is a heterogeneous disorder, frequently with indolent behavior.
- Sézary syndrome is an aggressive variant of primary cutaneous lymphomas, characterized by erythroderma, lymph node enlargement, and peripheral blood involvement by neoplastic cells.
- Other less frequent cutaneous T-cell lymphomas include adult T-cell leukemia/lymphoma, primary cutaneous CD30-positive lymphoproliferative disorders, subcutaneous panniculitis-like T-cell lymphoma, primary cutaneous γ/δ T-cell lymphoma, primary cutaneous aggressive epidermotropic

J. A. Sanches (✉) · D. Miyashiro
Dermatology, Faculdade de Medicina da Universidade de São Paulo, São Paulo, São Paulo, Brazil

J. C. Martins
Dermatology, Faculdade de Medicina da Universidade de São Paulo, São Paulo, São Paulo, Brazil

Instituto do Cancer do Estado de São Paulo—ICESP, São Paulo, São Paulo, Brazil

J. Pereira
Division of Hematology, Faculdade de Medicina da Universidade de São Paulo, São Paulo, São Paulo, Brazil

C. R. C. M. de Oliveira
Hospital Sirio-Libanês, São Paulo, São Paulo, Brazil

C. M. Z. Abdalla et al. (eds.), *Oncodermatology*,
https://doi.org/10.1007/978-3-031-29277-4_20

CD8-positive T-cell lymphoma (provisional), primary cutaneous CD4+ small/medium T-cell lymphoproliferative disorder (provisional), primary cutaneous acral CD8+ T-cell lymphoma (provisional), and primary cutaneous peripheral T-cell lymphoma, not otherwise specified.
- Primary cutaneous B-cell lymphomas are represented by primary cutaneous marginal zone lymphoma; primary cutaneous follicle center; primary cutaneous diffuse large B-cell lymphoma, leg type; EBV-positive mucocutaneous ulcer (provisional); and intravascular large B-cell lymphoma.
- Extranodal NK-/T-cell lymphoma, nasal type, may be derived from cytotoxic T cells or NK cells.

Cutaneous Lymphomas

Lymphomas constitute a group of neoplasms derived from the lymphoreticular system. They are divided into Hodgkin's and non-Hodgkin's lymphoma. Hodgkin's lymphoma accounts for 15% of lymphomas [1] and affects cervical, mediastinal, supraclavicular, and axillary lymph nodes in adult individuals [2]. Its absolute incidence has not changed over the years, in contrast to the evident increase in the incidence of non-Hodgkin's lymphomas [3]. The latter can be nodal, when they primarily affect lymph nodes, or extranodal. Extranodal lymphomas account for about 30% of non-Hodgkin's lymphomas [4]. The skin is the second most involved organ, after the gastrointestinal tract, comprising approximately 19% of these lymphomas [3]. Primary cutaneous lymphomas differ significantly from the equivalent nodal forms in clinical behaviors and prognoses [5].

In the past, cutaneous lymphomas were not recognized as a separate entity but as secondary involvement of the skin by nodal lymphoma. Initially, only mycosis fungoides (MF), a cutaneous T-cell lymphoma (CTCL), was recognized as a primary cutaneous lymphoma. The first reports of primary cutaneous lymphomas, excluding MF, were published in the 1960s and 1970s. Based on the immunophenotypic characteristics of neoplastic cells, in the late 1970s, lymphomas were divided into two groups according to their origins: T-cell and B-cell lymphomas. In the 1980s and 1990s, the concept of primary and secondary cutaneous lymphomas emerged. Then several classifications were proposed [6, 7]. In 2005, conferences between the World Health Organization (WHO) and the European Organization for Research and Treatment of Cancer (EORTC) proposed a classification that brought uniformity to the diagnosis and treatment of primary cutaneous lymphoproliferative processes [5]. Following this joint publication, WHO published two more updates of the classification of both cutaneous and extracutaneous lymphoid neoplasms [8, 9], and in 2018, the WHO-EORTC association reconvened and published an update in 2019, described in Table 20.1 [10].

Table 20.1 Classification of primary cutaneous lymphomas, relative frequency, and prognosis [10]

WHO-EORTC classification		
Cutaneous T-cell lymphomas	Frequency (%)	5-year DSS (%)
Mycosis fungoides		
Mycosis fungoides variants	39	88
• Folliculotropic MF	5	75
• Pagetoid reticulosis	<1	100
• Granulomatous slack skin	<1	100
Sézary syndrome	2	36
Adult T-cell leukemia/lymphoma	<1	NDA
Primary cutaneous CD30-positive lymphoproliferative disorders		
• Primary cutaneous anaplastic large cell lymphoma	8	95
• Lymphomatoid papulosis	12	99
Subcutaneous panniculitis-like T-cell lymphoma	1	87
Extranodal NK-/T-cell lymphoma, nasal type	<1	16
Chronic active EBV infection	<1	NDA
Primary cutaneous peripheral T-cell lymphoma, rare subtypes		
• Primary cutaneous γ/δ T-cell lymphoma	<1	11
• Primary cutaneous aggressive epidermotropic CD8-positive T-cell lymphoma (provisional)	<1	31
• Primary cutaneous CD4+ small/medium T-cell lymphoproliferative disorder (provisional)	6	100
• Primary cutaneous acral CD8+ T-cell lymphoma (provisional)	<1	100
Primary cutaneous peripheral T-cell lymphoma, not otherwise specified	2	15
Cutaneous B-cell lymphomas		
Primary cutaneous marginal zone lymphoma	9	99
Primary cutaneous follicle center lymphoma	12	95
Primary cutaneous diffuse large B-cell lymphoma, leg type	4	56
EBV-positive mucocutaneous ulcer (provisional)	<1	100
Intravascular large B-cell lymphoma	<1	72

DSS disease-specific survival, *NDA* no data available

Epidemiology

An annual incidence of 0.3–10.7 cases of cutaneous lymphomas per 1,000,000 population is estimated [3, 4, 11, 12]. Approximately 70–82% of primary cutaneous lymphomas are CTCL, with annual incidences between 3.4 and 7.7 per 1,000,000 population [3, 11, 12], and absolute predominance of MF and its variants, which correspond to approximately 50% of cases of cutaneous lymphomas [5]. Cutaneous B-cell lymphomas (CBCL) represent approximately 20–30% of all primary cutaneous lymphomas. The annual incidence of CBCL ranges from 0.3 to 3.9 cases per 1,000,000 population [3, 12, 13].

Studies show an increase in the incidence of cutaneous lymphomas, currently with an incidence three times higher than the epidemiological studies carried out in the early 1980s [3].

Pathophysiology

The pathophysiology of cutaneous lymphomas is not entirely understood. The most plausible hypothesis is the activation of B cells or T cells by antigen-presenting cells, leading to the gradual accumulation of mutations that lead to neoplastic cell development. However, the triggering antigen is unknown, and it could vary between patients [14, 15].

Bacterial, viral, fungal, and mycobacterial infections, medications, and low vitamin D levels have already been studied regarding the origin of cutaneous lymphoproliferative processes [16–22]. The analysis of regional groupings of patients with cutaneous lymphomas suggests exposure to unknown environmental factors and even occupational exposure (benzene and trichloroethylene) [23–26]. However, none of these factors has been shown to be consistently associated with the genesis of cutaneous lymphomas, and most of these studies are restricted to series and case reports.

Clinical Aspects

Different types of cutaneous lymphomas present with varied clinical manifestations, and they will be described in each specific section [5].

Histopathology

The diagnostic confirmation of cutaneous lymphoma is not easy. Diagnosis of malignancy is usually suggested by experienced pathologists through the evaluation of the cytomorphology and the architectural arrangement of the infiltrate. For the classification of cutaneous lymphomas, it is essential to carry out an immunohistochemical study, whose antibody panel is rationalized according to the histological findings [27].

Molecular Biology

The search for T-cell receptor (TCR) gene rearrangement, demonstrating monoclonal T lymphocyte proliferation in the skin, lymph nodes, and/or peripheral blood, can help in the diagnosis of T-cell lymphomas. For B-cell lymphomas, clonality is accessed by analyzing immunoglobulin heavy chain and kappa rearrangements since lambda gene rearrangements are limited. These molecular biology studies are performed by polymerase chain reaction (PCR), Southern blot, or next-generation sequencing (NGS) [28–31].

Evolutionary Aspects

Lymphomas that present primarily on the skin, without evidence of extracutaneous disease at the time of diagnosis, often have a more indolent clinical behavior and better prognoses than systemic lymphomas of similar histological subtype [5]. Within the WHO-EORTC classification, cutaneous lymphomas can be separated according to clinical behavior [10].

Indolent lymphomas include MF and its variants, primary cutaneous CD30-positive lymphoproliferative disorders, subcutaneous panniculitis-like T-cell lymphoma, primary cutaneous CD4+ small/medium T-cell lymphoproliferative disorder, primary cutaneous acral CD8+ T-cell lymphoma, primary cutaneous marginal zone lymphoma, primary cutaneous follicle center lymphoma, and EBV-positive mucocutaneous ulcer. Indolent lymphomas are characterized by a long natural history [10].

Primary cutaneous diffuse large B-cell lymphoma, leg type, is considered an intermediate behavior lymphoma, with a specific 5-year survival of 55% [5].

Aggressive lymphomas include SS; adult T-cell lymphoma/leukemia; extranodal NK-/T-cell lymphoma, nasal type; primary cutaneous γ/δ T-cell lymphoma; primary cutaneous aggressive epidermotropic CD8-positive T-cell lymphoma; and primary cutaneous peripheral T-cell lymphoma, not otherwise specified. These are characterized by poor prognosis; they usually have a rapid and aggressive course, with a high mortality rate despite treatment [5, 10].

Mycosis Fungoides

MF was described in 1806 by Jean-Louis-Marc Alibert, and later, Pierre-Antoine-Ernest Bazin described its evolution from patches to plaques and tumors. MF accounts for approximately 50% of cutaneous lymphomas and is characterized by the proliferation of small and medium epidermotropic T lymphocytes with convoluted nuclei. Neoplastic lymphocytes are commonly CD4 positive, but cases with proliferation of CD4-negative and CD8-positive lymphocytes are observed. The recent WHO-EORTC classification of cutaneous lymphomas recognizes the classic Alibert-Bazin MF and three variants (folliculotropic MF, pagetoid reticulosis, and granulomatous slack skin) [10].

There is a male predominance (53–73%) with median age at diagnosis between 54.0 and 73.0 years [32]. Time between symptom onset and MF diagnosis ranges between 2.0 and 4.2 years [33–35].

Clinical Aspects

MF is a polymorphic disease often called "the great imitator," and there is a wide range of differential diagnoses [36].

The classic Alibert-Bazin form of MF is an indolent disease, with lesions that initially appear on the skin of the buttocks, lower trunk, inguinal regions, and breasts, in variable numbers, spreading gradually. Initially, non-infiltrated patches are observed, and these lesions progressively become more infiltrated, forming erythematous-brownish plaques with well-defined borders (Fig. 20.1a, b). Tumors may appear over preexisting plaques or on areas of healthy skin. Patients have a combination of patches, plaques, and tumors concurrently (Fig. 20.1c). Infiltrated plaques and tumors may ulcerate, and erythroderma (erythema and scaling affecting more than 80% of the body surface area) may arise as the disease progresses (Fig. 20.1d) [5, 37]. Extracutaneous dissemination to lymph nodes, blood, or viscera is rare but has a significant negative impact on disease prognosis [38]. Pruritus is the most frequent symptom, present in almost all patients, with varying degrees of intensity. Systemic symptoms are rarely observed [39].

Folliculotropic MF is the most common variant (Fig. 20.2a). These cases may be divided into advanced folliculotropic MF, with infiltrated plaques and tumors in the cephalic region and a reserved prognosis, and early-stage folliculotropic MF, where there are patches and thin plaques with follicular accentuation in the trunk, with a favorable prognosis [40, 41].

Granulomatous slack skin is a rare variant of MF. Initially, there are sarcoid papules and plaques in the axillary and inguinal folds, which evolve with laxity (Fig. 20.2b). Histology shows granulomas and elastophagocytosis, in addition to atypical lymphocytes infiltrating the skin. This variant may be associated with other hematologic malignancies (Hodgkin's lymphoma, anaplastic large T-cell lymphoma) [42].

Pagetoid reticulosis is another rare variant, characterized by psoriasiform or hyperkeratotic lesions, affecting the extremities (Fig. 20.2c). Histology shows epidermal hyperplasia with a pagetoid proliferation of atypical lymphocytes [5].

Besides the classical Alibert-Bazin form and the three variants of MF, other clinicopathological subtypes of MF have been described.

Hypopigmented MF is characterized by hypochromic patches, and it affects younger patients (median age 32.2 years) and with a higher phototype (Fig. 20.2d). This is the most frequent type of MF in the pediatric population, comprising 50% of these patients [36, 43–45]. Poikilodermic MF is characterized by hypopigmented, hyperpigmented, atrophic lesions with telangiectasias, typically affecting the flexural areas and the trunk [46]. It can be divided into localized or generalized poikilodermic MF, when lesions affect more than 80% of the body surface area (Fig. 20.2e, f) [47].

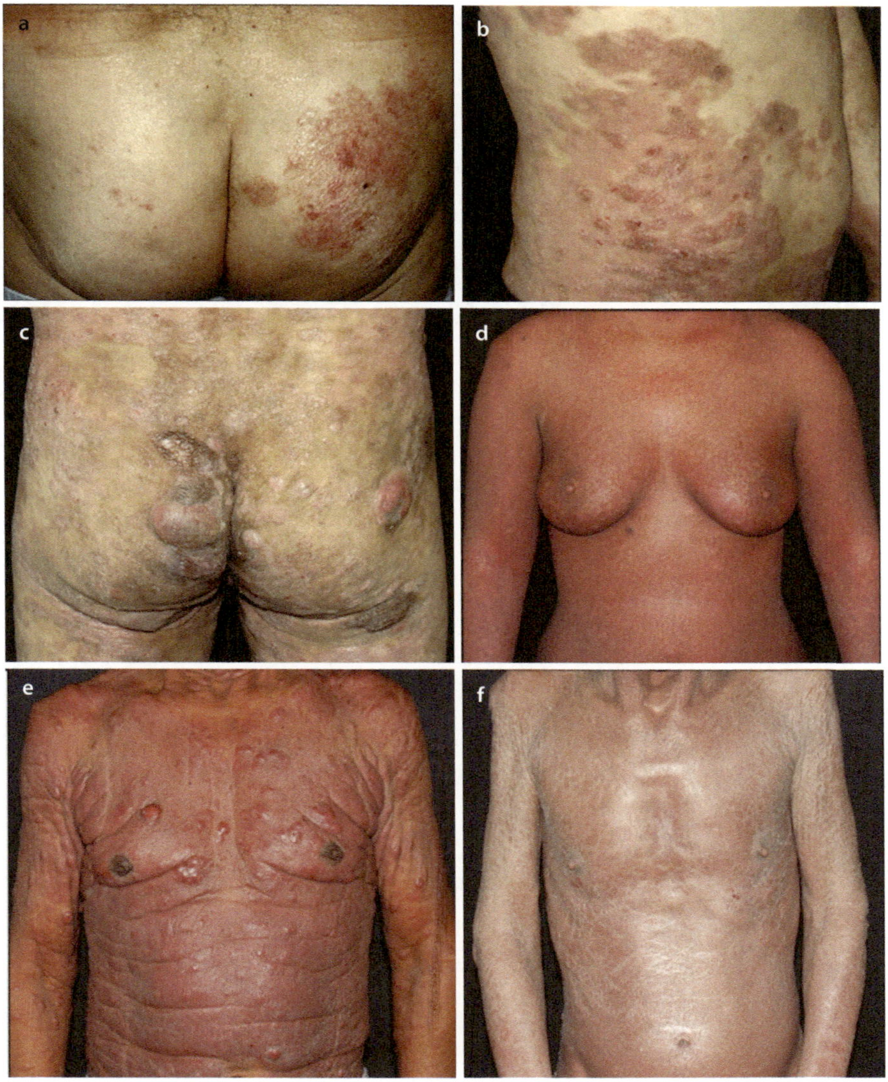

Fig. 20.1 Mycosis fungoides. Patches on the buttocks (**a**). Plaques on the abdomen (**b**). Patches, plaques, and tumors on the buttocks (**c**). Erythroderma (erythema and scaling ≥80% of the body surface area) in a patient with erythrodermic mycosis fungoides (**d**). Erythroderma and tumors (**e**). Erythroderma in a patient with Sézary syndrome (**f**)

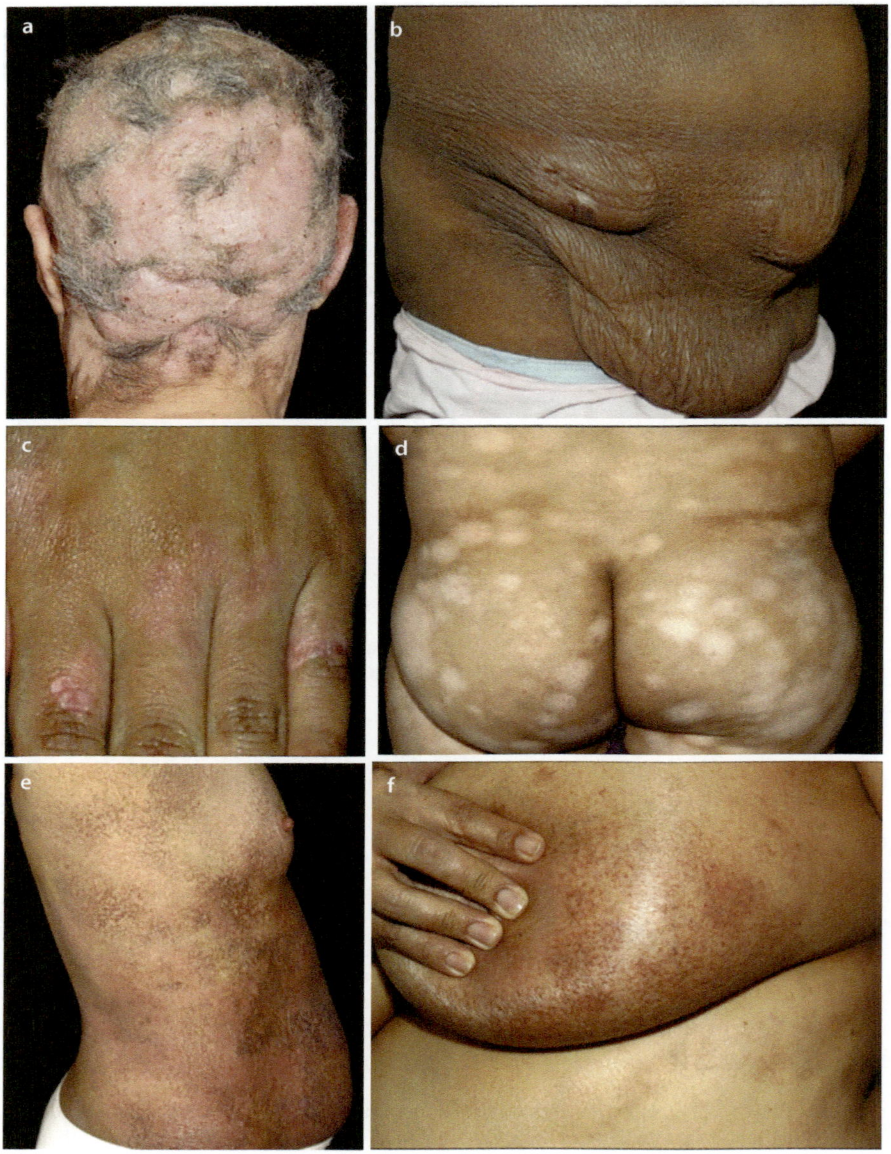

Fig. 20.2 Variants and subtypes of mycosis fungoides. Folliculotropic mycosis fungoides (**a**). Granulomatous slack skin (**b**). Pagetoid reticulosis (**c**). Hypopigmented mycosis fungoides (**d**). Generalized poikilodermic mycosis fungoides (**e**). Localized poikilodermic mycosis fungoides (**f**)

Histopathology

Histology shows epidermotropism of atypical lymphocytes with hyperchromatic and convoluted nuclei surrounded by a clear halo. These neoplastic cells may be isolated or aligned in the basal layer of the epidermis, and they may form Pautrier microabscesses (clustering of at least four lymphocytes around a Langerhans cell in the epidermis). Neoplastic cells are CD4-positive T cells with a memory phenotype (CD3+CD4+CD45RO+CD8−) with loss of expression of CD7 in approximately 70% of cases. MF neoplastic cells can be CD3+CD4−CD8+, especially in hypopigmented MF [37, 48, 49].

Molecular Biology

T-cell monoclonal population is observed in 50% of patch lesions, 73% of plaque lesions, and 83–100% of tumors, and the detection of the same clone in different skin biopsies favors the diagnosis of CTCL [50–52].

Diagnosis

There is no gold standard test for the diagnosis of MF, and it is based on clinical, histopathology, T-cell clonality, and follow-up data.

Staging

For MF and SS, the modified TNMB system (tumor, lymph nodes, visceral metastasis, blood) was adopted (Tables 20.2 and 20.3) [53].

Bone marrow biopsy is performed if there are hematological abnormalities that cannot be explained by other causes. Its involvement in MF/SS is rare and is considered visceral involvement (M1) [53, 54].

For patients in early stages (IA–IIA), chest X-ray and ultrasonography of the abdomen and lymph node chains can be performed. In advanced cases (IIB–IVB), computed tomography of the chest, abdomen, and pelvis or a positron emission tomography are indicated [53].

Table 20.2 MF/SS staging

T: Skin
T1: Limited papules, patches, and plaques <10% of the body surface area
T1a: Patches
T1b: Patches and plaques
T2: Generalized papules, patches, and plaques ≥10% of the body surface area
T2a: Patches
T2b: Patches and plaques
T3: One or more tumors (≥1 cm of diameter)
T4: Erythroderma (erythema and scaling affecting ≥80% of the body surface area)
N: Lymph nodes
N0: No clinically abnormal lymph nodes, no biopsy is required
N1: Clinically abnormal lymph node; dermatopathic lymphadenopathy
N1a: Negative clone[a]
N1b: Positive clone[a]
N2: Clinically abnormal lymph node; partial lymph node involvement by neoplastic cells, no architectural lymph node alteration
N2a: Negative clone[a]
N2b: Positive clone[a]
N3: Clinically abnormal lymph node; complete lymph node involvement by neoplastic cells, architectural lymph node alteration observed
Nx: Clinically abnormal lymph node, no histologic confirmation[b]
M: Viscera
M0: No visceral involvement
M1: Histologic confirmation of visceral involvement[c]
B: Blood
B0: No significant blood involvement: ≤5% of atypical lymphocytes (Sézary cells)
B0a: Negative clone[a]
B0b: Positive clone[a]
B1: Low blood tumor burden: >5% atypical lymphocytes (Sézary cells), no criteria for B2
B1a: Negative clone[a]
B1b: Positive clone[a]
B2: Monoclonal T-cell population on peripheral blood (positive clone)[a] and
≥1000 Sézary cells/L and/or
CD4/CD8 ≥ 10 and/or CD4+CD7− ≥ 40% and/or CD4+CD26− ≥ 30%

[a] TCR gene rearrangement analysis by polymerase chain reaction, Southern blot, or next-generation sequencing
[b] Clinically suspicious lymph nodes (≥1.5 cm, indurated, clustered, fixed to deep planes) should be biopsied
[c] Except for splenomegaly (no histologic confirmation required)

Table 20.3 MF/SS staging

	T	N	M	B
IA	1	0	0	0,1
IB	2	0	0	0,1
IIA	1,2	1,2	0	0,1
IIB	3	0–2	0	0,1
IIIA	4	0–2	0	0
IIIB	4	0–2	0	1
IVA_1	1–4	0–2	0	2
IVA_2	1–4	3	0	0–2
IVB	1–4	0–3	1	0–2

Prognosis

Patients with skin-limited disease respond well to topical treatments and have an overall survival similar to the healthy population. Only 2% of the patients with localized lesions (involvement of less than 10% of the body surface area) die after 32 years due to progression, and only 9% present progression to plaques and tumors with lymph node, blood, and visceral dissemination [34]. The 5-year overall survival is 91–97% for patients with localized patches and plaques (<10% of the skin surface), 81–85% for patients with generalized patches and plaques (≥10% of the skin surface), 44% for patients with tumors, and 20–30% for those with lymph node disease. Sepsis, especially caused by *Staphylococcus aureus*, represents one of the most frequent causes of death in advanced cases [54].

MF can progress with large-cell transformation, which is defined histologically by the presence of large cells (cells four times larger than normal lymphocyte size) in 25% or more of the dermal infiltrate or forming microscopic nodules. It can occur in tumoral lesions and, less frequently, in plaque and erythrodermic forms. These cells may or may not express CD30, and the possibility of coexistence between CD30-positive large T-cell anaplastic lymphoma and MF should be considered [53]. Transformed MF has a worse prognosis, with overall 5-year survival of 38.5% [38].

In addition to staging, other factors reported to be associated with a worse prognosis are older age, male gender, folliculotropism in histology, high expression of CD30, and high expression of Ki-67 [54–56]. The Cutaneous Lymphoma International Consortium (CLIC) study proposed a prognostic index based on age (≥60 years), increased lactate dehydrogenase, large cell transformation, and stage IV [38]. However, studies on prognostic factors are conflicting, and even the prognostic index proposed by the CLIC study was not applicable in all series [57]. Such prognostic studies are mostly retrospective observational studies. The PROCLIPI study (Prospective Cutaneous Lymphoma International Prognostic Index) is an international multicenter prospective study derived from the CLIC study. Its objective is to develop a prognostic index to better stratify and manage patients [58].

Treatment

Skin-directed therapies include topical treatments with corticosteroids, nitrogen mustard, bexarotene, phototherapy with narrowband UVB and PUVA, and radiotherapy (localized and total skin irradiation with an electron beam) [59].

Systemic treatments are used mainly in patients with advanced disease, and the most used therapeutic modalities are steroids and biological response modifiers (interferon-α, retinoids, histone deacetylase inhibitors). Alemtuzumab (anti-CD52), brentuximab-vedotin (anti-CD30), and mogamulizumab (anti-CCR4) may be used in some patients. Monochemotherapy (chlorambucil, methotrexate, pralatrexate, gemcitabine, pegylated liposomal doxorubicin) and polychemotherapy (CHOP, CVP, CHOEP) have high response rates, but with rapid recurrence, and are used in refractory advanced-stage disease [60].

Allogeneic bone marrow transplantation is an effective and potentially curative treatment in advanced cases [61]. Extracorporeal photopheresis (ECP) is indicated for erythrodermic forms (erythrodermic MF and SS) [62]. Surgery is reserved as a palliative treatment for localized nodular or tumoral lesions [63].

Sézary Syndrome

SS was described by Albert Sézary and Yves Bouvrain in 1938 [64]. It is a leukemic variant of CTCL and occurs almost exclusively in adults. The classic triad of SS includes erythroderma, lymphadenopathy, and circulating malignant cells. Males are more affected than females (2:1), and mean age at diagnosis is 66.2 years [50].

MF and SS were considered as poles of the same disease for many years. However, neoplastic cells in these two entities have distinct immunophenotypic profiles. In MF, cells strongly express CCR4 and CLA, which confer tropism to the skin, and are negative for CCR7 and L-selectin, receptors that confer tropism to lymph nodes. This immunophenotype is characteristic of resident skin memory T cells. On the other hand, SS cells express CCR7 and L-selectin, CD27 (a characteristic marker of central memory T cells), CCR4, and other skin-tropic receptors (CCR6, CCR10, CLA). These findings suggest that MF and SS are distinct diseases originating from different subtypes of T lymphocytes. Despite the description that the neoplastic cells of the two entities have different origins, cases of classic MF that evolve with erythroderma and peripheral blood involvement are occasionally observed, with a clinical-laboratory and evolutionary picture identical to those patients with SS. Therefore, whether MF and SS are distinct poles of the same disease, different diseases remains to be defined [65].

Clinical Aspects

Besides erythroderma, diffuse non-scarring alopecia, palmoplantar hyperkeratosis, nail dystrophies, and leonine facies may be observed (Fig. 20.1f) [66].

Intense pruritus is the most frequent symptom, and it is associated with worsening quality of life [39, 50]. Systemic symptoms (fever, night sweats, weight loss) are present in 1.6% of the patients [67].

Histopathology

In SS, the histopathology of skin is identical to MF. However, in erythrodermic forms of cutaneous lymphomas (erythrodermic MF and SS), epidermotropism is less evident, and in up to one-third of SS cases, the histology may be nonspecific [50].

Molecular Biology

T-cell monoclonality on the skin is detected in 73.3–77.5% [50, 66]; on the blood, in 86.7–100% [50, 68]; and on the lymph nodes, in 77.8–88.2% of SS patients [50, 66, 69]. Studies evaluating clonality in the bone marrow are scarce, but one study demonstrated T lymphocyte clone in 53.6% (15/28) of patients with SS [50].

Diagnosis

Diagnostic criteria for SS are detailed in Table 20.4 [53].

Table 20.4 Sézary syndrome diagnostic criteria [53]

Sézary cells on peripheral blood smear	≥1000 Sézary cells/μL
Immunophenotyping of lymphocytes by flow cytometry	CD4/CD8 ≥ 10
	CD4+CD7− ≥ 40%
	CD4+CD26− ≥ 30%
TCR gene rearrangement analysis	Monoclonal population on skin and blood (same clone)

Circulating Sézary cells are detected by peripheral blood smear (large lymphocytes with a cerebriform nucleus) and immunophenotyping of lymphocytes by flow cytometry. Search for TCR gene rearrangement shows a monoclonal population of T cells on the blood, and the same clone is detected on skin infiltrate [5, 50, 53].

Staging

As a leukemic variant of CTCL, SS diagnostic criteria fulfill criteria for B2 stage. Thus, SS patients are classified as stage IVA1, IVA2, or IVB (Tables 20.2 and 20.3) [53].

Prognosis

Five-year survival rates range between 40% and 50% [38, 50].

Treatment

First-line treatment includes ECP, chlorambucil associated with prednisone, retinoids, or interferon-α combined with ECP or PUVA and low-dose methotrexate. Second-line treatment include chemotherapy (gemcitabine, pegylated liposomal doxorubicin, CHOP, and CHOP-like regimens), alemtuzumab, and allogeneic stem cell transplantation [59].

Adult T-Cell Leukemia/Lymphoma

Adult T-cell leukemia/lymphoma (ATLL) is an aggressive disorder associated with the human T-cell lymphotropic virus type-1 (HTLV-1) infection [70]. HTLV-1 is endemic in Japan, the Caribbean islands, sub-Saharan Africa, South America, including the northern and northeastern parts of Brazil, the northern part of Iran, and some regions of Central Europe (Romania) and Oceania [71]. It is transmitted through breastfeeding, transfusion of contaminated blood and blood products, and unprotected sexual intercourse. In addition to ATLL, the virus causes HTLV-1-associated myelopathy/tropical spastic paraparesis (HAM/TSP), infective dermatitis associated with HTLV-1 (IDH), and HTLV-1-associated uveitis. High HTLV-1 proviral DNA load is associated with an increased risk of developing ATLL and HAM/TSP [72, 73].

Among HTLV-1-infected individuals, 1–5% develop ATLL, usually after more than two decades of viral persistence. The HTLV-1-infected cells generate oligoclones in asymptomatic carriers. These premalignant cells, together with the immunosuppressive state observed in HTLV-1-infected individuals, predispose to the expansion of the predominant clone, originating the neoplastic cells in ATLL [74]. The average age at diagnosis is between 50 and 60 years, with a slight predominance among men [75].

In 1991, Shimoyama proposed a classification of ATLL in four different types based on clinical, laboratory, and prognostic characteristics: acute, lymphomatous, chronic, and smoldering (Table 20.5) [76].

More recently, a primary cutaneous tumoral ATLL has been described in Brazilian [78] and Japanese cohorts [79], in patients with tumoral lesions but with no evidence of ATLL in other organs.

Table 20.5 Shimoyama's classification (adapted from Verdonck et al.) [76, 77]

	Acute	Lymphomatous	Chronic	Smoldering
Proportion	55%	20%	20%	5%
Median survival	6 months	10 months	24 months	Not reported
4-year survival	5%	6%	27%	66%
Lymphocyte count	Not definitory	<4000 per mL	≥4000 per mL	<4000 per mL
Lactate dehydrogenase	Not definitory	Not definitory	<2.0× normal upper limit	<1.5× normal upper limit
Calcium, corrected	Not definitory	Not definitory	<5.5 mEqL	<5.5 mEq/L
Abnormal T-lymphocytes	≥5%	<1%	≥5%	≥5%
Flower cells	Yes	No	Occasionally	Occasionally
Skin and/or lung lesions	Not definitory	Not definitory	Not definitory	If abnormal lymphocyte <5%
Lymph node involvement	Not definitory	Yes	Not definitory	No
Liver or spleen involvement	Not definitory	Not definitory	Not definitory	No
Central nervous system involvement	Not definitory	Not definitory	No	No
Bone involvement	Not definitory	Not definitory	No	No
Ascites	Not definitory	Not definitory	No	No
Pleural effusion	Not definitory	Not definitory	No	No
Gastrointestinal tract involvement	Not definitory	Not definitory	No	No

Clinical Aspects

Skin lesions may be observed in 39–72% of ATLL patients and may be the first symptom of ATLL [74]. Skin lesions include patches, papules, plaques, nodules, tumors, erythroderma, purpura, and xerosis/ichthyosis [74]. Nodulotumoral lesions are the most frequent (29.5%), followed by multiple papules (25.0%) and plaques (25.0%). Less frequently, erythroderma (10.1%), patches (7.3%), purpuric (2.4%), and ichthyosis-like lesions (0.7%) are observed. Different types of skin lesions may be seen concomitantly (Fig. 20.3) [74]. Cutaneous involvement is more common in chronic and smoldering types [80]. Uncommon manifestations of ATLL include subcutaneous induration, erythema multiforme-like lesions, psoriasis-like lesions, parapsoriasis-like lesions, palmoplantar psoriasis, alopecia, folliculitis, ichthyosis, and prurigo [81].

Differential diagnoses include MF, SS, dermatophytosis, eczematous dermatitis, lichen planus, psoriasis, atopic dermatitis, bullous pemphigoid, eruptive xanthomas, furuncle, granulomatous rosacea, histiocytosis, infected eczematoid dermatitis, leprosy, parapsoriasis, pityriasis rosea, pseudolymphoma, scabies, and urticaria [74, 82].

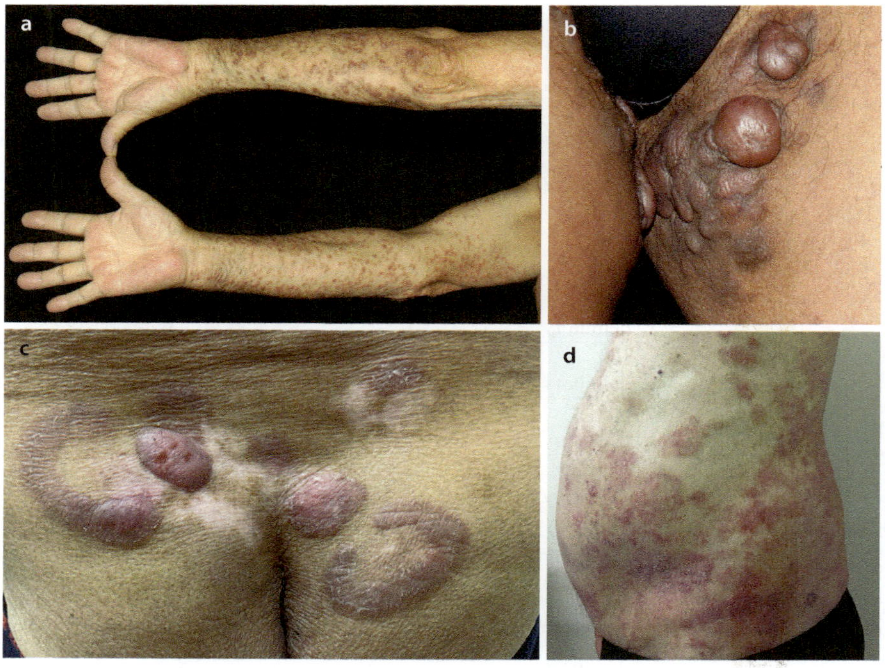

Fig. 20.3 Adult T-cell leukemia/lymphoma. Multiple infiltrated papules (**a**). Nodulotumoral lesions (**b**). Infiltrated arciform plaques and ulcerated tumors (**c**). Multiple infiltrated plaques (**d**)

Histopathology

The skin histopathology findings reflect the heterogeneity of skin lesions. Patches and plaques show perivascular or diffuse infiltration in the upper dermis of small- to medium-sized atypical lymphocytes. Papules, nodules, and tumors show nodular or diffuse infiltration from the dermis to the subcutaneous tissue of medium- to large-sized atypical lymphocytes with moderate to severe atypia [74, 80, 81, 83]. Neoplastic cells are mature, activated, post-thymic CD3+CD4+CD7−CD25+ cells [83]. The CD25 expression is sensitive but nonspecific for ATLL, and its positivity ranges from 71.0% to 93.3% [74].

Prognosis

The 4-year survival time of the acute, lymphoma, chronic, and smoldering types are 5%, 6%, 27%, and 66%, respectively [74, 77].

Advanced performance status, high blood lactate dehydrogenase level, older age (≥40 years), more than three involved sites, hypercalcemia, hepatosplenomegaly, and lymphadenopathy are associated with poorer prognosis [76, 84]. The presence of skin lesions are associated with a worse prognosis in the acute, chronic, and smoldering types but not in lymphomatous type, where the prognosis is poor independently of the presence of skin lesions [85, 86]. The type of skin lesion is also associated with prognosis, with worse survival in patients with nodulotumoral and erythrodermic presentation [86].

Treatment

Smoldering and chronic ATLL may be managed with "watch and wait" and skin-directed therapies (topical steroids, phototherapy, local radiotherapy) when cutaneous lesions are present. If multiple lesions are observed, systemic steroids, oral retinoids, interferon-α (IFN-α), antiretrovirals (zidovudine), or single-agent chemotherapy may be used [80, 87].

Acute and lymphomatous ATLL have poor prognoses. For acute ATLL, zidovudine + IFN-α and chemotherapy are indicated. For maintenance therapy, zidovudine + IFN-α are used [88]. For lymphomatous ATLL, intensive chemotherapy is followed by zidovudine + IFN-α in maintenance therapy [89]. Treatments with zidovudine + IFN-α or chemotherapy followed allo-HSCT for nonresponders are indicated. Skin-directed therapies are used for localized disease and radiotherapy for symptom control [88]. Chemotherapy regimens include CHOP (cyclophosphamide, vincristine, doxorubicin, prednisone), CHOEP (etoposide, cyclophosphamide, vincristine, doxorubicin, prednisone), DA-EPOCH (dose-adjusted etoposide, cyclophosphamide, vincristine, doxorubicin, prednisone), hyper-CVAD (cyclophosphamide, vincristine, doxorubicin, dexamethasone, alternated with high-dose cytarabine and methotrexate), IVAC (ifosfamide, etoposide, cytarabine) and VCAP-AMP-VECP (VACP: vincristine, cyclophosphamide, doxorubicin, prednisone; AMP: doxorubicin, ranimustine, prednisolone; VECP: vindesine, etoposide, carboplatin, prednisolone) [88, 89]. Mogamulizumab (anti-CCR4 monoclonal antibody) was approved in combination with VCAP-AMP-VECP [90], and lenalidomide was approved for relapsed or refractory ATLL [91]. Brentuximab vedotin (antibody-drug conjugate with anti-CD30 monoclonal antibody) associated with CHP (cyclophosphamide, doxorubicin, and prednisone) showed significant improvements in overall survival and progression-free survival in ATLL treatment [92].

In addition to symptoms related to the neoplastic condition, patients with ATLL are immunocompromised due to the immune dysregulation caused by HTLV-1. Dermatophyte infection and infestation by *Strongyloides stercoralis* are frequent and must be appropriately addressed [93, 94].

Primary Cutaneous CD30-Positive Lymphoproliferative Disorders

Epidemiology

Primary cutaneous CD30-positive lymphoproliferative disorders are the second most common group of primary cutaneous lymphomas, accounting for approximately 25% of cases. This group comprises a spectrum of diseases ranging from lymphomatoid papulosis (Lyp) to primary cutaneous anaplastic large cell lymphoma (PC-ALCL). There are cases of overlap between the two entities when they are called "borderline" [5]. The key feature of this group is the prominent expression of CD30. The mean age is 61 years, with a slight predominance in male and white patients [95].

Risk Factors/Genetic Determinants

Unlike systemic anaplastic lymphoma, almost all primary cutaneous CD30-positive lymphoproliferative disorders do not present the ALK gene translocation. Thus, the expression of ALK in anaplastic lymphoma should lead to suspicion of secondary cutaneous involvement of systemic anaplastic lymphoma [96].

DUSP22 (dual-specificity phosphatase 22) is a tyrosine/threonine/serine phosphatase that can act as a tumor suppressor. Its inactivation may be associated with the emergence of primary cutaneous CD30-positive lymphoproliferative disorders [97].

Diagnosis (Dermatologic Assessment/Biopsy/Pathology)

Lymphomatoid papulosis presents as erythematous, infiltrated papules with typical relapses and spontaneous remissions (Fig. 20.4). They can be generalized or grouped in some parts of the body and coexist in different stages of evolution. Typically, there is central ulceration with a subsequent resolution with a varioliform scar and residual hyperpigmentation. The papules usually take 3–8 weeks to resolve, and the disease can evolve with outbreaks for decades.

On the other hand, PC-ALCL presents more frequently as nodules measuring more than 2 cm or tumors that ulcerate in the course of evolution (Fig. 20.5). There is a multifocal or generalized disease in up to 20% of cases, and there may be tumor reduction or even spontaneous resolution. The most frequently affected skin sites are, in order of frequency: legs and hip (25.7%), head and neck (22.2%), arms and shoulder (18.6%), and trunk (17.9%) [95]. There are, however, patients who present with clinical features of lymphomatoid papulosis and PC-ALCL concomitantly and are classified as borderline cases.

Histopathology of lymphomatoid papulosis and PC-ALCL may be indistinguishable. For this reason, clinical correlation is essential for the correct classification of the disease.

The histopathological findings of lymphomatoid papulosis vary according to the evolutionary phase of the clinical lesion. In early lesions, there is a perivascular lymphocytic infiltrate with some large and atypical lymphocytes. However, in more advanced lesions, there is a dermal infiltrate composed of large cells similar to immunoblasts. There may be an inflammatory infiltrate associated with neutrophils and eosinophils. Six histopathological types of lymphomatoid papulosis are described and are summarized in Table 20.6.

There may be an aberrant T lymphocyte phenotype with loss of expression of common T antigens (CD3, CD2, CD5, or CD7).

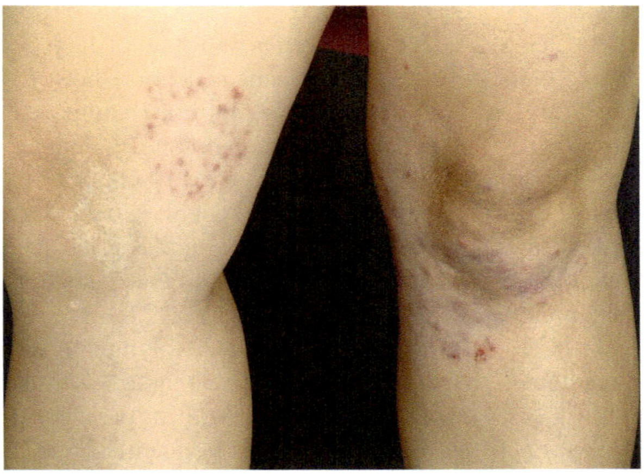

Fig. 20.4 Lymphomatoid papulosis. Grouped erythematous, infiltrated papules located in a patient legs

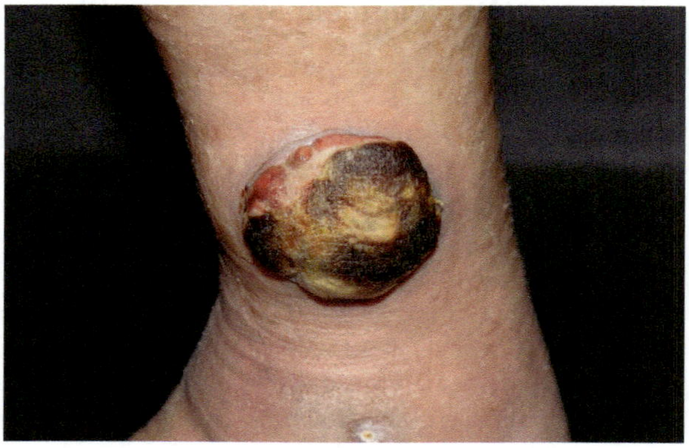

Fig. 20.5 Primary cutaneous anaplastic large cell lymphoma. Large ulcerated tumor in the ankle

Table 20.6 Histology types of lymphomatoid papulosis [98]

Lyp type (% frequency)	Characteristics	Predominant phenotype
Type A (>80%)	Wedge-shaped infiltrate of scattered or clustered large atypical CD30+ cells, intermingled with numerous inflammatory cells, such as small lymphocytes, neutrophils, eosinophils, and histiocytes	CD4+, CD8−
Type B (<5%)	Epidermotropic infiltrate of small atypical lymphocytes. These cells can be CD30+ or CD30−	CD4+, CD8−
Type C (10%)	Dermal clusters or sheets of large atypical CD30+ cells with few inflammatory cells	CD4+, CD8−
Type D (<5%)	Pagetoid infiltrate of epidermotropic small- to medium-sized atypical CD8+ and CD30+ lymphocytes	CD4−, CD8+
Type E (<5%)	Dermal angiocentric infiltrates of small, medium or large pleomorphic cells CD30+	CD4−, CD8+
Lyp with DUSP22-IRF4 rearrangement (<5%)	Small- to medium-sized epidermotropic cerebriform lymphocytes or large pleomorphic dermal lymphocytes CD30+	CD4−, CD8+ orCD4−,CD8−

In PC-ALCL, a dense dermal infiltrate of large CD30+ lymphocytes is found. These cells have pale cytoplasm and horseshoe-shaped nucleus with prominent nucleoli. Ulceration and reactive infiltrate composed of lymphocytes, histiocytes, eosinophils, and neutrophils are common. By definition, at least 75% of large cells must express CD30. In addition, primary cutaneous CD30-positive lymphoproliferative disorders, it is usually CD4+ with variable loss of expression of CD2, CD3, and CD5. There are rare cases of anaplastic CD8+ lymphoma. Unlike systemic anaplastic lymphoma, the expression of anaplastic lymphoma kinase (ALK) is very uncommon in the cutaneous form [95].

It is essential to distinguish CD30+ lymphoproliferative disorders from other lymphomas that may express such a marker as transformed mycosis fungoid and adult T-cell lymphoma/leukemia. Both in papulosis and PC-ALCL a clonal rearrangement of the TCR gene occurs frequently.

Risk Stratification and Staging and Molecular Classification

Patients with lymphomatoid papulosis have an increased risk of developing a second hematologic malignancy, especially mycosis fungoides, cutaneous or systemic anaplastic lymphoma, and even Hodgkin's lymphoma. The presence of lymph node enlargement or B symptoms (fever, weight loss, primary cutaneous CD30-positive lymphoproliferative disorders, or night sweats) should prompt the physician to consider this possibility [99].

Overall, the prognosis for primary cutaneous CD30-positive lymphoproliferative disorders is excellent. Patients with lymphomatoid papulosis that do not develop a second malignancy have a regular life expectancy for their age [99]. After a 5-year follow-up, more than 80% of patients with PC-ALCL remain alive. Adverse prognostic factors are age >60 years, tumor located in the leg or hip, male gender, and use of chemotherapy [95].

When diagnosing a primary cutaneous CD30-positive lymphoproliferative disorder, palpation of the lymph node chains should be performed in search of lymph node enlargement and palpation of the abdomen to assess visceromegaly. Laboratory tests require blood count, LDH, metabolic panel, and HTLV serology. In PC-ALCL, a CT scan with contrasts or whole-body PET/CT is indicated. If lymph node or visceral involvement is suspected, a biopsy is indicated. For cases of typical lymphomatoid papulosis and without suspicion of a second hematologic neoplasm, imaging tests are not necessary.

Treatment of Localized Disease

Patients with lymphomatoid papulosis with localized or asymptomatic lesions can be treated with topical corticosteroid therapy. The use of nitrogen mustard is also a possibility. When the lesions are more widespread or symptomatic, phototherapy (preferably UVB) can be used. Systemic treatment options are methotrexate (10–35 mg/week), systemic retinoids, or doxycycline. For localized PC-ALCL cases, surgical excision or radiotherapy can be performed [100].

Treatment of Advanced Disease

In very extensive, symptomatic, and refractory lymphomatoid papulosis cases, a therapeutic option is brentuximab vedotin. Multifocal cases of PC-ALCL are treated preferentially with brentuximab vedotin or methotrexate monotherapy. In cases where there is multiple relapse therapy failure, bexarotene, pralatrexate, gemcitabine, liposomal doxorubicin, or interferon-α can be used [100].

In cases where there is secondary nodal involvement, recommended treatment regimens include brentuximab vedotin associated with CHP (cyclophosphamide, doxorubicin, and prednisone), methotrexate or pralatrexate associated with radiotherapy (of the lymph node ± skin lesion), or CHOP or CHOEP associated with radiotherapy (lymph node ± skin lesion). Allogeneic bone marrow transplantation may be considered for patients who experience disease progression despite systemic therapy [100].

Follow-Up

Patients with primary cutaneous CD30-positive lymphoproliferative disorders should be systematically monitored to assess the treatment and evolution of skin lesions. Relapses are frequent, but for the most part, retreatment is entirely satisfactory. In addition, it is always essential to assess the appearance of B symptoms, lymph node enlargement, or visceromegaly to detect early the possible appearance of a hematologic neoplasm [95, 96].

Subcutaneous Panniculitis-Like T-Cell Lymphoma

Subcutaneous panniculitis-like T-cell lymphoma is a rare form of primary cutaneous lymphoma, accounting for approximately 1% of cases. The average age of onset is 46 years with a slight predominance in females, but there are reported cases in children. There is a clear relationship with autoimmune diseases (systemic lupus erythematosus, Sjogren's syndrome, juvenile idiopathic arthritis) since up to 20% of patients have one of these diseases at diagnosis [101].

It is a lymphoma derived from CD8+ cytotoxic T cells that predominantly affects the subcutaneous cellular tissue. It is postulated that this tropism occurs because neoplastic lymphocytes express CCR5, whose ligands (CCL3, CCL4, and CCL5) are expressed by adipocytes [102]. Studies have shown a loss-of-function mutation in the HAVCR2 gene, which encodes the TIM3 immunological checkpoint protein. These mutations maintain a constant immune activation and were strongly associated with the development of the hemophagocytic syndrome.

Clinical Features

Clinically, patients have multiple nodules or deeply infiltrated plaques of varying sizes (0.5–20 cm). In many cases, the lesions present in relapses and remissions. The overlying skin may present an erythematous or more violaceous color, and when there is regression, an area of lipoatrophy becomes permanent. Ulceration may occur, but this is not a common finding. Lesions are located mainly in the lower limbs, but they can also affect the trunk, upper limbs, and face [101].

In addition to skin lesions, patients may have systemic symptoms such as fever, weight loss, and myalgia, in addition to laboratory alterations such as anemia, leukopenia, lymphopenia, thrombocytopenia, and pancytopenia; increased LDH, ESR, and beta-2-microglobulin; and positive FAN. Such findings should make the physician suspect the possibility of a secondary hemophagocytic syndrome, a complication that occurs in about 18% of patients [101].

Diagnosis

Histopathology

For an adequate histopathological sample, a deep biopsy that includes a significant representation of the subcutaneous tissue is necessary. Typically, atypical lymphocytes infiltrate in the subcutaneous fat lobes, which may also surround the sweat glands and hair follicles. There is no involvement of the septa, dermis, or epidermis. Atypical lymphocytes characteristically surround, or rim, individual adipocytes and exhibit a hyperchromatic nucleus and pale cytoplasm. There may be fat necrosis and karyorrhexis.

Immunohistochemistry

The phenotype of neoplastic lymphocytes is positive for CD3, CD8, and T cell receptor alpha/beta. There is a strong expression of granzyme B, TIA-1, and perforin but negativity for CD56. There may be a loss of expression of CD2, CD5, and CD7. The presence of T lymphocyte receptor gene rearrangement is common. Currently, lymphomas that affect the hypodermis and express gamma/delta are not considered subcutaneous panniculitis-like T-cell lymphoma but primary cutaneous gamma/delta T-cell lymphoma [5].

The disease is restricted to the skin in most of the cases. If extracutaneous involvement is suspected, a PET/CT scan can be performed. Bone marrow biopsy is not routinely performed, as the involvement is not frequent except in cases of hemophagocytic syndrome.

Treatment

The prognosis is good, with an overall survival higher than 80% in 5 years, but the presence of hemophagocytic syndrome reduces life expectancy. Therefore, treatment is usually performed with systemic corticosteroids or immunosuppressive agents such as etoposide, cyclosporine, methotrexate, chlorambucil, and bexarotene. In rare, aggressive cases, multidrug therapy based on doxorubicin and even allogeneic bone marrow transplantation may be necessary [101].

Extranodal NK-/T-Cell Lymphoma, Nasal Type

Extranodal NK-/T-cell lymphoma, nasal type, is a rare, highly aggressive cytotoxic lymphoma associated with EBV infection. The skin is the second most affected site after the nasal cavity/nasopharynx. Cutaneous involvement can be primary or secondary (contiguity involvement) [5].

This lymphoma is more common in Asia, Central America, and South America and predominantly affects adults. Clinically, it may present as a destructive ulcerated mass or lesion in the nasal region or as cutaneous plaques and tumors located mainly on the trunk or extremities. Some patients may present with persistent facial swelling, particularly on the eyelids. There may be systemic symptoms such as fever and weight loss, and, in some cases, this may progress to the hemophagocytic syndrome [5].

From a histopathological point of view, there is a dense infiltrate involving the dermis and hypodermis. There is often angiodestruction and necrosis. Lymphocytes are pleomorphic and of varying sizes (small, medium, and large). The phenotype is mostly cytotoxic NK cells (CD2+, CD56+, cytoplasmic CD3, TIA-1+, granzyme B+, and perforin+). In rare cases, there may be a cytotoxic T lymphocyte phenotype, including the presence of monoclonal TCR rearrangement. In practically all cases, EBV is demonstrated through in situ hybridization in neoplastic cells. Immunohistochemistry for latent membrane protein (LMP) may be negative [5, 103].

The prognosis is poor, with a disease-specific 5-year survival of only 16% [10]. Due to the severity of the disease, the treatment of choice is chemotherapy. Allogeneic bone marrow transplantation can be performed for eligible patients [5].

Chronic Active EBV Infection

The current WHO-EORTC classification contains a section on childhood EBV+ lymphoproliferative disease. This section includes hypersensitivity reactions to mosquito bites and hydroa vacciniforme-like lymphoproliferative disease (HV-like LPD). The latter covers the cases formerly called hydroa vacciniforme and the hydroa vacciniforme-like T-cell lymphoma. Both conditions are more frequent in children and adolescents from Asia or an indigenous population from Mexico, Central America, and South America [103]. The pathophysiology involves a clonal expansion of cytotoxic T or NK cells secondary to genomic anomalies due to EBV infection [10].

Clinical Features

In hypersensitivity reactions to mosquito bites, the patient has an intense local inflammatory reaction with the appearance of erythema, blisters, ulcers, and scarring. Later, it may present with fever, lymphadenopathy, and liver dysfunction [12]. In HV-like LPD cases, there is a papulovesicular eruption in sun-exposed areas, especially on the face, earlobes, and back of the hands. There may be edema, ulcers, blisters, crusts, and scars. It is usually accompanied by fever, lymphadenopathy, hepatosplenomegaly, and increased liver enzymes. It is a severe disease with a 2-year survival rate of 36% [10, 103].

Diagnosis

Histopathology

Histopathology shows an infiltrate of small and medium T lymphocytes located in the dermis and hypodermis. Occasionally, there may be angiotropism and epidermotropism.

Immunohistochemistry

Immunohistochemistry shows that neoplastic lymphocytes are CD3+ and CD8+ and EBV+ is detected by in situ hybridization [10].

Treatment

The treatment is difficult, and immunosuppressive agents such as cyclosporine or corticosteroids have been tried. Hematopoietic stem cell transplantation alone is a curative treatment for the disease, although the incidence of transplantation-related complications is high [103].

Primary Cutaneous Gamma-Delta T-Cell Lymphoma

Primary cutaneous gamma-delta lymphoma is a rare and highly aggressive entity resulting from cytotoxic V-delta-2 gamma/delta T-cell clonal proliferation. It corresponds to less than 1% of primary cutaneous lymphomas, predominantly affecting adults around 60 years [104, 105].

Clinical Features

Clinically, it is heterogeneous and may present with patches (mycosis fungoides-like), plaques, nodules, or tumors located preferentially in the extremities. In most cases, these lesions quickly ulcerate or present areas of necrosis. B symptoms are frequently present, and the involvement of mucous membranes and extranodal sites is not uncommon [105].

Diagnosis

Histopathology

Histopathology is also heterogeneous, and there may be epidermotropism, dermal, or hypodermic infiltrate of small, medium, or large lymphocytes. On some occasions, the involvement may be exclusive to the hypodermis and simulate a subcutaneous panniculitis-like T-cell lymphoma. There is often epidermal necrosis, angiocentrism, angiodestruction, and dermal necrosis.

Immunohistochemistry

Immunohistochemistry reveals the phenotype of lymphocytes with an expression of the gamma/delta T-cell receptor, CD3+, CD2+, and CD56+. Most of the time, they are CD4− and CD8−, but sometimes they can be CD8+. There is also often a strong expression of cytotoxic proteins. In most cases, it is possible to demonstrate TCR-gamma and TCR-delta rearrangement gene monoclonality [5, 105].

Treatment

The prognosis is poor, with 5-year disease-specific survival of only 11%. Due to the severity of the disease, most patients are treated with multidrug therapy and, when possible, allogeneic bone marrow transplantation. There are cases of partial remission with brentuximab vedotin in CD30-positive cases.

Primary Cutaneous Aggressive Epidermotropic CD8-Positive T-Cell Lymphoma

The primary cutaneous aggressive epidermotropic CD8-positive T-cell Lymphoma is characterized by a clonal proliferation of CD8+ cytotoxic T lymphocytes and has a reserved prognosis. It is rare, accounting for less than 1% of primary cutaneous lymphomas, and is included as a provisional entity in the 2018 WHO classification. It mainly affects adults around the sixth to seventh decades of life, with a similar proportion between men and women [10].

So far, there is no specific genetic alteration for this disease. One study detected many copy number alterations (CNAs) with gains of functions in regions 7q, 8q24.3, and 17q and loss of 9p21.3 (CDKN2A–CDKN2B) [106].

Clinical Features

The clinical presentation of these patients is remarkable and characteristic. Typically, within weeks or a few months, there is a disseminated appearance of plaques, nodules, or tumors that rapidly evolve with areas of ulceration and central necrosis (Fig. 20.6). Mucosal involvement (both oral and genital) is not uncommon. Spread to the central nervous system, lungs, and testis occur in a significant number of patients, whereas lymph node involvement is uncommon [107].

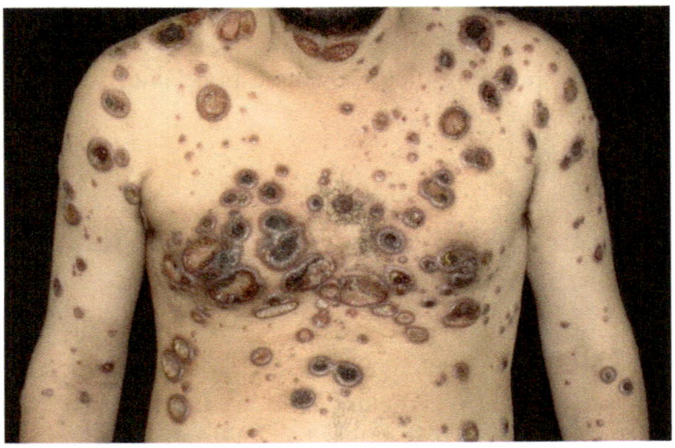

Fig. 20.6 Primary cutaneous aggressive epidermotropic CD8-positive T-cell lymphoma. Generalized plaques and tumors with areas of ulceration and central necrosis

Diagnosis

Histopathology

Histopathology is also remarkable. There is a pagetoid epidermotropism of pleomorphic lymphocytes. In more developed lesions, there is a lichenoid infiltrate associated with diffuse infiltration of a hyperplastic epidermis. There is often epidermal necrosis, ulceration, and destruction of the adnexa, and angiocentricity and angioinvasion can occur.

Immunohistochemistry

The cell phenotype demonstrated by immunohistochemistry is CD3+, CD8+, granzyme B+, perforin+, TIA-1+, CD45RA+/−, and CD45RO−. There may be a loss of expression of CD2, CD5, and CD7, and CD30 may be expressed in some cases. Clonal genetic rearrangement of the T lymphocyte receptor is expected [107].

Treatment

The prognosis is poor, with a disease-specific 5-year survival of 31% [5]. Due to the rarity of the disease, there are no controlled studies to evaluate treatments. Most cases are treated in the first line with polychemotherapy for aggressive lymphomas (CHOP, EPOCH). There are reports of treatment with gemcitabine, pralatrexate, brentuximab, alemtuzumab, and total skin electron beam radiotherapy. If the patient is eligible, allogeneic bone marrow transplantation may increase survival [108].

Primary Cutaneous CD4+ Small/Medium T-Cell Lymphoproliferative Disorder

The primary cutaneous CD4+ small/medium T-cell lymphoproliferative disorder is included in the WHO classification 2018 as a provisional entity and corresponds to 6% of the cases. It is defined as a lymphoproliferation of CD4 pleomorphic small/medium cell without prior or concurrent patches and plaques typical of MF [10]. It predominantly affects adults with a mean age of 59 years and presents similar proportion of men and women [109]. There are no genetic alterations characteristic of this entity.

Clinically, a solitary plaque or nodule is located on the head, neck, or upper trunk. Less commonly, it may present with more than one lesion. Histopathology is marked by a dense and diffuse dermal infiltrate of small and medium CD4+ lymphocytes, and there may be a small proportion (<30%) of large and pleomorphic cells. The phenotype of these lymphocytes is follicular T lymphocyte with a frequent expression of the following markers: PD1, BCL6, ICOS, and CXCL13. The proliferation rate is usually low (maximum 20%), and there is often a reactive infiltrate of CD8+ lymphocytes, B lymphocytes, and histiocytes [10].

The prognosis is excellent, and the average 5-year survival is 100%. As there is practically no extracutaneous dissemination, staging with imaging exams is not recommended. Lesions can spontaneously regress after biopsy, and in cases where this does not occur, it can be treated with topical corticosteroids, intralesional corticosteroids, surgical excision, or radiotherapy [10, 109].

Primary Cutaneous Acral CD8+ T-Cell Lymphoma

It is a rare and highly indolent clinical-pathological entity. It affects adults and has a slight male predominance. So far, there are no genetic alterations characteristic of this disease. Typically there is a solitary plaque or nodule in the ear or, less commonly, in other acral sites such as the nose, hands, or feet [10]. Histopathology is marked by a diffuse dermal infiltrate of medium-sized blast cells with a clear Grenz zone. Neoplastic cells express CD3+ and CD8+. There is positivity for TIA-1, but other cytotoxic markers such as granzyme B and perforin are negative. There may be a loss of expression of CD2, CD5, and CD7. CD68 often shows positive Golgi dot-like staining, and the proliferative index is usually very low (<10%). The neoplastic T cells of primary cutaneous acral CD8+ T-cell lymphoma show clonal T-cell receptor gene rearrangements [10].

As the prognosis is excellent, staging with imaging exams is not recommended. Treatment can be performed with surgical excision or radiotherapy, and aggressive treatments are not indicated [10].

TNM Staging of Cutaneous Lymphoma Other than MF/SS

As we have seen, non-mycosis fungoid/Sezary primary cutaneous lymphomas form a heterogeneous group of diseases with different clinical, histopathological, molecular, and prognostic presentations. Despite this, they have a common staging system (Table 20.7).

Table 20.7 TNM staging of cutaneous lymphoma other than MF/SS

T: Skin
T1: Solitary skin involvement
T1a: A solitary lesion <5 cm diameter
T1b: A solitary >5 cm diameter
T2: Regional skin involvement: multiple lesions limited to 1 body region or 2 contiguous body regions
T2a: All-disease-encompassing in a <15-cm-diameter circular area
T2b: All-disease-encompassing in a >15-and-<30-cm-diameter circular area
T2c: All-disease-encompassing in a >30-cm-diameter circular area
T3: Generalized skin involvement
T3a: Multiple lesions involving 2 noncontiguous body regions
T3b: Multiple lesions involving ≥3 body regions
N: Lymph nodes
N0: No clinical or pathologic lymph node involvement
N1: Involvement of 1 peripheral lymph node region that drains an area of current or prior skin involvement
N2: Involvement of 2 or more peripheral lymph node regions or involvement of any lymph node region that does not drain an area of current or prior skin involvement
N3: Involvement of central lymph nodes
M: Viscera
M0: No evidence of extracutaneous non-lymph node disease
M1: Extracutaneous non-lymph node disease present

Cutaneous B-Cell Lymphomas

Opposed to what is seen on systemic lymphomas, where the majority of cases are from B-cell origin, primary cutaneous B-cell lymphomas (PCBCL) represent only 20–25% of all cases of primary cutaneous lymphomas [5]. It has an incidence of about four cases per million persons (based on the Surveillance, Epidemiology, and End Results—SEER), affecting more adults, males (2:1), around 50 years [3, 110]. They usually differ from their nodal counterpart in clinical behavior, prognosis, immunohistochemical markers, and therapy.

B-cell lymphomas are classified into three main groups, two indolent forms—primary cutaneous follicle center lymphoma (PCFCL) and primary cutaneous marginal zone lymphoma (PCMZL)—and an intermediate aggressiveness form, primary cutaneous diffuse large B-cell lymphoma, leg type (PCDLBCL-LT). Other rare variants include EBV-positive mucocutaneous ulcer (provisional) and intravascular large B-cell lymphoma, accounting for less than 1% of cases of primary cutaneous lymphomas [10, 111].

For diagnosis, a punch or excisional biopsy of the cutaneous lesion is indicated. Main differences on immunohistochemical panels and clinical characteristics are summarized on Table 20.8. Cells are usually clonal for immunoglobulin light- or heavy-chain gene rearrangement [27]. For staging purposes, a complete

Table 20.8 Primary cutaneous B-cell lymphomas (major subtypes): main characteristics [110, 111, 115]

Lymphoma subtype	PCMZL	PCFCL	PCDLBCL-LT
Sex	Female = male	Female = male	Female > male
Age (median, in years)	55	60	76
Lesions	Solitary or multiple reddish papules, plaques, or nodules	Solitary or multiple reddish papules, plaques, or nodules	Solitary or multiple plaques or tumors, rapid growing, might ulcerate
Frequent location	Trunk and limbs	Head and neck, trunk	Legs
Cutaneous relapses	Frequent	Frequent	Frequent
Extracutaneous dissemination	Very rare	Rare (5–10%)	Frequent
5-year disease survival	>95%	>90%	<60%
Cell morphology	Small B cells, lymphoplasmacytoid, and plasma cells	Centrocytes and centroblasts	Centroblasts and immunoblasts
Immunohistochemistry			
CD20, CD79A, PAX5	+	+	+
BCL2	+	−/+ (weak)	++
BCL6	−	+	+
CD10	−	+/−	−
MUM-1	−	−	+
Genetic alterations	t(14;18) absent	t(14;18) in a minority of cases	• t(14;18) absent • Somatic MYD88 L265P mutations are the most common • C-myc translocations are rare

PCFCL primary cutaneous follicle center lymphoma, *PCMZL* primary cutaneous marginal zone lymphoma, *PCDLBCL-LT* primary cutaneous diffuse large B-cell lymphoma, leg type

history (including B-symptoms) and physical examination is mandatory. Imaging with either computed tomography (neck, chest, abdomen, pelvis) or PET-CT is indicated to exclude secondary involvement by a systemic lymphoma. Other exams include complete blood count and lactate dehydrogenase (LDH) level. Bone marrow biopsy is indicated for PCDLBCL-LT, but it is still a matter of debate for the indolent forms, with most authors not recommending this procedure on PCMZL and PCFCL, although 10% of PCFCL might present marrow involvement, with decrease in disease-specific survival [110]. TNM staging is similarly used for non-MF/SS CTCL and describes the extent of the disease as shown on Table 20.7.

Treatment recommendations are based mainly on retrospective studies or institutional experiences, since randomized controlled trials are not available. They will be described for each main subtype of PCBCL [110].

Primary Cutaneous Follicle Center Lymphoma

PCFCL is the most common form of cutaneous B-cell lymphoma, accounting for approximately 50–60% of cases [112, 113]. Opposed to systemic follicular lymphomas, the majority of PCFCL do not harbor the t(14;18) translocation involving the bcl-2 locus and do not strongly express bcl-2 by immunohistochemistry [110]. It has an excellent prognosis with a 5-year survival of more than 95%. If left untreated, lesions increase in size over the years, but dissemination to extracutaneous sites is rare. Recurrences are though frequent [5].

Clinical Features

PCFCL are usually characterized by solitary red to violaceous plaques, nodules, or tumors involving the head or scalp or on the trunk (Fig. 20.7). Particularly on the trunk, these tumors may be surrounded by erythematous papules and plaques, which may precede the development of tumorous lesions for months or years. In the past, this type of manifestation was referred to as "Crosti lymphoma" or "reticulohistiocytoma of the dorsum." Multifocal skin lesions are less common [5, 110].

Diagnosis

Histopathology

It presents as a dermal nodular or diffuse infiltrate with almost constant sparing of the epidermis. It is composed of small- to intermediate-sized cells, usually centrocytes admixed with variable numbers of centroblasts. It might present as a follicular, a follicular and diffuse, or a diffuse growth pattern [5, 27].

Immunohistochemistry

PCFCL is positive for pan-B-cell markers (CD20, CD79, PAX5); it usually expresses BCL6, and CD10 expression is variable; opposed to systemic FCL, BCL2 is either negative or positive, but faint or only in a subset of cells; MUM-1 is negative [27].

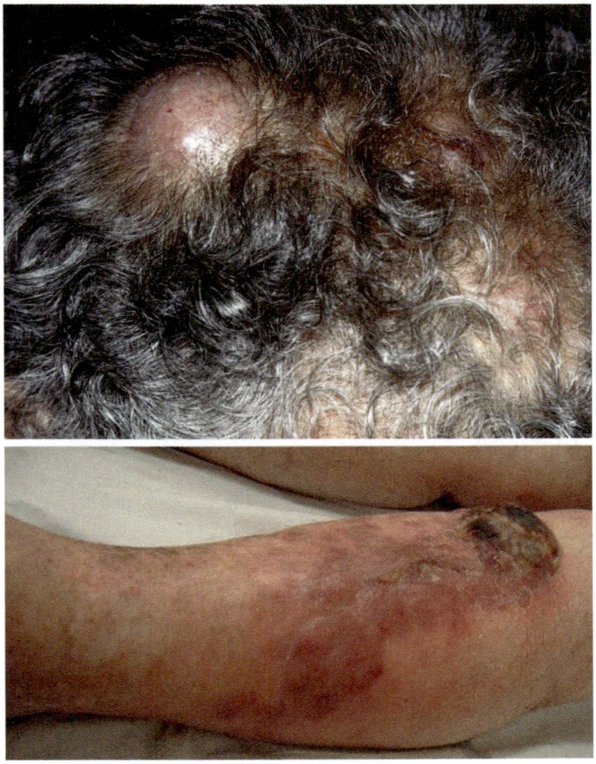

Fig. 20.7 B-cell lymphoma. PCFCL: infiltrated erythematous nodule on the scalp; PCDLBCL-LT: infiltrated erythematous plaques with rapid growing tumor on the lower leg

Treatment

For patients with solitary or localized lesions, low-dose radiation therapy is safe and highly effective. Surgical excision, clinical observation ("watch and wait") and topical treatments (intralesional corticosteroids or rituximab) might also be indicated.

For multiple lesions that can be included on multiple radiation fields, low-dose radiation is still an effective option, but for more extensive skin involvement, single-agent rituximab might be an alternative.

About 30% of patients will recur after either radiotherapy or rituximab, but recurrences are usually confined to the skin.

Primary Cutaneous Marginal Zone Lymphoma

PCMZL is an indolent lymphoma thought to be of post-germinal center marginal zone B cells. It has an excellent prognosis with a 5-year survival of about 100%. An association with *Borrelia burgdorferi* infection has been reported in a minority of

European cases but not in Asian or United States [5, 110]. They have a tendency to recur on the skin, but dissemination to extracutaneous sites is extremely rare.

Clinical Features

PCMZLs present with solitary or multifocal red to violaceous nodules, plaques, or papules that are usually localized on the trunk or extremities, especially the arms. Opposed to what is seen in PCFCL, presentation with multifocal skin lesions is frequent. Spontaneous resolution of the skin lesions may be observed, sometimes leaving areas of anetoderma on the areas of preexisting lesions. Skin relapses are common, but extracutaneous dissemination is rare [5, 114].

Diagnosis

Histopathology

Neoplastic infiltrate is composed of small- to medium-sized B cells, on a nodular or diffuse pattern. Cells include marginal zone (centrocyte-like) cells, lymphoplasmacytoid cells, and plasma cells. Many lesions present a small lymphoid cell infiltrate with no specific morphology, indicating a plasmacytic differentiation. Germinal centers might be evident but may also be absent, distorted, atrophic, or completely absent [27, 114].

Immunohistochemistry

PCMZL is positive for pan-B-cell markers (CD20, CD79, PAX5), positive for BCL2 and lack the expression of CD10 and BCL6. Ki67 is usually not very high. CD21 stain is useful in highlighting the follicular dendritic cells of lymphoid follicles that might be infiltrated by marginal zone cells (BCL2+, BCL6−), being a useful clue for the diagnosis. A population of reactive CD3+ T cells is usually noted [27, 114].

Treatment

Management is similar to PCFCL, with one difference: for PCMZL in European countries (but not in North America), an initial intent with antibiotics for *Borrelia burgdorferi* is recommended [110].

Diffuse Large B-Cell Lymphoma, Leg Type

PCDLBCL, LT is a more aggressive form of PCBCL. In contrast to the indolent forms (PCFCL and PCMZL), PCDLBCL, LT is associated with a 5-year disease-specific survival of approximately 50% with dissemination to extracutaneous sites occurring more often. Prognostic factors associated to a worse survival include dual bcl-2 and c-myc expression, presence of a somatic MYD88L265P mutation, and involvement of multiple sites, on one or both legs [110].

Clinical Features

PCDLBCL, LT usually affects elderly females and presents as rapidly growing red to violaceous tumors on one or both (lower) legs (Fig. 20.7). Ulceration might occur. Other sites other than the leg might occur but are less frequent.

Diagnosis

Histopathology

Neoplastic infiltrate is composed of a monomorphic population of large centroblasts and immunoblasts with few admixed cells, with a diffuse infiltrate, that often extend into the deep dermis and subcutaneous tissue. Mitotic figures are frequent [5, 27].

Immunohistochemistry

PCDLBCL, LT is positive for pan-B-cell markers (CD20, CD79, PAX5). Cells usually have a strong BCL2 expression; Bcl-6 is expressed by most cases, whereas CD10 staining is generally absent; MUM-1/IRF4 shows positivity. The strong BCL2 and MUM-1 expression helps in distinguishing it from a PCFCL with large cell transformation [5, 27].

Treatment

As a more aggressive lymphoma, the gold standard for therapy is R-CHOP (rituximab plus polychemotherapy—cyclophosphamide, doxorubicin, vincristine and prednisolone) with or without radiotherapy. In elderly patients that are not candidate for R-CHOP, R-miniCHOP might be used. Single-agent rituximab or radiotherapy alone might be used as palliative measures for patients not able to receive more aggressive therapies [110].

Blastic Plasmacytoid Dendritic Cell Neoplasm

Blastic plasmacytoid dendritic cell neoplasm (BPDCN) is a rare, aggressive hematopoietic neoplasm originating from plasmacytoid dendritic cell precursors, with a high frequency of cutaneous involvement and with an overall survival of less than a year if left untreated. Even though it is now classified on the myeloid neoplasm, it belonged for years to the cutaneous lymphoma classification. It has an incidence of 0.04/100,000 people and affects older males, with a 2–3.3:1 male to female ratio and a median age of 53–68 years [116, 117].

Clinical Features

The skin is affected in 60–100% of the cases, being the first manifestation in about 90% of the cases, but with rapid systemic involvement. Skin involvement is the most common, followed by the bone marrow and peripheral blood in 60–90% and lymph nodes in about 40–50% of the cases. The central nervous system (CNS) might be involved in 30% of the cases [116–118].

Cutaneous lesions are heterogeneous, can be single or more often generalized, with variable size and shapes, and can manifest as erythematous or purplish papules, plaques, nodules, or tumors, frequently with a bruise-like appearance. Mucosal involvement might also be present (Fig. 20.8) [117, 119].

Diagnosis

Histopathology

BPDCN is usually characterized by a diffuse, monomorphous infiltrate of medium- to large-sized blasts (resembling myeloid sarcoma) on the entire dermis and often extending to the subcutis, sparing the epidermis. Mitotic figures are common [116, 117].

Immunohistochemistry

Cells should be positive for at least three of five markers: CD4, CD123, CD56, TCL1, CD303; and negative for other lineage markers such as CD3, CD20, CD34, MPO, EBV. Ki-67 is usually high [116, 117, 119].

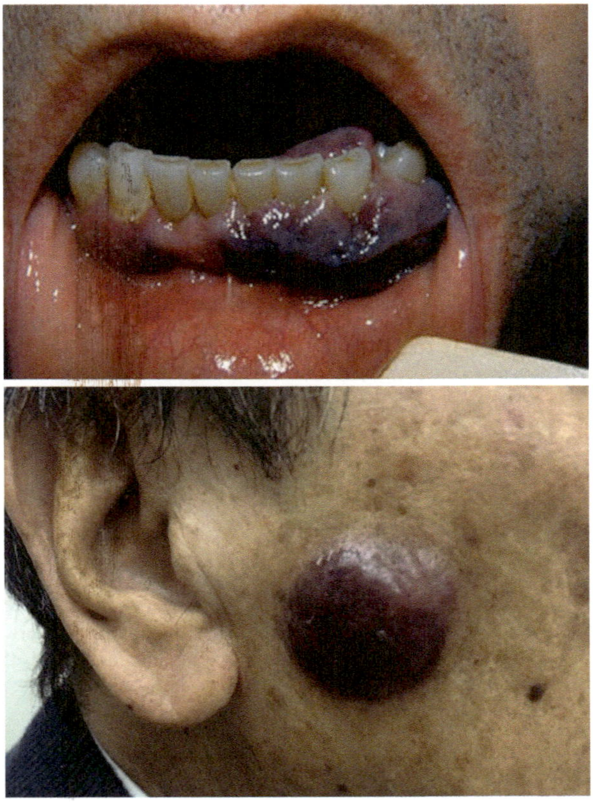

Fig. 20.8 BPDCN. Purplish nodule (bruise-like appearance) on the oral mucosa and face

Treatment

Target therapies are being developed, with an anti-CD123 drug already approved. If not available, data support the use of acute lymphoid leukemia-like regimen, associated to CNS prophylaxis, followed by allogenic HSCT on selected cases [116, 120].

References

1. Smith A, Crouch S, Lax S, Li J, Painter D, Howell D, et al. Lymphoma incidence, survival and prevalence 2004–2014: sub-type analyses from the UK's Haematological Malignancy Research Network. Br J Cancer. 2015;112(9):1575–84.
2. Ansell SM. Hodgkin lymphoma: 2014 update on diagnosis, risk-stratification, and management. Am J Hematol. 2014;89(7):771–9.
3. Bradford PT, Devesa SS, Anderson WF, Toro JR. Cutaneous lymphoma incidence patterns in the United States: a population-based study of 3884 cases. Blood. 2009;113(21):5064–73.
4. Newton R, Ferlay J, Beral V, Devesa S. The epidemiology of non-Hodgkin's lymphoma: comparison of nodal and extra-nodal sites. Int J Cancer. 1997;72(6):923–30.

5. Willemze R, Jaffe ES, Burg G, Cerroni L, Berti E, Swerdlow SH, et al. WHO-EORTC classification for cutaneous lymphomas. Blood. 2005;105(10):3768–85.
6. Willemze R, Beljaards RC, Meijer CJ, Rijlaarsdam JR. Classification of primary cutaneous lymphomas. Historical overview and perspectives. Dermatology. 1994;189(Suppl 2):8–15.
7. Slater DN. The new World Health Organization-European Organization for Research and Treatment of Cancer classification for cutaneous lymphomas: a practical marriage of two giants. Br J Dermatol. 2005;153(5):874–80.
8. Swerdlow S, Campo E, Harris N, Jaffe E, Pileri S, Stein H, et al. WHO classification of tumours of haematopoietic and lymphoid tissues. Lyon, France: IARC Press; 2008.
9. Swerdlow SH, Campo E, Pileri SA, Harris NL, Stein H, Siebert R, et al. The 2016 revision of the World Health Organization classification of lymphoid neoplasms. Blood. 2016;127(20):2375–90.
10. Willemze R, Cerroni L, Kempf W, Berti E, Facchetti F, Swerdlow SH, et al. The 2018 update of the WHO-EORTC classification for primary cutaneous lymphomas. Blood. 2019;133(16):1703–14.
11. Criscione VD, Weinstock MA. Incidence of cutaneous T-cell lymphoma in the United States, 1973–2002. Arch Dermatol. 2007;143(7):854–9.
12. Riou-Gotta MO, Fournier E, Mermet I, Pelletier F, Humbert P, Danzon A, et al. Primary cutaneous lymphomas: a population-based descriptive study of 71 consecutive cases diagnosed between 1980 and 2003. Leuk Lymphoma. 2008;49(8):1537–44.
13. Smith BD, Smith GL, Cooper DL, Wilson LD. The cutaneous B-cell lymphoma prognostic index: a novel prognostic index derived from a population-based registry. J Clin Oncol. 2005;23(15):3390–5.
14. Litvinov IV, Shtreis A, Kobayashi K, Glassman S, Tsang M, Woetmann A, et al. Investigating potential exogenous tumor initiating and promoting factors for Cutaneous T-Cell Lymphomas (CTCL), a rare skin malignancy. Oncoimmunology. 2016;5(7):e1175799.
15. Nicolay JP, Wobser M. Cutaneous B-cell lymphomas - pathogenesis, diagnostic workup, and therapy. J Dtsch Dermatol Ges. 2016;14(12):1207–24.
16. Rijlaarsdam U, Scheffer E, Meijer CJ, Kruyswijk MR, Willemze R. Mycosis fungoides-like lesions associated with phenytoin and carbamazepine therapy. J Am Acad Dermatol. 1991;24(2 Pt 1):216–20.
17. Magro CM, Crowson AN. Drugs with antihistaminic properties as a cause of atypical cutaneous lymphoid hyperplasia. J Am Acad Dermatol. 1995;32(3):419–28.
18. Jahan-Tigh RR, Huen AO, Lee GL, Pozadzides JV, Liu P, Duvic M. Hydrochlorothiazide and cutaneous T cell lymphoma: prospective analysis and case series. Cancer. 2013;119(4):825–31.
19. Peck JR, Frank MP, Peck LR. Was treatment the trigger? Mycosis fungoides. Am J Med. 2013;126(12):1048–9.
20. Talpur R, Cox KM, Hu M, Geddes ER, Parker MK, Yang BY, et al. Vitamin D deficiency in mycosis fungoides and Sezary syndrome patients is similar to other cancer patients. Clin Lymphoma Myeloma Leuk. 2014;14(6):518–24.
21. Abrams JT, Balin BJ, Vonderheid EC. Association between Sézary T cell-activating factor, Chlamydia pneumoniae, and cutaneous T cell lymphoma. Ann N Y Acad Sci. 2001;941:69–85.
22. Mirvish JJ, Pomerantz RG, Falo LD Jr, Geskin LJ. Role of infectious agents in cutaneous T-cell lymphoma: facts and controversies. Clin Dermatol. 2013;31(4):423–31.
23. Moreau JF, Buchanich JM, Geskin JZ, Akilov OE, Geskin LJ. Non-random geographic distribution of patients with cutaneous T-cell lymphoma in the Greater Pittsburgh Area. Dermatol Online J. 2014;20(7):13030/qt4nw7592w.
24. Litvinov IV, Tetzlaff MT, Rahme E, Habel Y, Risser DR, Gangar P, et al. Identification of geographic clustering and regions spared by cutaneous T-cell lymphoma in Texas using 2 distinct cancer registries. Cancer. 2015;121(12):1993–2003.
25. Ghazawi FM, Netchiporouk E, Rahme E, Tsang M, Moreau L, Glassman S, et al. Comprehensive analysis of cutaneous T-cell lymphoma (CTCL) incidence and mortality in Canada reveals changing trends and geographic clustering for this malignancy. Cancer. 2017;123(18):3550–67.

26. Clough L, Bayakly AR, Ward KC, Khan MK, Chen SC, Lechowicz MJ, et al. Clustering of cutaneous T-cell lymphoma is associated with increased levels of the environmental toxins benzene and trichloroethylene in the state of Georgia. Cancer. 2020;126(8):1700–7.
27. Dewar R, Andea AA, Guitart J, Arber DA, Weiss LM. Best practices in diagnostic immunohistochemistry: workup of cutaneous lymphoid lesions in the diagnosis of primary cutaneous lymphoma. Arch Pathol Lab Med. 2015;139(3):338–50.
28. Ponti R, Fierro MT, Quaglino P, Lisa B, Paola F, Michela O, et al. TCRgamma-chain gene rearrangement by PCR-based GeneScan: diagnostic accuracy improvement and clonal heterogeneity analysis in multiple cutaneous T-cell lymphoma samples. J Invest Dermatol. 2008;128(4):1030–8.
29. Schafernak KT, Variakojis D, Goolsby CL, Tucker RM, Martinez-Escala ME, Smith FA, et al. Clonality assessment of cutaneous B-cell lymphoid proliferations: a comparison of flow cytometry immunophenotyping, molecular studies, and immunohistochemistry/in situ hybridization and review of the literature. Am J Dermatopathol. 2014;36(10):781–95.
30. Sufficool KE, Lockwood CM, Abel HJ, Hagemann IS, Schumacher JA, Kelley TW, et al. T-cell clonality assessment by next-generation sequencing improves detection sensitivity in mycosis fungoides. J Am Acad Dermatol. 2015;73(2):228–36.e2.
31. van Dongen JJ, Langerak AW, Bruggemann M, Evans PA, Hummel M, Lavender FL, et al. Design and standardization of PCR primers and protocols for detection of clonal immunoglobulin and T-cell receptor gene recombinations in suspect lymphoproliferations: report of the BIOMED-2 Concerted Action BMH4-CT98-3936. Leukemia. 2003;17(12):2257–317.
32. Mourad A, Gniadecki R. Overall survival in mycosis fungoides: a systematic review and meta-analysis. J Invest Dermatol. 2020;140(2):495–7.e5.
33. Quaglino P, Pimpinelli N, Berti E, Calzavara-Pinton P, Alfonso Lombardo G, Rupoli S, et al. Time course, clinical pathways, and long-term hazards risk trends of disease progression in patients with classic mycosis fungoides: a multicenter, retrospective follow-up study from the Italian Group of Cutaneous Lymphomas. Cancer. 2012;118(23):5830–9.
34. Kim YH, Liu HL, Mraz-Gernhard S, Varghese A, Hoppe RT. Long-term outcome of 525 patients with mycosis fungoides and Sezary syndrome: clinical prognostic factors and risk for disease progression. Arch Dermatol. 2003;139(7):857–66.
35. Scarisbrick JJ, Quaglino P, Prince HM, Papadavid E, Hodak E, Bagot M, et al. The PROCLIPI international registry of early-stage mycosis fungoides identifies substantial diagnostic delay in most patients. Br J Dermatol. 2019;181(2):350–7.
36. Hodak E, Amitay-Laish I. Mycosis fungoides: a great imitator. Clin Dermatol. 2019;37(3):255–67.
37. Guitart J, Kennedy J, Ronan S, Chmiel J, Hsiegh Y, Variakojis D. Histologic criteria for the diagnosis of mycosis fungoides: proposal for a grading system to standardize pathology reporting. J Cutan Pathol. 2001;28(4):174–83.
38. Scarisbrick JJ, Prince HM, Vermeer MH, Quaglino P, Horwitz S, Porcu P, et al. Cutaneous Lymphoma International Consortium Study of outcome in advanced stages of mycosis fungoides and Sezary syndrome: effect of specific prognostic markers on survival and development of a prognostic model. J Clin Oncol. 2015;33(32):3766–73.
39. Molloy K, Jonak C, Woei AJF, Guenova E, Busschots AM, Bervoets A, et al. Characteristics associated with significantly worse quality of life in mycosis fungoides/Sezary syndrome from the Prospective Cutaneous Lymphoma International Prognostic Index (PROCLIPI) study. Br J Dermatol. 2020;182(3):770–9.
40. Hodak E, Amitay-Laish I, Atzmony L, Prag-Naveh H, Yanichkin N, Barzilai A, et al. New insights into folliculotropic mycosis fungoides (FMF): a single-center experience. J Am Acad Dermatol. 2016;75(2):347–55.
41. Mitteldorf C, Stadler R, Sander CA, Kempf W. Folliculotropic mycosis fungoides. J Dtsch Dermatol Ges. 2018;16(5):543–57.
42. Kempf W, Ostheeren-Michaelis S, Paulli M, Lucioni M, Wechsler J, Audring H, et al. Granulomatous mycosis fungoides and granulomatous slack skin: a multicenter study of the

Cutaneous Lymphoma Histopathology Task Force Group of the European Organization For Research and Treatment of Cancer (EORTC). Arch Dermatol. 2008;144(12):1609–17.
43. Furlan FC, Pereira BA, Sotto MN, Sanches JA. Hypopigmented mycosis fungoides versus mycosis fungoides with concomitant hypopigmented lesions: same disease or different variants of mycosis fungoides? Dermatology. 2014;229(3):271–4.
44. Valencia Ocampo OJ, Julio L, Zapata V, Correa LA, Vasco C, Correa S, et al. Mycosis fungoides in children and adolescents: a series of 23 cases. Actas Dermo-Sifiliográficas (Engl Ed). 2020;111(2):149–56.
45. Rodney IJ, Kindred C, Angra K, Qutub ON, Villanueva AR, Halder RM. Hypopigmented mycosis fungoides: a retrospective clinicohistopathologic study. J Eur Acad Dermatol Venereol. 2017;31(5):808–14.
46. Abbott RA, Sahni D, Robson A, Agar N, Whittaker S, Scarisbrick JJ. Poikilodermatous mycosis fungoides: a study of its clinicopathological, immunophenotypic, and prognostic features. J Am Acad Dermatol. 2011;65(2):313–9.
47. Vasconcelos Berg R, Valente NYS, Fanelli C, Wu I, Pereira J, Zatz R, et al. Poikilodermatous mycosis fungoides: comparative study of clinical, histopathological and immunohistochemical features. Dermatology. 2020;236(2):117–22.
48. Furmanczyk PS, Wolgamot GM, Kussick SJ, Sabath DE, Olerud JE, Argenyi ZB. Diagnosis of mycosis fungoides with different algorithmic approaches. J Cutan Pathol. 2010;37(1):8–14.
49. Ahn CS, ALSayyah A, Sangueza OP. Mycosis fungoides: an updated review of clinicopathologic variants. Am J Dermatopathol. 2014;36(12):933–48; quiz 49–51.
50. Kubica AW, Davis MD, Weaver AL, Killian JM, Pittelkow MR. Sezary syndrome: a study of 176 patients at Mayo Clinic. J Am Acad Dermatol. 2012;67(6):1189–99.
51. Vega F, Luthra R, Medeiros LJ, Dunmire V, Lee SJ, Duvic M, et al. Clonal heterogeneity in mycosis fungoides and its relationship to clinical course. Blood. 2002;100(9):3369–73.
52. Jawed SI, Myskowski PL, Horwitz S, Moskowitz A, Querfeld C. Primary cutaneous T-cell lymphoma (mycosis fungoides and Sezary syndrome): Part I. Diagnosis: clinical and histopathologic features and new molecular and biologic markers. J Am Acad Dermatol. 2014;70(2):205.e1–16; quiz 21–2.
53. Olsen E, Vonderheid E, Pimpinelli N, Willemze R, Kim Y, Knobler R, et al. Revisions to the staging and classification of mycosis fungoides and Sezary syndrome: a proposal of the International Society for Cutaneous Lymphomas (ISCL) and the cutaneous lymphoma task force of the European Organization of Research and Treatment of Cancer (EORTC). Blood. 2007;110(6):1713–22.
54. Agar NS, Wedgeworth E, Crichton S, Mitchell TJ, Cox M, Ferreira S, et al. Survival outcomes and prognostic factors in mycosis fungoides/Sezary syndrome: validation of the revised International Society for Cutaneous Lymphomas/European Organisation for Research and Treatment of Cancer staging proposal. J Clin Oncol. 2010;28(31):4730–9.
55. Talpur R, Singh L, Daulat S, Liu P, Seyfer S, Trynosky T, et al. Long-term outcomes of 1,263 patients with mycosis fungoides and Sezary syndrome from 1982 to 2009. Clin Cancer Res. 2012;18(18):5051–60.
56. Benner MF, Jansen PM, Vermeer MH, Willemze R. Prognostic factors in transformed mycosis fungoides: a retrospective analysis of 100 cases. Blood. 2012;119(7):1643–9.
57. Sanz-Bueno J, Lora D, Monsalvez V, Maronas-Jimenez L, Postigo C, Rodriguez-Peralto JL, et al. The new Cutaneous Lymphoma International Prognostic index (CLIPi) for early mycosis fungoides failed to identify prognostic groups in a cohort of Spanish patients. Br J Dermatol. 2016;175(4):794–6.
58. Scarisbrick JJ. Survival in mycosis fungoides and Sezary syndrome: how can we predict outcome? J Invest Dermatol. 2020;140(2):281–3.
59. Trautinger F, Eder J, Assaf C, Bagot M, Cozzio A, Dummer R, et al. European Organisation for Research and Treatment of Cancer consensus recommendations for the treatment of mycosis fungoides/Sezary syndrome - update 2017. Eur J Cancer. 2017;77:57–74.

60. Sanches JA, Cury-Martins J, Abreu RM, Miyashiro D, Pereira J. Mycosis fungoides and Sezary syndrome: focus on the current treatment scenario. An Bras Dermatol. 2021;96(4):458–71.
61. Iqbal M, Reljic T, Ayala E, Sher T, Murthy H, Roy V, et al. Efficacy of allogeneic hematopoietic cell transplantation in cutaneous T cell lymphoma: results of a systematic review and meta-analysis. Biol Blood Marrow Transplant. 2020;26(1):76–82.
62. Knobler R, Berlin G, Calzavara-Pinton P, Greinix H, Jaksch P, Laroche L, et al. Guidelines on the use of extracorporeal photopheresis. J Eur Acad Dermatol Venereol. 2014;28(Suppl 1):1–37.
63. Gilson D, Whittaker SJ, Child FJ, Scarisbrick JJ, Illidge TM, Parry EJ, et al. British Association of Dermatologists and U.K. Cutaneous Lymphoma Group guidelines for the management of primary cutaneous lymphomas 2018. Br J Dermatol. 2019;180(3):496–526.
64. Sézary A, Bouvrain Y. Érythrodermie avec présence de cellules monstrueuses dans le derme et le sang circulant. Bull Soc Fr Dermatol Syph. 1938;45:254–60.
65. Campbell JJ, Clark RA, Watanabe R, Kupper TS. Sezary syndrome and mycosis fungoides arise from distinct T-cell subsets: a biologic rationale for their distinct clinical behaviors. Blood. 2010;116(5):767–71.
66. Miyashiro D, Sanches JA. Erythroderma: a prospective study of 309 patients followed for 12 years in a tertiary center. Sci Rep. 2020;10(1):9774.
67. Morris L, Tran J, Duvic M. Non-classic signs of Sezary syndrome: a review. Am J Clin Dermatol. 2020;21(3):383–91.
68. Boonk SE, Zoutman WH, Marie-Cardine A, van der Fits L, Out-Luiting JJ, Mitchell TJ, et al. Evaluation of immunophenotypic and molecular biomarkers for Sezary syndrome using standard operating procedures: a multicenter study of 59 patients. J Invest Dermatol. 2016;136(7):1364–72.
69. Fraser-Andrews EA, Mitchell T, Ferreira S, Seed PT, Russell-Jones R, Calonje E, et al. Molecular staging of lymph nodes from 60 patients with mycosis fungoides and Sezary syndrome: correlation with histopathology and outcome suggests prognostic relevance in mycosis fungoides. Br J Dermatol. 2006;155(4):756–62.
70. Dittus C, Sloan JM. Adult T-cell leukemia/lymphoma: a problem abroad and at home. Hematol Oncol Clin North Am. 2017;31(2):255–72.
71. Gessain A, Cassar O. Epidemiological aspects and world distribution of HTLV-1 infection. Front Microbiol. 2012;3:388.
72. Yamano Y, Nagai M, Brennan M, Mora CA, Soldan SS, Tomaru U, et al. Correlation of human T-cell lymphotropic virus type 1 (HTLV-1) mRNA with proviral DNA load, virus-specific CD8(+) T cells, and disease severity in HTLV-1-associated myelopathy (HAM/TSP). Blood. 2002;99(1):88–94.
73. Okayama A, Stuver S, Matsuoka M, Ishizaki J, Tanaka G, Kubuki Y, et al. Role of HTLV-1 proviral DNA load and clonality in the development of adult T-cell leukemia/lymphoma in asymptomatic carriers. Int J Cancer. 2004;110(4):621–5.
74. Miyashiro D, Sanches JA. Cutaneous manifestations of adult T-cell leukemia/lymphoma. Semin Diagn Pathol. 2020;37(2):81–91.
75. Cartier L, Castillo JL, Cabrera ME, Araya F, Matutes E, Ford AM, et al. HTLV-I positive progressive spastic paraparesis (TSP) associated with a lymphoid disorder in three Chilean patients. Leuk Lymphoma. 1995;17(5–6):459–64.
76. Shimoyama M. Diagnostic criteria and classification of clinical subtypes of adult T-cell leukaemia-lymphoma. A report from the Lymphoma Study Group (1984–87). Br J Haematol. 1991;79(3):428–37.
77. Verdonck K, González E, Van Dooren S. Human T lymphotropic virus 1: recent knowledge about an ancient infection. Lancet Infect Dis. 2007;7:266–81.
78. Bittencourt AL, Barbosa HS, Vieira MD, Farre L. Adult T-cell leukemia/lymphoma (ATL) presenting in the skin: clinical, histological and immunohistochemical features of 52 cases. Acta Oncol. 2009;48(4):598–604.

79. Shimizu S, Yasui C, Koizumi K, Ikeda H, Tsuchiya K. Cutaneous-type adult T-cell leukemia/lymphoma presenting as a solitary large skin nodule: a review of the literature. J Am Acad Dermatol. 2007;57(5 Suppl):S115–7.
80. Hurabielle C, Battistella M, Ram-Wolff C, Fite C, Meignin V, Rivet J, et al. Cutaneous presentation of adult T-cell leukemia/lymphoma (ATLL). Single-center study on 37 patients in metropolitan France between 1996 and 2016. Ann Dermatol Venereol. 2018;145(6–7):405–12.
81. Setoyama M, Katahira Y, Kanzaki T. Clinicopathologic analysis of 124 cases of adult T-cell leukemia/lymphoma with cutaneous manifestations: the smouldering type with skin manifestations has a poorer prognosis than previously thought. J Dermatol. 1999;26(12):785–90.
82. Marchetti MA, Pulitzer MP, Myskowski PL, Dusza SW, Lunning MA, Horwitz SM, et al. Cutaneous manifestations of human T-cell lymphotrophic virus type-1-associated adult T-cell leukemia/lymphoma: a single-center, retrospective study. J Am Acad Dermatol. 2015;72(2):293–301.
83. Yamaguchi T, Ohshima K, Karube K, Tutiya T, Kawano R, Suefuji H, et al. Clinicopathological features of cutaneous lesions of adult T-cell leukaemia/lymphoma. Br J Dermatol. 2005;152(1):76–81.
84. Lymphoma Study Group. Major prognostic factors of patients with adult T-cell leukemia-lymphoma: a cooperative study. Lymphoma Study Group (1984–1987). Leuk Res. 1991;15(2–3):81–90.
85. Tokura Y, Sawada Y, Shimauchi T. Skin manifestations of adult T-cell leukemia/lymphoma: clinical, cytological and immunological features. J Dermatol. 2014;41(1):19–25.
86. Sawada Y, Hino R, Hama K, Ohmori S, Fueki H, Yamada S, et al. Type of skin eruption is an independent prognostic indicator for adult T-cell leukemia/lymphoma. Blood. 2011;117(15):3961–7.
87. Ishitsuka K, Tamura K. Human T-cell leukaemia virus type I and adult T-cell leukaemia-lymphoma. Lancet Oncol. 2014;15(11):e517–26.
88. Cook LB, Phillips AA. How I treat adult T-cell leukemia/lymphoma. Blood. 2021;137(4):459–70.
89. Cook LB, Fuji S, Hermine O, Bazarbachi A, Ramos JC, Ratner L, et al. Revised adult T-cell leukemia-lymphoma International Consensus Meeting Report. J Clin Oncol. 2019;37(8):677–87.
90. Ishida T, Jo T, Takemoto S, Suzushima H, Suehiro Y, Choi I, et al. Follow-up of a randomised phase II study of chemotherapy alone or in combination with mogamulizumab in newly diagnosed aggressive adult T-cell leukaemia-lymphoma: impact on allogeneic haematopoietic stem cell transplantation. Br J Haematol. 2019;184(3):479–83.
91. Ogura M, Imaizumi Y, Uike N, Asou N, Utsunomiya A, Uchida T, et al. Lenalidomide in relapsed adult T-cell leukaemia-lymphoma or peripheral T-cell lymphoma (ATLL-001): a phase 1, multicentre, dose-escalation study. Lancet Haematol. 2016;3(3):e107–e18.
92. Horwitz S, O'Connor OA, Pro B, Illidge T, Fanale M, Advani R, et al. Brentuximab vedotin with chemotherapy for CD30-positive peripheral T-cell lymphoma (ECHELON-2): a global, double-blind, randomised, phase 3 trial. Lancet. 2019;393(10168):229–40.
93. Okajima R, Oliveira AC, Smid J, Casseb J, Sanches JA Jr. High prevalence of skin disorders among HTLV-1 infected individuals independent of clinical status. PLoS Negl Trop Dis. 2013;7(11):e2546.
94. Yamaguchi K, Matutes E, Catovsky D, Galton DA, Nakada K, Takatsuki K. Strongyloides stercoralis as candidate co-factor for HTLV-I-induced leukaemogenesis. Lancet. 1987;2(8550):94–5.
95. Sarfraz H, Gentille C, Ensor J, et al. Primary cutaneous anaplastic large-cell lymphoma: a review of the SEER database from 2005 to 2016. Clin Exp Dermatol. 2021; https://doi.org/10.1111/ced.14777.
96. Melchers RC, Willemze R, van de Loo M, et al. Clinical, histologic, and molecular characteristics of anaplastic lymphoma kinase-positive primary cutaneous anaplastic large cell lymphoma. Am J Surg Pathol. 2020;44(6):776–81.

97. Karai LJ, Kadin ME, Hsi ED, et al. Chromosomal rearrangements of 6p25.3 define a new subtype of lymphomatoid papulosis. Am J Surg Pathol. 2013;37(8):1173–81.
98. Kempf W, Kazakov DV, Schärer L, et al. Angioinvasive lymphomatoid papulosis: a new variant simulating aggressive lymphomas. Am J Surg Pathol. 2013;37(1):1–13.
99. Melchers RC, Willemze R, Bekkenk MW, et al. Frequency and prognosis of associated malignancies in 504 patients with lymphomatoid papulosis. J Eur Acad Dermatol Venereol. 2020;34(2):260–6.
100. National Comprehensive Cancer Network. Primary cutaneous lymphomas (Version2.2021). https://www.nccn.org/professionals/physician_gls/pdf/primary_cutaneous.pdf. Accessed 10 Sept 2021.
101. López-Lerma I, Peñate Y, Gallardo F, et al. Subcutaneous panniculitis-like T-cell lymphoma: clinical features, therapeutic approach, and outcome in a case series of 16 patients. J Am Acad Dermatol. 2018;79(5):892–8.
102. Fujii K. New therapies and immunological findings in cutaneous T-cell lymphoma. Front Oncol. 2018;8:198.
103. Sangueza-Acosta M, Sandoval-Romero E. Epstein-Barr virus and skin. An Bras Dermatol. 2018;93(6):786–99.
104. Daniels J, Doukas PG, Escala MEM, et al. Cellular origins and genetic landscape of cutaneous gamma delta T cell lymphomas. Nat Commun. 2020;11(1):1806.
105. Guitart J, Weisenburger DD, Subtil A, et al. Cutaneous γδ T-cell lymphomas: a spectrum of presentations with overlap with other cytotoxic lymphomas. Am J Surg Pathol. 2012;36(11):1656–65.
106. Fanoni D, Corti L, Alberti-Violetti S, et al. Array-based CGH of primary cutaneous CD8+ aggressive EPIDERMO-tropic cytotoxic T-cell lymphoma. Genes Chromosomes Cancer. 2018;57(12):622–9.
107. Robson A, Assaf C, Bagot M, et al. Aggressive epidermotropic cutaneous CD8+ lymphoma: a cutaneous lymphoma with distinct clinical and pathological features. Report of an EORTC Cutaneous Lymphoma Task Force Workshop. Histopathology. 2015;67(4):425–41.
108. Cyrenne BM, Gibson JF, Subtil A, et al. Transplantation in the treatment of primary cutaneous aggressive epidermotropic cytotoxic CD8-Positive T-cell lymphoma. Clin Lymphoma Myeloma Leuk. 2018;18(1):e85–93.
109. Beltzung F, Ortonne N, Pelletier L, et al. Primary cutaneous CD4+ small/medium T-cell lymphoproliferative disorders: a clinical, pathologic, and molecular study of 60 cases presenting with a single lesion: a multicenter study of the French Cutaneous Lymphoma Study Group. Am J Surg Pathol. 2020;44(7):862–72.
110. Wilcox RA. Cutaneous B-cell lymphomas: 2019 update on diagnosis, risk stratification, and management. Am J Hematol. 2018;93(11):1427–30.
111. Lima M. Cutaneous primary B-cell lymphomas: from diagnosis to treatment. An Bras Dermatol. 2015;90(5):687–706.
112. Hope CB, Pincus LB. Primary cutaneous B-cell lymphomas with large cell predominance-primary cutaneous follicle center lymphoma, diffuse large B-cell lymphoma, leg type and intravascular large B-cell lymphoma. Semin Diagn Pathol. 2017;34(1):85–98.
113. Subramaniyam S, Magro CM, Gogineni S, Tam W, Mathew S. Primary cutaneous follicle center lymphoma associated with an extracutaneous dissemination: a cytogenetic finding of potential prognostic value. Am J Clin Pathol. 2015;144(5):805–10.
114. Gibson SE, Swerdlow SH. How I diagnose primary cutaneous marginal zone lymphoma. Am J Clin Pathol. 2020;154(4):428–49.
115. Malachowski SJ, Sun J, Chen PL, Seminario-Vidal L. Diagnosis and Management of Cutaneous B-Cell Lymphomas. Dermatol Clin. 2019;37(4):443–54.
116. Venugopal S, Zhou S, El Jamal SM, Lane AA, Mascarenhas J. Blastic plasmacytoid dendritic cell neoplasm-current insights. Clin Lymphoma Myeloma Leuk. 2019;19(9):545–54.
117. Sapienza MR, Pileri A, Derenzini E, Melle F, Motta G, Fiori S, et al. Blastic plasmacytoid dendritic cell neoplasm: state of the art and prospects. Cancers (Basel). 2019;11(5):595.

118. Pileri A, Delfino C, Grandi V, Agostinelli C, Pileri SA, Pimpinelli N. Blastic plasmacytoid dendritic cell neoplasm (BPDCN): the cutaneous sanctuary. G Ital Dermatol Venereol. 2012;147(6):603–8.
119. Pagano L, Valentini CG, Grammatico S, Pulsoni A. Blastic plasmacytoid dendritic cell neoplasm: diagnostic criteria and therapeutical approaches. Br J Haematol. 2016;174(2):188–202.
120. Taylor J, Haddadin M, Upadhyay VA, Grussie E, Mehta-Shah N, Brunner AM, et al. Multicenter analysis of outcomes in blastic plasmacytoid dendritic cell neoplasm offers a pretargeted therapy benchmark. Blood. 2019;134(8):678–87.

Chapter 21
Dermatologic Manifestations of Internal Malignancies and Paraneoplastic Syndromes

José Antonio Sanches and Denis Miyashiro

Key Points

- Internal malignancies may cause cutaneous lesions by direct infiltration of the skin by neoplastic cells (cutaneous metastases) or by indirect inflammatory changes induced by cytokines and inflammatory cells (paraneoplastic dermatoses).
- The skin is the second most affected organ by paraneoplastic disorders, and it may be the first manifestation of internal malignancy.
- Paraneoplastic dermatoses are heterogeneous and are associated with different types of cancer. Early recognition of these disorders allows a prompt search for the underlying malignancy.

Overview

The skin is the most accessible organ of the body, and patients with internal malignancies may exhibit cutaneous lesions. In paraneoplastic disorders, inflammatory skin lesions are caused by cytokines produced by tumor or tumor microenvironment cells. These cytokines alter cellular activity causing damage without the direct action of the tumor [1]. The skin is the second organ most affected by paraneoplastic disorders, behind the endocrine system [2].

Paraneoplastic dermatoses present varied clinical aspects, and each condition is associated with different malignancies. Recognizing these changes allows the

J. A. Sanches (✉) · D. Miyashiro
Dermatology, Faculdade de Medicina da Universidade de São Paulo, São Paulo, São Paulo, Brazil

C. M. Z. Abdalla et al. (eds.), *Oncodermatology*,
https://doi.org/10.1007/978-3-031-29277-4_21

Table 21.1 Criteria for paraneoplastic skin conditions (modified from Curth) [3]

Skin lesions and neoplasm begin simultaneously
They run parallel courses
The dermatosis is not associated with a genetic syndrome
A specific dermatosis accompanies a specific tumor
The cutaneous disease is uncommon in the general population
There is a high frequency of association between the dermatosis and the neoplasm

screening and diagnosis of internal cancer as early as possible, reducing the risk of progression and increasing the chances of cure. Recurrence of paraneoplastic dermatoses is also indicative of cancer relapse and should be promptly recognized [3, 4]. Criteria proposed for paraneoplastic skin conditions (modified from Curth) are shown in Table 21.1 [3].

Acrokeratosis Paraneoplastica (Bazex Syndrome)

Acrokeratosis paraneoplastica was first described by Gougerot and Grupper in 1922, but only in 1965, Bazex et al. recognized the skin lesions as a paraneoplastic entity in a patient with laryngeal carcinoma [5, 6].

Clinical Aspects

Erythematous and violaceous scaly plaques with hyperkeratosis in a honeycomb appearance affect ear helices, nasal tip, fingers, toes, and nails (nail thickening, onycholysis, longitudinal ridging, subungual hyperkeratosis, discoloration, onychomadesis, and nail plate loss) (Fig. 21.1). Palmar and plantar lesions occur predominantly on pressure points. Penis, chest, and back may rarely be affected. When the onset of the lesions is acute, within days, vesicles may appear [7–10].

Bazex and Griffiths described three stages of the disease. First, lesions affect the fingers, toes, nose, and ear helices, and the neoplasm has no clinical manifestations (precede cancer symptoms by 2–6 months). In the second stage, lesions spread centrifugally, affecting the palms, soles, and other areas of the face, and the neoplasm starts to manifest initial symptoms. In the third stage, lesions spread to the knees, elbows, and trunk, and the neoplasm is highly symptomatic [11].

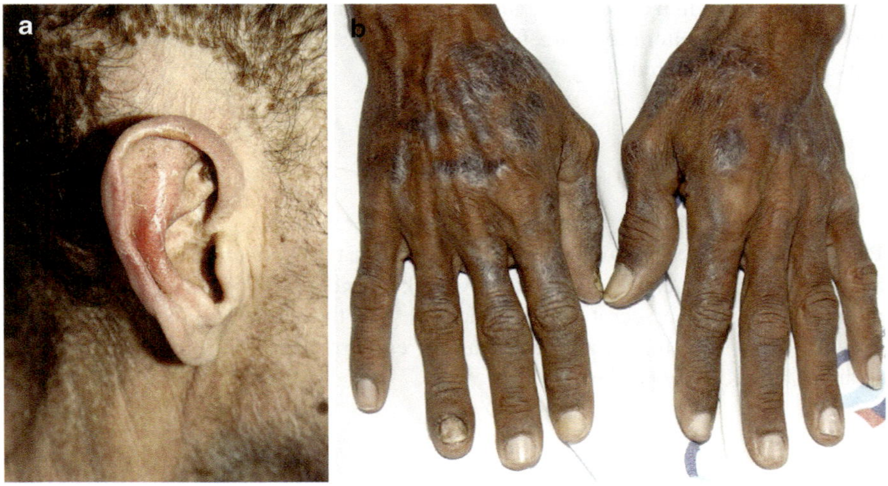

Fig. 21.1 Acrokeratosis paraneoplastica (Bazex syndrome). Erythematous and violaceous scaly plaques on the ear helix (**a**) and hands and fingers (**b**)

Histology

Hyperkeratosis, focal parakeratosis, acanthosis, mild spongiosis, apoptotic keratinocytes, and varying degrees of vacuolar degeneration of the basal cell layer are observed. In the dermis, there is a perivascular infiltrate with lymphocytes, histiocytes, and eosinophils. Direct immunofluorescence may show positivity for C3 and fibrin in the basement membrane zone [7, 12].

Associated Neoplasms

Upper aerodigestive tract squamous cell carcinomas (oral cavity, pharynx, larynx, esophagus) correspond to half of the associated malignancies. Other malignancies include lung (small cell carcinoma and adenocarcinoma), gastric, colon, and prostate adenocarcinoma; vulvar, uterine, and bladder carcinoma; hepatocarcinoma; thymoma; cutaneous squamous cell carcinoma; and hematological malignancies (Hodgkin's disease, T-cell lymphomas, multiple myeloma) [7]. Acrokeratosis paraneoplastica precedes cancer diagnosis in 47–67% with an average of 11 months; in 18%, they are concurrent; and in 15%, skin lesions occur after the diagnosis of cancer [13, 14].

After the diagnosis of Bazex syndrome, search for an occult malignancy should include detailed anamnesis with complete physical examination, including ear, nose, and throat evaluation, complete blood count, erythrocyte sedimentation rate, basic chemistry profile, tumor markers, stool guaiac test, chest X-ray, colonoscopy, upper gastrointestinal endoscopy, and computed tomography of the chest, abdomen, and pelvis. If no alterations are found, clinical reevaluation and basic laboratory tests should be repeated every 3 months [7].

Pathogenesis

Pathogenesis is unclear, but the hypotheses include the production of autoantibodies against tumor antigens cross-reacting with keratinocyte antigens of the basement membrane zone; the secretion of epidermal growth factor, TGF-α or insulin-like growth factor 1 by malignant cells causing epidermal proliferation; and zinc and vitamin A deficiency [15, 16].

Treatment

Treatment of the underlying malignancy is essential for skin improvement. Palliative treatments include topical corticosteroids, keratolytic, photochemotherapy with psoralen-UVA, and oral retinoids. Rarely, skin lesions persist after successful treatment of cancer, and careful follow-up is necessary [9, 14, 17].

Acquired Ichthyosis

The term "ichthyosis" comes from the ancient Greek word "ichthys," which means "fish" because of the clinical aspect of the skin, similar to the scales from a fish. It can be congenital or acquired. Acquired ichthyosis (AI) can be a manifestation of numerous conditions, such as malignancies, inflammatory disorders, and malnutrition. Malignancies correspond to half of the causes of AI [18, 19].

Clinical Aspects

AI is characterized by scaling affecting extremities and trunk, more prominent on the extensor surfaces of the limbs, with varying color and size of scales (Fig. 21.2). Palmoplantar keratoderma and ectropion may be present. Usually, patients with AI associated with malignancies have associated weight loss, fever, and lymphadenopathy [20].

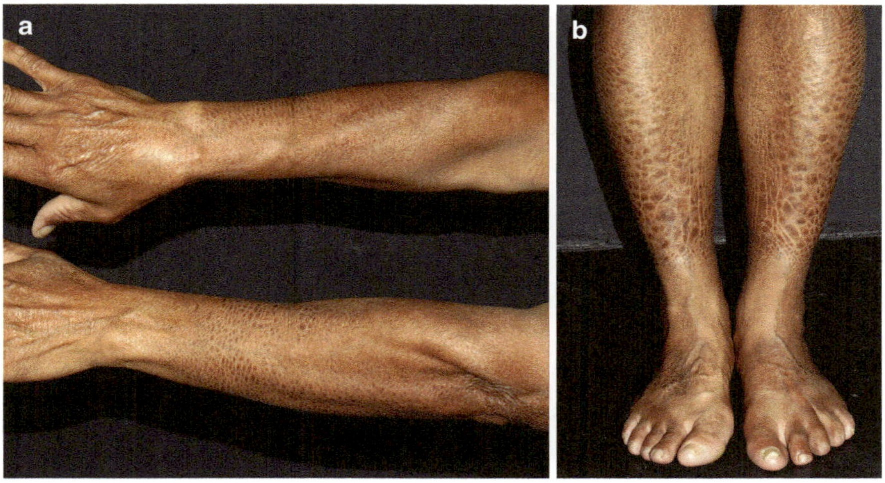

Fig. 21.2 Acquired ichthyosis. Scaling on the forearms (**a**), legs, and feet (**b**)

Histology

Hyperkeratosis, compact orthokeratosis, absence of the granular cell layer, reduced granular cell layer, and lack of spongiosis are common features. No or mild perivascular infiltrate of lymphocytes may be seen in the papillary dermis. Cutaneous T-cell lymphomas, mainly mycosis fungoides, and sarcoidosis are disorders associated with AI. The histological aspect shows epidermotropism of atypical lymphocytes (in MF) and granulomas (in sarcoidosis), raising the question of whether these diseases have an ichthyotic specific manifestation or AI is an associated condition [19].

Associated Neoplasms

Most associated malignancies are lymphoproliferative disorders, but solid neoplasms have been described. Half of the cases have Hodgkin's disease. Adult T-cell leukemia/lymphoma (ATLL), lymphomatoid papulosis, multiple myeloma, and carcinomas of the breast and lung may cause AI. Inflammatory disorders associated with AI are lupus erythematosus, dermatomyositis, sarcoidosis, and eosinophilic fasciitis [16, 19, 21].

Pathogenesis

Pathogenesis is unclear, but some authors suggest the role of metabolites produced by neoplastic cells that alter the function of the complex pool of enzymes necessary to normal keratinization of the stratum corneum. Deficiency in vitamin A absorption and altered lipid profile are other proposed pathogenic mechanisms [19].

Treatment

Treatment must be directed to the underlying disorder, but the use of humectants (glycolic acid) and keratolytics (salicylic acid) may relieve dryness [19].

Dermatomyositis

Dermatomyositis (DM) is an autoimmune disease characterized by polymyositis and inflammatory skin lesions. It is divided into adult-onset or juvenile DM [22, 23]. Stertz, in 1916, described a patient with inflammatory myositis and gastric cancer [24]. Since then, the association of DM and polymyositis with malignancies has been discussed. The incidence of cancer ranges between 7% and 30% of the patients with adult-onset DM [22]. The association of juvenile DM and malignant diseases is considered anecdotal [25]. Some patients may present typical DM skin lesions in the absence of clinical and laboratory myositis findings, a condition called amyopathic dermatomyositis [16].

Clinical Aspects

Clinical findings of paraneoplastic DM resemble those from classical DM, with violaceous and poikilodermatous rash in sun-exposed areas (face, upper trunk, extensor surfaces of the upper limbs), heliotrope (erythema and edema around the eyelids), and Gottron papules (Fig. 21.3). Pruritus, skin necrosis, and nail involvement (onychodystrophy, overgrowth cuticles, periungual erythema, and telangiectasia) can also be observed. Cutaneous vasculitis (palpable purpura, necrosis, ulcerations), calcinosis cutis (indurated nodules on elbows, knees, and buttocks), and erythroderma have been described [23, 26].

Myopathy is characterized by difficulties climbing the stairs and combing the hair, due to symmetrical proximal weakness, with or without creatine kinase (CK) elevation. Swallowing difficulties sometimes may also be present [25, 27]. Electromyography and magnetic resonance imaging show nonspecific alterations but are useful to indicate myopathic changes, guide muscle biopsy, and monitor disease activity [28].

Older age, male sex, dysphagia, and cutaneous necrosis were associated with increased risk of cancer, whereas arthritis and interstitial lung disease were associated with decreased risk [29]. There is no difference in the incidence of malignancies DM and amyopathic DM [28]. It is hypothesized that interstitial lung disease decreases the risk of neoplasm in DM patients due to the severity of this condition, which may lead to death before the onset or diagnosis of cancer [30]. Antinuclear

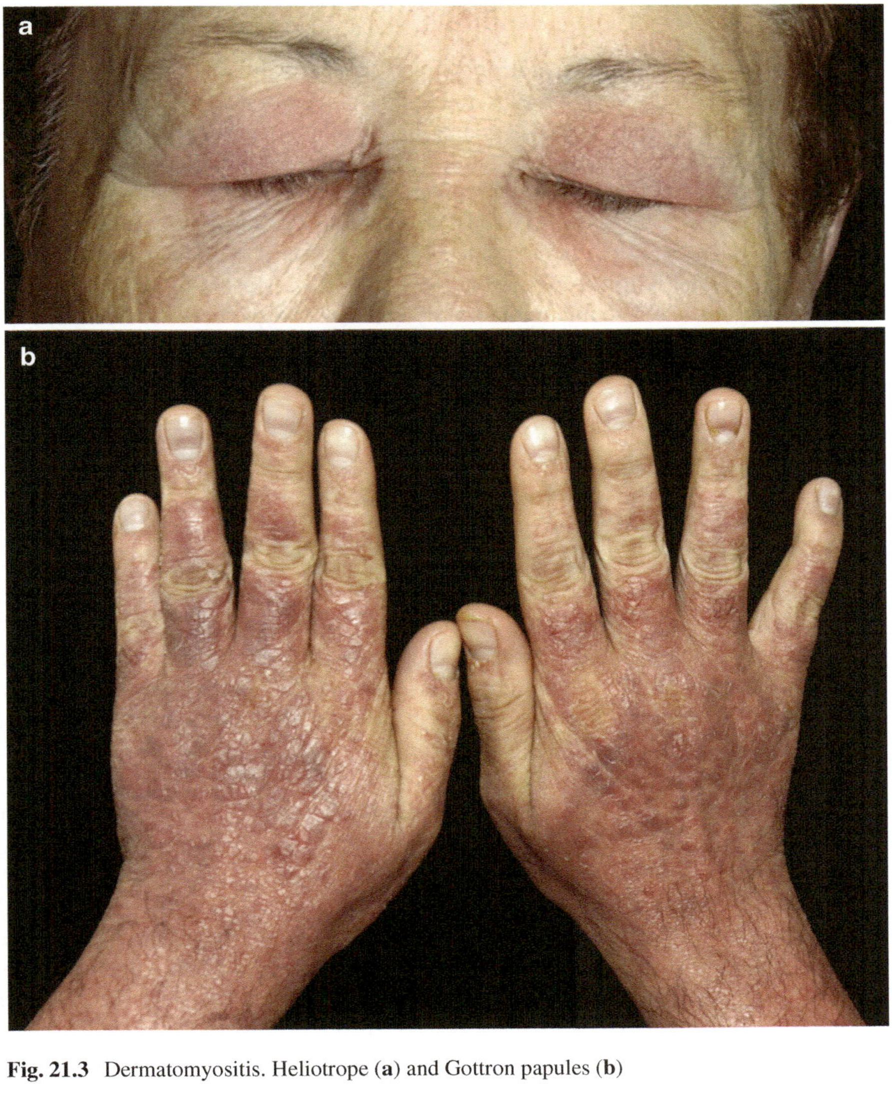

Fig. 21.3 Dermatomyositis. Heliotrope (**a**) and Gottron papules (**b**)

antibody test (ANA) has a 40–60% sensitivity, low specificity, and no correlation with cancer [29]. Myositis-associated markers, such as anti-Jo-1 and anti-Mi-2, are not associated with increased cancer risk [28]. Anti-p155 has 78% sensitivity and 89% specificity for diagnosing cancer-associated DM, with positive and negative predictive values of 58% and 95%, respectively [31]. Anti-MDA5 (melanoma differentiation-associated protein 5) antibody has been associated with increased risk of interstitial lung disease and lower risk of malignancy [32].

Histology

DM histology shows epidermal atrophy, interface dermatitis with vacuolar degeneration of the basal layer, apoptotic keratinocytes, melanin incontinence, edematous papillary dermis, dilated blood vessels in the superficial dermis, lymphocytic perivascular infiltrate, and mucin deposition [33]. Direct immunofluorescence shows deposits of IgG and C3 at the dermal-epidermal junction in 5–67% of patients [28]. These findings are identical to lupus erythematosus; thus, histopathology and immunopathology are not diagnostic tests; instead, they should be used to support the diagnosis when clinical aspects suggest DM [28]. Muscle biopsy is the gold standard diagnostic test to inflammatory myopathies. DM patients show loss of capillaries, altered morphology of capillaries, capillary necrosis, muscle infarcts, perifascicular atrophy, lymphocytic infiltrate, and complement deposition in the vessel wall [33].

Associated Neoplasms

Most malignancies associated with DM are breast and ovarian cancer in women and lung, prostate, and rectum cancer in men [22]. In Asian countries, a higher frequency of nasopharyngeal carcinomas is reported [34, 35]. Other associations are liver, bladder, and kidney carcinomas, non-Hodgkin lymphomas, gastric and pancreatic adenocarcinomas, and uterine cervix squamous cell carcinoma [30]. Prognosis is related to the underlying neoplasm, and sometimes, cancer is diagnosed already with metastatic disease [33].

DM can precede (40%), be concomitant (26%), or follow diagnosis of cancer (34%) [27]. In adult-onset DM, an extensive work-up is needed, including detailed anamnesis and physical examination and laboratory investigation with tumorous markers, such as CA125 for women and PSA for men; transvaginal ultrasonography; mammography; chest X-ray; computed tomography scan of the thorax, abdomen, and pelvis; colonoscopy; and gastroscopy. If no malignancy is detected, it is recommended to repeat the screening once a year for the first 3 years, as the highest risk of cancer occurs during the first year after diagnosis of DM [25, 35].

Pathogenesis

Hypotheses to the development of DM in patients with underlying malignancies are crossover immunity due to common antigens expressed by cancer, skin, and muscle tissues; altered immune system causing myositis and onset of cancer; bioactive products from neoplastic cells stimulating immune reactions against skin and muscle; carcinogenic antigens which trigger immune reactions and induce malignancy; and changes in the extracellular matrix surrounding the tumor, causing changes in the extracellular matrix of nontumoral tissues, with mucin deposition, edema, and atrophy [36].

Treatment

Treatment of paraneoplastic DM requires treatment of the underlying malignancy [33]. Systemic corticosteroids in the dosage of 1 mg/kg/day are usually the first choice for DM without malignancy. Methotrexate, azathioprine, mycophenolate mofetil, rituximab, and intravenous immunoglobulin may be used if there is no response to systemic corticosteroids or prolonged treatment is required. Topical treatment with steroids, emollients, and sunscreens may be associated. These treatments have little impact on the improvement of the disease but may result in symptomatic relief. Recurrence of skin eruption and muscle weakness may be early indications of cancer relapse [23, 33].

Erythema Gyratum Repens

Erythema gyratum repens (EGR) was described in 1952 by Gammel in a woman who presented a skin eruption with a "knotty cypress wood grain" appearance and metastatic breast cancer. Skin lesions disappeared after successful treatment of cancer [37]. EGR is classified with figurate erythemas. "Gyratum" means coiled or winding around a central point, and "repens," from the Latin, means to crawl or creep [38, 39].

Clinical Aspects

Multiple erythematous and serpiginous concentric bands, with a hyperkeratotic scale at one edge, resembling a geographical map or a wood grain, are the typical cutaneous presentation (Fig. 21.4). These lesions migrate centrifugally, with new lesions appearing within the existing ones. More pronounced in intertriginous areas

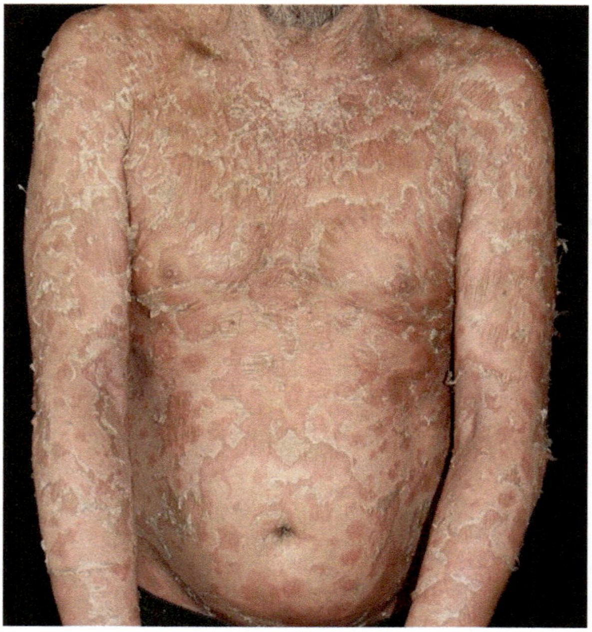

Fig. 21.4 Erythema gyratum repens. Serpiginous scaly plaques on the trunk and arms

of axillae and groin, it may affect the trunk and extremities, often sparing the face. Palmoplantar keratosis, onychodystrophy, and ichthyosis may be present [38, 40, 41]. Severe pruritus may be a debilitating symptom [42]. Cases evaluating erythroderma have been described [43].

Histology

Histopathology shows nonspecific findings, but it is useful to rule out other differential diagnoses. Hyperkeratosis, focal parakeratosis, acanthosis, mild spongiosis, and superficial perivascular lymphocytic infiltrate are seen. Direct immunofluorescence shows granular deposits of IgG, C3, and fibrin in the basement membrane zone and IgM deposition in colloid bodies. Indirect immunofluorescence is negative. IgG and C3 deposits at the basement membrane zone of lung epithelium may be present [41, 42].

Associated Neoplasms

Seventy percent of EGR patients have an underlying neoplasm, and 30% have other conditions that may mimic EGR clinically. Of the malignant diseases, bronchial cancer is the most prevalent (46.5%), followed by gastric (8.6%), esophagus (6.9%), breast cancer (5.2%), and unknown primary site (5.2%) [42]. Other described neoplasms are cervix, pharynx, kidney, anus, tongue, bowel, pancreas, bladder, prostate, uterus, multiple myeloma, Hodgkin's lymphoma, and essential thrombocythemia [40]. EGR precedes the diagnosis of malignancy in 87.9% of the patients, with a mean time of 7 months; it is concurrent in 8.6% and is diagnosed after malignancy in 3.4% of the cases [42]. Other diseases that may mimic EGR are lupus erythematosus, mycosis fungoides, bullous dermatoses (linear IgA dermatosis, bullous pemphigoid, pemphigus vulgaris), urticarial vasculitis, neutrophilic dermatoses, leukocytoclastic vasculitis, erythrokeratodermia variabilis, erythema annulare centrifugum, erythema annulare of infancy, and Sjogren's syndrome [44]. Two cases of EGR associated with interferon-α for chronic hepatitis C, a case associated with azathioprine, and a case of EGR lesions in a patient with psoriasis treated with acitretin were described [42, 45].

Pathogenesis

The deposition of IgG and C3 in the basement membrane zone of the skin and bronchial epithelium of the tumor raises the hypothesis of an immune reaction. Skin antigens may be the target of antibodies produced against tumor antigens or altered molecules from the tumor stroma in a cross-reaction process. Molecules produced by neoplastic cells or immunocomplexes made by the interaction of tumor antigens and antibodies may selectively deposit on the skin, leading to the inflammatory reaction [40, 41].

Treatment

Treatment of tumors leads to the resolution of skin lesions. In metastatic disease, lesions may persist despite appropriate treatment if the tumor is unresponsive to chemotherapy or radiotherapy. Topical and systemic steroids may be associated with partial and transient relief of skin lesions and pruritus [38, 40, 41].

Erythroderma

Erythroderma was described by Hebra in 1868, and it is characterized by diffuse erythema and scaling affecting more than 80% of the body surface area. It is an inflammatory condition caused by several etiologies. Classically, it is associated with preexisting dermatoses (psoriasis, eczema, pityriasis rubra pilaris, pemphigus foliaceous), drug reactions (carbamazepine, phenytoin, phenobarbital, allopurinol), cutaneous lymphomas (mycosis fungoides, Sézary syndrome, adult T-cell leukemia/lymphoma), and infections (dermatophytosis, crusted scabies). Rarely, it may represent a paraneoplastic condition associated with solid tumors [46].

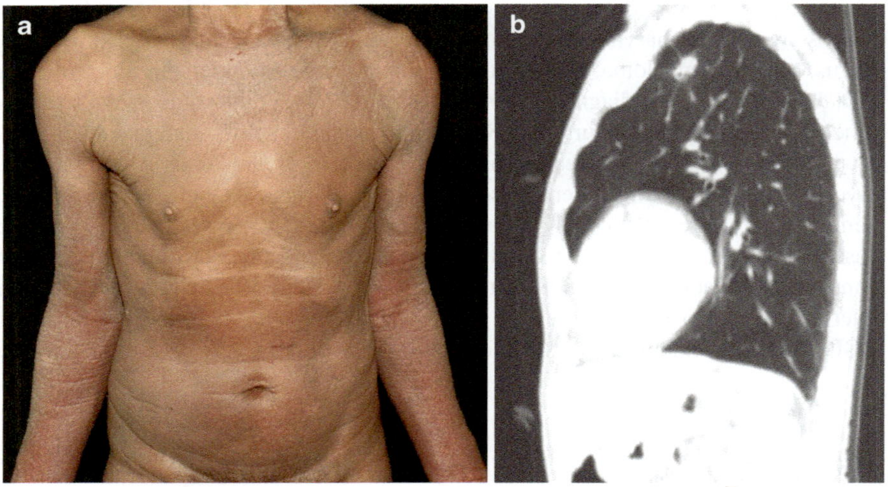

Fig. 21.5 Erythroderma. Erythema and scaling affecting more than 80% of the body surface area (**a**). Computed tomography showing a nodule on the upper lobe, which biopsy confirmed a lung adenocarcinoma (**b**)

Clinical Aspects

Generalized erythema and scaling may be associated with palmoplantar keratoderma, onychodystrophy, diffuse non-scarring alopecia, lower limb edema, weight loss, pruritus, and lymph node enlargement (Fig. 21.5). Erythroderma is a potentially severe condition due to alteration in skin barrier function [47]. Extensive investigation, comprehensive anamnesis and clinical examination, laboratory work-up, and histopathology evaluation are required. Search for T-cell receptor gene rearrangement and immunophenotyping of peripheral blood lymphocytes by flow cytometry are essential to diagnosing erythroderma caused by cutaneous lymphomas [46]. Papuloerythroderma of Ofuji, described by Ofuji in 1984, is a distinct clinical entity characterized by coalescent papules, leading to erythroderma. It typically spares skinfold areas ("deck chair" sign). Often associated with hematological malignancies (cutaneous T-cell lymphomas, non-epidermotropic peripheral T-cell lymphoma, Hodgkin's disease, acute myeloid leukemia), patients with this condition should undergo extensive work-up to find associated neoplasm, similar to erythrodermic patients [16, 48].

Histology

Skin histopathology of paraneoplastic erythroderma shows nonspecific features. Hyperkeratosis, parakeratosis, acanthosis, spongiosis, and mild perivascular lymphohistiocytic infiltrate in the upper dermis are common findings. Eosinophils may be present [49].

Associated Neoplasms

Due to the rarity of paraneoplastic erythroderma, studies report isolated cases associated with Hodgkin's lymphoma, diffuse large B-cell lymphoma, and anaplastic large T-cell lymphoma; renal cell carcinoma; breast cancer; gallbladder adenocarcinoma; lung and tongue Langerhans cell histiocytosis; carcinoma of the colon, prostate, thyroid, fallopian tubes, larynx, esophagus, and liver; acute and chronic leukemia; and sarcoma. Erythroderma may precede or be concomitant to cancer diagnosis, and recurrence of erythroderma is associated with recurrence of malignancy [46, 50–54].

Pathogenesis

Pathogenesis of erythroderma is unknown, but evidence suggests a Th2 cytokine profile leading to generalized skin inflammation, with eosinophilia and increased serum IgE levels [55]. Interaction of interleukins 1, 2, and 8, intercellular adhesion molecule-1, and TNF may also act in erythroderma pathogenesis, increasing epidermal turnover rate [51].

Treatment

Treatment is directed to the underlying tumor, but topical and systemic corticosteroids may relieve symptoms [54].

Hypertrichosis Lanuginosa Acquisita

Hypertrichosis lanuginosa acquisita (HLA) was described by Turner in 1865 in a female patient with breast cancer [56].

Clinical Aspects

Hypertrichosis is the increase of lanugo, vellus, or terminal hair. The increase of lanugo hair can be congenital or acquired. Lanugo-type hair is observed in utero, with thin, nonpigmented hair, shed during the last month of pregnancy. Hypertrichosis lanuginosa congenita occurs in premature neonates [57]. In HLA, mature hair follicle produces this embryonic hair [58]. HLA may be secondary to endocrine

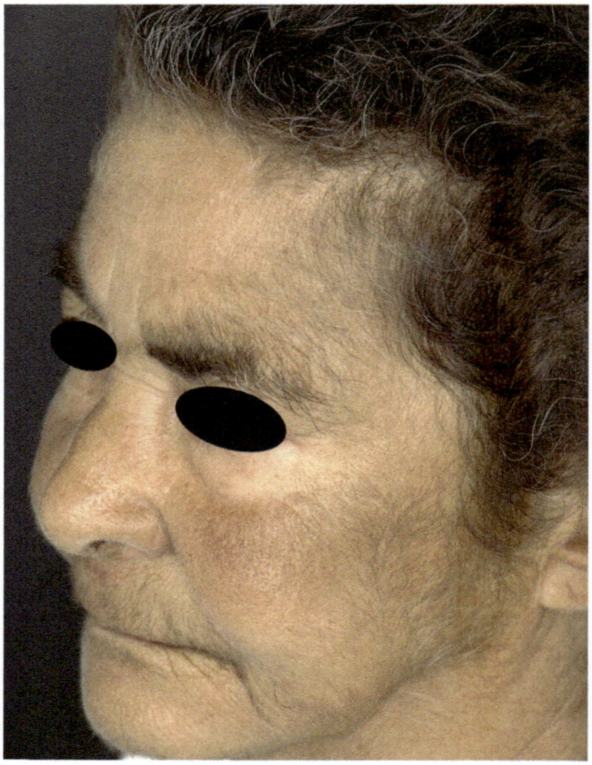

Fig. 21.6 Hypertrichosis lanuginosa acquisita. Multiple fine hairs on the face

disorders and adverse drug reactions (ciclosporin, penicillamine, psoralens, glucocorticosteroids, diazoxide, interferon, minoxidil, phenytoin, cetuximab) and may be a sign of internal malignancy [57].

Paraneoplastic HLA is characterized by the sudden and progressive appearance of multiple fine, long, and nonpigmented hair, initially affecting the face, progressing to the neck, shoulders, chest, and limbs (Fig. 21.6). Other associated symptoms are hypersensitivity on the tongue, erythema and fissures, dysgeusia, weight loss, and diarrhea. It affects women 2–3 times more frequently than men, with a range of 40–70 years [59]. Cases of HLA may be underreported since clinicians may be unfamiliar with this condition and because the increase in lanugo-type hair in men is less obvious. Search for signs of virilization and hirsutism is important, as there are reports of association of hypertrichosis and hirsutism in androgen-producing tumors [57].

Associated Neoplasms

The most common associated malignancies in women are colon, lung, and breast cancer, and in men, they are lung and colon cancer. Isolated reports show the association with prostate, bladder, kidney, uterus, ovary, stomach, pancreas, gallbladder, liver, rectum, and parotid gland cancer, lymphoma, leukemia, Ewing's sarcoma, and melanoma [57, 59]. Malignancy can be diagnosed before, concomitantly, or after skin eruption, and the prognosis is usually poor. The malignancy is usually diagnosed in the metastatic phase. Work-up should include a detailed anamnesis and physical examination, blood tests, chest X-ray, colonoscopy, and mammography [57, 59].

Pathogenesis

Pathogenesis is unclear, but the production of a nonrecognized humoral factor by tumoral cells, causing a prolongation of the anagen phase of vellus hair follicles, is the most accepted theory [59]. Other laboratory alterations, such as elevated cortisol and other hormones, were reported, but no consistent association with HLA was observed. The association of HLA and acanthosis nigricans suggests the involvement of TNF-α and insulin-like growth factor [60].

Treatment

Successful treatment of malignancy leads to the resolution of HLA within weeks [58].

Hypertrophic Osteoarthropathy

Digital clubbing, Hippocratic fingers, watch-glass nails, or drumstick fingers, was described by Hippocrates in a patient with empyema in 400 BC. Hypertrophic osteoarthropathy (HOA), or pachydermoperiostitis, is characterized by digital clubbing, periostitis of tubular bones, and arthritis. Primary HOA is an autosomal-dominant disease. Secondary HOA has been associated with malignant, cardiac, and congenital diseases [61, 62].

Clinical Aspects

Primary HOA starts in childhood with clubbing, periostitis, thickening of the skin of the face and scalp, coarsening of facial features, hyperhidrosis, and seborrhea [61]. In secondary HOA, unilateral digital clubbing is associated with neurologic or vascular diseases; if bilateral, there is a strong association with pulmonary neoplasms. First, periungual erythema occurs, with a spongy sensation on palpation due to softening of the nail bed. Then, an increase in the 160° angle between the nail bed and proximal nail fold occurs. This leads to increasing convexity of the nail. In malignancy-associated HOA, periostitis of lower extremities is common, associated with the knees and ankles synovitis. Incomplete forms may show isolated findings [61].

Histology

Histology of fingertip skin lesions shows vascular alterations: endothelial hyperplasia with partial occlusion of the capillary lumen by platelet clusters, pericapillary lymphohistiocytic infiltrate, thickening of collagen fibers, and sebaceous and eccrine hypertrophy. Vasculitis of small vessels and arteries may be present [61].

Associated Neoplasms

HOA is associated with primary or metastatic lung cancer in 80% of cases. Other associated malignancies are intrathoracic Hodgkin's disease, nasopharyngeal carcinoma, mesothelioma, pleural tumors, kidney, esophageal, gastric, and pancreatic cancer, breast phyllodes tumor, melanoma, thyroid cancer, osteosarcoma, and intestinal lymphoma. Cystic fibrosis, tuberculosis, endocarditis, syphilis, AIDS, congenital heart diseases, hepatic cholestatic diseases, and inflammatory bowel disease are other diseases associated with HOA. In primary lung cancer, HOA is present in 4–32% of the cases [61]. Periostitis and HOA can precede malignancy by several months [62].

Pathogenesis

Megakaryocytes are usually fragmented into platelets in the lungs. Disruption of normal pulmonary circulation would allow whole megakaryocytes to enter the systemic circulation. Due to their large size, they would impact distal fingertip circulation, leading to the release of platelet-derived growth factor (PDGF), promoting growth, vascular permeability, and monocyte and neutrophils chemotaxis, increasing the number of vascular smooth muscle cells and fibroblasts. Vascular endothelial growth factor (VEGF) is also increased in lung cancer and HOA patients, contributing to vascular hyperplasia [61]. Prostaglandin E is a potent bone formation stimulator, and its use has been associated with the development of periostitis and clubbing [62].

Treatment

Treatment of cancer with surgery or chemotherapy may improve digital clubbing. Pain can be relieved by nonsteroidal anti-inflammatory drugs. Some studies report a reduction of pain with pamidronate, probably due to its antitumor and anti-inflammatory actions. Octreotide inhibits the production of VEGF, decreasing endothelial proliferation and relieving pain. Gefitinib and colchicine may be used for periostitis [62].

Leser-Trélat Sign

The sign of Leser-Trélat, described by Holländer in 1900, refers to the eruption of multiple seborrheic keratoses. Leser, a German surgeon, and Trélat, a French surgeon, reported multiple eruptive angiomas in patients with underlying malignancies. Posteriorly, its association was found to be untrue, with seborrheic keratosis as the lesions associated with cancer. Due to the historical importance of the first authors, the name of the sign persists. Sign and syndrome of Leser-Trélat should be distinguished. "Sign" should be used when there are multiple eruptive lesions of seborrheic keratosis, with or without association with malignancy. On the other hand, "syndrome" should be used when diagnosing underlying malignancy with skin lesions [63].

Clinical Aspects

The association of eruptive seborrheic keratosis and malignancies is still controversial, as some authors argue that seborrheic keratosis lesions are extremely common and occur predominantly in the elderly when the risk of cancer is increased. This hypothesis is weakened, as there are some reports of lesions occurring in young adults [64]. Multiple seborrheic keratoses may develop in erythrodermic patients, and investigation of the cause of erythroderma is imperative, as lymphoproliferative diseases may be associated with Leser-Trélat sign and erythroderma [65]. Involvement of the trunk is found in 76% of the patients, followed by extremities in 38%. Christmas tree pattern has been described. In a person with numerous seborrheic keratosis, Leser-Trélat sign must be considered if there is a rapid increase in size and number of the lesions, and it has been associated with TP in 10% of the cases. Nonmalignant disorders may present multiple eruptive seborrheic keratoses: HIV infection, heart transplant, and acromegaly [66].

Histology

Histopathology is consistent with seborrheic keratosis, hyperkeratosis, acanthosis, and papillomatosis in the epidermis. Sometimes, pseudohorn cysts are found [66].

Associated Neoplasms

It is most often associated with adenocarcinomas of the stomach and colon, leukemia, and lymphomas and rarely with cancers of the breast, lung, esophagus, liver, pancreas, bladder, and kidney and melanoma. Most cases have more advanced stage neoplasms, with metastases. The sign may occur before, concomitantly, or after the diagnosis of cancer [64, 65].

Pathogenesis

Immunohistochemistry shows an elevated expression of epidermal growth factor receptor (EGFR) in all epidermis layers, except in the stratum corneum, in the seborrheic keratosis lesions of patients with associated malignancies. In normal skin, EGFR is expressed only in the basal keratinocytes. Transforming growth factor-α (TGF-α) has also been implicated as an important mechanism in Leser-Trélat sign. TGF-α induces epidermal changes in different cutaneous regions. Thus, flexural areas would develop acanthosis nigricans, whereas exposed cutaneous surfaces would respond with the development of seborrheic keratoses lesions [63, 67].

Treatment

Treatment of cancer leads to a decrease and disappearance of the lesions [63].

Malignant Acanthosis Nigricans, Tripe Palms, and Florid Cutaneous Papillomatosis

Acanthosis nigricans is a skin condition often associated with endocrinopathies, particularly obesity and insulin resistance [68, 69]. The term "acanthus," from the Greek, means "thorn"; and "nigricans," from the Latin, means "becoming black." Pollitzer and Janovsky independently described the first reports of acanthosis nigricans in patients with digestive tract cancers [70]. These cases associated with malignancies are called malignant acanthosis nigricans (MAN). Tripe palms (TP) and florid cutaneous papillomatosis (FCP) are variants of MAN that affect the palms and soles, lips, and oral cavity, respectively [71, 72].

Clinical Manifestations

MAN shows brownish discoloration, thickening, and velvety hyperpigmented surface on skinfolds of axillary, groin, and cervical regions, similar to benign acanthosis nigricans. Overlying acrochordons may be present, as well as pruritus in varying degrees of intensity. MAN can be the first sign of malignancy and must be suspected if atypical topography is observed (nipples, periumbilical, orbicular, labial), if the appearance of the lesions is sudden, and if extensive areas of the skin are affected, especially in the elderly with no obesity and endocrinologic disorders [68, 73, 74].

TP and FCP may occur in association with MAN or alone. In TP, a velvety appearance of the palmar surface, skin ridging, and sharp demarcation of dermatoglyphics are found. FCP is similar to warts, with diffuse and extensive verrucous papules on the lips and oral cavity (tongue, palate, and retrocomissural areas) (Fig. 21.7). The presence of these conditions must raise the suspicion of occult malignancy, and appropriate investigation is imperative, especially if they occur in

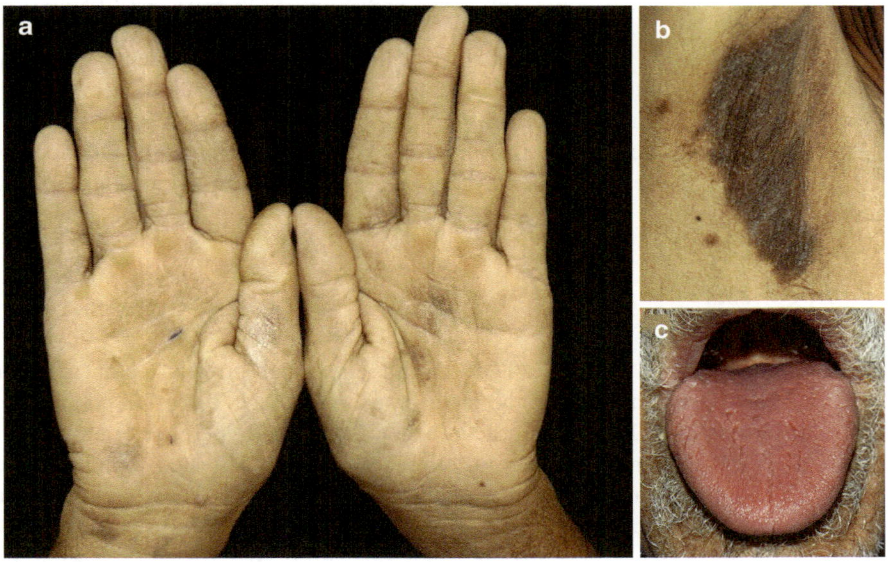

Fig. 21.7 Tripe palms, malignant acanthosis nigricans, florid cutaneous papillomatosis. Velvety appearance of the palms (**a**), hyperpigmented velvety plaque on the axillae (**b**), multiple papules on the tongue (**c**). These lesions were observed in the same patient, who was diagnosed with colon adenocarcinoma

elderly patients with a history of weight loss and familiar history of cancer [68, 75]. Rarely, the esophagus, larynx, eyes, and anal and genital mucosa may be involved [66].

Histology

Skin biopsy is characterized by basket-woven hyperkeratosis, papillomatosis with "fingerlike" projections of rete ridges, mild acanthosis, and basal layer hyperpigmentation. Differential diagnosis includes HPV infections [66, 76].

Associated Neoplasms

Gastrointestinal adenocarcinomas correspond to 90% of the malignancies associated with MAN, and half of these cases correspond to gastric adenocarcinomas. Rarely, it may be associated with ovarian, endometrial, breast, prostatic, pancreatic, and lung adenocarcinomas, epithelial carcinomas, and hematologic malignancies. Usually, the underlying neoplasm is in advanced metastatic stage [68, 73].

Skin lesions appear concomitantly with the diagnosis of the neoplasm in 60% of the cases, but occasionally they can occur before (20%) or after (20%) cancer is diagnosed [16, 76].

TP is associated with lung cancer, followed by gastric adenocarcinoma. Nonmalignant conditions have also been associated with TP: bullous pemphigoid, psoriasis, erythroderma, and pruritus [66, 71].

Most FCP cases are associated with gastric adenocarcinoma, with some reports of association with breast, bladder, ovarian, uterine, prostate, and lung cancer [16].

Pathogenesis

Transforming growth factor-α (TGF-α) and epidermal growth factor receptor (EGFR) play important roles in the pathogenesis of MAN. Tumoral cells secrete large quantities of TGF-α, which acts in keratinocytes' hyperproliferation, as it binds to EGFR, leading to the activation of the mitogen-activated protein kinase (MAPK) and the extracellular-signal-regulated kinase (ERK). These pathways are implicated in keratinocytes proliferation and differentiation. EGFR is constitutively expressed in the basal cell layer of the epidermis, but in MAN, it was shown to be present in basal and suprabasal keratinocytes. Also, ERK activity was increased within keratinocytes from MAN skin samples. Production of insulin-like growth factor 1, fibroblast growth factor, and α-melanocyte-stimulating hormone by neoplastic cells leads to melanocyte pigmentation, explaining the hyperpigmentation of the lesions [60, 77, 78].

Treatment

Treatment of the neoplasm leads to remission of skin lesions. The course of skin lesions has a parallel course with the malignancy. When skin lesions do not improve after cancer treatment, or when they recur, search for unresponsive, progressive, or recurrent disease must be done [73, 76]. Pruritus is treated with antihistamines, photochemotherapy with psoralen plus ultraviolet A (PUVA), systemic retinoids, or gabapentin, with varying degrees of response [79].

Multicentric Reticulohistiocytosis

Multicentric reticulohistiocytosis (MRH) is a rare non-Langerhans cell histiocytosis of unknown etiology that affect the skin and synovium. In 25–30% of the cases, an underlying malignancy is observed [80, 81].

Clinical Aspects

Skin lesions are characterized by reddish-brown papules and nodules on the face, hands, and arms. Small papules around nail folds in a coral-bead appearance is observed in 30% of the patients [82].

Besides skin lesions, MRH may affect the joints, causing severe symmetrical inflammatory polyarthritis especially involving interphalangeal joints of the hands that can be rapidly progressive and destructive [16, 82].

Histology

Dermal infiltrate of histiocytes and multinucleated giant cells containing eosinophilic cytoplasm with ground-glass appearance. These cells express CD68 and CD163 and, sometimes, are factor XIIIa positive [16, 82].

Associated Neoplasms

A variety of types of malignancies of different cell lineages have been associated with MRH: melanoma, carcinomas (breast, gastrointestinal tract), sarcomas, leukemias, and lymphomas [16, 80]. MRH lesions may precede cancer diagnosis in 70% of the patients [81].

Pathogenesis

The pathogenesis of MRH is unknown, but it has been hypothesized that cytokines may play a role in the uncontrolled macrophage activation leading to skin lesions and mutilating polyarthritis [81].

Treatment

Treatment of MRH is challenging. Spontaneous remission may occur after years, but joint lesions may persist. Immunosuppressants and immunomodulators are often contraindicated if a malignant neoplasm is diagnosed. Bisphosphonates are effective on skin and joint lesions. In paraneoplastic MRH, complete remission of skin lesions may be achieved with treatment of the underlying malignancy [16, 82].

Necrolytic Migratory Erythema

Becker et al. described a patient with skin eruption and pancreatic cancer in 1942 [83]. In 1966, McGavran et al. reported a female patient with bullous and eczematoid lesions, elevated glucagon levels, and functional alpha-cell pancreatic neoplasm [84]. But only in 1977, Mallinson et al. defined the glucagonoma syndrome, characterized by necrolytic migratory erythema (NME), stomatitis, weight loss, anemia, and diabetes mellitus, in nine patients with pancreatic tumors [85].

Clinical Aspects

The characteristic features of NME are annular erythematous plaques, with scaling, erosions, and crusted borders, hypopigmented centers that migrate, extending centrifugally. It has a predilection for the intertriginous areas of the perineum, inguinal and axillary folds, lower abdomen, and thighs (Fig. 21.8). Intense pruritus is a common symptom. Angular cheilitis, glossitis, and conjunctivitis may be present [86]. Nail involvement with onycholysis and onychoschizia and hair thinning are

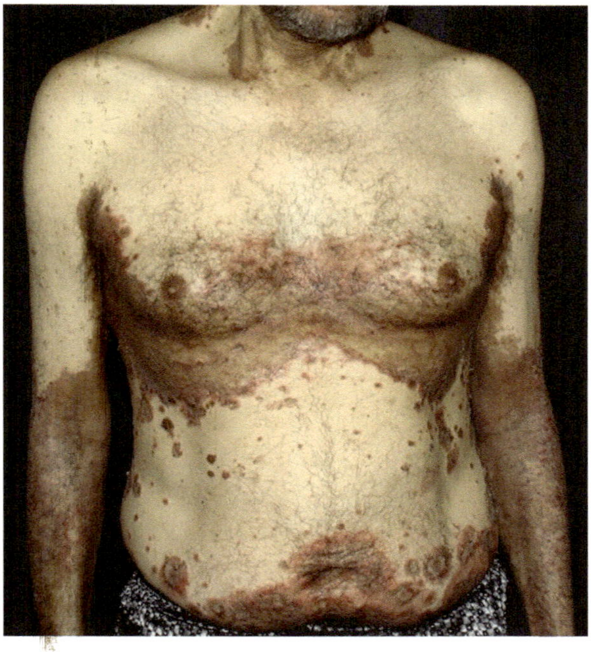

Fig. 21.8 Necrolytic migratory erythema. Annular plaques with crusted borders and hyperpigmented centers

associated features [87]. Besides NME, stomatitis, weight loss, diabetes mellitus or glucose intolerance, normocytic anemia, thromboembolic disease, and psychiatric disorders may be observed, and glucagonoma syndrome must be considered [88, 89]. Patients usually have an initial diagnosis of eczema, with a poor and transient response to conventional treatment with topical steroids, contributing to the delay in the diagnosis of NME and the search for pancreas neoplasm [88].

Histology

Skin histopathology shows a pale aspect of the superior layers of the epidermis (necrolysis), acanthosis, confluent parakeratosis, spongiosis, vacuolar degeneration of superficial epidermal keratinocytes, and mild perivascular infiltrate in the superficial dermis composed mainly of lymphocytes and few neutrophils. Intraepidermal cleft and subcorneal pustules may be present [86, 90].

Differential Diagnoses

Differential diagnoses include zinc deficiency (acrodermatitis enteropathica), biotin deficiency, pellagra, pemphigus vulgaris, psoriasis, seborrheic dermatitis, and contact dermatitis [86].

Associated Neoplasms

The underlying neoplasm is, commonly, an alpha-cell pancreatic adenocarcinoma. Most of the patients have a metastatic disease by the time of diagnosis. Skin lesions usually appear before the diagnosis of malignancy, and identification of NME must raise the suspicion of a pancreatic neoplasm [88].

Association with other conditions was described, but it is very rare. These conditions include neuroendocrine hepatic tumors, jejunal and rectal adenocarcinoma, myelodysplastic syndromes, inflammatory bowel disease, celiac disease, chronic pancreatitis, hepatic cirrhosis, and malabsorption disorders, and these conditions are termed “pseudoglucagonoma syndrome” [16, 91].

Pathogenesis

The pathogenesis of NME is unknown. Glucagon is a catabolic hormone and acts in glucose, fat, and protein metabolism. It promotes hepatic gluconeogenesis and glycogenolysis; proteolysis of muscle tissue, increasing the source of alanine and glutamine, necessary to hepatic gluconeogenesis; and lipolysis of triglyceride due to lipase activation, increasing free fatty acid delivery for hepatic ketogenesis. When a functional tumor of the pancreas secretes glucagon, diabetes mellitus is observed, as well as important weight loss and cachexia, due to an increase in serum glucose with depletion of glycogen stores, muscle tissue, and fat mass [92].

Evidence supports the role of glucagon in the pathogenesis of NME lesions. Improvement of skin rash is rapidly achieved when successful treatment of the malignancy is done, with a rapid decrease in glucagon levels. Even in metastatic disease, treatment with somatostatin analogs, a glucagon inhibitor, leads to significant improvement [92]. Evidence suggests the role of glucagon in releasing inflammatory cytokines, such as arachidonic acid, which lead to superficial necrolysis of the skin [93]. Hyperglucagonemia causes nutrients and vitamin B deficiencies, probably contributing to the appearance of skin lesions. Thus, the association of hyperglucagonemia, nutrient deficiency (zinc, amino acids, fatty acids, vitamins), cytokine release, and liver dysfunction may lead to pathogenesis of NME [94].

Treatment

There is a good association between the resolution of skin lesions and the decrease in glucagon concentrations [92]. Thus, excision of pancreatic cancer leads to rapid resolution of skin lesions within few days. Postinflammatory hyperpigmentation persists for a few months [89]. When metastatic disease is diagnosed, palliative treatment with somatostatin (glucagon inhibitor) and interferon-α is effective [92]. A transient improvement of skin lesions and pruritus is achieved with topical or systemic steroids, but rapid relapse occurs when the drug is withdrawn [86]. Supplementation with zinc, amino acids, and essential fatty acids are adjuvant treatments [16, 95].

Paraneoplastic Pemphigus

In 1990, Anhalt et al. described the paraneoplastic pemphigus (PNP), and [96] in 2001, Nguyen et al. proposed the term paraneoplastic autoimmune multi-organ syndrome due to the presence of autoantibodies in multiple organs [97].

Clinical Aspects

PNP affects mucosa and skin. Mucosal lesions are reported in 94% of the patients. Severe oral lesions, with painful erosions affecting more than 10% of the mucosal area, are characteristic features (Fig. 21.9a). These erosions may extend to the pharyngeal, laryngeal, esophageal, and bronchial mucosa. Ocular and genital lesions are observed in 80% and 66% of the patients, respectively [98, 99].

Skin lesions are polymorphic. Lichenoid and target-like lesions, resembling erythema multiforme, are the most common findings, but blistering lesions (pemphigus-like, bullous pemphigoid-like, and linear IgA dermatosis-like) may also be present (Fig. 21.9b). Acral lesions on the palms, soles, and nails, with

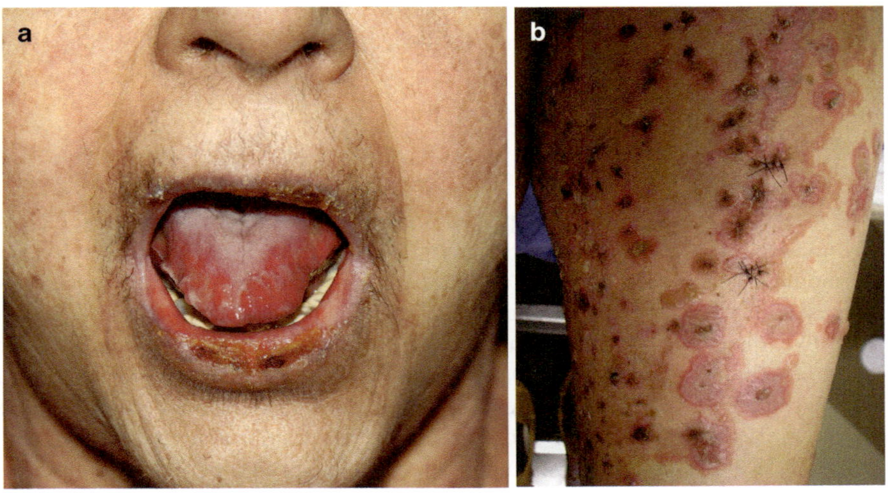

Fig. 21.9 Paraneoplastic pemphigus. Erosions on the tongue (**a**). Targetoid plaques and bullae similar to erythema multiforme on the thighs (**b**)

paronychia, are observed. Some patients may develop only mucous lesions; most develop mucous and skin lesions, and rarely, only skin lesions are found [100–102]. Children and adolescents may be affected by PNP, with similar clinical features from adult PNP. However, lichenoid lesions are more frequent in children, with few blisters, contrasting with the common association of blistering and lichenoid lesions in adults.[86] Lung involvement has been reported with variable frequencies, from 17% to 93% of patients. Bronchiolitis obliterans is the most frequent cause of respiratory symptoms, with dry cough and dyspnea [100].

Histology

Histopathology is characterized by erythema multiforme and pemphigus vulgaris features. There is lichenoid infiltrate, with vacuolar degeneration of the basal cell layer, apoptotic keratinocytes, band-like infiltrate of lymphocytes in the superficial dermis, and melanophages; suprabasilar acantholysis with cleft formation is present [16, 103]. Direct immunofluorescence shows IgG and C3 in epidermal intercellular spaces, along the basement membrane zone, or both. Indirect immunofluorescence using monkey esophagus or rat bladder epithelium shows the same pattern observed in direct immunofluorescence but may be negative in 20–25% of cases [100]. Immunoblotting, immunoprecipitation, and ELISA are used to identify the target antigens. Envoplakin (lower band of 210 kDa), periplakin (190 kDa), desmoplakin 1 (250 kDa), desmoplakin 2 (upper band of 210 kDa), bullous pemphigoid antigen 1 (230 kDa), α2-macroglobulin-like-1 molecule (170 kDa), desmoglein 1 (160 kDa), and desmoglein 3 (130 kDa) are the recognized antigens [104].

Associated Neoplasms

The most common associated neoplasms are lymphoproliferative disorders, including non-Hodgkin's lymphoma, chronic lymphocytic leukemia, Castleman's disease, thymoma, and follicular dendritic cell sarcoma. Associations with carcinomas, sarcomas, melanoma, and other hematologic disorders (Hodgkin's disease, myeloproliferative disorders, Waldenström disease, dysglobulinemia) may be found. In children and adolescents, Castleman's disease is the most frequent associated neoplasm [96]. One-third of the cases of PNP show mucocutaneous manifestations before the diagnosis of cancer; two-thirds show PNP lesions after diagnosis of cancer [101]. Rarely, cases with no tumor detected have been reported, and close follow-up is recommended [16].

Pathogenesis

It is suggested that a cytotoxic lichenoid eruption promotes exposure of self-antigens, leading to the development of humoral autoimmunity with the production of autoantibodies. Thus, lesions would be caused by the association between lichenoid reaction/interface dermatitis and anti-plakin family members' antibodies [99, 104]. Antibodies against plakin family antigens are produced by Castleman's tumor cells. This was not observed in thymoma and follicular dendritic cell sarcoma cells, suggesting different autoimmune mechanisms. Epitope spreading is another proposed explanation for the wide distribution of epitopes in plakin family members in PNP [104].

Treatment

Treatment of neoplastic disease is essential to the improvement of PNP. High-dose systemic corticosteroids (1–1.5 mg/kg/day) and immunosuppressive drugs (azathioprine, rituximab) are used. Topical corticosteroids may be associated. Spontaneous remission has been described [98].

Paraneoplastic Vasculitis

Vasculitis is a specific pattern of inflammation of the blood vessel wall, and it may be caused by drugs, systemic infections, and connective tissue diseases. In 3.8–8% of the cases, vasculitis is associated with internal malignancies. The association of malignancy and cutaneous vasculitis was made by Longley et al. in 1986, who suggested that malignant neoplasms might produce antigens and consequently cause paraneoplastic vasculitis [105].

Clinical Aspects

As cutaneous involvement occurs almost exclusively with vasculitis of small and medium vessels, the major clinical feature is palpable purpura on the legs. Urticarial vasculitis and erythema elevatum diutinum are less commonly observed. Fever, arthralgia, malaise, hematuria, abdominal pain, oral ulcers, pericarditis, and polyneuropathy due to vasculitis in other organs are reported [16, 105]. Cytopenias and immature peripheral blood cells are present in hematologic malignancies associated with cutaneous vasculitis. Antinuclear antibodies (ANA), rheumatoid factor, and cryoglobulins may be present at low titles [105, 106].

Comparing paraneoplastic vasculitis and other cutaneous vasculitides, older age, longer duration of skin lesions, and constitutional symptoms were more frequent in patients with underlying malignancy. In patients with unexplained vasculitis, especially with advancing age, investigation for the presence of neoplasm is mandatory. Death occurs due to neoplasm complications rather than vasculitis [105, 106].

Histopathology

Histopathology shows small-vessel neutrophilic vasculitis, leukocytoclasia, erythrocyte extravasation, and fibrinoid necrosis into the vessel walls. Most patients show histologic features consistent with small-vessel leukocytoclastic vasculitis, and rarely medium-sized vessels are involved [16, 106].

Associated Neoplasms

Hematologic disorders are the most common associated neoplasms: myelodysplastic syndrome, plasma cell myeloma, B-cell lymphoma, chronic lymphoid leukemia, multiple myeloma, acute myelogenous leukemia, Hodgkin's lymphoma, and non-Hodgkin's lymphoma. Less commonly, solid tumors are associated: non-small-cell lung cancer, prostate, colon, renal, bladder, breast, gastric, head and neck, and endometrial cancer [16, 106]. Skin lesions are commonly the first clinical manifestation of malignancy, preceding 2–4 years the clinical manifestations of the tumor [105].

Pathogenesis

In leukocytoclastic vasculitis, circulating antigens bind to immunoglobulins, causing the formation of immune complexes, which deposit within vascular walls. In paraneoplastic vasculitis, the antigens are derived from tumor or tumor microenvironment cells. The immune complexes fix complement, activate neutrophils, and interact with lymphocytes provoking the release of cytokines, causing vascular tissue damage. Moreover, the immune complexes interact with the endothelium through their Fc receptor, which induces the release of tissue plasminogen activator (t-PA), which causes the activation of the fibrinolytic system, increasing vasodilation and vascular permeability. Fibrinolysis is increased in the early phases of the disease and reduced in the late phases. The reduction of endothelial t-PA release and the increased levels of plasminogen activator inhibitors (PAI-1 and PAI-2) causes the reduction of fibrinolytic activity, leading to intravascular deposition of fibrin, with consequent microvascular thrombosis and necrosis, increasing tissue damage.

Other proposed mechanisms for the pathogenesis of paraneoplastic vasculitis are the production of immunoglobulins directed to the abnormal tumor cells and the normal endothelium; release of cytokines, causing endothelial injury; and the induction of a delayed hypersensitivity reaction to deposition of cancer proteins on vessel walls. Concomitant precipitating events (drugs, infections) may also cause an immune complex-mediated disorder observed even at the beginning of the neoplastic disease. All pathogenetic mechanisms lead to vascular permeability and vasodilation, with erythema and edema, endothelial cell dysfunction, neutrophilic infiltrate, platelet aggregation, and fibrin deposition, characteristics of cutaneous vasculitis [105].

Treatment

Successful treatment of the underlying malignancy leads to the resolution of skin lesions in the majority of patients. Systemic treatments available are corticosteroids, nonsteroidal anti-inflammatory drugs, colchicine, dapsone, stanazolol (fibrinolytic agent), immunosuppressive drugs such as cyclophosphamide, methotrexate, azathioprine, and cyclosporine A; intravenous immunoglobulin; and recombinant tissue plasminogen activator (rt-PA) [105].

Paraneoplastic Pruritus/Prurigo

Patients with chronic pruritus without concomitant skin changes have a higher incidence of renal, liver, and thyroid disease, diabetes, depression, and anxiety. Chronic pruritus may also be associated with hematological malignancies and cholangiocarcinoma [107].

Clinical Aspects

Patients with paraneoplastic pruritus, by definition, have varying degrees of pruritus but with no direct action of neoplastic cells in the skin by invasion or compression. Thus, most patients exhibit only excoriations and, less frequently, ichthyosiform or eczematous lesions. Severe paraneoplastic pruritus significantly decreases patient's quality of life [108].

Prurigo nodularis is characterized by a hyperkeratotic nodule, with a predilection for extensor surfaces of the limbs. Crusting and excoriations, with postinflammatory hyperpigmented and hypopigmented macules may be present. Prurigo nodularis may be considered a pathological reaction secondary to pruritus and scratching and may be present in patients with paraneoplastic pruritus [109].

If lymph node enlargement, hepatosplenomegaly, and B symptoms (fever, night sweats, weight loss) are present, search for hematological malignancies is mandatory. If jaundice, weight loss, and abdominal pain are detected, cholangiocarcinoma must be investigated [107].

Associated Neoplasms

Hematological malignancies and cholangiocarcinomas are the associated neoplasms. Thirty percent of patients with Hodgkin's lymphoma have chronic pruritus [107].

Pathogenesis

Malignant cells in hematological malignancies may release histamine, leukopeptidases, bradykinin, and IL-31, leading to pruritus. In cholangiocarcinoma, pruritus occurs due to hyperbilirubinemia [107].

Treatment

First-line agents include oral antihistamines, oral antidepressants such as doxepin, and corticosteroids. Second-line agents include UV light exposure (UVB or PUVA) and capsaicin (induces itch and burning sensation). Third-line includes cyclosporine, thalidomide, and naltrexone [109]. Off-label use of aprepitant, a neurokinin 1 receptor antagonist, has been described to reduce pruritus in a patient with Hodgkin's lymphoma [108].

Pyoderma Gangrenosum

Pyoderma gangrenosum (PG) is a neutrophilic dermatosis commonly associated with systemic disorders such as rheumatoid arthritis and inflammatory bowel disease. PG may be part of autoinflammatory syndromes, and sometimes it may be associated with internal malignancies [110].

Clinical Aspects

There are six clinical variants of PG: ulcerative, bullous, pustular, vegetative, peristomal, and postoperative [111].

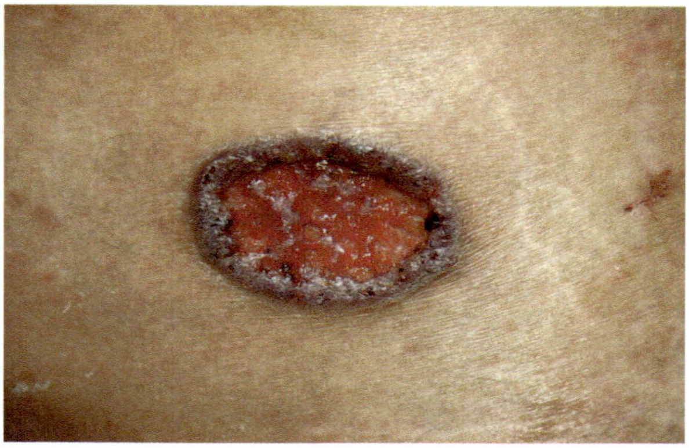

Fig. 21.10 Pyoderma gangrenosum. Ulcer with undermined borders

The ulcerative type is the most common. It starts with pustules or nodules that rapidly evolve to ulcers with violaceous and undermined borders that heal with cribriform scars (Fig. 21.10). It affects most commonly the lower extremities and the trunk [110, 111]. Pathergy phenomenon may be present [16].

The bullous type shows a painful bulla that progresses to an ulcer and affects the face and upper extremities. This type is the most frequently associated with myeloproliferative disorders [111].

Histology

Histopathology shows dermal edema, suppurative inflammation, and abscess formation, and no evidence of infection or vasculitis is observed. At the periphery of the lesion, a perivascular or periadnexal lymphocytic infiltrate may be present [111].

Associated Neoplasms

PG is diagnosed before malignancy in 78.9% of the cases. Acute myeloid leukemia, myelodysplastic syndromes, multiple myeloma, polycythemia vera, and monoclonal gammopathy are the most frequent associated diseases [111]. Less frequently, PG may be associated with solid organ tumors: breast, rectal, gastric, renal, lung, ileum, hypopharyngeal, and colon cancers [110].

Pathogenesis

Tumor cells may release cytokines, especially granulocyte colony-stimulating factors (G-CSF) that increase neutrophil levels in the blood, which may infiltrate the dermis [110].

Treatment

If a malignancy is detected, treatment of the tumor is essential to the healing of PG lesions. As palliative measures, in an attempt to control inflammation and reduce pain in PG patients, topical or systemic steroids, dapsone, colchicine, thalidomide, cyclosporine, methotrexate, azathioprine, mycophenolate mofetil, anti-TNF-α, anti-IL-12/23, anti-IL-23, anti-IL-17, anti-IL-1, and anti-IL-6 inhibitors have been used [110, 111].

Pityriasis Rotunda

Pityriasis rotunda is a rare skin condition that has been described in East Asia, Africa, and the Middle East [112]. It was described by Toyama et al. in 1906. There are two types of pityriasis rotunda. Type I is observed in Asian and black patients, associated with underlying malignancy (gastric or hepatocellular carcinoma). Type II is familial and has not been associated with malignancies [112, 113].

Clinical Aspects

Pityriasis rotunda is characterized by scaly ovoid patches, sharply defined, with pink or light brown coloration (Fig. 21.11). Lesions affect the buttocks, thighs, abdomen, trunk, and extremities [112].

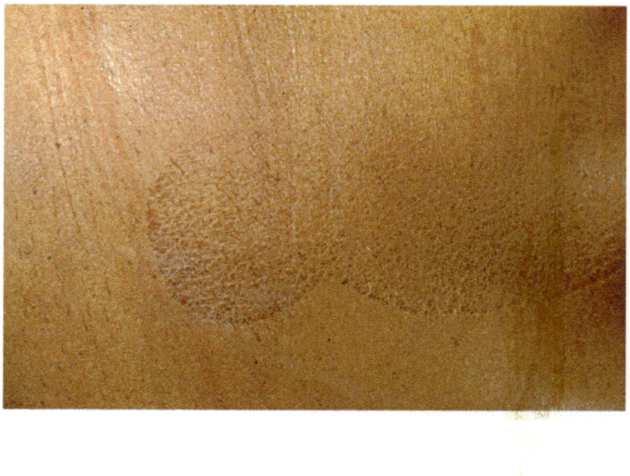

Fig. 21.11 Pityriasis rotunda. Ovoid scaly patches

Histopathology

Histopathology includes compact orthokeratosis, hypogranulosis, lack of spongiosis, mimicking ichthyosis vulgaris [16].

Associated Neoplasms

Associated neoplasms include gastric or hepatocellular carcinoma [16].

Pathogenesis

The pathogenesis is unclear.

Treatment

Skin lesions have a chronic course, with periods of remission and exacerbation. Improvements may be observed with emollients and keratolytic agents, besides treatment of the underlying malignancy [112].

Sweet's Syndrome

Sweet's syndrome was described by Robert Douglas Sweet in 1964, and it was defined as an acute febrile neutrophilic dermatosis [114]. There are three types of Sweet's syndrome: classical, malignancy associated, and drug induced [115]. Here, we will focus on the malignancy-associated Sweet's syndrome.

Clinical Aspects

Skin lesions are characterized by the sudden appearance of painful erythematous and edematous papules and plaques affecting the face, neck, and upper extremities (Fig. 21.12). Vesicles and ulceration be present. Fever is a common feature and is frequently accompanied by leukocytosis and neutrophilia. Pyoderma gangrenosum, swelling of the tongue, and periorbital cellulitis are associated with cutaneous findings. Anemia is present in 82–83% of malignancy-associated Sweet's syndrome and is rare in the classical type [116].

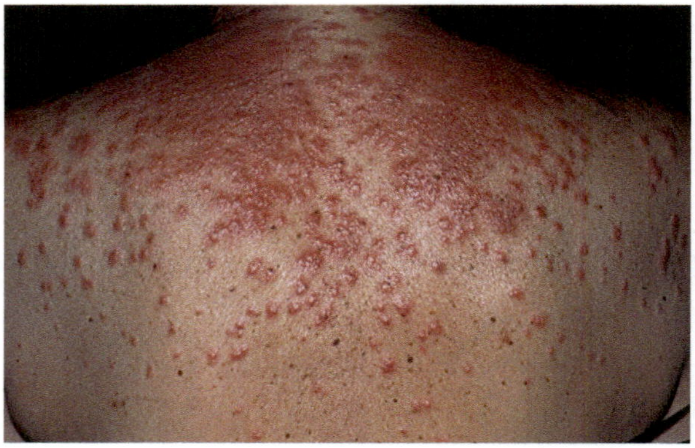

Fig. 21.12 Sweet's syndrome. Multiple erythematous and edematous papules and plaques on the upper back

Histology

The classical histopathological picture shows dense neutrophilic infiltrate in the dermis, with papillary dermal edema. Neutrophils infiltrating the epidermis (subcorneal pustules or neutrophilic spongiotic vesicles) and leukocytoclasis may be present, but leukocytoclastic vasculitis is typically absent. Subcutaneous neutrophilic inflammation is not common, but it suggests the presence of an underlying malignancy [16, 116].

Associated Neoplasms

The most common underlying neoplasms are acute myeloid or myelomonocytic leukemia, but other hematologic diseases have been implicated: myeloproliferative neoplasms, diffuse large B-cell lymphoma, Hodgkin's lymphoma, myelodysplastic syndrome, myelofibrosis, and polycythemia vera. Eighty-five percent of associated neoplasms are hematological disorders. Solid malignancies correspond to 15%, commonly carcinomas of the breast, gastrointestinal or genitourinary tracts, lung, prostate, and uterine cervix [116]. Sweet's syndrome has a good correlation with the course of malignancy, as skin eruption indicates recurrence or onset of a new malignancy. It is important to review all medications once many drugs commonly used for oncologic treatments are associated with Sweet's syndrome (granulocyte-colony-stimulating factor, antineoplastic agents, immunomodulating drugs, differentiation-inducing agents) [116].

Pathogenesis

Pathogenesis is unknown, but the hypothesis for Sweet's syndrome associated with malignancies is the overproduction of cytokines (IL 1, IL-3, IL-6, IL-8, GCSF, GM-CSF) or a hypersensitivity reaction against tumor antigens [116].

Treatment

Treatment of the underlying malignancy can result in complete remission of skin lesions. Systemic corticosteroids, 1 mg/kg/day, is the gold standard treatment. If there are few lesions, topical or intralesional corticosteroids may be used. Potassium iodine and colchicine are other effective agents. Dapsone and cyclosporine are second-line agents and may be associated with systemic corticosteroids in refractory cases. Indomethacin, clofazimine, chlorambucil, cyclophosphamide, antimetabolites, immunoglobulins, interferon-α, infliximab, and thalidomide are used if other agents did not reach a good response [116].

Trousseau's Syndrome

First described by Armand Trousseau in 1865, superficial migratory thrombophlebitis or Trousseau's syndrome is a paraneoplastic syndrome characterized by recurrent, migrant thrombophlebitis. After 2 years of the first description, Dr. Trousseau diagnosed the syndrome on himself due to gastric cancer [105].

Clinical Aspects

Recurrent erythematous nodules or cords over the course of a superficial vein, with migratory and tender aspects, are the typical features of migratory thrombophlebitis. Less frequently, disseminated intravascular coagulation, pulmonary embolism, thrombotic endocarditis, and diffuse bleeding are present [105].

Histology

Thrombosis at the dermal-subcutaneous interface vein, with neutrophilic inflammatory infiltrate, followed by lymphocytes and granulomatous elements [16].

Associated Neoplasms

Most associated neoplasms are pancreatic, lung, stomach, prostate, or hematogenic malignancies [16, 105].

Pathogenesis

The hypercoagulability and thromboembolic states in patients with tumors may be caused by several pathogenetic mechanisms: inflammatory cytokines produced by neoplastic cells that activate the endothelium and induce the expression of adhesive molecules such as V-CAM and E-selectin, high concentrations of tissue factor (a primary cellular initiator of fluid-phase blood coagulation), and activation of factor X of coagulation by products from the malignant cells are some proposed hypotheses [105].

Treatment

Treatment of the underlying malignancy is imperative. Anticoagulant therapy must be used for embolic symptoms. If tissue factor (TF) is increased, anti-TF agents, including recombinant tissue factor pathway inhibitors, are being tested [105].

Conclusions

Studies of paraneoplastic dermatoses are essential to disseminate knowledge of these disorders for the population of dermatologists, clinical oncologists, hematologists, and general practitioners to perform the initial suspicion and the proper screening tests.

More studies are needed to better understand its pathogenesis and treatment, especially in cases where the cancer is at an advanced stage, when remission of paraneoplastic skin disease is very difficult since the treatment of malignant disease becomes palliative.

References

1. Yuste-Chaves M, Unamuno-Pérez P. Cutaneous alerts in systemic malignancy: part I. Actas Dermosifiliogr. 2013;104(4):285–98.
2. Silva JA, Mesquita KC, Igreja AC, Lucas IC, Freitas AF, Oliveira SM, et al. Paraneoplastic cutaneous manifestations: concepts and updates. An Bras Dermatol. 2013;88(1):9–22.
3. Ramos ESM, Carvalho JC, Carneiro SC. Cutaneous paraneoplasia. Clin Dermatol. 2011;29(5):541–7.
4. Miyashiro D, Sanches JA. Paraneoplastic skin disorders: a review. G Ital Dermatol Venereol. 2016;151(1):55–76.
5. Gougerot H, Grupper C. Dermatose érythémato-squameuse avec hyperkératose palmoplantaire, porectasies digitales et cancer de la langue latent. Paris Med. 1922;24:234–7.

6. Bazex A, Salvador R, Dupré A, Christol B. Syndrome paranéoplasique á type d'hyperkératose des extrémités. Guérison aprés le traitement de l'épithélioma laryngé. Bull Soc Fr Dermatol Syphiligr. 1965;72:182–5.
7. Valdivielso M, Longo I, Suarez R, Huerta M, Lazaro P. Acrokeratosis paraneoplastica: Bazex syndrome. J Eur Acad Dermatol Venereol. 2005;19(3):340–4.
8. Graves MS, Hardin ME, Davis LS. A case of Bazex syndrome with genital involvement. JAMA Dermatol. 2014;150(12):1368–70.
9. Humphrey SR, Hussain AS, Chandran R, Wilson B, George B. Acute onset of acrokeratosis paraneoplastica (Bazex syndrome). JAMA Dermatol. 2015;151(6):677–8.
10. Roy B, Lipner SR. A review of nail changes in acrokeratosis paraneoplastica (Bazex syndrome). Skin Appendage Disord. 2021;7(3):163–72.
11. Bazex A, Griffiths A. Acrokeratosis paraneoplastica—a new cutaneous marker of malignancy. Br J Dermatol. 1980;103(3):301–6.
12. Rio Ramirez MT, Casado Lopez ME, Peiron Puyal MJ, Penas Herrero JM. Pulmonary adenocarcinoma and Bazex syndrome (paraneoplastic acrokeratosis). Arch Bronconeumol. 2007;43(1):46–8.
13. Bolognia JL. Bazex syndrome: acrokeratosis paraneoplastica. Semin Dermatol. 1995;14(2):84–9.
14. Eckstein J, Healy E, Jain A, Hawkins D, Ho QA, Agrawal A, et al. A series of typical and atypical cases of Bazex syndrome: identifying the red herring to avoid delaying cancer treatment. Clin Case Rep. 2020;8(11):2259–64.
15. Strobel ES, Bouveret C, Kohl PK. Acrokeratosis paraneoplastica of Bazex as an indicator for underlying squamous cell carcinoma of the lung. J Cancer Res Clin Oncol. 2006;132(6):376–8.
16. Wick MR, Patterson JW. Cutaneous paraneoplastic syndromes. Semin Diagn Pathol. 2019;36(4):211–28.
17. Fasanmade A, Farrell K, Perkins CS. Bazex syndrome (acrokeratosis paraneoplastica): persistence of cutaneous lesions after successful treatment of an associated oropharyngeal neoplasm. Br J Oral Maxillofac Surg. 2009;47(2):138–9.
18. Milagres SP, Sanches JA Jr, Milagres ACP, Valente NYS. Histopathological and immunohistochemical assessment of acquired ichthyosis in patients with human T-cell lymphotropic virus type I-associated myelopathy. Br J Dermatol. 2003;149(4):776–81.
19. Patel N, Spencer LA, English JC III, Zirwas MJ. Acquired ichthyosis. J Am Acad Dermatol. 2006;55(4):647–56.
20. Patsatsi A, Kyriakou A, Karavasilis V, Tsatsou F, Lazaridis G, Kalabalikis D, et al. Acquired ichthyosis triggered by an osseous hemangiopericytoma: a case report and review of the literature. Case Rep Dermatol. 2014;6(1):10–5.
21. Miyashiro D, Sanches JA. Cutaneous manifestations of adult T-cell leukemia/lymphoma. Semin Diagn Pathol. 2020;37(2):81–91.
22. Di Rollo D, Abeni D, Tracanna M, Capo A, Amerio P. Cancer risk in dermatomyositis: a systematic review of the literature. G Ital Dermatol Venereol. 2014;149(5):525–37.
23. Didona D, Fania L, Didona B, Eming R, Hertl M, Di Zenzo G. Paraneoplastic dermatoses: a brief general review and an extensive analysis of paraneoplastic pemphigus and paraneoplastic dermatomyositis. Int J Mol Sci. 2020;21(6):2178.
24. Stertz G. Polymyositis. Berl Klin Wochenschr. 1916;53:489.
25. Requena C, Alfaro A, Traves V, Nagore E, Llombart B, Serra C, et al. Paraneoplastic dermatomyositis: a study of 12 cases. Actas Dermosifiliogr. 2014;105(7):675–82.
26. Miyashiro D, Arnone M, Ferreira PS, Romiti R, Sanches JA. Extensive cutaneous involvement by dermatomyositis: report of six cases and review of the literature. Autoimmun Rev. 2020;19(12):102680.
27. Kumar S, Mahajan BB, Kaur S, Singh A. Paraneoplastic dermatomyositis with carcinoma cervix: a rare clinical association. Case Rep Dermatol Med. 2014;2014:836246.
28. Gerami P, Schope JM, McDonald L, Walling HW, Sontheimer RD. A systematic review of adult-onset clinically amyopathic dermatomyositis (dermatomyositis sine myositis): a

missing link within the spectrum of the idiopathic inflammatory myopathies. J Am Acad Dermatol. 2006;54(4):597–613.
29. Wang J, Guo G, Chen G, Wu B, Lu L, Bao L. Meta-analysis of the association of dermatomyositis and polymyositis with cancer. Br J Dermatol. 2013;169(4):838–47.
30. Chen YJ, Wu CY, Shen JL. Predicting factors of malignancy in dermatomyositis and polymyositis: a case-control study. Br J Dermatol. 2001;144(4):825–31.
31. Trallero-Araguas E, Rodrigo-Pendas JA, Selva-O'Callaghan A, Martinez-Gomez X, Bosch X, Labrador-Horrillo M, et al. Usefulness of anti-p155 autoantibody for diagnosing cancer-associated dermatomyositis: a systematic review and meta-analysis. Arthritis Rheum. 2012;64(2):523–32.
32. Fiorentino D, Chung L, Zwerner J, Rosen A, Casciola-Rosen L. The mucocutaneous and systemic phenotype of dermatomyositis patients with antibodies to MDA5 (CADM-140): a retrospective study. J Am Acad Dermatol. 2011;65(1):25–34.
33. Bursac DS, Sazdanic-Velikic DS, Tepavac AP, Secen NM. Paraneoplastic dermatomyositis associated with adenocarcinoma of the lung. J Cancer Res Ther. 2014;10(3):730–2.
34. Ungprasert P, Leeaphorn N, Hosiriluck N, Chaiwatcharayut W, Ammannagari N, Raddatz DA. Clinical features of inflammatory myopathies and their association with malignancy: a systematic review in Asian population. ISRN Rheumatol. 2013;2013:509354.
35. Hsu JL, Liao MF, Chu CC, Kuo HC, Lyu RK, Chang HS, et al. Reappraisal of the incidence, various types and risk factors of malignancies in patients with dermatomyositis and polymyositis in Taiwan. Sci Rep. 2021;11(1):4545.
36. Stone OJ. Dermatomyositis/polymyositis associated with internal malignancy: a consequence of how neoplasms alter generalized extracellular matrix in the host. Med Hypotheses. 1993;41(1):48–51.
37. Gammel JA. Erythema gyratum repens; skin manifestations in patient with carcinoma of breast. AMA Arch Derm Syphilol. 1952;66(4):494–505.
38. Rojo Sanchez S, Suarez Fernandez R, de Eusebio Murillo E, Lopez Bran E, Sanchez de Paz F, Robledo Aguilar A. Erythema gyratum repens: another case of a rare disorder but no new insight into pathogenesis. Dermatology. 1996;193(4):336–7.
39. De La Torre-Lugo EM, Sanchez JL. Erythema gyratum repens. J Am Acad Dermatol. 2011;64(5):e89–90.
40. Bakos N, Krasznai G, Begany AA. Erythema gyratum repens an immunological paraneoplastic dermatosis. Pathol Oncol Res. 1997;3(1):59–61.
41. Votquenne N, Richert B. Erythema gyratum repens. JAMA Dermatol. 2020;156(8):912.
42. Rongioletti F, Fausti V, Parodi A. Erythema gyratum repens is not an obligate paraneoplastic disease: a systematic review of the literature and personal experience. J Eur Acad Dermatol Venereol. 2014;28(1):112–5.
43. Müller CSL, Lorenz MT, Tilgen W, Rass K. Primary manifestation of erythema gyratum repens as a transient erythroderma in a patient with bronchial carcinoma. Int J Dermatol. 2010;49(6):676–8.
44. Eubanks LE, McBurney E, Reed R. Erythema gyratum repens. Am J Med Sci. 2001;321(5):302–5.
45. Bryan ME, Lienhart K, Smoller BR, Johnson SM. Erythema gyratum repens in a case of resolving psoriasis. J Drugs Dermatol. 2003;2(3):315–7.
46. Miyashiro D, Sanches JA. Erythroderma: a prospective study of 309 patients followed for 12 years in a tertiary center. Sci Rep. 2020;10(1):9774.
47. Rothe MJ, Bernstein ML, Grant-Kels JM. Life-threatening erythroderma: diagnosing and treating the "red man". Clin Dermatol. 2005;23(2):206–17.
48. Wong CL, Houghton JB, Andrew S, Griffiths CEM. Papuloerythroderma of Ofuji associated with acute myeloid leukaemia. Clin Exp Dermatol. 2003;28(3):277–9.
49. Protopsaltis I, Drossou A, Katsantonis I, Roussos N, Manoludaki K, Arvanitis M, et al. Breast cancer presenting as paraneoplastic erythroderma: an extremely rare case. Case Rep Med. 2014;2014:351065.

50. Pal S, Haroon TS. Erythroderma: a clinico-etiologic study of 90 cases. Int J Dermatol. 1998;37(2):104–7.
51. Sehgal VN, Srivastava G, Sardana K. Erythroderma/exfoliative dermatitis: a synopsis. Int J Dermatol. 2004;43(1):39–47.
52. Akhyani M, Ghodsi ZS, Toosi S, Dabbaghian H. Erythroderma: a clinical study of 97 cases. BMC Dermatol. 2005;5:5.
53. Hanafusa T, Igawa K, Takagawa S, Yahara H, Harada J, Tani M, et al. Erythroderma as a paraneoplastic cutaneous disorder in systemic anaplastic large cell lymphoma. J Eur Acad Dermatol Venereol. 2012;26(6):710–3.
54. Li J, Zheng HY. Erythroderma: a clinical and prognostic study. Dermatology. 2012;225(2):154–62.
55. Stinco G, Errichetti E. Erythrodermic psoriasis - current and future role of biologicals. BioDrugs. 2015;29(2):91–101.
56. Turner M. Case of a woman whose face and body in two or three weeks became covered with a thick crop of short and white downy hair. Med Time Gaz. 1865;2:507.
57. Slee PH, van der Waal RI, Schagen van Leeuwen JH, Tupker RA, Timmer R, Seldenrijk CA, et al. Paraneoplastic hypertrichosis lanuginosa acquisita: uncommon or overlooked? Br J Dermatol. 2007;157(6):1087–92.
58. Wyatt JP, Anderson HF, Greer KE, Cordoro KM. Acquired hypertrichosis lanuginosa as a presenting sign of metastatic prostate cancer with rapid resolution after treatment. J Am Acad Dermatol. 2007;56(2 Suppl):S45–7.
59. Perez-Losada E, Pujol RM, Domingo P, Matias-Guiu X, Lenti J, Lopez-Pousa A, et al. Hypertrichosis lanuginosa acquisita preceding extraskeletal Ewing's sarcoma. Clin Exp Dermatol. 2001;26(2):182–3.
60. Torley D, Bellus GA, Munro CS. Genes, growth factors and acanthosis nigricans. Br J Dermatol. 2002;147(6):1096–101.
61. Spicknall KE, Zirwas MJ, English JC III. Clubbing: an update on diagnosis, differential diagnosis, pathophysiology, and clinical relevance. J Am Acad Dermatol. 2005;52(6):1020–8.
62. Yao Q, Altman RD, Brahn E. Periostitis and hypertrophic pulmonary osteoarthropathy: report of 2 cases and review of the literature. Semin Arthritis Rheum. 2009;38(6):458–66.
63. Heaphy MR Jr, Millns JL, Schroeter AL. The sign of Leser-Trelat in a case of adenocarcinoma of the lung. J Am Acad Dermatol. 2000;43(2 Pt 2):386–90.
64. Siedek V, Schuh T, Wollenberg A. Leser-Trelat sign in metastasized malignant melanoma. Eur Arch Otorhinolaryngol. 2009;266(2):297–9.
65. Ikari Y, Ohkura M, Morita M, Seki K, Kubota Y, Mizoguchi M. Leser-Trelat sign associated with Sezary syndrome. J Dermatol. 1995;22(1):62–7.
66. Moore RL, Devere TS. Epidermal manifestations of internal malignancy. Dermatol Clin. 2008;26(1):17–29, vii.
67. Ellis DL, Kafka SP, Chow JC, Nanney LB, Inman WH, McCadden ME, et al. Melanoma, growth factors, acanthosis nigricans, the sign of Leser-Trelat, and multiple acrochordons. A possible role for alpha-transforming growth factor in cutaneous paraneoplastic syndromes. N Engl J Med. 1987;317(25):1582–7.
68. Costa MC, Martinez NS, Belicha MG, Leal F. Acanthosis nigricans and "tripe palm" as paraneoplastic manifestations of metastatic tumor. An Bras Dermatol. 2012;87(3):498–500.
69. Zhang R, Jiang M, Lei W, Wang A. Malignant acanthosis nigricans with recurrent bladder cancer: a case report and review of literature. Onco Targets Ther. 2021;14:951–7.
70. Kuner N, Hartschuh W. First descriptions in the "international atlas of rare skin diseases" of 1886. Hautarzt. 2003;54(1):67–72.
71. Cohen PR, Grossman ME, Silvers DN, Kurzrock R. Tripe palms and cancer. Clin Dermatol. 1993;11(1):165–73.
72. Janniger EJ, Schwartz RA. Florid cutaneous papillomatosis. J Surg Oncol. 2010;102(6):709–12.
73. Mekhail TM, Markman M. Acanthosis nigricans with endometrial carcinoma: case report and review of the literature. Gynecol Oncol. 2002;84(2):332–4.

74. Kebria MM, Belinson J, Kim R, Mekhail TM. Malignant acanthosis nigricans, tripe palms and the sign of Leser-Tre'lat, a hint to the diagnosis of early stage ovarian cancer: a case report and review of the literature. Gynecol Oncol. 2006;101(2):353–5.
75. McGinness J, Greer K. Malignant acanthosis nigricans and tripe palms associated with pancreatic adenocarcinoma. Cutis. 2006;78(1):37–40.
76. Pentenero M, Carrozzo M, Pagano M, Gandolfo S. Oral acanthosis nigricans, tripe palms and sign of leser-trélat in a patient with gastric adenocarcinoma. Int J Dermatol. 2004;43(7):530–2.
77. Haase I, Hunzelmann N. Activation of epidermal growth factor receptor/ERK signaling correlates with suppressed differentiation in malignant acanthosis nigricans. J Invest Dermatol. 2002;118(5):891–3.
78. Popa M-L, Popa A, Tanase C, Gheorghisan-Galateanu A-A. Acanthosis nigricans: to be or not to be afraid (review). Oncol Lett. 2018;17:4133.
79. Lazzarini R, Simone K, Queiroz G, Courral I, Magliari ME, Feder CK, et al. Malignant acanthosis nigricans: report of a case. Dermatol Online J. 2014;20(4):22377.
80. Tan BH, Barry CI, Wick MR, White KP, Brown JG, Lee A, et al. Multicentric reticulohistiocytosis and urologic carcinomas: a possible paraneoplastic association. J Cutan Pathol. 2011;38(1):43–8.
81. Teo HY, Goh BK. Multicentric reticulohistiocytosis in association with nasopharyngeal carcinoma. Clin Exp Dermatol. 2009;34(7):e347–8.
82. Dell'Antonia M, Atzori L, Pilloni L, Ferreli C. Multicentric reticulohistiocytosis revealing breast cancer: report of a case with dermoscopic, radiological and therapeutic aspects. Australas J Dermatol. 2021;62:527.
83. Becker SW, Kahn D, Rothman S. Cutaneous manifestations of internal malignant tumors. Arch Dermatol Syphilol. 1942;45:1069–80.
84. McGavran MH, Unger RH, Recant L, Polk HC, Kilo C, Levin ME. A glucagon secreting alpha-cell carcinoma of the pancreas. N Engl J Med. 1966;274:1408–13.
85. Mallinson CN, Bloom SR, Warin AP, Salmon PR, Cox B. A glucagonoma syndrome. Lancet. 1974;2(7871):1–5.
86. Dal Coleto CC, de Mello AP, Piquero-Casals J, Lima FR, Vilela MA, Festa-Neto C, et al. Necrolytic migratory erythema associated with glucagonoma syndrome: a case report. Rev Hosp Clin Fac Med Sao Paulo. 2001;56(6):183–8.
87. Nightingale KJ, Davies MG, Kingsnorth AN. Glucagonoma syndrome: survival 24 years following diagnosis. Dig Surg. 1999;16(1):68–71.
88. Lobo I, Carvalho A, Amaral C, Machado S, Carvalho R. Glucagonoma syndrome and necrolytic migratory erythema. Int J Dermatol. 2010;49(1):24–9.
89. Kovacs RK, Korom I, Dobozy A, Farkas G, Ormos J, Kemeny L. Necrolytic migratory erythema. J Cutan Pathol. 2006;33(3):242–5.
90. Liu JW, Qian YT, Ma DL. Necrolytic migratory erythema. JAMA Dermatol. 2019;155(10):1180.
91. Schwartz RA. Glucagonoma and pseudoglucagonoma syndromes. Int J Dermatol. 1997;36(2):81–9.
92. van Beek AP, de Haas ER, van Vloten WA, Lips CJ, Roijers JF, Canninga-van Dijk MR. The glucagonoma syndrome and necrolytic migratory erythema: a clinical review. Eur J Endocrinol. 2004;151(5):531–7.
93. Peterson LL, Shaw JC, Acott KM, Mueggler PA, Parker F. Glucagonoma syndrome: in vitro evidence that glucagon increases epidermal arachidonic acid. J Am Acad Dermatol. 1984;11(3):468–73.
94. Tierney EP, Badger J. Etiology and pathogenesis of necrolytic migratory erythema: review of the literature. MedGenMed. 2004;6(3):4.
95. Alexander EK, Robinson M, Staniec M, Dluhy RG. Peripheral amino acid and fatty acid infusion for the treatment of necrolytic migratory erythema in the glucagonoma syndrome. Clin Endocrinol. 2002;57(6):827–31.

96. Anhalt GJ, Kim SC, Stanley JR, Korman NJ, Jabs DA, Kory M, et al. Paraneoplastic pemphigus. An autoimmune mucocutaneous disease associated with neoplasia. N Engl J Med. 1990;323(25):1729–35.
97. Nguyen VT, Ndoye A, Bassler KD, Shultz LD, Shields MC, Ruben BS, et al. Classification, clinical manifestations, and immunopathological mechanisms of the epithelial variant of paraneoplastic autoimmune multiorgan syndrome: a reappraisal of paraneoplastic pemphigus. Arch Dermatol. 2001;137(2):193–206.
98. Leger S, Picard D, Ingen-Housz-Oro S, Arnault JP, Aubin F, Carsuzaa F, et al. Prognostic factors of paraneoplastic pemphigus. Arch Dermatol. 2012;148(10):1165–72.
99. Ohyama M, Amagai M, Hashimoto T, Nousari HC, Anhalt GJ, Nishikawa T. Clinical phenotype and anti-desmoglein autoantibody profile in paraneoplastic pemphigus. J Am Acad Dermatol. 2001;44(4):593–8.
100. Choi Y, Nam KH, Lee JB, Lee JY, Ihm CW, Lee SE, et al. Retrospective analysis of 12 Korean patients with paraneoplastic pemphigus. J Dermatol. 2012;39(12):973–81.
101. Yuste-Chaves M, Unamuno Perez P. Cutaneous manifestations of systemic malignancies: Part 2. Actas Dermosifiliogr. 2013;104(7):543–53.
102. Dong Y, Wang M, Nong L, Wang L, Cen X, Liu W, et al. Clinical and laboratory characterization of 114 cases of Castleman disease patients from a single centre: paraneoplastic pemphigus is an unfavourable prognostic factor. Br J Haematol. 2015;169(6):834–42.
103. Mimouni D, Anhalt GJ, Lazarova Z, Aho S, Kazerounian S, Kouba DJ, et al. Paraneoplastic pemphigus in children and adolescents. Br J Dermatol. 2002;147(4):725–32.
104. Zhang B, Zheng R, Wang J, Bu D, Zhu X. Epitopes in the linker subdomain region of envoplakin recognized by autoantibodies in paraneoplastic pemphigus patients. J Invest Dermatol. 2006;126(4):832–40.
105. Buggiani G, Krysenka A, Grazzini M, Vasku V, Hercogova J, Lotti T. Paraneoplastic vasculitis and paraneoplastic vascular syndromes. Dermatol Ther. 2010;23(6):597–605.
106. Loricera J, Calvo-Rio V, Ortiz-Sanjuan F, Gonzalez-Lopez MA, Fernandez-Llaca H, Rueda-Gotor J, et al. The spectrum of paraneoplastic cutaneous vasculitis in a defined population: incidence and clinical features. Medicine (Baltimore). 2013;92(6):331–43.
107. Fett N, Haynes K, Propert KJ, Margolis DJ. Five-year malignancy incidence in patients with chronic pruritus: a population-based cohort study aimed at limiting unnecessary screening practices. J Am Acad Dermatol. 2014;70(4):651–8.
108. Villafranca JJ, Siles MG, Casanova M, Goitia BT, Dominguez AR. Paraneoplastic pruritus presenting with Hodgkin's lymphoma: a case report. J Med Case Rep. 2014;8:300.
109. Lee MR, Shumack S. Prurigo nodularis: a review. Australas J Dermatol. 2005;46(4):211–18; quiz 9–20.
110. Shah M, Sachdeva M, Gefri A, Jfri A. Paraneoplastic pyoderma gangrenosum in solid organ malignancy: a literature review. Int J Dermatol. 2020;59(2):154–8.
111. Maverakis E, Marzano AV, Le ST, Callen JP, Bruggen MC, Guenova E, et al. Pyoderma gangrenosum. Nat Rev Dis Primers. 2020;6(1):81.
112. Al-Refu K, Al-Tarawneh A, Odeibat H. Pityriasis rotunda. A clinical study in Jordan: experience of 10 years. Int J Dermatol. 2018;57(7):759–62.
113. Batra P, Cheung W, Meehan SA, Pomeranz M. Pityriasis rotunda. Dermatol Online J. 2009;15(8):14.
114. Sweet RD. An acute febrile neutrophilic dermatosis. Br J Dermatol. 1964;76:349–56.
115. Raza S, Kirkland RS, Patel AA, Shortridge JR, Freter C. Insight into Sweet's syndrome and associated-malignancy: a review of the current literature. Int J Oncol. 2013;42(5):1516–22.
116. Paydas S. Sweet's syndrome: a revisit for hematologists and oncologists. Crit Rev Oncol Hematol. 2013;86(1):85–95.

Chapter 22
Cutaneous Metastases

Camila Cristina Tormena, Jade Cury-Martins, Denis Miyashiro, and José Antonio Sanches

Key Points

- Cutaneous metastases are characterized by skin infiltration by neoplastic cells originating from a distant organ.
- Skin infiltration by cancer can occur by hematogenous or lymphatic embolization, direct contiguous tissue invasion, and direct iatrogenic implantation during surgical procedures.
- Melanoma and breast cancer are the most frequent tissue of origin of cutaneous metastases.
- Breast and lung cancers frequently metastasize to the chest wall, whereas cancers of the bowel, ovary, and bladder most often metastasize to the abdomen.
- Melanoma metastasis site depends upon the topography of the primary lesion.
- Cutaneous metastasis may be the first sign of internal malignancy, and prompt recognition and confirmation by histopathology and immunohistochemistry are essential to institute early treatment.

Overview

Metastasis is defined as a neoplastic lesion arising from another neoplasm with which it is no longer in continuity [1] or in proximity within the same tissue [2]. It's a complex process and remains an enigma in many cases. Cutaneous metastases

C. C. Tormena · J. Cury-Martins (✉) · D. Miyashiro · J. A. Sanches
Hospital das Clínicas, Faculdade de Medicina da Universidade de São Paulo, Instituto do Câncer do Estado de São Paulo, São Paulo, Brazil

C. M. Z. Abdalla et al. (eds.), *Oncodermatology*,
https://doi.org/10.1007/978-3-031-29277-4_22

(CMs) are characterized by infiltration of the dermis and/or subcutaneous tissue by proliferating cells from distant cancers. The cell spread can occur at any time of the neoplastic process, and the importance of prompt recognition is highlighted by the fact that it can be the first manifestation of a new internal tumor or recurrence of an already diagnosed malignancy [3]. According to Lookingbill [4], they may arise before the identification of a primary neoplasm or concomitantly in 25.1% of cases, but in general later in the course of the disease. The diagnosis of cutaneous metastases usually leads to a change in the staging of tumor disease, with therapeutic and prognostic implications.

The skin does not appear to be a preferred target organ for the development of metastases [5]. Usually, when the skin is affected, other organs have already been involved [6].

Early recognition of CM can facilitate prompt and accurate diagnosis resulting in early treatment and possibly a prolonged life expectancy; however, they are generally indicative of a poor prognosis. With the advance of immunohistochemical and molecular techniques, identification of the primary tumor from the metastasis has been greatly facilitated [7]. Also, some tumors have a predilection to metastasize to specific areas. Recognition of these patterns provides information that can guide the search for underlying tumor or the possible initial immunohistochemical panel to be used [8].

Incidence

Although primary skin cancers comprise most cancerous lesions of the skin, the true incidence of cutaneous metastases may vary according to the biological characteristics of cancers among populations, but the skin remains a relatively uncommon destination for internal tumor metastasis considering its massive surface area. It remains an often overlooked yet highly relevant contributor, particularly as total cancer incidence increases, and more cancer survivors require surveillance for relapse [9].

There are several studies of CM, most of which are not uniform in their data inclusion. Most are retrospective, often using the results of postmortem examination, and sometimes include lesions believed to be a cutaneous metastasis, but without histologic confirmation [7].

Some studies include metastasis from primary skin cancer (melanomas) and from hematological malignancies (lymphomas, and leukemias); others include only CM from solid tumors.

The incidence appears to be higher in some recent studies than with historical series, although this may be due to higher rates of biopsy and diagnosis rather than a true increase in the incidence. The prevalence varies between 0.7% and 10% of patients with internal tumors, depending on the series (Table 22.1) [4, 10, 12, 14, 16–18]. In 22% of all cases, CMs can lead to the diagnosis of an internal malignance [19].

Table 22.1 Summary of reported cutaneous metastases from primary visceral malignancies

Investigators	Total cutaneous metastases (*n*)	Total primary malignancies (*n*)	%
Gates [10]	64	2.298	2.3
Ulker Gu [11]	15	1287	1.16
McDonald et al. [12]	33	11.265	0.3
Abrams et al. [13]	44	1.000	4.4
Reingold [14]	36	2.300	1.6
Held and Johnson [15]	1.046	46.929	2.2
Brady et al. [16]	100	2.992	3.3
Spencer and Helm [17]	679	7.518	9.0
Lookingbill et al. [4]	367	7.316	5.0
Enticknap [18]	14	512	2.0
Total	2398	83.417	3.12

Table 22.2 Origin of the most frequent skin metastases according to gender

Men	Women
Lung	Breast
Colon	Colon
Melanoma	Melanoma
Carcinoma squamous cell	Ovary
Kidney	Lung
Stomach	

Although any type of cancer may cause CM, in some types, it occurs more frequently, as highlighted by gender, on Table 22.2 [20].

Cutaneous metastases from urologic tumors occur in 1% of patients with advanced disease. Urologic skin metastases are the most common from renal tumors, followed by those of the bladder and then prostate. Mueller et al. identified an incidence of cutaneous metastases from the kidney, bladder, prostate, and testes as 3.4%, 0.84%, 0.36% and 0.4%, respectively [21].

These lesions have the potential to invade nearly every segment of the skin. Skin metastases most frequently occur in the vicinity of the primary tumor. Regarding the area of occurrence, by sex, in women the most common site of CMs is the thorax, followed by the abdomen, the back, the upper limbs, the scalp, and the neck; in men, the thorax (Fig. 22.1) is also the area most commonly affected, followed by the abdomen, the back, the scalp, the neck, the face, the upper and lower limbs, and the pelvis [8].

Breast and lung cancers frequently metastasize to the chest wall, whereas cancers of the bowel, ovary, and bladder most often metastasize to the abdomen. Umbilical nodules are a frequently described (but infrequently seen) manifestation of metastatic intraabdominal carcinoma. This sign, the Sister Joseph nodule, is attributed to the nun who made the clinical observation while working in St. Mary's Hospital at the Mayo Clinic [22]. In contrast, the back, buttock, pelvis-perineum, and extremities are each involved in less than 10% of metastases [23, 24].

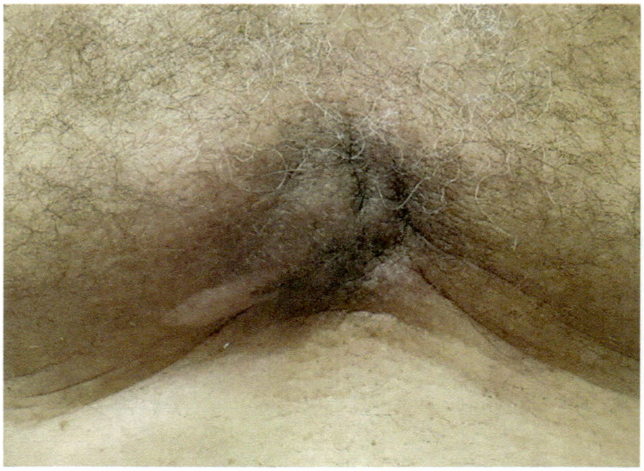

Fig. 22.1 Cutaneous metastases of neuroendocrine adenocarcinoma on the chest

Cutaneous metastases are very rare in children, probably because carcinoma uncommonly occurs in this age group. The most common primary tumors that produce CMs in this age group are rhabdomyosarcoma and neuroblastoma [25]. Leukemia can also be a cause of skin metastases in children [4].

Breast carcinoma is the second most common cancer in women and the most common tumor leading to the appearance of skin metastasis [26]. A review published in 2013 observed that women previously treated for breast carcinoma need constant evaluation and require a skin biopsy on the slightest suspicion of a lesion [27].

Prognosis

The median survival after skin metastasis of non-skin squamous cell carcinoma of the head and neck was 8.8 months; cutaneous squamous cell carcinoma, 6.5 months; carcinoma of esophagus, 4.7 months; colorectal cancer, 4.4 months; pancreatic cancer, 3.3 months; stomach cancer, 1.2 months; and liver and gall bladder carcinoma, >1 month. The authors found that 50% of patients with skin metastasis die within the first 6 months after the diagnosis [28].

Biological Aspects of Cutaneous Metastases

One of the most striking and disheartening qualities of cancer is the relentlessness of its spread throughout the organism [13]. Skin infiltration by cancer can occur by several different pathways: hematogenous, lymphatic embolization, direct contiguous tissue invasion, and direct iatrogenic implantation during surgical procedures [29].

Sánchez-García [30] described one of the most recently hypotheses of the metastases production, which predicts that protein expression that regulate the epithelial-mesenchymal transition promotes oncogenesis, concomitant with metastatic dissemination. In the alternative model, cell diffusion of the primary tumor can occur at any time during cancer development. They compared with the classical model where the development of cancer metastases corresponds to the final stage of the metastatic cascade. First, the primary tumor must be large enough to release enough neoplastic cells to the circulatory or lymphatic system. These cells, in turn, would need to have certain properties, such as cell suspension and an adequate index to survive. The development of metastatic clone is initially aided by the activation of specific oncogenes and the loss of tumor suppressor genes. To establish themselves, neoplastic cells found in the circulatory system must penetrate through the vessel walls. Once adhesion occurs, a thrombus forms around the neoplastic cells due to endothelial cell injury. This thrombus serves as protection for neoplastic cells. Metastasis is established and obtained initially nutrition through diffusion phenomena and subsequently forms its own vessels (angiogenesis). In this classic model described for the development of cancer, metastases correspond to the final stage of the metastatic cascade.

Clinical Presentation

The three typical patterns of presentation seen in cutaneous metastases are mechanical tumor stasis, site-specific metastasis, and nonselective spread.

In mechanical tumor stasis, the metastatic disease appears in close anatomic proximity to the initial tumor. This presentation commonly occurs when cells spread through the lymphatic route or through direct invasion [31]. Breast carcinoma and squamous cell carcinoma of the head and neck are examples of malignancies that often spread to the skin by direct invasion. Site-specific metastasis arises when neoplastic cells have a predilection for specific organs (Table 22.3). Finally,

Table 22.3 Differential diagnosis of causative internal malignancy by anatomic location of skin lesion

Location	Common primary malignancies
Head-neck	Breast, hematological malignancies, lung
Chest	Breast, lung
Abdomen	Breast, colorectum, gastric
Umbilicus	Ovary, gastric
Pelvis-perineum	Colorectum
Back and buttock	Breast, lung
Extremities	Heme-lymph, lung
Surgical scar	Breast, ovary, uterus

nonselective metastasis occurs when the neoplastic cells metastasize without a specific organ preference [32].

Clinically, nodular appearance is the most common form. They vary in size from "miliary lesions" to large tumors. Lookingbill [4] found that solitary cutaneous metastases were most frequently associated with lung carcinoma. In their patients with skin metastases from lung cancer, metastases were solitary in 53%. The next most common cause of solitary metastases was cancer from an unknown primary site; this occurred in 35% of those patients. Melanoma metastases may be pigmented and was noted in 36% of the cases [4].

The color of the lesion might provide useful information; metastases from renal cell carcinoma, for example, are frequently red or purple and may mimic hemangiomas.

A case series published in 2014 reviewed high-quality dermoscopic images of 20 outpatients with biopsy-proven cutaneous metastases and observed that visible vascular structures within a cutaneous nodule in patients with a known cancer diagnosis should raise suspicion for cutaneous metastasis. The high prevalence (88%) of vascular structures among cutaneous metastases may suggest a role for angiogenesis in their pathogenesis. Pigmentation in such lesions, in the absence of a history of melanoma, suggests a primary breast carcinoma. The study supports the use of dermoscopy in the evaluation of suspected skin metastases or in assessment of lesions of unknown origin in patients with cancer [33].

Metastases of breast cancer frequently are inflammatory, mimicking cellulitis. When the inflammation is acute and localized to the breast, it can be difficult to distinguish from a mastitis. Therefore, any persistent inflammation without response to conventional therapy must be carefully evaluated to rule out metastatic infiltration, especially in the absence of fever and leukocytosis [34]. From other sites, we can find inflammatory metastases with cancers of the pancreas, rectum, lung, ovary, and parotid glands [21]. Cancer patients with atypical or unusual inflammatory dermatoses should undergo skin biopsy to rule out metastases.

Paget's disease of the nipple and areola is the cutaneous manifestation of an underlying breast adenocarcinoma in 100% of cases. It is an epidermotropic cutaneous metastases by extension of an intraductal tumor through milk ducts to overlying skin [35].

A review published in 2004 identified infiltrated plaques and nodules as the most common presentation of cutaneous metastases from primary genitourinary malignancies. Most cases displayed clinical features that mimicked common skin disorders [10].

Other common unique morphologic presentations include sessile acrochordon-type lesions with metastatic colon cancer; kidney, liver, and neuroblastoma presenting as ulcers; flushing or a pellagra-like presentation with carcinoid tumors; and lastly larynx and breast cancer presenting as sclerodermoid plaques.

Other rare presentations include bullous, carcinoma erysipeloides, neoplastic alopecia, erythema annular-like, zosteriform, or target-like lesions.

Zosteriform pattern is a rarely seen subtype, and there have been less than a 100 cases reported on the literature [36]. This pattern might present as two different aspects: either with a morphology mimicking herpetic vesicles or with lesions on a zosteriform distribution. The latter may be associated with breast, colon, or squamous cell carcinomas. The zosteriform skin metastases usually develop near to and on the same side of the primary tumor. Nonetheless, some zosteriform skin metastases develop on the opposite side of the body or on an area distant from the primary carcinoma. The mechanism of zosteriform distribution remains unknown; however, proposed theories include lymphatic spread, koebnerization at the site of previous zoster infection, surgical implantation of tumor cells, or neural spread via the dorsal ganglia [37–39].

Another rare expression is cicatricial metastases, where the lesions have the aspect of a scar. When these occur in the scalp, they can be clinically confused with other causes of scarring alopecia. Carcinoma *en cuirasse* is another fibrotic metastatic process that affects the trunk and results in an appearance of encasement in armor. Both presentations are usually due to breast cancer [4].

Although in most cases the lesions are asymptomatic, patients can report pain, especially in certain locations, such as subungual metastases [40]. The differential diagnosis are infectious processes, especially acute paronychia or glomus tumors. There are reports of painless dactylitis as the manifestation of CM [40].

Histopathology and Immunohistochemical Markers

The histology of the metastatic tumors can be broadly classified as adenocarcinoma; squamous cell carcinoma; undifferentiated carcinoma, or in a miscellaneous category that includes tumors of the liver, endometrium, kidney, or bladder; and small cell carcinomas [41]. The diagnosis of metastatic adenocarcinoma or squamous cell carcinoma does not determine the site of the primary tumor; however, sometimes clues suggest a primary site. For example, signet ring cells were frequently seen in metastasis from adenocarcinomas of the stomach or gastrointestinal tract. However, signet ring cells have also been described in other tumors, including metastatic bladder carcinoma and melanoma [42]. The tumors in the miscellaneous histologic category did have certain features or patterns that were suggestive of the site of origin. For example, metastatic renal cell carcinomas frequently are composed of lobules of clear-staining cells containing glycogen in a highly vascular stroma. Metastatic ovarian carcinoma has a characteristic papillary pattern; however, a papillary pattern can also be seen in metastatic thyroid, stomach, and lung cancers [43, 44].

Ultrastructural studies can be useful in the identification of certain undifferentiated tumors. The presence of desmosomes in carcinomas, cytoplasmic lumens in adenocarcinomas, melanosomes in melanoma, and neurosecretory granules in neuroendocrine tumors can help resolve the diagnosis. However, they are lengthy and expensive techniques that are not available in most clinical centers and require a highly specialized staff and therefore are not used in clinical practice [45].

Summary of Findings Based on Primary Tumor Site

Breast Carcinoma

Cutaneous metastases from breast carcinoma can infrequently be the first sign of the disease. The most likely site for CMs in women is the chest wall. Less common sites include the scalp, neck, upper extremities (Fig. 22.2), abdomen, and back.

They may present as miliary-sized skin-colored solid papules and be either scattered or confluent on the side of the abdomen with typical zosteriform distribution consistent with the thoracic dermatomes. Histologically, CMs from the invasive ductal carcinoma are composed of malignant ductal epithelial cells arranged in syncytial sheets, cords, and glands or are diffusely infiltrative. Metastatic deposits from lobular carcinoma of the breast consist of monomorphic population of loosely cohesive malignant cells with regular nuclei, evenly distributed chromatin, and inconspicuous nucleoli. The tumor cells are positive for estrogen receptors, progesterone receptors, high-molecular-weight cytokeratin, and epithelial membrane antigens (Table 22.4) [46].

Lung Carcinoma

About 50% and 80% of non-small-cell and small-cell lung carcinomas, respectively, are metastatic at the time of diagnosis. The most common sites for CMs in men are the chest, abdomen, upper lip, and back.

Cutaneous metastasis from the small-cell carcinoma of the lung consists of mitotically active cells arranged in sheets, ribbons, clusters, and rosettes of small- to

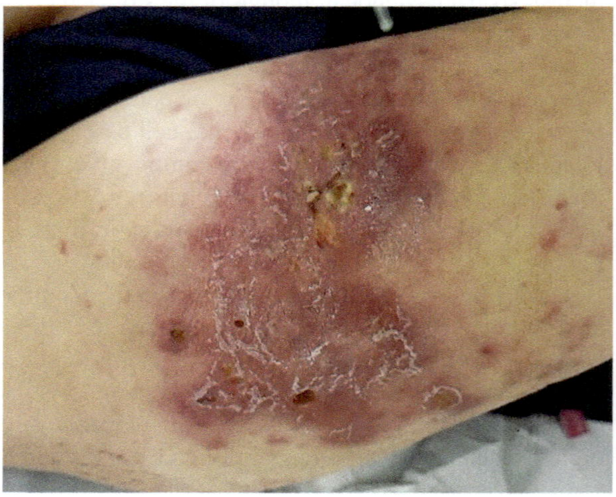

Fig. 22.2 Cutaneous metastasis from breast cancer on the right arm

Table 22.4 Immunohistochemical markers for cutaneous metastases

Origin	Histopathology	Immunohistochemical markers	
		Positive	Negative
Breast	Ductal Lobular	CK7, estrogen-R, progesterone-R, GCDFP-15, CEA, c-erbB-2, mammaglobin	CK20, CK5/6 (ductal) S100, E-cadherin, podoplanin, P63 (lobular)
	Telangiectatic	CD31	Podoplanin
	Mammary Paget disease	MUC1, CK7	MUC2, MUC5AC, CK20
Lung	Squamous cell carcinoma	CK5/6	CK7, CK20, TTF-1, CEA
	Adenocarcinoma	CK7, TTF-1, Ber-EP4, CEA, surfactant, apoprotein A	CK5/6, CK20
	Oat-cell carcinoma	TTF-1, CAM5.2, CK8/18, Ber-EP4, ENS	CK7, CK20, CD99
	Mesothelioma	CK5/6, calretinin, vimentin	CEA, TTF-1, S100, CD31
Colorectal	Adenocarcinoma	CK20, CEA, mucin, CDX2	CK7
Small intestine	SCC	CK20, EMA, AE1/AE3	CK7
	Adenocarcinoma	CEA, EMA	
Stomach	Adenocarcinoma	CK20, CEA, EMA, CDX2, HIK1083	CK7+/CK7−
Esophagus	SCC/ADC	CK5/6, Ber-EP4	CK7, CK20
Mouth	SCC	Ber-EP4	
Liver	HCC	Alpha-feto, polyclonal CEA, HepPar 1, arginase-1	All CKs, EMA, monoclonal CEA
Biliary system	Adenocarcinoma	CK7, CK20	CDX2
Pancreas	Adenocarcinoma	CA19.9, CK7, CK8, CK19	CK20
Kidney	RCC	AE1/AE3, MNF116, CD31, RCC-Ma, PAX8 vimentin, CD10, EMA, S100, adipophilin	Inhibin, melan-A, TTF-1, CK7, CK20
Bladder-urethra	Transitional carcinoma	CK7, CK19, CK20, CK14, thrombomodulin, uroplakin III, CD10	
Prostate	Adenocarcinoma	PSA, prostatic acid phosphatase, AMACR (p504s), ERG	CK7, CK20, thrombomodulin
Testis	Choriocarcinoma	Beta-HCG	
Ovary	Carcinoma	CA125, CK7, PAX8	CK20
Cervix/vagina	Carcinoma	CK7, EMA+/EMA−	CK20, CEA
Endometrium	Carcinoma	CK7, PAX8	CK20, P63, podoplanin

(continued)

Table 22.4 (continued)

Origin	Histopathology	Immunohistochemical markers	
		Positive	Negative
Thyroid	Papillary	Thyroglobulin, TTF-1, PAX8	
	Anaplastic	Thyroglobulin +/−	
	Medullary	Calcitonin	Thyroglobulin, PAX8
Carcinoid tumors	Enterochromaffin carcinoma	NSE, chromogranin, synaptophysin, ArgentaffinCDX2, TTF-1	CK5/6, CK7, CK20, p63
Neuroblastoma		NSE, chromogranin, synaptophysin	CD99, desmin, myogenin
Soft tissue sarcomas	Leiomyosarcoma	SMA, desmin	
	Rhabdomyosarcoma	MYOD1, vimentin, myogenin, CD45	Desmin, SMA
	Angiosarcoma	CD31, CD34, ERG transcription factor, podoplanin, CKs, EMA	
	Chondrosarcoma	CD99, vimentin, S100, podoplanin, YKL-40, SMA, desmin, CAM5.2	AE1/AE3, SMA, CD17
	Ewing sarcoma	Vimentin, NSE, CD99, LEU7/CD57, FL11	Podoplanin
	Osteosarcoma	EZRIN, SMA, c-*erb*B-2	
Salivary glands	Adenoid cystic carcinoma	CKs, CEA, S100, CD117/CKIT, SMA, vimentin	
	Mucoepidermoid	CK5/6, EMA, CEA	
Laryngeal and tracheal	Carcinoma	AE1/AE3, p53	
Nasopharynx	Carcinoma	RNA of EBV	
Glioblastoma		GFAP, EGFR+/EGFR−, vimentin YKL-40	Neurofilaments, HM45, melan-A, CKs, cocktail
Medulloblastoma		Synaptophysin NSE	Neurofilaments
Meningioma		Vimentin, EMA, S100, progesterone-R, CKs, CEA	
Adrenocortical	Carcinoma	NSE, inhibin, synaptophysin, A103, chromogranin, calretinin	Melan-A, CD10

Adapted from Alcaraz L. et al.
AMACR alpha-methylacyl-CoA racemase, *beta-HCG* beta-human chorionic gonadotropin, *Hep Par 1* hepatocyte paraffin 1, *CEA* carcinoembryonic antigen, *EMA* epithelial membrane antigen, *GCDFP* gross cystic disease fluid protein, *NSE* neuron-specific enolase, *PSA* prostate-specific antigen, *RCC-ma* renal cell carcinoma marker, *SMA* smooth muscle actin

medium-sized round/oval cells with nuclear molding. The neoplastic cells have scant cytoplasm, salt-and-pepper chromatin, and indistinct nucleoli. They lack reactivity for the lymphoid markers (CD3, CD20, CD45) and CD99/MIC2 (Table 22.4). Non-small-cell carcinoma of the lung consists of malignant cells arranged in solid, nesting (squamous cell carcinoma, positive for CK20) or glandular patterns (adenocarcinoma).

Gastrointestinal Carcinomas

Carcinomas of the esophagus, pancreas, stomach, biliary tract, intestine, and liver can metastasize to the skin of the abdomen and pelvis. The CM of gastric carcinoma may be in the form of cutaneous nodules, cellulitis, carcinoma *en cuirasse*, infiltrated skin plaques, carcinoma erysipeloides, nodules or a large cauliflower-like papillomatous mass (Fig. 22.3). The carcinoma cells are seen in the middle and lower dermis, forming glands, clusters, or strands of neoplastic cells in an abundance of fibrous stroma. Some gastric and pancreaticobiliary carcinomas are positive for both CK20 and CK7.

Cutaneous metastasis from colon cancer commonly appears on the skin of the abdomen and the pelvis, but they occasionally involve the facial skin or the sites of the old scars. They may also appear as single or multiple nodules at the umbilicus "Sister Mary Joseph's nodules." Interestingly, CMs from colorectal carcinomas carry a better prognosis in comparison to those of other carcinomas. The positive stains include CK20, mucin, carcinoembryonic antigen, and CDX2. The tumor cells lack reactivity for CK7 (Table 22.4).

Cutaneous metastases from hepatocellular carcinomas present usually as multiple reddish-blue, firm, painless, and nonulcerative papules or nodules over the fingers, face, palms, toes, soles, and backs. Metastases may rarely appear as cauliflower, angiomatous, or granuloma telangiectatic-like lesions.

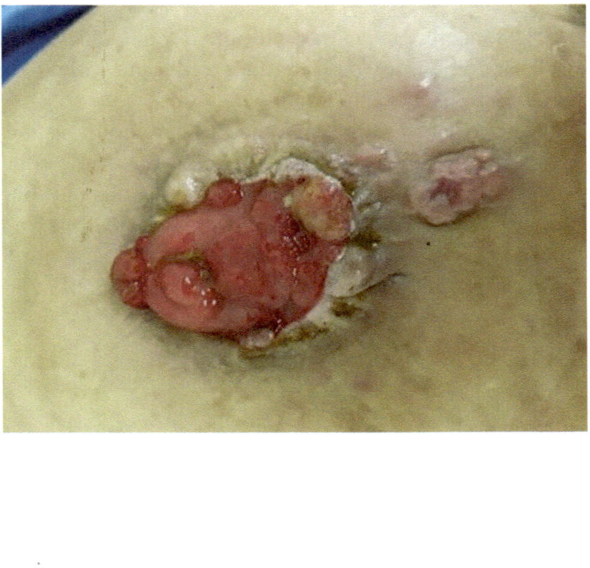

Fig. 22.3 Extensive cutaneous metastasis from sigmoid adenocarcinoma

Urothelial, Prostatic, and Renal Cell Carcinomas

Their CMs develop either by iatrogenic implantation of the tumor cells or by vascular spread. The skin lesions usually involve the scrotum, the pubic/inguinal regions, and the lower limbs. The patients usually present with solitary or multiple skin nodules, red to violaceous papules, indurated plaques, contact dermatitis, and cellulitis-like pictures. Occasionally, extensive skin metastasis may be the primary complaint in patients with urothelial carcinoma. The tumor cells resembling transitional cells are usually seen arranged in nests, solid patterns, or grouped inside dilated dermal lymphatic vessels. The tumor cells are reactive for blood group antigens (variable), CK7, CK20 (minority are negative for CK20), thrombomodulin, and uroplakin III (Table 22.4).

Cutaneous metastasis from cancer prostate usually appears as skin nodules over the abdomen and back. The neoplastic deposits are usually seen in the dermis and consist of malignant cells arranged in glands (small, medium sized, or cribriform) or in diffuse single-cell infiltration with necrosis. They are usually reactive for CK903/34 beta E12/high-molecular-weight cytokeratin, prostate-specific antigen/prostatic acid phosphatase and P504S/alpha-methylacyl-CoA racemase (AMACR) (Table 22.4).

Renal cell carcinoma represents about 2% of all cancers and is the primary tumor in about 6% of skin metastasis. The metastatic deposits are composed of cells with clear cytoplasm and sharp borders arranged in compact, tubulocystic, alveolar, or papillary architectures. Positive stains include keratin, epithelial membrane antigen, RCC-Ma,164 CD10, vimentin, and S100. Negative stains include CK7, CK20, inhibin, melan-A (A103), calretinin, and thyroid transcription factor-1 (Table 22.4).

Gynecologic Cancers

The lesions may appear as multiple dermal and subcutaneous nodules on the chest, back, abdomen, lower extremity, axilla, neck, and scalp. The nodules are usually firm, tender, and nonulcerative.

Metastases from the endometrial carcinoma usually appear as multiple pruritic skin nodules on the lower abdomen, groin, or the upper thigh.

CM of ovarian carcinoma may present as nodular carcinoma, carcinoma erysipelatous, or as large cauliflower-like lesions in the lower abdominal wall. These lesions are indicative of aggressive behavior and dismal outcome. Female genital tract carcinomas are usually positive for CA125, CK7, and CK20 (Table 22.4).

Thyroid and Salivary Gland Carcinomas

The thyroid follicular carcinoma has a greater preponderance than papillary carcinoma for sending CMs. The latter are usually localized to the head and neck regions and appear as single or multiple reddish nodules. Histologically, CMs are identical to the primary tumors. Immunostaining usually reveals reactivity to thyroid transcription factor and thyroglobulins (Table 22.4).

Metastases from adrenal cortical carcinoma were reported in the skin of the cheek.

Laryngeal Carcinoma and Meningioma

Cutaneous metastases from the laryngeal cancer appear as solitary or multiple nodules on the head and neck region. Occasionally, CMs from epidermoid carcinoma of the larynx may appear as erythematous infiltrating plaques on the supraclavicular and infraclavicular regions. The tumor is composed of malignant squamous cells arranged in solid/nesting patterns and is reactive for cytokeratin cocktail (AE1/AE3) and p53 (Table 22.4). The metastatic tumor cells may be seen inside dilated lymphatic vessels.

Meningiomas occasionally send metastases to the lung or mediastinum. CMs can appear as nodules at scar of the previous incisions. The tumor is composed of whorled clusters of spindle cells with intranuclear pseudo inclusions and psammoma bodies. The tumor cells stain positively for vimentin, epithelial membrane antigens, S100, progesterone receptors, cytokeratin, and carcinoembryonic antigen (Table 22.4).

Malignant Melanoma

The CMs of the malignant melanoma appear as pigmented or nonpigmented, sometimes angiomatous subcutaneous nodules. They may simulate the blue nevi and may be epidermotropic or simulate primary cutaneous melanoma. Occasionally, these lesions may present as cutaneous hemorrhagic lesions. In men, the metastatic nodules occur on the chest, extremities, and back. In women, metastases to the lower extremities are common.

Monitoring CMs with total-body photography may be apply for patients with many nevi to identify and reliably document small, rapidly growing, disseminated skin metastases also in the presence of multiple nevi. The first case of a precise analysis of eruptive epidermotropic melanoma metastases under immuno and targeted therapy using total-body 3D photography using the VECTRA 360WB 3D imaging system was published and valuable tool for early recognition of skin cancer and surveillance of cutaneous metastases [47].

Melanoma metastatic to the skin differs from a primary melanoma by the absence of junctional activity and tumor infiltrating lymphocytes. In epidermotropic metastatic melanoma, the tumor cells are initially localized in the papillary dermis and then involve the overlying epidermis. Most of these lesions occur in the regions distal to the side of the primary melanoma. The tumor cells may be spindled or epithelioid and arranged in nesting, bundle, or solid patterns. The cells may show marked atypia, frequent mitosis, large eosinophilic nucleoli, melanin pigment, or intranuclear inclusions. Melanoma cells are positive for S100, HMB45, Fontana-Masson (detects melanin granules), vimentin, melan-A/Mart-1, tyrosinase, and microphthalmia transcription factor.

Hematological Malignancies

Skin involvement (leukemia cutis) occurs in 5% of patients with chronic myeloid leukemia, 8% of patients with chronic lymphocytic leukemia, and 10% of patients with monocytic leukemia [48]. The skin lesions in patients with leukemia cutis appear as macules, papules, plaques, nodules, and skin ulcers. On histology, dermal infiltrates with nodular, interstitial, and perivascular distribution are observed. They are composed of a range of myelocytic differentiation from myeloblasts to segmented neutrophils. The blasts have distinct cytoplasmic borders, dispersed chromatin, and small nucleoli. Some eosinophilic myelocytes are also seen. The precise identification of the neoplastic cells in most of the cases requires ancillary studies including immunophenotypic stains, cytochemistry, and cytogenetic studies. The negative reactivity for epithelial markers (cytokeratins) helps rule out the possibility of poorly differentiated carcinomas. The negative reactivity for leukocyte common antigen, CD20, CD3, CD45RO, and CD45RA rules out obvious lymphoid malignancies (Table 22.4). The nearly perfect reticular pattern throughout a lesion together with the presence of eosinophilic myelocytes favors the diagnosis of leukemic infiltrates.

Soft Tissue Sarcomas

Sarcomas with reported CM include Ewing's sarcoma/primitive or peripheral neuroectodermal tumor, osteosarcoma, leiomyosarcoma, chondrosarcoma, epithelioid sarcoma, and angiosarcoma. They appear as solitary or multiple nodules overlying the site of the primary tumor or on the scalp. On histology, the basic structures and components of the metastatic lesions are identical to those of the primary malignancies. CMs are usually reactive for CD99 (O13, MIC2), PAS+ diastase sensitive (glycogen), neuron-specific enolase, Leu7/CD57, FLI1 protein and vimentin [49].

Similarly, only few cases of skin metastases of angiosarcoma (infiltrating, freely anastomosing channels lined by markedly atypical spindled to epithelioid endothelial cells with positive reactivity for factor VIII-related antigen, CD34, and CD31) were reported (Table 22.4). The patients usually present with erythematotelangiectatic nodules.

Cutaneous metastases from chordoma can occur by lymph vascular invasion. They usually appear as solitary or multiple nodules on the nose, back, scalp, and thigh [11]. The cells stain positively for S100, keratins (CK8/18, CK19), cytokeratin cocktail (AE1/AE3), epithelial membrane antigen, 5′ nucleotidase, glycogen, and neural-type cadherin [11]. Metastatic lesions of chordomas may be confused with chondroid syringoma. However, the presence of physaliferous cells and the coexpression of low-molecular-weight keratins and S100 protein help confirm the diagnosis of chordoma (Table 22.4).

Management

Cutaneous involvement portends a very poor prognosis and often flares up simultaneously with other metastases; majority occurred as a late event in the course of the disease. Most patients had known stage IV cancer. In an article by Kovács et al., 38 of 80 patients with skin metastasis from nonhematologic or no breast sources had inoperable primary tumors [50].

Interventions focused on the level of the skin represent increasingly relevant priorities for managing pain, tumor burden, and quality of life.

A review article by Wong et al. [51] in 2013 recommended excision of cutaneous metastases when surgically feasible and when it will result in a significant decrease in total tumor burden, will improve quality of life, or increase functionality. Using metastatic melanoma as a model, the investigators suggested 1-cm excision margins, with the caveat that no great data exists regarding excision margins of metastatic disease [36].

In general, treatment follows the regimen appropriate for the primary malignancy. However, systemic therapy appears to have limited efficacy. Therefore, skin-directed therapies have been developed to treat skin metastases. Skin-directed therapies are forms of localized treatment that have been shown to illicit a greater response than systemic therapy alone [52].

A meta-analysis by Spratt et al. [53] reported high response rates and low recurrence rates following skin-directed therapy. The modalities of skin-directed therapies include electrochemotherapy, photodynamic therapy, radiotherapy, intralesional therapy, and topical therapy, of which electrochemotherapy appears to have the most efficacy [54]. Electrochemotherapy functions via the application of pulsed electricity to a tumor-specific area to increase cell permeability [55, 56]. It has been shown to significantly increase the cytotoxicity of cisplatin and bleomycin [36]. Another efficacious skin-directed therapy is radiotherapy, which is a highly accurate modality that has also long been associated with the abscopal effect [5].

Imiquimod, a toll-like receptor-7 agonist applied topically as a 5% cream, has been linked to regression of tumor size and surrounding pain in extramammary Paget disease and in case reports of metastatic ductal carcinoma and highly vascular cancers including renal cell carcinoma [57–59]. Certainly, conventional techniques such as excision and radiation remain to be the mainstays of therapy for such lesions [60]. The immunomodulatory therapies used in advanced visceral and primary skin cancer treatment likely have a role in treating cutaneous metastases; however, they are yet to be investigated [61].

In summary, dermatologists might be aware of the possibility of cutaneous metastases, since they have a wide clinical spectrum and might mimic other benign conditions. A careful dermatological examination, with skin biopsy, when indicated, is important for the early detection.

References

1. Alcaraz I, Cerroni L, Rütten A, Kutzner H, Requena L. Cutaneous metastases from internal malignancies. Am J Dermatopathol. 2012;34(4):347–93. https://doi.org/10.1097/dad.0b013e31823069cf.
2. Lambert WC, Schwartz RA. Metastasis. J Am Acad Dermatol. 1992;27:131–3.
3. Strickley JD, Jenson AB, Jung JY. Cutaneous metastasis. Hematol Oncol Clin North Am. 2019;33(1):173–97. https://doi.org/10.1016/j.hoc.2018.08.008. PMID: 30497674
4. Lookingbill DP, Spangler N, Sexton FM. Skin involvement as the presenting sign of internal carcinomas. J Am Acad Dermatol. 1990;22:19–26.
5. Bittencourt MJS, Carvalho AH, Nascimento BAM, Freitas LKM, Parijós AM. Cutaneous metastasis of a breast cancer diagnosed 13 years before. An Bras Dermatol. 2015;90(3 Suppl 1):S134–7.
6. Sittart JA, Senise M. Cutaneous metastasis from internal carcinomas: a review of 45 years. An Bras Dermatol. 2013;88:541–4.
7. Schwartz RA. Cutaneous metastatic disease. J Am Acad Dermatol. 1995;33(2 Pt 1):161–85., ISSN 0190-9622. https://doi.org/10.1016/0190-9622(95)90231-7.
8. Fernández-Antón Martinez MC, et al. Metástasis cutâneas de origen visceral. Actas Dermosifiliogr. 2013;(10):841–53.
9. U.S. Cancer Statistics Working Group. U.S. Cancer Statistics data visualizations tool, based on 2020 submission data (1999–2018): U.S. Department of Health and Human Services, Centers for Disease Control and Prevention and National Cancer Institute. www.cdc.gov/cancer/dataviz. Released June 2021.
10. Gates O. Cutaneous metastases of malignant disease. Am J Cancer. 1937;30:718–30.
11. Gül U, Kiliç A, Gönül M, Çakmak S, Erinçkan C. Spectrum of cutaneous metastases in 1287 cases of internal malignancies: a study from Turkey. Acta Derm Venereol. 2007;87(2):160–2. https://doi.org/10.2340/00015555-0199.
12. McDonald JH, Heckel NJ, Kretschmer HL. Cutaneous metastases secondary to carcinoma of the urinary bladder. Arch Dermatol Syphilol. 1950;61:276–84.
13. Abrams HL, Spiro R, Goldstein N. Metastases in carcinoma. Analysis of 1000 autopsied cases. Cancer. 1950;3:74–85. https://doi.org/10.1002/1097-0142(1950)3:1<74::AID-CNCR2820030111>3.0.CO;2-7.
14. Reingold IM. Cutaneous metastases from internal carcinoma. Cancer. 1966;19(2):162–8. https://doi.org/10.1002/1097-0142(196602)19:2<162::aid-cncr2820190204>3.0.co;2-a. PMID: 5948332

15. Held B, Johnson DE. Cutaneous metastases from malignant genitourinary disease. South Med J. 1972;65(5):569–71. https://doi.org/10.1097/00007611-197205000-00012.
16. Brady KL, Scott GA, Gilmore ES. Cutaneous metastasis from penile squamous cell carcinoma resembling carcinoma en cuirasse. Dermatol Online J. 2014;21(3):13030/qt2c8085xm. PMID: 25780971
17. Spencer PS, Helm TN. Skin metastases in cancer patients. Cutis. 1987;39(2):119–21. PMID: 3829718
18. Enticknap JB. An analysis of 1,000 cases of cancer with special reference to metastasis. Guys Hosp Rep. 1952;101(4):273–9. PMID: 12999050
19. Nashan D, Muller ML, Braun-Falco M, et al. Cutaneous metastases of visceral tumours: a review. J Cancer Res Clin Oncol. 2009;135:1–14.
20. Quatresooz P, Piérard-Franchimont C, Rorive A, Piérard GE. Comment j'explore… une métastase cutanée. Qui es-tu, d'où viens-tu? [How I explore… a cutaneous metastasis. What are you, from where are you coming from?]. Rev Med Liege. 2008;63(9):559–63. French. PMID: 19051512
21. Mueller TJ, Wu H, Greenberg RE, Hudes G, Topham N, Lessin SR, Uzzo RG. Cutaneous metastases from genitourinary malignancies. Urology. 2004;63(6):1021–6. https://doi.org/10.1016/j.urology.2004.01.014.
22. Schwartz IS. Sister Mary Joseph's nodule. N Engl J Med. 1987;316:1348–9.
23. Handa U, Kundu R, Dimri K. Cutaneous metastasis: a study of 138 cases diagnosed by fine-needle aspiration cytology. Acta Cytol. 2017;61:47–54. https://doi.org/10.1159/000453252.
24. El Khoury J, Khalifeh I, Kibbi A-G, Abbas O. Cutaneous metastasis: clinicopathological study of 72 patients from a tertiary care center in Lebanon. Int J Dermatol. 2014;53:147–58.
25. Wesche WA, Khare VK, Chesney TM, Jenkins JJ. Non-hematopoietic cutaneous metastases in children and adolescents: thirty years experience at St. Jude Children's Research Hospital. J Cutan Pathol. 2000;27:485–92.
26. Alcaraz I, Cerroni L, Rütten A, Kutzner H, Requena L. Cutaneous metastases from internal malignancies: a clinicopathologic and immunohistochemical review. Am J Dermatopathol. 2012;34:347–93.
27. Tschen EH, Apisarnthanarax P. Inflammatory metastatic carcinoma of the breast. Arch Dermatol. 1981;117:120–1.
28. Schoenlaub P, Sarraux A, Grosshans E, Heid E, Cribier B. Survival after cutaneous metastasis: a study of 200 cases. Ann Dermatol Venereol. 2001;128:1310.
29. Hu SC, Chen GS, Wu CS, Chai CY, Chen WT, Lan CC. Rates of cutaneous metastases from different internal malignancies: experience from a Taiwanese medical center. J Am Acad Dermatol. 2009;60(3):379–87. https://doi.org/10.1016/j.jaad.2008.10.007. Epub 2008 Dec 3. PMID: 19056145
30. Sánchez-García I. The crossroads of oncogenesis and metastasis. N Engl J Med. 2009;360(3):297–9. https://doi.org/10.1056/NEJMcibr0808031.
31. Ko C, McNiff J. Cutaneous metastases. In: Bolognia J, editor. Dermatology. 4th ed. New York: Elsevier; 2018. p. 2160–7.
32. Jaros J, Hunt S, Mose E, Lai O, Tsoukas M. Cutaneous metastases: a great imitator. Clin Dermatol. 2019; https://doi.org/10.1016/j.clindermatol.2019.1.
33. Chernoff KA, Marghoob AA, Lacouture ME, Deng L, Busam KJ, Myskowski PL. Dermoscopic findings in cutaneous metastases. JAMA Dermatol. 2014;150(4):429. https://doi.org/10.1001/jamadermatol.2013.850.
34. Hazelrigg DE, Rudolph AH. Inflammatory metastatic carcinoma. Carcinoma erysipelatoides. Arch Dermatol. 1977;113:69–70.
35. Requena L, Sangueza M, Sangueza OP, Kutzner H. Pigmented mammary Paget disease and pigmented epidermotropic metastases from breast carcinoma. Am J Dermatopathol. 2002;24:189–98.
36. Dagdelen D, Karadag AS, Akdeniz N, Ozkanli SS, Gurel MS. Zosteriform cutaneous metastasis: a case series. Dermatol Ther. 2020;33:e14137. https://doi.org/10.1111/dth.14137.

37. Bauza A, Redondo P, Idoate MA. Cutaneous zosteriform squamous cell carcinoma metastasis arising in an immunocompetent patient. Clin Exp Dermatol. 2002;27:199–201.
38. Damin DC, Lazzaron AR, Tarta C, Cartel A, Rosito MA. Massive zosteriform cutaneous metastasis from rectal carcinoma. Tech Coloproctol. 2003;7:105.
39. Shafqat A, Viehman GE, Myers SA. Cutaneous squamous cell carcinoma with zosteriform metastasis in a transplant recipient. J Am Acad Dermatol. 1997;37:1008.
40. Martorell-Calatayud A, Llombart-Cussac B, Requena-Caballero C, Guillén-Barona C. Dactilitis crónica indolora como hallazgo inicial de un adenocarcinoma pulmonar diseminado. Actas Dermosifiliogr. 2009;100:727–9.
41. Brownstein MH, Helwig EG. Spread of tumors to the skin. Arch Dermatol. 1973;107:80–6.
42. Schwartz RA, Rubinstein DJ, Raventos A, et al. Inflammatory metastatic carcinoma of the parotid. Arch Dermatol. 1984;120:796–7.
43. McKee PH. Cutaneous metastases. J Cutan Pathol. 1985;12:239–50.
44. Elgart GW, Patterson JW, Taylor R. Cutaneous metastasis from papillary carcinoma of the thyroid gland. J Am Acad Dermatol. 1991;25:404–8.
45. Seve P, Billotey C, Broussolle C, Dumontet C, Mackey JR. The role of 2-deoxy-2-[F-18]fluoro-D-glucose positron emission tomography in disseminated carcinoma of unknown primary site. Cancer. 2007;109(292–9):92.
46. Green AR, Young P, Krivinskas S, et al. The expression of ER alpha, ERbeta and PR in lobular carcinoma in situ of the breast determined using laser microdissection and real-time PCR. Histopathology. 2009;54:419.
47. Erdmann M, Heinzerling L, Schuler G, Berking C, Schliep S. Monitoring skin metastases during immuno- and targeted therapy using total-body 3D photography. J Eur Acad Dermatol Venereol. 2020;35:e61. https://doi.org/10.1111/jdv.16806.
48. Vishalakshi V, Torsekar RG, Shinde S. Aleukemic leukemia cutis. Indian J Dermatol Venereol Leprol. 2007;73:109.
49. Martínez MA, García RN, Galván JJ, Marrero OB, Castro IG. Ewing's sarcoma: histopathological and immunohistochemical study. Orthopedics. 2003;26:723–5.
50. Kovács KA, Kenessey I, Tímár J. Skin metastasis of internal cancers: a single institution experience. Pathol Oncol Res. 2013;19(3):515–20.
51. Wong CY, Helm MA, Kalb RE, et al. The presentation, pathology, and current management strategies of cutaneous metastasis. N Am J Med Sci. 2013;5(9):499–504.
52. Mole RH. Whole body irradiation; radiobiology or medicine? Br J Radiol. 1953;26(305):234–41.
53. Spratt DE, Gordon Spratt EA, Wu S, et al. Efficacy of skin-directed therapy for cutaneous metastases from advanced cancer: a meta-analysis. J Clin Oncol. 2014;32(28):3144–55.
54. Andtbacka RH, Kaufman HL, Collichio F, et al. Talimogene laherparepvec improves durable response rate in patients with advanced melanoma. J Clin Oncol. 2015;33(25):2780–8.
55. Cabula C, Campana LG, Grilz G, et al. Electrochemotherapy in the treatment of cutaneous metastases from breast cancer: a multicenter cohort analysis. Ann Surg Oncol. 2015;22(Suppl 3):S442–50.
56. Bourke MG, Salwa SP, Sadadcharam M, et al. Effective treatment of intractable cutaneous metastases of breast cancer with electrochemotherapy: ten year audit of single centre experience. Breast Cancer Res Treat. 2017;161(2):289–97.
57. Sanderson P, Innamaa A, Palmer J, et al. Imiquimod therapy for extramammary Paget's disease of the vulva: a viable non-surgical alternative. J Obstet Gynaecol. 2013;33(5):479–83.
58. Luyten A, Sörgel P, Clad A, et al. Treatment of extramammary Paget disease of the vulva with imiquimod: a retrospective, multicenter study by the German Colposcopy Network. J Am Acad Dermatol. 2014;70(4):644–50.
59. Henriques L, Palumbo M, Guay MP, et al. Imiquimod in the treatment of breast cancer skin metastasis. J Clin Oncol. 2014;32(8):e22–5.
60. Asakura M, Miura H. Imiquimod 5% cream for the treatment of nasal lesion of metastatic renal cell carcinoma. Dermatol Ther. 2011;24(3):375–7.
61. Okino T, Fujioka A, Nakajima H, et al. Effective treatment of metastatic renal cell carcinoma with topical imiquimod therapy. J Dtsch Dermatol Ges. 2014;12(2):155–7.

Chapter 23
Cutaneous Adverse Events from Systemic Anticancer Treatments

Jade Cury-Martins, Cristina Martinez Zugaib Abdalla, and José Antonio Sanches

Key Points

- Dermatologic adverse events (dAEs) have a high frequency and might cause an important impact on the patient's quality of life (QoL).
- Those skin toxicities might lead to dose reductions or even discontinuation of cancer therapy, with impact on the disease outcome.
- The National Cancer Institute's Common Terminology Criteria for Adverse Events (CTCAE) is a standardized tool used in oncology trials to document and grade toxic effects of oncologic therapies.
- Patients and professionals must deal with the chronic aspects of the toxicities.
- Preventive measures decrease occurrence and severity of dAE.

J. Cury-Martins (✉)
Dermatology, Faculdade de Medicina da Universidade de São Paulo, São Paulo, São Paulo, Brazil

Instituto do Cancer do Estado de São Paulo—ICESP, São Paulo, São Paulo, Brazil

C. M. Z. Abdalla
Hospital Sirio-Libanês, São Paulo, São Paulo, Brazil

Núcleo de Oncodermatologia Hospital Sírio-Libanês, São Paulo, São Paulo, Brazil

J. A. Sanches
Dermatology, Faculdade de Medicina da Universidade de São Paulo, São Paulo, São Paulo, Brazil

C. M. Z. Abdalla et al. (eds.), *Oncodermatology*, https://doi.org/10.1007/978-3-031-29277-4_23

Overview

Dermatologic adverse events (dAEs) became an important issue with the advance of cancer treatment, since they have a high frequency, are often symptomatic, may be disfiguring, and might cause an important impact on the patient's quality of life (QoL). Those skin toxicities might lead to dose reductions or even discontinuation of cancer therapy, with impact on the disease outcome.

It is important for dermatologists to know the most common types of reactions to be able to help patients and oncologists on the prevention and management of those toxicities [1, 2].

The National Cancer Institute's Common Terminology Criteria for Adverse Events (CTCAE) is a standardized tool used in oncology trials to document and grade toxic effects of oncologic therapies. It is available online with open access at https://ctep.cancer.gov/protocolDevelopment/electronic_applications/ctc.htm.

Class of Agents

Oncologic treatments might be divided into three main categories, regarding their mechanism of action:

Conventional Chemotherapeutic Drugs

Conventional cytotoxic chemotherapy still plays an important role in cancer treatment. It works primarily through the inhibition of cell division. It is associated with many adverse events (AE), especially in some systems that share with the tumor the property of rapid cell proliferation and therefore a high rate of cell division, such as the hematopoietic, gastrointestinal systems, and the skin [2, 3]. Examples of common effects are emesis, cytopenia, alopecia, mucositis, and nail changes. They are associated with dose, type of drug, and time of infusion and are in most cases reversible with the end of chemotherapy cycles.

The related cutaneous adverse events to this class, most frequent causing agents and management (with level of evidence) are summarized on Table 23.1.

Targeted Therapies and Immunomodulatory Agents ("Checkpoint" Inhibitors)

In the past few years, a huge development on oncologic treatments have occurred, with the emergence of numerous targeted agents and immune checkpoint-related agents. With those new mechanisms of action, a totally new scope of adverse reactions has

Table 23.1 Dermatologic adverse events of conventional chemotherapeutic agents

Dermatologic toxicity	Most frequent agents	Management	Level of evidence
Hyperpigmentation		• Photoprotective measures • Bleaching agents	IV
Diffuse	Busulfan ("tan" appearance); methotrexate; procarbazine, capecitabine		
Flagellate	Bleomycin		
Serpentine supravenous	5-FU, docetaxel, vincristine, vinorelbine		
Areas of pressure, flexural, under occlusive dressings	Ifosfamide, thiotepa, hydroxyurea, cisplatin, docetaxel		
Palms and soles	Hydroxyurea, doxorubicin, capecitabine		
Palmar creases	Ifosfamide, cyclophosphamide bleomycin, busulfan, doxorubicin		
Mucosa	Cyclophosphamide (gingiva), busulfan, doxorubicin, cisplatin, capecitabine		
Nail changes		*General measures to all patients*: reduction of contact to water, use of cotton gloves beneath plastic or rubber gloves for any wet work, avoidance of any damaging procedure (e.g., aggressive manicuring), and hydration with thick emollients	IV
Onycholysis	Taxanes, cyclophosphamide doxorubicin, capecitabine, etoposide	*Prevention*: Frozen gloves and socks during infusion (depending on the agent and type of infusion)	IIA
		Treatment: • Avoiding traumas (e.g., keeping nails short) and humidity • If green discoloration: topical antibiotic (tobramycin or ciprofloxacin eye drops)	IV

(continued)

Table 23.1 (continued)

Dermatologic toxicity	Most frequent agents	Management	Level of evidence
Paronychia	Taxanes, etoposide, capecitabine	• Topical corticosteroids • If secondary infection is suspected, culture guided antibiotics	IV
Nail discoloration	5-FU, taxanes, hydroxyurea, cyclophosphamide, doxorubicin, capecitabine	Might be diffuse or banding/streaking. No treatment needed	
Hand-foot syndrome (HFS)	Capecitabine, doxorubicin, citarabine, 5-FU, taxanes	*Prevention*:	
		• Regional cooling during chemotherapy infusion	IB
		• Nonsteroidal anti-inflammatory agent	IA
		• Use thick cotton gloves and/or socks; urea-based emollients; avoid irritants and tight clothing and shoes; avoid extremes of temperature, pressure, and friction	III
		Treatment: • Potent topical steroid • For relief of symptoms, cool compresses or emergence of hands and feet on cool water, topical anesthetics, and NSAIDs • Dose reduction or treatment interruption is sometimes necessary	III–IV
PATEO syndrome	Docetaxel	See measures for HFS above	
Chemotherapy-induced alopecia	Cyclophosphamide, doxorubicin, irinotecan and taxanes	*Prevention*: scalp cooling devices	I
		Treatment:	
		• Topical minoxidil 2%	IB
		• Topical minoxidil 5%, biotin containing oral supplements	IV
		• Topical bimatoprost (for eyelashes)	IIA

5-FU 5-fluorouracil, *PATEO* PeriArticular Thenar Erythema and Onycholysis arisen [4–7]. In one hand, those therapies were crucial for the improvement of survival. On the other hand, they created a new challenge: With the continuous and prolonged use of these drugs, patients and professionals must deal with the chronic aspects of the toxicities, not anymore related with a specific number of chemotherapy cycles, but lasting for months to years, with an important impact on quality of life.

Targeted Therapies inhibit specific molecules involved in tumor development and growth, having a more specific action than conventional chemotherapy, with greater efficacy and less toxicity. They might be monoclonal antibodies, large molecules that target extracellular components, or small molecule inhibitors that can enter cells, block receptor signaling, and interfere with downstream intracellular molecules (they will be referred as tyrosine kinase inhibitors—TKI) [8]. Many of those molecules are mutated or overexpressed on tumors but are also present in normal tissues such as the skin. The main agents on this class are epidermal growth factor receptor inhibitors (EGFRi) (e.g., cetuximab, panitumumab, gefitinib, erlotinib, lapatinib); antiangiogenic agents, such as inhibitors of vascular endothelial growth factor receptor (VEGFRi) (e.g., bevacizumab, sorafenib); inhibitors of the mitogen-activated protein kinase (MAPK) pathway, such as RAFi (e.g., vemurafenib, dabrafenib), MEKi (e.g., cobimetinib, trametinib); mTOR inhibitors (e.g., everolimus); multikinase inhibitors (e.g., vandetanib, pazopanib, sunitinib); Hedgehog pathway inhibitors (vismodegib); and more recently fibroblast growth factor receptor inhibitors (FGFRi) (e.g., erdafitinib, infigratinib, pemigatinib, rogaratinib) [9]. Related cutaneous adverse events to the agents on this class, their management, and levels of evidence are summarized in Table 23.2.

Immunotherapy More recently, the comprehension of the regulatory processes involved in the restriction of the immune response to cancer led to the development of a new promising group of agents, the "immune checkpoint"-targeted agents. They have the goal of releasing the immune system against tumor cells, blocking inhibitory receptors expressed on T cells such as cytotoxic T lymphocyte-associated antigen 4 (CTLA-4) or programmed death 1 (PD-1). This releasing of the immune system also affects normal cells, justifying the most common adverse events related to this class, the "immune-related adverse events" (irAE). On this group, we find the CTLA-4 inhibitor (ipilimumab), PD-1, and PD-1 ligand inhibitors (e.g., nivolumab, pembrolizumab, atezolizumab) [6, 10–14]. Related cutaneous adverse events to the agents on this class, their management, and levels of evidence are summarized in Table 23.3.

Table 23.2 Dermatologic adverse events of targeted therapies

Drug class	Agents	Dermatologic toxicities	Management	Level of evidence
EGFR inhibitors	• Monoclonal antibodies: cetuximab and panitumumab • TKI specific for EGFR: erlotinib and gefitinib • Less specific multikinase inhibitors: vandetanib	Papulopustular eruption (starts on the first 2 weeks)	*Prevention*: • Systemic antibiotics for the first 6–8 weeks (tetracyclines), sunscreen	IB
			Treatment:	
			• Low-potency topical steroids	III
			• Systemic antibiotics (tetracyclines)	IB
			• Systemic isotretinoin (low doses)	III
			• Culture-driven antibiotics if secondary infection	
		Xerosis	• Limited shower time, use of gentle cleansers (pH-neutral soaps or syndets), regular use of emollients • Topical steroid if eczematous lesions	III
		Paronychia and pyogenic granuloma-like lesions	*Prevention*:	
			• Systemic antibiotics (tetracyclines)	IB
			• Antiseptic solutions	III
			Treatment:	
			• Topical steroids	III
			• Systemic antibiotics (tetracyclines)	III
			• Culture-driven antibiotics if secondary infection	IB
		Fissures	Protective coverings (hydrocolloid, biological, or cyanoacrylate glue), barrier creams (petroleum jelly, zinc oxide cream), and thick emollients	IIB
		Hair changes	• Non-scarring alopecia: topical minoxidil	IB
			• Inflammatory and scarring alopecia: topical steroids	III
			• Trichomegaly: eyelash trimming	III
			• Hypertrichosis: laser hair reduction	IB
KIT and BCR-ABL inhibitors	Imatinib, nilotinib, dasatinib	Exanthema (rash)	Topical steroids or short courses of oral steroids	III
		Hypopigmentation	Reversible after treatment interruption	III

Drug class	Agents	Dermatologic toxicities	Management	Level of evidence
Antiangiogenic agents	• Selective VEGFR inhibitors: bevacizumab and ranibizumab • Nonselective multikinase inhibitors: sorafenib, pazopanib, sunitinib	Hand-foot skin reaction	*Prevention*:	
			• Use thick cotton gloves and/or socks; urea-based emollients; avoid irritants and tight clothing and shoes; avoid extremes of temperature, pressure, and friction	III
			• Pretreatment evaluation with a podiatrist with callosity chopping and the use of orthopedic shoe inserts when needed	III
			• Urea-based emollients	IB
			Treatment: • Keratolytic agents • Topical corticosteroids • Potent topical steroid • For relief of symptoms, cool compresses or emergence of hands and feet on cool water, topical anesthetics, and NSAIDs	III
			• Hydrocolloid dressings	IB
		Pigmentary changes	• Hypopigmentation of hair and skin (pazopanib and sunitinib), yellow discoloration of skin (sunitinib)—reversible after discontinuation	III
		Hair and scalp	• Seborrheic dermatitis-like rash: topical steroids	III
			• Non-scarring alopecia: topical minoxidil	IV

(continued)

Table 23.2 (continued)

Drug class	Agents	Dermatologic toxicities	Management	Level of evidence
RAF inhibitors	Vemurafenib and dabrafenib	Exanthema (rash)	• Oral antihistamines, topical or short courses of systemic steroids • Temporary treatment interruption might be necessary	III
		Photosensitivity	*Prevention*: photoprotective measures *Treatment*: topical or short courses of systemic steroids *Mostly vemurafenib, UVA induced	IIB III
		Keratosis pilaris-like eruption	Keratolytic and emollients, gentle skin care	III
		Seborrheic dermatitis-like	Topical steroids	III
		Hand-foot skin reaction	See above (antiangiogenic agents)	
		Keratoacanthomas and squamous cell carcinomas	• Frequent dermatological monitoring	III
			• If few lesions: surgical excision	III
			• If multiple lesions: 5-FU, systemic retinoids or photodynamic therapy *Association with a MEKi decreases lesions	IIA/B
		Warts and verrucal keratoses	• Destructive or surgical measures • Topical treatments: keratolytic, 5-FU, imiquimod	III
MEK inhibitors	Cobimetinibe, trametinibe, selumetinibe	Papulopustular eruption	See EGFR inhibitors above	
		Xerosis		
		Paronychia		
		Exanthema (rash)	• Oral antihistamines, topical or short courses of systemic steroids	III
mTOR inhibitors	Rapamycin, everolimus, sirolimus	Stomatitis	Antiseptic washes, topical steroids, and anesthetics	

Drug class	Agents	Dermatologic toxicities	Management	Level of evidence
FGFR inhibitors	Infigratinib, erdafitinib, derazantinib, pemigatinib, futibatinib	Nail changes (onycholysis, paronychia, nail dystrophy)	Antiseptic solutions; culture-driven antibiotics if secondary infection Same as for HFSR of VEGFRi	III–IV
		Stomatitis, dry mouth		
		Xerosis		
		Alopecia		
		Acral involvement		

NSAID **nonsteroidal anti-inflammatory drug**

Table 23.3 Dermatologic adverse events of immunotherapy (immune-related adverse events—irAE)

Drug class	Agents	Dermatologic toxicities	Management	Level of evidence
"Checkpoint" inhibitors	• CTLA-4 inhibitors: ipilimumab • PD-1 inhibitors: nivolumab, pembrolizumab • PD1l inhibitors: atezolizumab	Exanthema *(rash)*	• Mild (<30% BSA): oral antihistamines, topical steroids • Moderate (>30% BSA): oral steroids (1–2 mg/kg); hold immunotherapy • Severe (SSJ/TEN or necrotic, bullous or hemorrhagic complications): systemic steroid (1–2 mg/kg); permanently discontinue immunotherapy	IV
		Pruritus	*Prevention*: Limited shower time, use of gentle cleansers (pH-neutral soaps or syndets), regular use of emollients *Treatment*: • Oral antihistamines • Topical or oral steroids • GABA agonists (pregabalin, gabapentin)	IV
		Oral toxicity • Lichenoid lesions • Dry mouth	Topical steroids and anesthetics, good oral hygiene	IV
		Vitiligo	No definitive treatment	IV
		Others: • Lichenoid eruptions • Sarcoidosis • Autoimmune blistering diseases (bullous pemphigoid) • Psoriasis	Same as for exanthema Rituximab might be used for grade 3 Biologics[a] or retinoids might be used for grade 3	IV

[a] Dual-checkpoint blockade (anti-CTLA-4 + anti-PD1) is related to a higher grade of adverse events, including dermatologic toxicities. Case reports for severe irAE are available with the use of other immunomodulatory agents

BSA body surface area, *CTLA-4* cytotoxic T lymphocyte-associated antigen 4, *PD-1* programmed death 1, *PD-1l* programmed death 1 ligand, *SSJ* Steven-Johnson syndrome, *TEN* toxic epidermal necrolysis

Dermatological Adverse Events and Their Management

Daily Baseline Skin Care

Xerosis is a common dermatological condition in patients on cancer treatment, with incidences ranging from 1% to 84% and can collaborate to a decrease in QoL and to the occurrence of other dAE, such as infections, sensitization to allergens, and pruritus. It is even more frequent with the use of targeted therapies (for xerosis, RR 2.99, 95% CI 2.0–4.3, $p < 0.001$; for pruritus, RR 2.56, 95% CI 1.51–4.35, $p < 0.001$) [15, 16]. The skin also becomes more sensitive to the ultraviolet radiation and more prone to skin pigmentation. Therefore, it is fundamental to educate patients on preventive measures, even prior to the start of any therapy, that help maintain skin barrier function, possibly decreasing the occurrence and severity of dAE.

Some important measures to all cancer patients are listed below [1].

Routine measures to all oncologic patients
Avoidance of irritating products
Limited shower time
Use of gentle cleansers (pH-neutral soaps or syndets)
Regular use of emollients and sun-protective measures (e.g., broad-spectrum sunscreen—SPF30 or higher with a UVA-PF—protective clothes)

The use of deodorants is controversial, but some data show no evidence of harm, and therefore, patients might use those products to maintain their regular routine and improve their well-being [17]. The use of makeup or camouflage may also help on the self-esteem. Preference for noncomedogenic products is recommended.

The dAE will be divided in types of skin reactions and areas of involvement, more related to the dermatological exam, but in Tables 23.1, 23.2, and 23.3, readers can find the dAE grouped by class of agents.

Pigmentary Changes

Hyperpigmentation can occur at different sites and in different patterns. They can start days to months after initiation and most of the times fade months after discontinuation of therapy. It can occur on photo-distributed areas, preceded or not by photosensitivity signs, as a serpentine supravenous hyperpigmentation after peripheral chemotherapy infusion (e.g., fluorouracil, docetaxel) that might be preceded or not by erythema and inflammation (Fig. 23.1); in a diffuse pattern, sometimes reticulated (doxorubicin, hydroxyurea, methotrexate); localized in areas of pressure, flexural areas, or under occlusive dressings (ifosfamide, thiotepa); and as acral pigmentation (along the crease lines or macular, over the palms and soles) [3, 18].

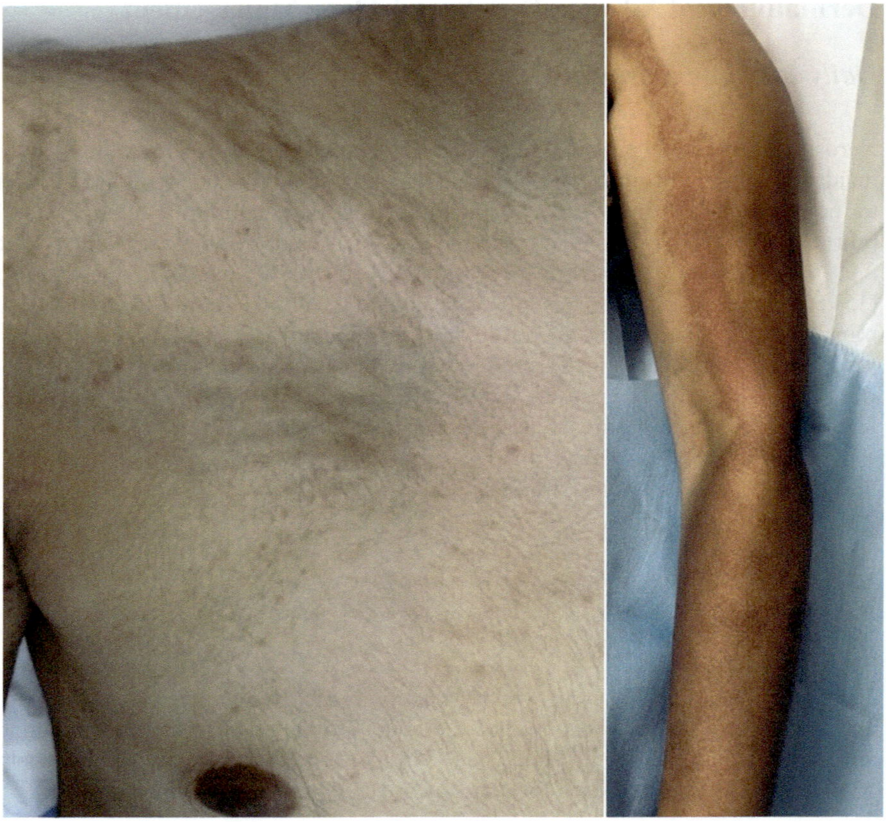

Fig. 23.1 Flagellate dermatitis (bleomycin) and supravenous hyperpigmentation. (Courtesy of Cristina Abdalla, MD)

Flagellate Dermatitis and pigmentation is related to bleomycin treatment (20–30% of patients) and occur as a pruritic erythematous linear streaks, followed by pigmentation (Fig. 23.1). Busulfan treatment can cause an "Addison-like" pigmentation, with a "tan" appearance [3].

Patients should be oriented to adhere to sun-protective measures, and bleaching agents might also be used to accelerate clearing.

Targeted Therapies can also cause pigmentary changes such as a yellow pigmentation on sunitinib-treated patients (VEGFRi). Hypopigmentation (diffuse or localized) is associated with c-kit inhibitors such as imatinib, especially in patients with darker skin, as c-kit also regulates melanocyte function. They are usually reversible with dose reduction or discontinuation [4].

Immunotherapy has been linked to vitiligo-like lesions, mainly but not only in melanoma-treated patients. Associated hair depigmentation can also be observed. No definitive treatment exists, and it usually persists after the completion of immunotherapy. Reports of white hair repigmentation are also available [10–12, 19].

Nail Changes

Nail alterations during cancer treatment are frequent, usually well tolerated and disappear under cessation of treatment. However, in some circumstances, they might be symptomatic and interfere with patient's daily activities [20].

Conventional chemotherapeutic agents are usually related to alterations such as melanonychia (diffuse, transverse, or longitudinal), leukonychia, onycholysis, Beau's lines, onychomadesis, and onychorrhexis.

Taxanes are associated with painful subungual hemorrhage, followed by onycholysis (Fig. 23.2) and sometimes subungual abscess formation that are quite symptomatic and might lead to dose reductions or treatment discontinuation. The use of frozen gloves and socks during infusion might reduce the severity of nail alterations, but they are usually not well tolerated (nail toxicity, one study, 45 patients, side-to-side, 11% vs. 51%, $p = 0.0001$) [2, 3, 18]. Drainage of hemorrhage and abscesses might be needed for symptom relief as well as culture-guided antibiotic treatments.

Both conventional and targeted treatments can cause nail plate alterations such as brittle nails, nail cracking, and onychoschizia. Those effects can be handled with preventive measures such as reduction of contact to water, use of cotton gloves beneath plastic or rubber gloves for any wet work, avoidance of any damaging procedure (e.g., aggressive manicuring), and hydration with thick emollients. Oral biotin and lacquers such as hydroxypropyl chitosan and poly-ureaurethane might be used, although no controlled study is yet available [20].

For onycholysis, avoiding traumas (e.g., keeping nails short) and humidity is important. If signs of pseudomonas colonization (green discoloration), a topical antibiotic might be used (we suggest ophthalmologic solutions such as tobramycin or ciprofloxacin eye drops twice daily).

VEGFRi are associated with asymptomatic splinter subungual hemorrhages (black, red, or brown longitudinal lines) in 25–70% of patients, with fingernails being mostly affected [4, 6].

EGFRi are related to frequent nail toxicities, occurring in around 17.2% of patients on a previous meta-analysis [21]. Periungual fissures, paronychia, and pyogenic

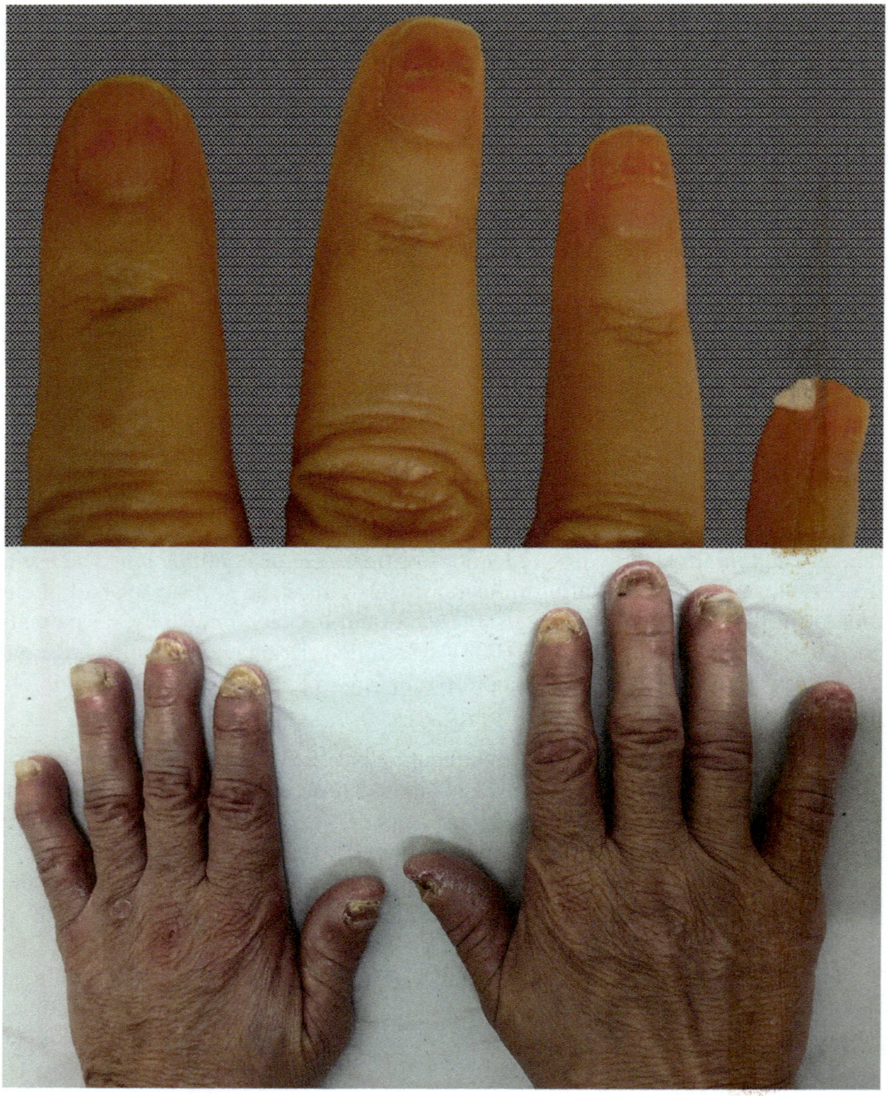

Fig. 23.2 Nail changes: Subungual hemorrhage and onycholysis due to taxanes (on the top); nail dystrophy, paronychia and onycholysis associated to FGFRi (bottom). (Courtesy of Cristina Abdalla, MD and Jade Cury-Martins, MD)

granuloma-like lesions start to develop 2 or more months after initiation of therapy, on both finger and toenails (Fig. 23.5). They are initially sterile, but secondary infection may occur. Preventive measures include the ones listed above and also the use of comfortable shoes, sometimes with cushioning inserts for the affected nails, adequate nail cutting, and the use of antiseptic solutions such as Burrow's solution soaks, white vinegar soaks (1:1), bleach soaks (1/4 cup bleach: approx. 10 L of water), chlorhexidine or povidone iodine [5, 22–24], or a solution of sodium hypochlorite 2.5%, sodium chloride 1.0%, and deionized water *qsp* 100 mL (5 drops/1 L). The use of oral tetracyclines is controversial as they were related to a decrease on the incidence of paronychia in some trials and showed no benefits on others [25]. For fissuring, protective coverings such as hydrocolloid, biological glue, or even cyanoacrylate glue to relieve pain and promote healing, barrier creams (petroleum jelly, zinc oxide cream) and thick emollients might be used. For granulomas, if secondary infection is suspected, culture is indicated, and proper antibiotics should be prescribed. For noninfected lesions, destructive measures such as trichloroacetic acid (70–90%) or cryotherapy might be used. Potent topical steroids, occlusive or not, are also indicated [26]. Sometimes surgical treatment might be necessary. Recently, the use of topical betaxolol was described for treating a pyogenic granuloma-like lesion induced by EGFRi [27].

FGFRi are also related to frequent nail toxicities, reported in 7–24% of patients. It usually starts 1–2 months after treatment initiation, can be prolonged and debilitating, and may lead to treatment discontinuation. The most important manifestation is onycholysis; other less frequent include paronychia, Beau's line/onychomadesis, onychoschizia, and nail dystrophy (Fig. 23.2). Counseling on the possible nail changes before treatment initiation is recommended. Preventive measures include avoidance of repeated trauma and prolonged contact with water. The use of protective gloves, emollients, and loose-fitting socks and footwear is also helpful. Avoid biting nails or cutting nails too short. For paronychia and onycholysis, the use of antiseptic solutions as listed above is recommended. For grades 2–3, obtaining cultures and use of 14-day course oral antibiotics, such as cefadroxil, are recommended [9].

Acral Reactions

Hand-foot syndrome (HFS), also known as palmoplantar erythrodysesthesia, is a dAE related to ***conventional chemotherapeutic drugs***, common with agents such as capecitabine, doxorubicin, cytarabine, and 5-FU. It is preceded by prodrome symptoms such as tingling or pain at the extremities, followed by a symmetric, sharply demarcated erythema and edema of the palms and soles (Fig. 23.3). Vesicles and bullae might also be present. Pain usually limits daily activities and might be a cause of dose reduction or discontinuation. Incidence is higher with prolonged infusions or oral agents [2, 3].

PATEO syndrome (**P**eri**A**rticular **T**henar **E**rythema and **O**nycholysis) is a variant of HFS, specific to the ***taxanes*** (docetaxel). It is characterized by scaly erythematous lesions with a distinct distribution to the dorsal aspects of the hands (overlying the joints) and thenar eminences. More rarely, it can also affect the dorsum

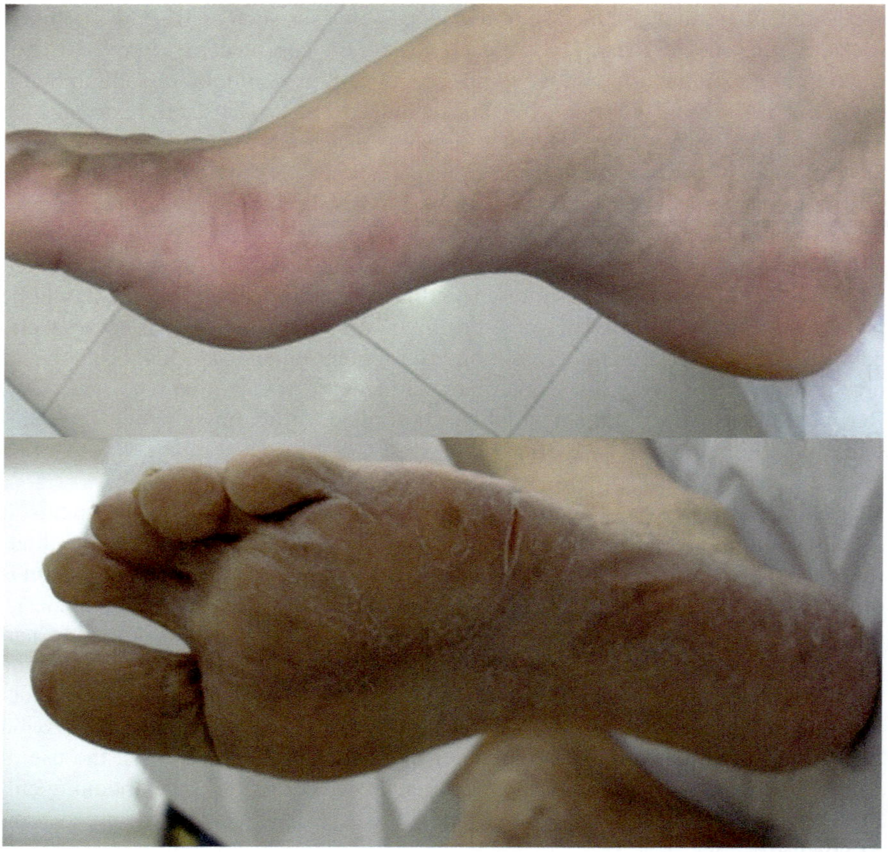

Fig. 23.3 Hand-foot syndrome (conventional chemotherapy) and Hand-foot skin reaction (targeted therapies). (Courtesy of Cristina Abdalla, MD)

of the feet. Although common, nails are not universally affected. It is usually bilateral, not necessarily symmetric. It may start on the first chemotherapy cycle or develop progressively. Burning sensation and pain are the most reported symptoms [18].

Hand-foot skin reaction (HFSR) is another variant of acral toxicity related to targeted therapies, with both monoclonal antibodies and small molecules tyrosine kinase inhibitors especially with those targeting VEGFR (bevacizumab, sorafenib, sunitinib) and BRAF (vemurafenib). Despite the similar palmoplantar distribution, dose dependency, and associated pain, HFSR develop on friction or trauma-prone areas (pressure areas), such as the heel and lateral aspects of the soles and web spaces. Lesions start 2–4 weeks after beginning of therapy and are characterized by hyperkeratosis, resembling skin calluses, occasionally with superficial blistering and erythematous halos (Fig. 23.3) [2, 4, 5, 28, 29]. Depending on the drug, lesions might improve or not over time [30].

Palmar-plantar erythrodysesthesia syndrome (PPES) is a recently described term for acral involvement related to FGFRi. It is reported in 18–21% of patients and has findings resembling both HFS and HFSR. For PPES, the ventral aspect of the distal digits and lateral aspects of the palms and soles are affected by erythema and pain. It often presents as a mild to moderate cutaneous edema, erythema, and hyperkeratosis that might evolve into painful digits impacting patient's QoL [9].

Prevention

HFS and PATEO On a prior systematic review, the only two evidence-based measures for prevention (to decrease incidence and/or severity) were the use of a nonsteroidal anti-inflammatory drug (NSAIDs: celecoxib) (for any grade, odds ratio, odds ratio (OR) 0.47, 95% CI 0.29–0.78, $p = 0.003$; for grade 2–3, OR 0.39, 95% CI 0.20–0.73, $p = 0.003$) and dose reduction. One study showed benefit with the use of regional cooling during chemotherapy infusion (incidence 36% × 7.1%, $p = 0.0097$). However, as prior discussed, frozen gloves and socks are usually not well tolerated by patients; regarding NSAIDs, the risks and benefits of their use must be weighted; regarding dose reductions, it has direct impact on disease outcome [31, 32]. The use of emollients seemed promising, but with no statistically significant difference. Pyridoxine was not effective for prevention [31–33]. A small RCT showed benefits with the use of an antioxidant-containing ointment when compared to placebo on pegylated liposomal doxorubicin-treated patients [34]. For **HFSR**, one RCT showed a decreased incidence in any grade and >grade 2 reaction with the use of urea 10% cream compared to "best supportive care" (for any grade, OR 0.457, 95% CI 0.34–0.60, $p < 0.001$; for ≥grade 2, OR 0.635, 95% CI 0.46–0.86, $p = 0.004$). Results might be questioned, though, because "best supportive care" was indeed no preventive care [35, 36].

Recommended preventive measures are listed below [2, 4–6, 28, 29, 37]:

Preventive measures for acral reactions
Educate patients of early signs and symptoms
Use thick cotton gloves and/or socks
Apply emollient creams (urea-based emollients in hyperkeratotic type) to hands and feet regularly
Avoid irritants such as alcohol, harsh cleansing agents, and tight clothing and shoes
Avoid extremes of temperature, pressure, and friction (e.g., repetitive activities, stressful manual work, etc.)
For **HFSR,** also include a pretreatment evaluation with a podiatrist with callosity chopping and the use of orthopedic shoe inserts when needed

Treatment Low evidence exists on treatment measures. Dose reductions are effective but interferes with disease-related outcomes. One small prospective noncomparative trial showed improvement in QoL and decrease in **HFS** symptoms with the use of a topical nonocclusive polymer for 8 weeks [38]. For **HFSR**, one small randomized phase II trial showed benefit with the treatment of grade 1 toxicity with a hydrocolloid dressing containing ceramide with a low-friction external surface when compared to urea 10% cream (grades 2–3, 29% vs. 69%, $p = 0.03$) [39].

Recently, a systematic review showed benefits of different Chinese herbs on the treatment of acral toxicities. However, most of the studies were not blinded and with a lower quality [40, 41]. One case report and a small case series suggest benefits on the use of topical henna for capecitabine HFS [42, 43]. Besides the already mentioned preventive measures, recommendations of this board for the treatment of those toxicities include the following [2, 4–6, 9, 28, 29, 37]:

- Continuing the use of preventive measures.
- Maintaining the use of emollients and, on the case of **HFSR** and **PPE**, including the use of keratolytic agents (e.g., urea 10–40%, salicylic acid, etc.).
- Add a potent topical steroid.
- For relief of symptoms, cool compresses or emergence of hands and feet on cool water, topical anesthetics, and NSAIDs might be used.
- Dose reduction or treatment interruption is sometimes necessary until symptoms decrease.

Skin "Rashes"

One of the problems of better defining the dAE in many oncology trials is that frequently investigators report the different types of cutaneous eruptions as a skin "rash." Yet, as we will see, there are different types of cutaneous eruptions, associated with different classes of drugs and with different treatment options.

Acute Hypersensitivity Reactions Those type I immunoglobulin E-mediated reactions may occur within minutes to hours of infusion. They manifest as regular hypersensitivity reactions to conventional drugs, as pruritus, flushing, urticaria, and even anaphylaxis. The difference relies though on the way we deal with it. With conventional drugs, patients are usually oriented to avoid re-exposure. When dealing with oncologic treatments, the chemotherapeutic agent is fundamental for disease-related survival. Therefore, we usually maintain the drug for the next cycles and manage the reaction with a slower infusion, a premedication with corticosteroids and antihistamines before every infusion, and a closer monitoring [3, 5, 6].

Exanthema Many treatments may be related to a nonspecific maculopapular rash or morbilliform eruption that starts gradually, sometimes weeks after the start of drug, with mild symptoms such as pruritus. Those dAEs can be handled with antihistamines and topical corticosteroids when limited or with short courses of oral corticosteroids when more disseminated. All class of agents might cause those kind of reactions, such as kinase inhibitors (e.g., BRAFi—vemurafenib/kit—and BCR-ABL inhibitors: imatinib, dasatinib), "checkpoint" inhibitors (ipilimumab, nivolumab), and conventional chemotherapeutic agents (bleomycin, carboplatin, etoposide, etc.) [3, 5, 6]. Only on rare occasions, severe reactions such as toxic epidermal necrolysis (TEN), Steven-Johnson syndrome (SSJ), or drug rash with eosinophilia and systemic symptoms (DRESS) might occur, but it must be remembered that a maculopapular rash may represent the first manifestation of those life-threatening conditions. Special attention should be given when using a *targeted therapy after the use of an immunotherapy* (e.g., melanoma patients treated with immunotherapy and then switched to a BRAFi) as it may be associated with a higher risk of severe skin toxicity (>grade 3 and SSJ/TEN). Some authors suggest at least a 4-week interval between treatments with those agents [6, 44–46].

When a patient is on immunotherapy, skin adverse events to conventional drugs (e.g., antibiotics) might be more intense, so it is always important to exclude other causative agents, before relating the rash to the "checkpoint" inhibitor.

Toxic Erythema of Chemotherapy (TEC) This term is suggested by some authors to unify different manifestations such as HFS, intertriginous eruption of chemotherapy, or other used histopathologic terms such as "eccrine squamous syringometaplasia," all related to a direct toxicity of the chemotherapeutic agent and not due to an allergic reaction. This type of dAE is characterized by overlapping features of bilateral painful erythema, edema, and even bullous lesions located on hands and feet (see hand-foot syndrome) and sometimes also affecting intertriginous areas such as axilla and groins (less frequently ears, knees, and elbows) (Fig. 23.4). It is important to distinguish, because those manifestations are usually

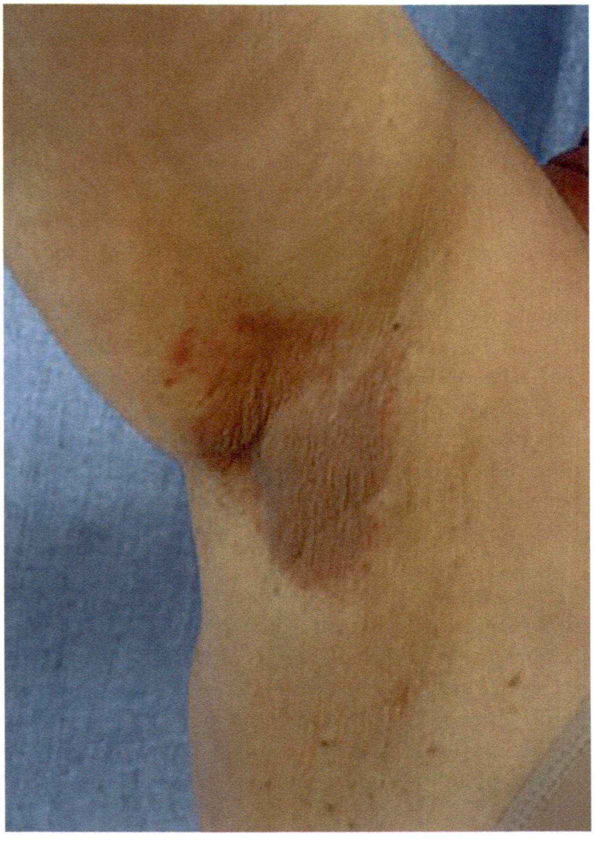

Fig. 23.4 Toxic erythema of chemotherapy or flexural eruption of chemotherapy on the axillar region. (Courtesy of Cristina Abdalla, MD)

self-limited, often resolving with desquamation and postinflammatory pigmentation and not demanding aggressive measures. In addition, lesions develop 2–3 weeks after the chemotherapy cycle, usually when patient's defenses are lower (e.g., neutropenia), being many times misdiagnosed as infections or graft-versus-host disease (GVHD). Treatment relies on topical corticosteroids and emollients and educating the patient about the nature of the manifestation. It often recrudesces on the subsequent cycles. It might be milder with dose reductions [18, 47].

Papulopustular Rash also known as "acne-like rash" or "folliculitis," is the most common dermatological toxicity of **EGFRi** treatment. It usually appears 1–2 weeks after initiation of therapy, starts with erythema, followed by the eruption of papules and pustules (sterile) on the face, scalp, upper chest, and back, with a lack of comedones (Fig. 23.5). Sometimes lesions extend to the limbs. Skin is usually dry, itchy, and sensible (patients refer sensation of burning, stinging, tenderness). This AE has a high impact on patient's QoL and on social aspects of daily living, being a cause of dose reduction or even treatment discontinuation. The rash tends to improve around the eighth week but usually persists as a milder eruption, with periods of improvement and worsening. Other features that are present, especially later on during treatment, are the already discussed paronychia, periungual fissures and granulomas, xerosis, pruritus and the yet to be discussed hair alterations such as trichomegaly, hypertrichosis, and non-scarring alopecia [5, 21–23, 48].

Prevention General daily baseline measures have already been discussed and are of great importance on this group of agents. They include the regular use of emollients, photoprotective measures (sun exposure might worsen the eruption), avoidance of irritating agents, limited shower time, and use of gentle cleansers. The use of systemic antibiotics (mostly tetracycline agents) on the first 6–8 weeks of treatment has been evaluated in some trials with discordant results. The available data suggest some benefit of the preventive treatment in decreasing the incidence and mainly the intensity of the papulopustular rash when compared to no treatment or even to the reactive treatment (started once the rash is already present) [24, 49, 50]. This is also the opinion of this expert panel. We suggest the use of oral tetracyclines (e.g., doxycycline 100 mg bid) during the first 6–8 weeks of treatment with EGFRi. On one randomized phase II trial, topical erythromycin was inferior to oral doxycycline for the prevention of EGFR skin toxicity [50]. Another trial showed some benefit with the preventive use of low-potency topical steroids, but we recommend their use only as a reactive treatment.

Treatment Despite the acne-like appearance*, topical agents used to treat acne* and acneiform eruptions such as benzoyl peroxide, retinoic acids, and salicylic acid containing products *are contraindicated*. If the rash occurs, preventive measures should be maintained, and to that, topical steroids can be added. If more pronounced and tetracycline was not started for prevention, it can now be initiated [5, 21, 22]. Sometimes dose reductions might be necessary. If there is excessive crusting or secretion, cultures are indicated to exclude secondary bacterial infection. In those

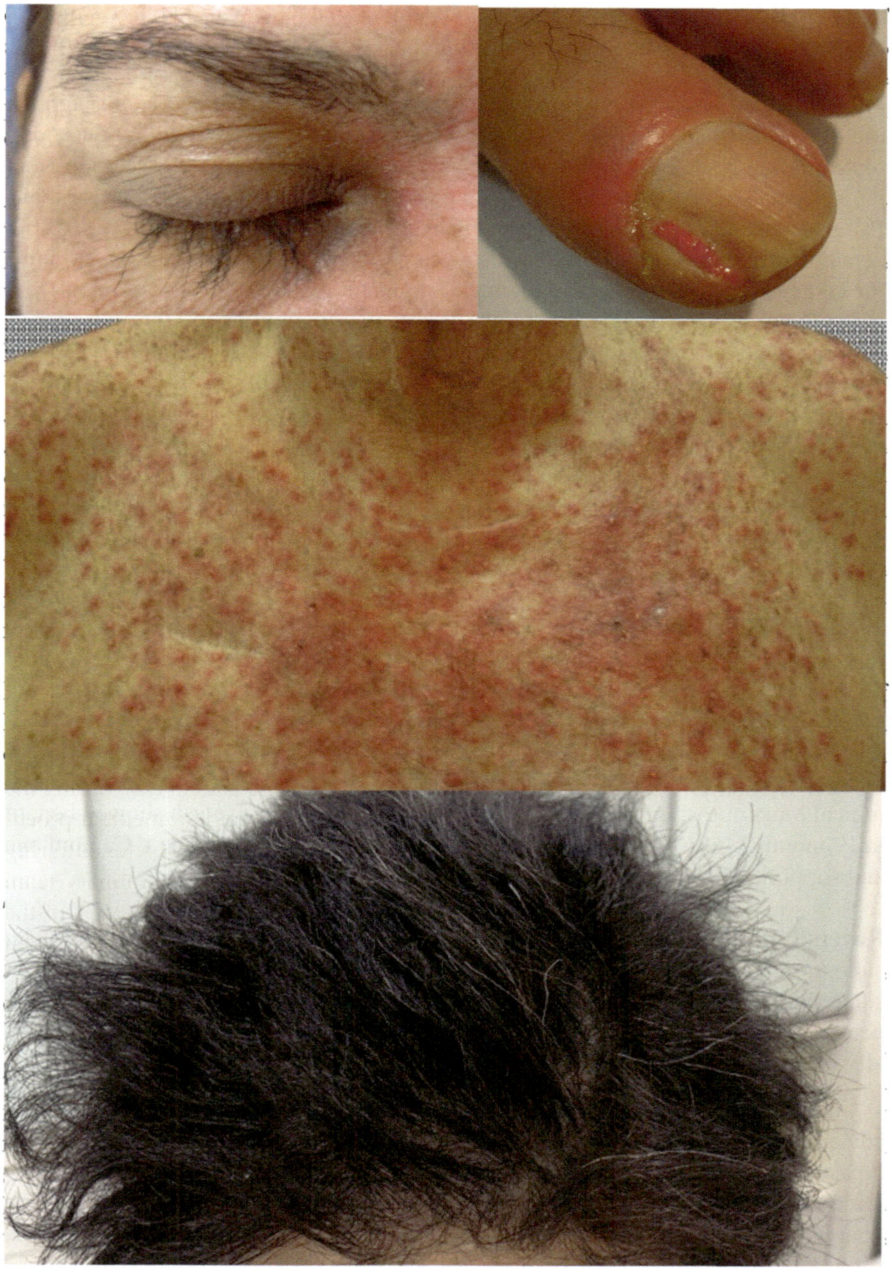

Fig. 23.5 EGFR-related adverse events: trichomegaly, paronychia, papulopustular eruption, and hair fragility. (Courtesy of Jade Cury-Martins, MD)

more prone to cause complete alopecia). Examples of agents with a high risk include cyclophosphamide, doxorubicin, irinotecan, and taxanes (docetaxel and paclitaxel).

Prevention A systematic review of preventive measures found no benefit with the use of topical minoxidil or scalp compression. Benefit was found with the use of a scalp cooling device (RR = 0.38, 95% CI 0.32–0.45, $p < 0.001$) [54–57]. Scalp cooling systems include static devices (cool caps) and dynamic scalp cooling systems. Patients should be warned that treatment efficacy is variable (around 50–80% depending on agent). Available data suggest that this technology is most effective for taxane-based chemotherapy regimens compared with anthracycline-based chemotherapy regimens [58]. Besides, the use of the cooling devices are not always well tolerated as they may cause symptoms like headache and scalp pain. Devices are also not reimbursable by insurance companies and might have a high cost. Recent studies have shown that the incidence of scalp metastasis is not increased in breast cancer patients with localized disease treated with scalp cooling [59, 60]. However, there are two reported cases of disease recurrence in patients with hematological malignancies (mycosis fungoides and acute myeloid leukemia) [61, 62]. Because of that, scalp cooling should be avoided in hematological malignancies [63].

Treatment Minoxidil was not effective in preventing CIA, but a small trial showed that minoxidil 2% was associated with a faster regrowth of hair (time to regrowth of 86 vs. 136 days on the placebo group) [64]. Other agents such as topical calcitriol are under investigation but still with no definitive results [2, 65]. Based on the studies and on authors' daily practice, we recommend the use of topical minoxidil 5% once daily after the end of the chemotherapy cycles. For eyebrows and eyelashes, topical bimatoprost might be used (one controlled study for eyelash showed benefit at 12 months) [66]. Biotin and other oral supplements might be added. Camouflage and support for patients are also important strategies.

Reversibility CIA is completely reversible in most of the cases. When incomplete/suboptimal hair regrowth occurs after 6 months of discontinuing therapy, it is considered a ***persistent CIA*** (pCIA). It has a usually diffuse, non-scaring pattern and occurs more often with pre-bone marrow transplantation high-dose regimens (usually busulfan and cyclophosphamide) or with taxanes [18, 67].

Another frequent pattern of persistent alopecia on cancer patients is described as ***endocrine therapy (ET)-induced alopecia***. For many hormone receptor-positive breast cancer survivors, selective estrogen receptor modulators (e.g., tamoxifen, toremifene), aromatase inhibitors (e.g., anastrozole, letrozole, exemestane), and gonadotropin-releasing hormone agonist (e.g., leuprolide) are usually administered for 5–10 years to reduce the risk of recurrence. This estrogen deprivation might lead to an androgenetic pattern alopecia. Topical minoxidil can be used. As for the use of systemic therapies for androgenic alopecia (e.g., spironolactone, finasteride), there is a putative risk of hormonal stimulation of endocrine receptor-positive tumors, so the use of these agents must be discussed with the oncologist and used with caution [63, 67].

Targeted Therapies Induced Hair Abnormalities Changes in hair quality, texture, and growth pattern might be seen around the second or third month of treatment.

- **Scalp**: Scalp hair grows slower and with a fragile quality (Fig. 23.5). A seborrheic dermatitis-like rash may develop (especially with VEGFRi and BRAFi). Also, the papulopustular rash affecting the face and trunk might involve the scalp (especially with EGFRi). Alopecia is usually mild and with an androgenetic pattern, but cases of inflammatory non-scarring alopecia have been described, as cases of erlotinib-induced cicatricial alopecia [4, 5].
- For those inflammatory changes, we suggest the use of anti-dandruff shampoos and topical corticosteroids (lotion or shampoo). If bacterial infection is suspected, culture-guided antibiotics are indicated.
- **Face, eyelashes, and eyebrow**: *Trichomegaly* (longer, thicker, and often curled eyelashes) (Fig. 23.5) and *hypertrichosis* are frequent. Inward eyelashes may result in keratitis; therefore, eyelash clipping is advised, and patients with ocular symptoms should be referred to an ophthalmologist. For hypertrichosis, topical, cosmetic interventions can be used (e.g., waxing or bleaching). When available laser and photoepilation treatments are most effective and are not contraindicated [65]. Creams for epilation should be avoided due to their sensitizing potential in those subjects that already have a skin barrier dysfunction.

Immunotherapy-Induced Hair Abnormalities Cases of alopecia with a clinical and histologic pattern consistent with *alopecia areata* (AA) have been reported. Patients should be treated similarly to non-oncologic AA cases. Also reports of hair depigmentation and repigmentation have been described. Even though we advise patients to avoid hair dyeing, it is not contraindicated, and if there is an important cosmetic concern, dyes might be used [65].

Changes in Melanocytic Nevi

BRAF Inhibitors might be associated to the appearance of eruptive melanocytic nevi (EMN), change of preexisting nevi (both the increase and acquisition of dermatoscopic structures, as well as the regression of nevi that have the BRAF mutation), and the appearance of new melanomas [68, 69]. Therefore, close dermatoscopic follow-up is recommended. The involution of BRAF inhibitor-induced EMN following the concomitant addition of MEK inhibitor has been described [70].

Immunotherapy Recently, regression of multiple melanocytic nevi after immunotherapy for melanoma has been described [71, 72].

Other Particular Toxicities

Epidermal Neoplasms Related to BRAF Inhibitors Keratoacanthomas, squamous cell carcinomas, and verrucal keratosis are common dAEs of BRAFi; they might also occur with some antiangiogenic agents. This is probably due to the paradoxical stimulation of the MAPK pathway in BRAF wild-type cells. When MEK inhibitors are used in association, this AE is much less frequent. Lesions can be treated with surgical excision (when only a few lesions are present), destructive treatments (cryotherapy, curettage, etc.), topical treatments (keratolytics, 5-FU, imiquimod), or photodynamic therapy [6].

Stomatitis

Stomatitis is the most common AE related to **mTOR inhibitors (rapamycin, everolimus, sirolimus)** and might be severe leading to dose adjustments. Different from conventional chemotherapy mucositis (broad ulceration with pseudo membrane formations), mTOR-related stomatitis manifests as discrete aphthae on non-keratinized epithelium. They can be handled with antiseptic washes, topical steroids, and anesthetics [6]. It has also been described more recently with FGFRi, occurring in about 12–58% [9].

Other Eruptions Related to Immunotherapy A nonspecific maculopapular rash, as reported above, represents the most prevalent type of immune-related adverse events (irAE) to this class of agents. However, peculiar types of reactions have been described and include the following [14]:

- Lichenoid reactions: Those eruptions can develop on both skin and/or mucosae (oral and genital). Oral involvement might also include xerostomia and taste change.
- Psoriasiform rash: These agents might induce exacerbation or new onset of psoriasis; for grade 3 or more, biologics or systemic retinoids might be added.
- Autoimmune bullous diseases: The development of autoimmune blistering disorders, especially bullous pemphigoid, have been reported (Fig. 23.6). For grade 3 or more, rituximab might be used.
- Sarcoidosis: Also reports of sarcoidosis (new onset or reactivation) are being recently published.
- Vitiligo: Immunotherapy has been linked to vitiligo-like lesions, mainly but not only in melanoma-treated patients [60].

A point of discussion is about whether the use of corticosteroids may antagonize the efficacy of immunotherapy. Current clinical data is limited and controversial. In some retrospective analyses, it was not associated with inferior responses to the oncologic treatment. A recent systematic review concluded that it "may not necessarily lead to poorer clinical outcomes" [73]. On the other hand, retrospective

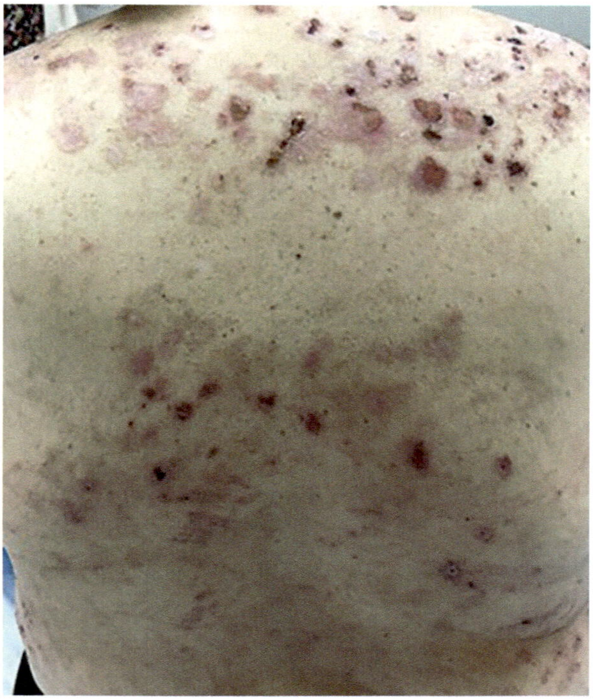

Fig. 23.6 Bullous eruption after immunotherapy. (Courtesy of Cristina Abdalla, MD)

analysis on lung cancer patients using corticosteroids at baseline or for irAE suggested a possible deleterious effect [74, 75]. Most of the current guidelines and expert panels do not contraindicate its use [6, 10–13]. As there are no definitive conclusions, we suggest that corticosteroids should be used with caution and always discussing its use with the rest of the team, especially the oncologists. For steroid-refractory cases, other immunomodulatory agents, such as mycophenolate, infliximab, methotrexate, and others, and also rituximab for blistering diseases might be necessary, and a few reports with their use have been published.

References

1. Bensadoun RJ, Humbert P, Krutman J, Luger T, Triller R, Rougier A, Seite S, Dreno B. Daily baseline skin care in the prevention, treatment, and supportive care of skin toxicity in oncology patients: recommendations from a multinational expert panel. Cancer Manag Res. 2013;5:401–8.
2. Balagula Y, Rosen ST, Lacouture ME. The emergence of supportive oncodermatology: the study of dermatologic adverse events to cancer therapies. J Am Acad Dermatol. 2011;65(3):624–35.
3. Reyes-Habito CM, Roh EK. Cutaneous reactions to chemotherapeutic drugs and targeted therapies for cancer: Part I. Conventional chemotherapeutic drugs. J Am Acad Dermatol. 2014;71(2):203.e1–203.e12.

4. Reyes-Habito CM, Roh EK. Cutaneous reactions to chemotherapeutic drugs and targeted therapy for cancer: Part II. Targeted therapy. J Am Acad Dermatol. 2014;71(2):217.e1–217.e11.
5. Macdonald JB, Macdonald B, Golitz LE, LoRusso P, Sekulic A. Cutaneous adverse effects of targeted therapies: Part I: Inhibitors of the cellular membrane. J Am Acad Dermatol. 2015;72(2):203–18.
6. Macdonald JB, Macdonald B, Golitz LE, LoRusso P, Sekulic A. Cutaneous adverse effects of targeted therapies: Part II: Inhibitors of intracellular molecular signaling pathways. J Am Acad Dermatol. 2015;72(2):221–36.
7. Tischer B, Huber R, Kraemer M, Lacouture ME. Dermatologic events from EGFR inhibitors: the issue of the missing patient voice. Support Care Cancer. 2017;25(2):651–60.
8. Gerber DE. Targeted therapies: a new generation of cancer treatments. Am Fam Physician. 2008;77(3):311–9.
9. Lacouture ME, Sibaud V, Anadkat MJ, et al. Dermatologic adverse events associated with selective fibroblast growth factor receptor inhibitors: overview, prevention, and management guidelines. Oncologist. 2021;26:e316–26.
10. Friedman CF, Proverbs-Singh TA, Postow MA. Treatment of the immune-related adverse effects of immune checkpoint inhibitors: a review. JAMA Oncol. 2016;2(10):1346–53.
11. Puzanov I, Diab A, Abdallah K, Bingham CO III, Brogdon C, Dadu R, Hamad L, Kim S, Lacouture ME, LeBoeuf NR, Lenihan D, Onofrei C, Shannon V, Sharma R, Silk AW, Skondra D, Suarez-Almazor ME, Wang Y, Wiley K, Kaufman HL, Ernstoff MS, Society for Immunotherapy of Cancer Toxicity Management Working Group. Managing toxicities associated with immune checkpoint inhibitors: consensus recommendations from the Society for Immunotherapy of Cancer (SITC) Toxicity Management Working Group. J Immunother Cancer. 2017;5(1):95.
12. Rapoport BL, van Eeden R, Sibaud V, Epstein JB, Klastersky J, Aapro M, Moodley D. Supportive care for patients undergoing immunotherapy. Support Care Cancer. 2017;25(10):3017–30.
13. Lacouture ME, Wolchok JD, Yosipovitch G, Kähler KC, Busam KJ, Hauschild A. Ipilimumab in patients with cancer and the management of dermatologic adverse events. J Am Acad Dermatol. 2014;71(1):161–9.
14. Geisler AN, Phillips GS, Barrios DM, et al. Immune checkpoint inhibitor related dermatologic adverse events. J Am Acad Dermatol. 2020;83:1255–68.
15. Valentine J, Belum VR, Duran J, Ciccolini K, Schindler K, Wu S, Lacouture ME. Incidence and risk of xerosis with targeted anticancer therapies. J Am Acad Dermatol. 2015;72(4):656–67.
16. Santoni M, Conti A, Andrikou K, Bittoni A, Lanese A, Pistelli M, Pantano F, Vincenzi B, Armento G, Massari F, Tonini G, Cascinu S, Santini D. Risk of pruritus in cancer patients treated with biological therapies: a systematic review and meta-analysis of clinical trials. Crit Rev Oncol Hematol. 2015;96(2):206–19.
17. Chan RJ, Webster J, Chung B, Marquart L, Ahmed M, Garantziotis S. Prevention and treatment of acute radiation-induced skin reactions: a systematic review and meta-analysis of randomized controlled trials. BMC Cancer. 2014;14:53.
18. Sibaud V, Lebœuf NR, Roche H, Belum VR, Gladieff L, Deslandres M, Montastruc M, Eche A, Vigarios E, Dalenc F, Lacouture ME. Dermatological adverse events with taxane chemotherapy. Eur J Dermatol. 2016;26(5):427–43.
19. Yin ES, Totonchy MB, Leventhal JS. Nivolumab-associated vitiligo-like depigmentation in a patient with acute myeloid leukemia: a novel finding. JAAD Case Rep. 2017;3(2):90–2.
20. Robert C, Sibaud V, Mateus C, Verschoore M, Charles C, Lanoy E, Baran R. Nail toxicities induced by systemic anticancer treatments. Lancet Oncol. 2015;16(4):e181–9.
21. Garden BC, Wu S, Lacouture ME. The risk of nail changes with epidermal growth factor receptor inhibitors: a systematic review of the literature and meta-analysis. J Am Acad Dermatol. 2012;67(3):400–8.
22. Burtness B, Anadkat M, Basti S, Hughes M, Lacouture ME, McClure JS, Myskowski PL, Paul J, Perlis CS, Saltz L, Spencer S. NCCN Task Force Report: Management of dermatologic and

other toxicities associated with EGFR inhibition in patients with cancer. J Natl Compr Cancer Netw. 2009;7(Suppl 1):S5–21.
23. Melosky B, Leighl NB, Rothenstein J, Sangha R, Stewart D, Papp K. Management of EGFR TKI-induced dermatologic adverse events. Curr Oncol. 2015;22(2):123–32.
24. Lacouture ME, Anadkat M, Jatoi A, Garawin T, Bohac C, Mitchell E. Dermatologic toxicity occurring during anti-EGFR monoclonal inhibitor therapy in patients with metastatic colorectal cancer: a systematic review. Clin Colorectal Cancer. 2018;17(2):85–96.
25. Dsouza PC, Kumar S. Role of systemic antibiotics in preventing epidermal growth factor receptor: tyrosine kinase inhibitors-induced skin toxicities. Asia Pac J Oncol Nurs. 2017;4(4):323–9.
26. Wnorowski AM, de Souza A, Chachoua A, Cohen DE. The management of EGFR inhibitor adverse events: a case series and treatment paradigm. Int J Dermatol. 2012;51(2):223–32.
27. Yen CF, Hsu CK, Lu CW. Topical betaxolol for treating relapsing paronychia with pyogenic granuloma-like lesions induced by epidermal growth factor receptor inhibitors. J Am Acad Dermatol. 2018;78:e143–4.
28. Lacouture ME, Wu S, Robert C, Atkins MB, Kong HH, Guitart J, Garbe C, Hauschild A, Puzanov I, Alexandrescu DT, Anderson RT, Wood L, Dutcher JP. Evolving strategies for the management of hand-foot skin reaction associated with the multitargeted kinase inhibitors sorafenib and sunitinib. Oncologist. 2008;13(9):1001–11.
29. Anderson R, Jatoi A, Robert C, Wood LS, Keating KN, Lacouture ME. Search for evidence-based approaches for the prevention and palliation of hand-foot skin reaction (HFSR) caused by the multikinase inhibitors (MKIs). Oncologist. 2009;14(3):291–302.
30. Flaherty KT, Brose MS. Sorafenib-related hand-foot skin reaction improves, not worsens, with continued treatment. Clin Cancer Res. 2009;15(24):7749.
31. Macedo LT, Lima JP, dos Santos LV, Sasse AD. Prevention strategies for chemotherapy-induced hand-foot syndrome: a systematic review and meta-analysis of prospective randomized trials. Support Care Cancer. 2014;22(6):1585–93.
32. Huang XZ, Chen Y, Chen WJ, Zhang X, Wu CC, Wang ZN, Wu J. Clinical evidence of prevention strategies for capecitabine-induced hand-foot syndrome. Int J Cancer. 2018;142(12):2567–77.
33. Yap YS, Kwok LL, Syn N, Chay WY, Chia JWK, Tham CK, Wong NS, Lo SK, Dent RA, Tan S, Mok ZY, Koh KX, Toh HC, Koo WH, Loh M, Ng RCH, Choo SP, Soong RCT. Predictors of hand-foot syndrome and pyridoxine for prevention of capecitabine-induced hand-foot syndrome: a randomized clinical trial. JAMA Oncol. 2017;3(11):1538–45.
34. Jung S, Sehouli J, Chekerov R, Kluschke F, Patzelt A, Fuss H, Knorr F, Lademann J. Prevention of palmoplantar erythrodysesthesia in patients treated with pegylated liposomal doxorubicin (Caelyx®). Support Care Cancer. 2017;25(11):3545–9.
35. Ren Z, Zhu K, Kang H, Lu M, Qu Z, Lu L, Song T, Zhou W, Wang H, Yang W, Wang X, Yang Y, Shi L, Bai Y, Guo X, Ye SL. Randomized controlled trial of the prophylactic effect of urea-based cream on sorafenib-associated hand-foot skin reactions in patients with advanced hepatocellular carcinoma. J Clin Oncol. 2015;33(8):894–900.
36. Negri FV, Porta C. Urea-based cream to prevent sorafenib-induced hand-and-foot skin reaction: which evidence? J Clin Oncol. 2015;33(28):3219–20.
37. von Moos R, Thuerlimann BJ, Aapro M, Rayson D, Harrold K, Sehouli J, Scotte F, Lorusso D, Dummer R, Lacouture ME, Lademann J, Hauschild A. Pegylated liposomal doxorubicin-associated hand-foot syndrome: recommendations of an international panel of experts. Eur J Cancer. 2008;44(6):781–90.
38. Fabbrocini G, Cristaudo A, Ionescu MA, Panariello L, Robert G, Pellicano M, Ayala F. Topical non-occlusive polymers in hand-foot syndrome. G Ital Dermatol Venereol. 2018;153(2):165–71.
39. Shinohara N, Nonomura N, Eto M, Kimura G, Minami H, Tokunaga S, Naito S. A randomized multicenter phase II trial on the efficacy of a hydrocolloid dressing containing ceramide with a low-friction external surface for hand-foot skin reaction caused by sorafenib in patients with renal cell carcinoma. Ann Oncol. 2014;25(2):472–6.
40. Deng B, Sun W. Herbal medicine for hand-foot syndrome induced by fluoropyrimidines: a systematic review and meta-analysis. Phytother Res. 2018;32:1211.

41. Tian A, Zhou A, Bi X, Hu S, Jiang Z, Zhang W, Huang Z, Shi H, Yang B, Chen W. Efficacy of topical compound danxiong granules for treatment of dermatologic toxicities induced by targeted anticancer therapy: a randomized, double-blind, placebo-controlled trial. Evid Based Complement Alternat Med. 2017;2017:3970601.
42. Yucel I, Guzin G. Topical henna for capecitabine induced hand-foot syndrome. Investig New Drugs. 2008;26(2):189–92.
43. Ilyas S, Wasif K, Saif MW. Topical henna ameliorated capecitabine-induced hand-foot syndrome. Cutan Ocul Toxicol. 2014;33(3):253–5.
44. Harding JJ, Pulitzer M, Chapman PB. Vemurafenib sensitivity skin reaction after ipilimumab. N Engl J Med. 2012;366(9):866–8.
45. Johnson DB, Wallender EK, Cohen DN, Likhari SS, Zwerner JP, Powers JG, Shinn L, Kelley MC, Joseph RW, Sosman JA. Severe cutaneous and neurologic toxicity in melanoma patients during vemurafenib administration following anti-PD-1 therapy. Cancer Immunol Res. 2013;1(6):373–7.
46. Ludlow SP, Pasikhova Y. Cumulative dermatologic toxicity with ipilimumab and vemurafenib responsive to corticosteroids. Melanoma Res. 2013;23(6):496–7.
47. Bolognia JL, Cooper DL, Glusac EJ. Toxic erythema of chemotherapy: a useful clinical term. J Am Acad Dermatol. 2008;59(3):524–9.
48. Chanprapaph K, Vachiramon V, Rattanakaemakorn P. Epidermal growth factor receptor inhibitors: a review of cutaneous adverse events and management. Dermatol Res Pract. 2014;2014:734249.
49. Lacouture ME, Keefe DM, Sonis S, Jatoi A, Gernhardt D, Wang T, Doherty JP, Giri N, Nadanaciva S, O'Connell J, Sbar E, Piperdi B, Garon EB. A phase II study (ARCHER 1042) to evaluate prophylactic treatment of dacomitinib-induced dermatologic and gastrointestinal adverse events in advanced non-small-cell lung cancer. Ann Oncol. 2016;27(9):1712–8.
50. Kripp M, Prasnikar N, Vehling-Kaiser U, Quidde J, Al-Batran SE, Stein A, Neben K, Hannig CV, Tessen HW, Trarbach T, Hinke A, Hofheinz RD. AIO LQ-0110: a randomized phase II trial comparing oral doxycycline versus local administration of erythromycin as preemptive treatment strategies of panitumumab-mediated skin toxicity in patients with metastatic colorectal cancer. Oncotarget. 2017;8(62):105061–71.
51. Requena C, Llombart B, Sanmartín O. Acneiform eruptions induced by epidermal growth factor receptor inhibitors: treatment with oral isotretinoin. Cutis. 2012;90(2):77–80.
52. Woods JA, Ferguson JS, Kalra S, Degabriele A, Gardner J, Logan P, Ferguson J. The phototoxicity of vemurafenib: an investigation of clinical monochromator phototesting and in vitro phototoxicity testing. J Photochem Photobiol B. 2015;151:233–8.
53. Zimmer L, Vaubel J, Livingstone E, Schadendorf D. Side effects of systemic oncological therapies in dermatology. J Dtsch Dermatol Ges. 2012;10(7):475–86.
54. Shin H, Jo SJ, Kim DH, Kwon O, Myung SK. Efficacy of interventions for prevention of chemotherapy-induced alopecia: a systematic review and meta-analysis. Int J Cancer. 2015;136(5):E442–54.
55. Vasconcelos I, Wiesske A, Schoenegg W. Scalp cooling successfully prevents alopecia in breast cancer patients undergoing anthracycline/taxane-based chemotherapy. Breast. 2018;40:1–3.
56. Shah VV, Wikramanayake TC, DelCanto GM, van den Hurk C, Wu S, Lacouture ME, Jimenez JJ. Scalp hypothermia as a preventative measure for chemotherapy-induced alopecia: a review of controlled clinical trials. J Eur Acad Dermatol Venereol. 2018;32(5):720–34.
57. Nangia J, Wang T, Osborne C, Niravath P, Otte K, Papish S, Holmes F, Abraham J, Lacouture M, Courtright J, Paxman R, Rude M, Hilsenbeck S, Osborne CK, Rimawi M. Effect of a scalp cooling device on alopecia in women undergoing chemotherapy for breast cancer: the SCALP randomized clinical trial. JAMA. 2017;317(6):596–605.
58. Kruse M, Abraham J. Management of chemotherapy-induced alopecia with scalp cooling. J Oncol Pract. 2018;14(3):149–54.
59. Rugo HS, Klein P, Melin SA, et al. Association between use of a scalp cooling device and alopecia after chemotherapy for breast cancer. JAMA. 2017;317(6):606–14.

60. Rugo HS, Voigt J. Scalp hypothermia for preventing alopecia during chemotherapy. A systematic review and meta-analysis of randomized controlled trials. Clin Breast Cancer. 2018;18(1):19–28.
61. Witman G, Cadman E, Chen M. Misuse of scalp hypothermia. Cancer Treat Rep. 1981;65(5–6):507–8.
62. Forsberg SA. Scalp cooling therapy and cytotoxic treatment. Lancet. 2001;357(9262):1134.
63. Rubio-Gonzalez B, Juhász M, Fortman J, Mesinkovska NA. Pathogenesis and treatment options for chemotherapy-induced alopecia: a systematic review. Int J Dermatol. 2018;57:1417.
64. Yeager CE, Olsen EA. Treatment of chemotherapy-induced alopecia. Dermatol Ther. 2011;24(4):432–42.
65. Freites-Martinez A, Shapiro J, Goldfarb S, Nangia J, Jimenez JJ, Paus R, Lacouture ME. CME Part 1: Hair disorders in cancer patients. J Am Acad Dermatol. 2019;80(5):1179–96.
66. Glaser DA, Hossain P, Perkins W, Griffiths T, Ahluwalia G, Weng E, Beddingfield FC. Long-term safety and efficacy of bimatoprost solution 0.03% application to the eyelid margin for the treatment of idiopathic and chemotherapy-induced eyelash hypotrichosis: a randomized controlled trial. Br J Dermatol. 2015;172(5):1384–94.
67. Freites-Martinez A, Shapiro J, van den Hurk C, Goldfarb S, Jimenez J, Rossi AM, Paus R, Lacouture ME. CME Part 2: Hair disorders in cancer survivors persistent chemotherapy-induced alopecia, persistent radiotherapy-induced alopecia, and hair growth disorders related to endocrine therapy or cancer surgery. J Am Acad Dermatol. 2018; https://doi.org/10.1016/j.jaad.2018.03.056.
68. Göppner D, Müller J, Krüger S, et al. High incidence of naevi-associated BRAF wild-type melanoma and dysplastic naevi under treatment with the class I BRAF inhibitor vemurafenib. Acta Derm Venereol. 2014;94(5):517–20.
69. Perier-Muzet M, Thomas L, Poulalhon N, et al. Melanoma patients under vemurafenib: prospective follow-up of melanocytic lesions by digital dermoscopy. J Invest Dermatol. 2014;134(5):1351–8.
70. Chen FW, Tseng D, Reddy S, Daud AI, Swetter SM. Involution of eruptive melanocytic nevi on combination BRAF and MEK inhibitor therapy. JAMA Dermatol. 2014;150(11):1209–12.
71. Libon F, Arrese JE, Rorive A, Nikkels AF. Ipilimumab induces simultaneous regression of melanocytic naevi and melanoma metastases. Clin Exp Dermatol. 2013;38(3):276–9.
72. Burillo-Martinez S, Morales-Raya C, Prieto-Barrios M, Rodriguez-Peralto JL, Ortiz-Romero PL. Pembrolizumab-induced extensive panniculitis and nevus regression: two novel cutaneous manifestations of the post-immunotherapy granulomatous reactions spectrum. JAMA Dermatol. 2017;153(7):721–2.
73. Garant A, Guilbault C, Ekmekjian T, et al. Concomitant use of corticosteroids and immune checkpoint inhibitors in patients with hematologic or solid neoplasms: a systematic review. Crit Rev Oncol Hematol. 2017;120:86–92.
74. Arbour KC, Mezquita L, Long N, et al. Impact of baseline steroids on efficacy of programmed cell death-1 and programmed death-ligand 1 blockade in patients with non-small-cell lung cancer. J Clin Oncol. 2018;36(28):2872–8.
75. Scott SC, Pennell NA. Early use of systemic corticosteroids in patients with advanced NSCLC treated with nivolumab. J Thorac Oncol. 2018;13(11):1771–5.

Chapter 24
Cutaneous Malignancies in the Immunocompromised Patient

Walmar Roncalli Pereira de Oliveira, Marcela Soares Pincelli, Isadora Zago Miotto, and Paula Yume Sato Serzedello Correa

Key Points

- Immunosuppressed patients are at a higher risk for aggressive cutaneous malignancies with worse outcomes.
- Cutaneous cancer is the most frequent malignancy posttransplantation, 95% of which correspond to nonmelanoma skin cancer (NMSC), especially squamous cell carcinoma (SCC) and basal cell carcinoma (BCC).
- Immunosuppressed patients should be routinely evaluated and screened for preneoplastic lesions and should be oriented regarding strict daily sun protection.
- Immunosuppressed hosts are unable to mount an adequate immune response and therefore are more prone to developing HPV-associated neoplasms.
- Multiple factors may contribute to the increased incidence of malignancy in patients infected with HIV: immunosuppression, direct effects of the HIV virus itself, coinfection with oncogenic viruses, environmental factors, and possibly the use of antiretroviral therapy.

W. R. P. de Oliveira (✉) · M. S. Pincelli · I. Z. Miotto · P. Y. S. S. Correa
Dermatology, University of São Paulo Medical School, São Paulo, Brazil
e-mail: walmar.roncalli@hc.fm.usp.br

C. M. Z. Abdalla et al. (eds.), *Oncodermatology*,
https://doi.org/10.1007/978-3-031-29277-4_24

Introduction

The immunosuppressed population is a peculiar high-risk group for aggressive cutaneous malignancies with worse outcomes. This population comprises a variety cohort of patients comprising solid organ transplant recipients (SOTRs) as well as patients with chronic lymphoid malignancies, patients infected with human immunodeficiency virus (HIV)/acquired immunodeficiency syndrome (AIDS), and autoimmune diseases. Immunosuppressed patients present clinical distinct forms of skin cancers compared to immunocompetent individuals with greater morbidity and mortality. The most common skin cancers are keratinocyte carcinomas, which often present with more aggressive features and have a greater rate of metastasis. The incidence of malignant melanoma, Merkel cell carcinoma, and Kaposi sarcoma are also higher in the immunosuppressed patient's cohort [1]. Most tumors with strongly increased incidence rates in immunocompromised patients have been found to have a viral etiology; among these are Kaposi sarcoma, Merkel cell carcinoma, B-cell lymphomas, and squamous cell carcinomas [2]. The American Joint Committee on Cancer Staging eighth edition now acknowledges the poorer prognosis of cutaneous squamous cell carcinoma in the immunosuppressed population, but further studies are necessary to fully delineate the impact of immune status on prognosis [3].

Skin Cancer in Solid Organ Transplant Recipients

SOTRs are at a higher risk of skin malignancies due to their long-term immunosuppressive state. As the number of these patients is increasing, as well as their life expectancy, skin cancer has been recognized as an important problem. Cutaneous cancer is the most frequent malignancy posttransplantation, 95% of which correspond to nonmelanoma skin cancer (NMSC), especially squamous cell carcinoma (SCC) and basal cell carcinoma (BCC). Indeed, SOTRs are very sensitive to sun damage due to their lifelong immunosuppression, which results in field cancerization with numerous lesions such as actinic keratosis (AK), in situ SCC, and Bowen's disease [4, 5]. SOTRs also present a high risk for development of other skin tumors such as malignant melanoma, Kaposi sarcoma, Merkel cell carcinoma, atypical fibroxanthoma, and cutaneous B- and T-cell lymphomas. Many elements are considered to be at play in the evolution of skin cancers in transplant recipients: immunosuppressive therapy, lifespan since transplantation, the role of oncogenic viruses, duration and intensity of exposure to ultraviolet radiation (UVR) prior to transplantation, fair skin complexion, male gender, and age at transplantation [4–6].

Long-term immunosuppression in SOTRs leads to decreased tumor immunosurveillance and development of malignancies. A delicate balance between intensity of immunosuppression, allograft function, and risk of complications must be maintained [7].

Actinic Keratosis (AK) and Field Cancerization (FC)

Actinic keratosis are common sun-induced lesions that result from the proliferation of atypical keratinocytes. AKs represent early lesions on a continuum with SCC that present as erythematous and scaly macules or papules, mostly detected in adults with fair skin [8].

The term field cancerization is used to describe the presence of multifocal clinical and subclinical atypical lesions, including AKs and SCCs, in a skin area with chronic ultraviolet radiation exposure. Sun damage indicative of field cancerization is clinically identified by the presence of skin atrophy, dyspigmentation, telangiectasia, and sandpaper-like texture (Figs. 24.1 and 24.2) [9].

Risk factors for developing AK, FC, and SCC are similar and include exposure to ultraviolet radiation, increasing age, fair skin, male gender, and immunosuppression [9]. SOTRs are at a high risk for the development of AKs, and the likelihood of an AK lesion progressing to invasive SCC is higher in SOTRs than in the general population, although the exact progression rates have not been identified. Decreased immunosurveillance allows for high rates of skin tumorigenesis [9, 10].

A cohort of over 450 SOTRs showed a 17% prevalence rate of FC, which increased with the length of immunosuppression. Furthermore, SOTRs who present with FC are four times more likely to develop SCCs than those with isolated AKs [9, 11]. Given the confluent nature of actinic damage, patients with FC are at a higher risk of SCC development compared to patients with multiple yet isolated AKs [9]. The overall transformation rate of a single AK to SCC ranges between 0% and 0.075% per year and up to 0.5% in patients with a previous history of skin cancer [11].

Gene mutations caused by chronic ultraviolet radiation are the main driver of FC, with p53 being identified in more than 90% of specimens. P53 plays critical roles in both apoptosis and cell cycle arrestment after DNA damage. These mutations can be found in clinically normal sun-exposed skin, as well as in photodamaged skin and AKs, but are nearly absent in sun-protected areas [9].

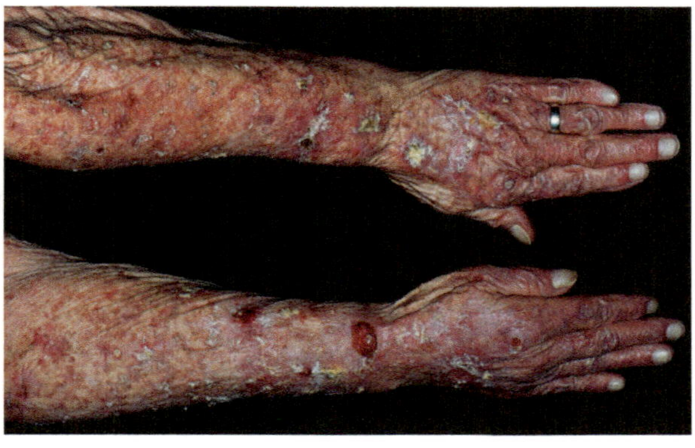

Fig. 24.1 Field cancerization on the forearms: multiple actinic keratoses and squamous cell carcinomas in an area with extensive chronic ultraviolet radiation exposure. (Courtesy of Walmar Roncalli Pereira de Oliveira, MD)

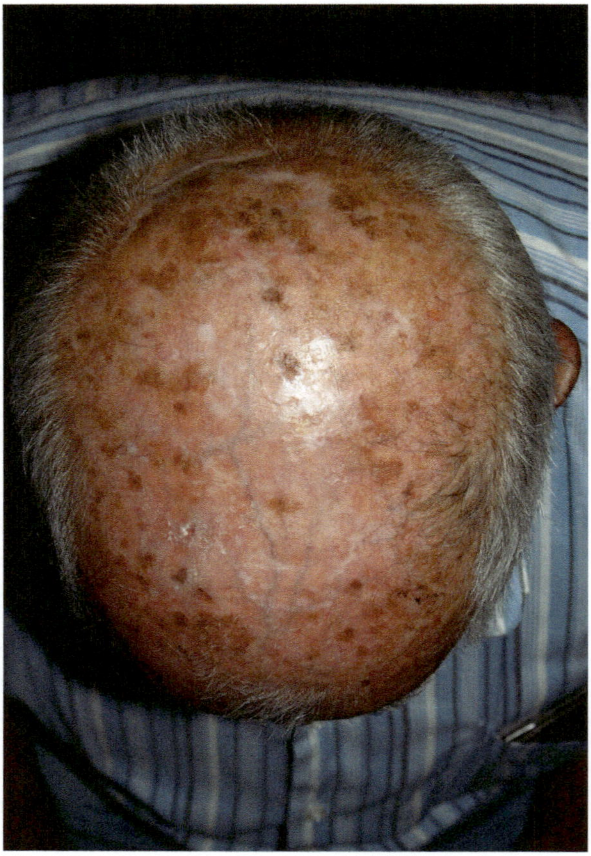

Fig. 24.2 Extensive sun-induced skin damage on the scalp of an elderly patient. (Courtesy of Walmar Roncalli Pereira de Oliveira, MD)

Management: AK, Field Cancerization, and In Situ SCC

Immunosuppressed patients should be routinely evaluated and screened for preneoplastic lesions and should be oriented regarding strict daily sun protection. Large areas of extensive actinic damage may represent subclinical lesions of epidermal dysplasia and should be frequently biopsied [7]. Recognition and treatment of FC before transformation to SCC leads to significant morbidity reduction [9].

Individual AK lesions are most commonly treated with liquid nitrogen cryotherapy [7]. In patients with multiple lesions or involvement of a large skin area (cancerization field), topical therapies such as 5-fluorouracil (5-FU) and imiquimod should be considered [7, 11].

5-FU inhibits thymidylate synthetase, which subsequently interferes with DNA synthesis and leads to cell death. It can be used either alone or in combination with topical tretinoin or alpha-hydroxy acids in order to decrease the thickness of the stratum corneum and increase drug penetration [12]. In a study of kidney transplant recipients treated with 5-FU twice daily for 3 weeks, the mean AK clearance rate was 98% at 8 weeks and 79% at 12 months [8].

Imiquimod is an immunomodulatory agent that has both antitumor and antiviral properties. It activates Toll-like receptor 7 and stimulates innate immune response [12]. The use of imiquimod was initially limited in SOTRs due to a concern about the drug's potential of inducing allograft rejection. However, recent studies have suggested that it is relatively safe and effective in this population [10, 13]. One study has shown that when applied to limited areas (less than 100 cm^2), imiquimod is able to achieve an AK clearance rate of 62%, without deterioration of graft function [14].

For SOTRs with involvement of a large skin area, photodynamic therapy (PDT) may be a suitable option. This therapeutic modality involves the administration of a precursor of photosensitizer protoporphyrin IX that is activated by light and attacks malignant cells [4]. A study of kidney transplant recipients showed a complete AK clearance rate of 71% after two sessions [15]. The most limiting aspects of PDT are pain and prolonged photosensitivity [7, 16].

Squamous Cell Carcinoma (SCC)

SOTRs are 65–200 times more likely to develop SCC when compared to general population. Tumors tend to be more aggressive and are more commonly poorly differentiated on histological analysis [7]. A study showed a local recurrence rate of 14.1% within the first 19 months and a risk of metastases of 3–8% in this population [17, 18].

SCC can develop on any cutaneous surface, and in fair-skinned individuals, it is more common in sun-exposed sites. In situ SCC (Bowen's disease) usually presents as an asymptomatic erythematous scaly patch or plaque that tends to grow slowly, over the course of years. The clinical appearance of invasive SCC correlates to the tumor differentiation level. Well-differentiated lesions usually appear as firm hyperkeratotic papules, plaques, or nodules, whereas poorly differentiated lesions tend to be fleshy and less hyperkeratotic, often resembling pyogenic granuloma, and may present with ulceration, hemorrhage, and areas of necrosis (Figs. 24.3 and 24.4) [7, 19].

Pretransplantation SCC is the strongest predictor of posttransplant SCC risk. Other significant factors include the presence of actinic keratosis and human papillomavirus infection. Some observational studies suggest a higher risk of squamous cell carcinoma in the heart, lung, and combined pancreas-kidney transplant recipients, when compared with liver and kidney transplant recipients. Elderly patients and patients with lighter skin (Fitzpatrick skin phototypes I to III) are at the highest risk of keratinocyte carcinoma, due to the prolonged sun exposure. Patients must be educated about sunlight avoidance and sunscreen use [7].

Duration, intensity, and choice of immunosuppression are also important factors. Patients treated with cyclosporine in a three-drug combination are at a higher risk of

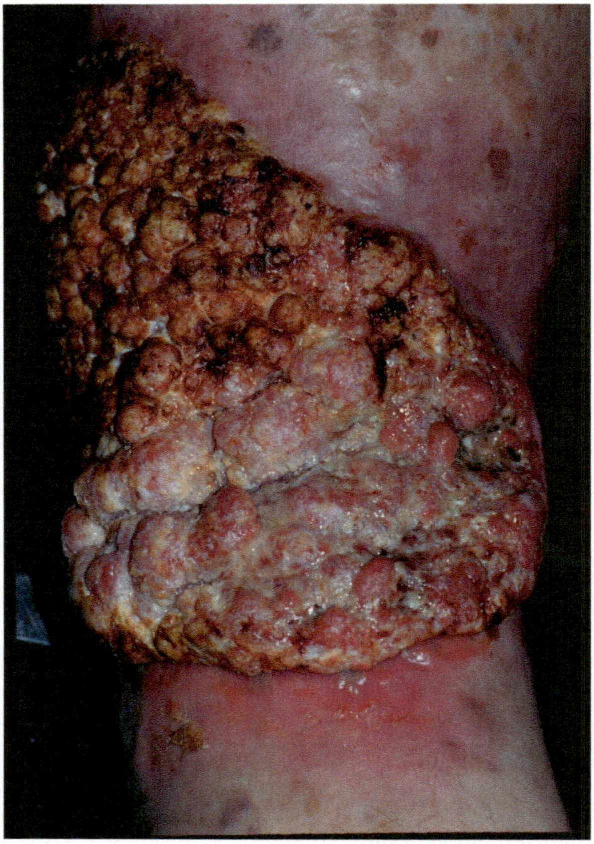

Fig. 24.3 Invasive squamous cell carcinoma: a large exophytic growing tumor on the leg of an immunosuppressed patient. (Courtesy of Walmar Roncalli Pereira de Oliveira, MD)

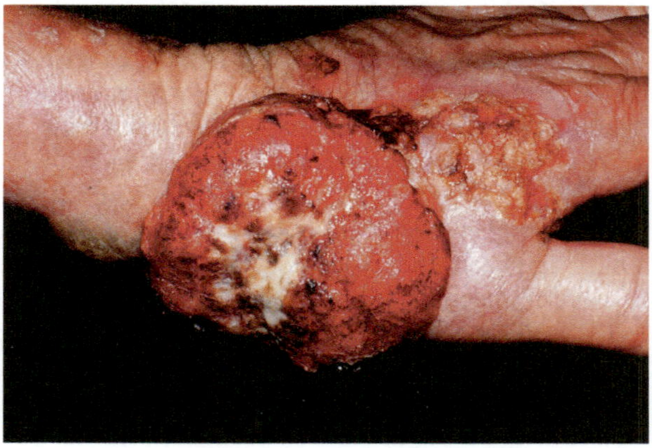

Fig. 24.4 Invasive squamous cell carcinoma: an extensive ulcerated tumor on the hand. (Courtesy of Walmar Roncalli Pereira de Oliveira, MD)

developing SCC, but the impact of specific immunosuppressive regimen remains unclear [7]. Some studies have demonstrated that a conversion from calcineurin inhibitors to sirolimus led to a reduction of SCC development risk [20, 21].

The pathogenesis of SCC in SOTRs is complex and involves multiple factors. Ultraviolet radiation is a potent carcinogen that causes both local and systemic immunosuppression. When combined with the chronic pharmacologic immunosuppression used in SOTRs, it leads to a significantly reduced capacity for immune-mediated tumor surveillance and an increased risk of carcinogenesis [7].

The immunosuppressive agents used after transplantation also contribute to the initiation and promotion of skin cancers. One mechanism is through the inhibition of the calcineurin pathway that results in activation of transcription factor 3, a member of the activation protein-1 (AP-1) family, which plays an important role in suppressing p53-mediated cell death and leads to carcinogenesis [7].

Cyclosporine causes resistance to UV-induced apoptosis in human keratinocytes. Normally, keratinocyte mitochondria respond to oxidative stress caused by UV radiation by opening mitochondrial permeability transition pores (MPTP). Studies have shown that cyclosporine inhibits MPTPs from opening and allows toxic insults to propagate [7]. Cyclosporine may also be involved in tumor growth and invasion by inducing the production of growth factors, such as TGF-β [7].

Azathioprine has been shown to worsen UV-induced damage through the incorporation of metabolites into DNA and the generation of reactive oxygen species. In contrast, mycophenolate mofetil (MMF) and tacrolimus have a lower relative risk of skin cancer [7].

Management: Invasive SCC

Lesions suspicious for invasive SCC should be promptly biopsied. Before surgery, patients with high-risk SCCs should be evaluated as to their metastatic potential, once tumors tend to be more aggressive and to have a worse treatment outcome in immunosuppressed patients [12]. For deep tumors in high-risk areas, additional imaging scans (computed tomographic/magnetic resonance) may be performed to evaluate deep extension and nodal involvement [4]. The most effective treatment options for invasive SCC include Mohs micrographic surgery (MMS), surgical excision with intraoperative frozen sections and margin control, and surgical excision with wide margins [7].

MMS has the highest cure rate, given its capacity of evaluating 100% of peripheral and deep margins. When surgical excision is performed, the recommendations for margins depend on the presence of high-risk tumor features (poor differentiation, perineural invasion, and high-risk anatomical locations). Margins of 6–10 mm and resection into the subcutaneous fat are recommended for immunosuppressed patients with high-risk features. However, in certain anatomical locations such as the face or the hands, margins of 6–10 mm may be impractical and smaller margins may are justified [4, 7].

Adjuvant radiation therapy is indicated in high-risk tumors, inoperable or partially excised tumors, tumors with an extensive perineural invasion, and in patients unable to tolerate surgery [12].

As the incidence of SCCs in SOTRs is directly related to the intensity and duration of immunosuppressive therapy, a reduction may be considered in case of the development of multiple or high-risk and life-threatening tumors [7, 22]. Immunosuppression can be modified by a dose reduction or a switch of drug class. For patients with stable graft function, a conversion from calcineurin inhibitors to inhibitors of the mammalian target of rapamycin (mTOR inhibitors) may be considered, once the latter confer a lower carcinogenic risk and have the ability to partially reverse the oncogenic effects of other immunosuppressive agents [12, 23].

Patients who develop multiple SCCs (more than 5 per year) or who develop aggressive or early-onset tumors may be evaluated for chemoprophylaxis [4, 7]. Systemic retinoids can reduce and delay the recurrence of SCCs and should be considered as a long-term treatment, once its preventive effects are lost, and once the drug is discontinued. Thus, it is important to counsel patients regarding long-term side effects of retinoids that may reduce life quality, including disorders of the musculoskeletal system [24, 25].

Nicotinamide, a vitamin B3 analogue, is another drug currently being considered for SCC and AK chemoprophylaxis in SOTRs. It enhances DNA repair and decreases ultraviolet-induced inflammation [7, 12]. A phase 3 randomized trial showed a reduction in the SCC rate of 30% related to the drug intake [26]. However, a recent trial in kidney transplant recipients demonstrated no significant SCC and AK reduction [27]. Given the conflicting data, further studies are needed in order to access the effectiveness of nicotinamide in SOTRs [28].

Capecitabine is an oral chemotherapy prodrug that metabolizes to 5-FU. It is recommended for SOTRs who develop more than two SCCs in 6 months or at least 10 new AKs in 12 months. It can also be used in patients who develop further NMSCs despite treatment with oral retinoids, PDT, and optimization of immunosuppressive therapy [7, 12].

In patients with metastatic cutaneous SCC, systemic chemotherapy is recommended. Cisplatin and 5-FU have shown clinical efficacy [7]. Immunotherapy with cetuximab, a monoclonal antibody that competitively inhibits the epidermal growth factor, is a therapeutic option. However, most studies were conducted in nontransplant populations, and clinical experience in SOTRs is limited [7, 29].

Checkpoint inhibitors, including anti-cytotoxic T lymphocyte-associated protein 4 (anti-CTLA-4) and anti-programmed death 1 (anti-PD-1), such as cemiplimab, have been shown to be effective against solid tumors in SOTRs and should be considered for advanced or metastatic disease [30]. Although these therapies are promising, they should be used with caution, given the potential risk of graft rejection related to PD-1 inhibitors [12].

Human Papillomavirus (HPV) Infection and Cutaneous Malignancies

HPVs are double-strained DNA viruses with over 100 serotypes described, which infect keratinocytes of the skin and mucosa. The virus carcinogenicity properties are mostly related to the capacity of its oncoproteins (especially E6 and E7) to inhibit the function of human tumor suppressor proteins p53 and pRb [31, 32].

A balance between viral infectivity and host response is maintained by the host immune system. An antigen-dependent response is essential to control viral infections and virally transformed cells that may evolve into malignancies. Immunosuppressed hosts are unable to mount an adequate immune response and therefore are more prone to developing HPV-associated neoplasms [31].

Alpha-papillomaviruses are mostly associated with anogenital or oropharyngeal lesions and can be divided into low-risk and high-risk types regarding their malignant potential. Almost 100% of cervix cancers, 85% of anal cancers, 70% of oropharyngeal cancers, and 50% of cancers of the vagina, vulva, and penis are attributable to α-HPVs (Fig. 24.5) [31].

Beta-papillomaviruses are ubiquitous commensals that can cause widespread asymptomatic infections. β-HPVs tend to cause preneoplastic and neoplastic skin lesions, especially in immunosuppressed hosts. β-HPV DNA is detectable in up to 90% of SCCs in SOTRs, in contrast to 30% from immunocompetent individuals. Positive correlations between β-HPV viral load and time since transplantation are consistent with a direct causal role of these HPV subtypes in posttransplant cutaneous SCCs [7, 31, 32].

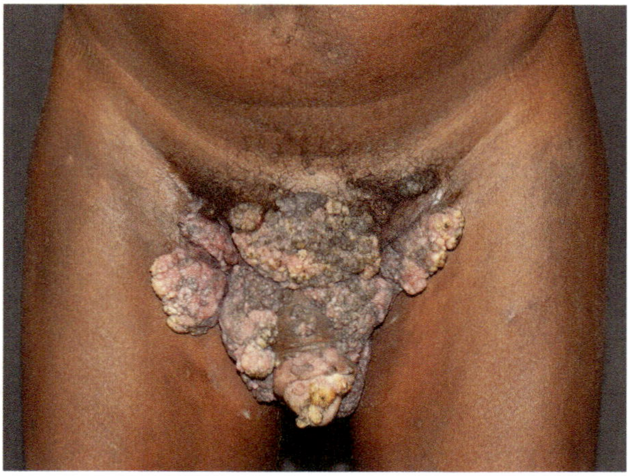

Fig. 24.5 Squamous cell carcinoma related to HPV infection in an immunosuppressed host: an extensive tumor with exophytic growth on the genital area. (Courtesy of Walmar Roncalli Pereira de Oliveira, MD)

Current HPV vaccines target α-HPV serotypes that cause anogenital and oropharyngeal tumors, and suboptimal responses have been shown on the immunogenicity of HPV vaccines in SOTRs. Novel vaccines that could potentially offer cross-reactivity against β-HPV could lead to better outcomes in this population, especially if administrated pretransplantation [12].

Epidermodysplasia Verruciformis-Like Syndrome

Epidermodysplasia verruciformis (EV) is a rare genodermatosis characterized by β-HPV infection (mostly HPV types 5 and 8) of the skin. The disease is clinically manifested by the presence of extensive flat warts and scaly erythematous macules that resemble pityriasis versicolor. Lesions are more frequently observed in sun-exposed sites and may transform into SCC in about 30% of cases [32, 33].

An EV-like syndrome may occur in immunosuppressed patients, such as SOTRs and HIV carriers, who have an acquired predisposition to HPV infection. The same dermatological findings that characterize the genodermatosis are found in this population (Fig. 24.6). The viral carcinogen potential combined with ultraviolet radiation exposure is related to an elevated risk of development of premalignant and malignant skin lesions, such as AK and SCC [32, 33].

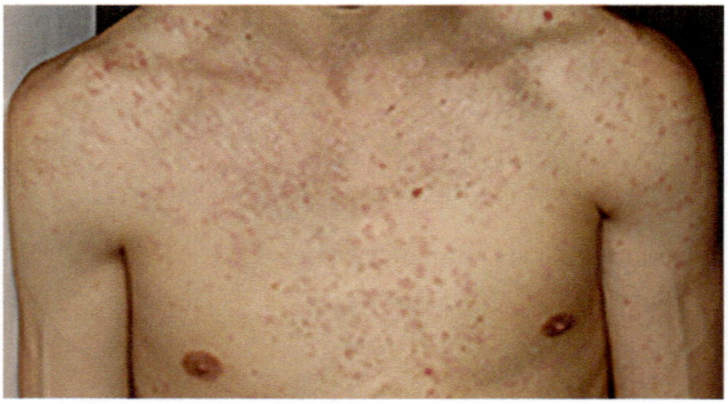

Fig. 24.6 Epidermodysplasia verruciformis-like syndrome: multiple flat warts on the chest of an immunosuppressed patient. (Courtesy of Walmar Roncalli Pereira de Oliveira, MD, PhD)

Basal Cell Carcinoma (BCC)

BCC accounts for 80% of all NMSC and is the most common malignancy in humans, with an increasing incidence related to chronic sun exposure and to the elderly [34]. Compared to the general population, SOTRs are 10–16 times more likely to develop BCC. Also, patients who develop BCC after transplantation are at a higher risk of developing additional lesions during follow-up [7, 35].

BCC is more common in individuals with fair skin complexion, and lesions are more frequent on sun-exposed areas. Although SOTRs are at a higher risk of developing BCC, tumors do not appear to be more aggressive in this population [7, 12].

Tumors may present as pink and pearly papules, nodules, or scar-like plaques that occur predominantly on the face, trunk, and upper limbs (Fig. 24.7). BCCs are indolent malignancies that rarely metastasizes but can be locally destructive and cause great morbidity [7].

Management

The current standard therapies for BCC in immunosuppressed patients are similar to those used in the general population. Surgical excision with wide margins, surgical excision with intraoperative frozen sections, and MMS are commonly performed and remain the treatment of choice in most cases [7].

Nonsurgical interventions and destructive methods such as cryotherapy, PDT, electrodessication after curettage, and topical treatments including 5-FU and imiquimod cream are also beneficial, especially for the treatment of low-risk BCCs, like the superficial variant [34, 36].

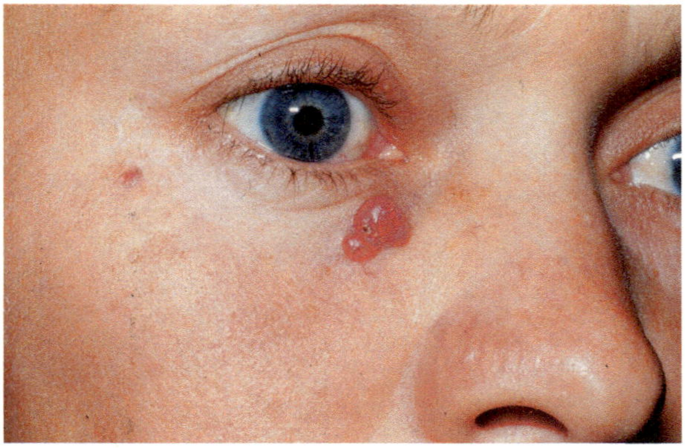

Fig. 24.7 Basal cell carcinoma: a pink pearly ulcerated nodule on the lower eyelid. (Courtesy of Walmar Roncalli Pereira de Oliveira, MD)

Novel targeted systemic therapies that inhibit the Sonic hedgehog pathway, such as vismodegib and sonidegib, are promising therapeutic options for patients with locally advanced or metastatic tumors. Although experience with the use of pathway inhibitors is limited in SOTRs, case reports revealed efficacy without graft compromise [7, 37].

Kaposi Sarcoma (KS)

Kaposi sarcoma (KS) is a vascular neoplasm, derived from lymphatic endothelium associated with human herpes-virus type 8 (HHV-8) that arises in immunosuppressed patients.

KS develops on the skin and mucosa and is characterized by purple-red macules, papules, plaques, or nodules that usually begin in the lower limbs and can ulcerate and bleed (Figs. 24.8 and 24.9) [38, 39].

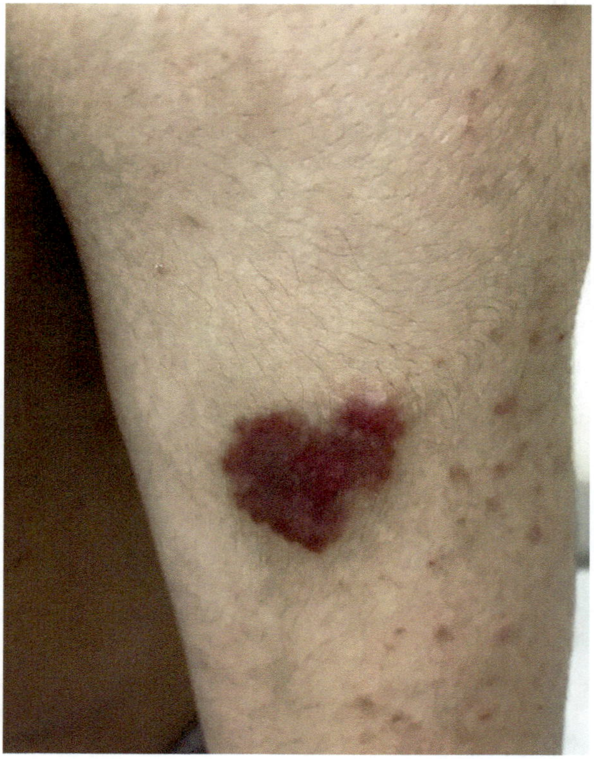

Fig. 24.8 Kaposi sarcoma: A violaceous infiltrated plaque on the leg of an immunosuppressed patient. (Courtesy of Walmar Roncalli Pereira de Oliveira, MD)

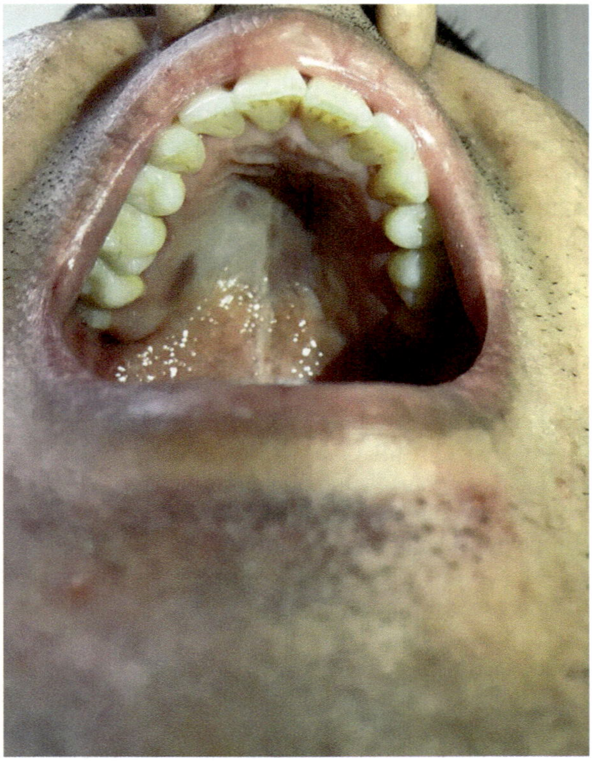

Fig. 24.9 Kaposi sarcoma: A violaceous infiltrated plaque on the hard palate of an immunosuppressed patient. (Courtesy of Walmar Roncalli Pereira de Oliveira, MD)

SOTRs have 200-fold increased risk for KS than the general population [40]. The mean time to development of KS after transplant is approximately 13 months. Dissemination to the lungs, gastrointestinal tract, and lymphoid tissue is common in those patients. Considering SOTRs who are affected by KS after transplantation, 25–30% of kidney and 50% of heart and liver transplant recipients develop visceral involvement of the neoplasm [7, 41].

Risk factor for KS in SOTRs is a pretransplant seropositivity for HHV-8, which has higher incidence in areas of Mediterranean, African, or Arabic origin. Immunosuppressive drugs, such as calcineurin inhibitors (tacrolimus and cyclosporine) seem to be associated with a higher risk for developing KS, at least after kidney transplantation [42].

Diagnosis is made with a skin biopsy that shows atypical endothelial proliferation and positivity for HHV-8 on immunohistochemistry [40].

Management of KS in SOTRs is based on immunosuppression reduction and conversion to mTOR inhibitors, which can induce an adequate response in more than 80% of the patients. Chemotherapy is required in cases of extensive or symptomatic visceral KS and can be combined with mTOR conversion with an increase of the response rates [40].

Merkel Cell Carcinoma (MCC)

Merkel cell carcinoma (MCC, neuroendocrine carcinoma of the skin) is a rare, aggressive tumor that affects mostly sun-damaged skin. It is named so because of its histological differentiation for Merkel cells, which are normal components of the basal layer of the skin and have a role in touch reception. It has a high rate of recurrence and metastases, including regional node metastases [43]. Pathogenesis of MCC is unclear, although it is known that a polyomavirus (Merkel cell polyoma virus, MCPyV) has an oncogenic role in this neoplasm [44].

SOTRs have higher risk of acquiring the tumor—24-fold compared to the general population—once they must be pharmacologically immunosuppressed to prevent graft-rejection [7, 45, 46]. Other risk factors include light exposure, other types of immunosuppression (iatrogenic, autoimmune diseases, HIV/AIDS, lymphocytic leukemia), and advanced age [47].

Incidence of MCC in SOTRs is higher in males than in females (2:1), and the mean age of transplant recipients affected is 53 years old, compared to the 70 years in overall population. Furthermore, the incidence is increased after 10 or more years of the transplant procedure [48].

MCC in SOTRs is mostly linked with kidney, liver, and heart transplantation. The organ type appears to not affect the incidence of posttransplant MCC. Instead, the different immunosuppressive regimens (e.g., cyclosporine/azathioprine) are associated with higher MCC risk [46, 48].

Clinically, MCC manifests as a firm raised painless erythematous to violaceous dome-shaped nodule (Fig. 24.10). The tumor may grow to a considerable size in just a few months and be locally invasive with high metastatic potential [45]. The most affected areas are head and neck (51%) and the upper extremities (26%) [7]. The presence or absence of lymph node metastatic spread is the most important prognostic marker [45].

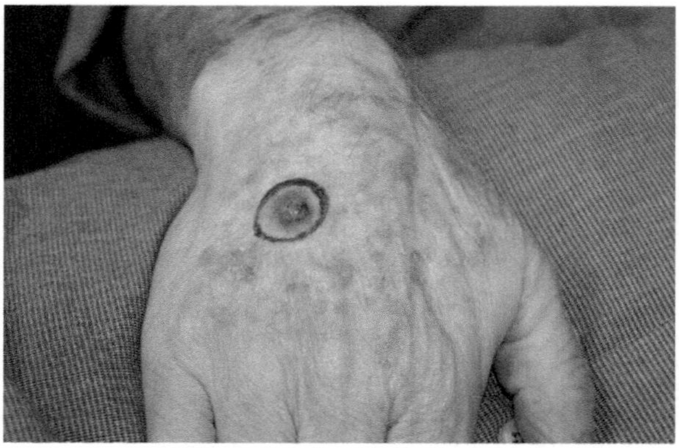

Fig. 24.10 Merkel cell carcinoma: A firm erythematous nodule on the hand of a solid organ transplant recipient. (Courtesy of Walmar Roncalli Pereira de Oliveira, MD)

Management

Management of SOTRs with suspicion for MCC includes, firstly, a complete skin check with lymph node palpation. Then, a skin biopsy with histopathological examination is paramount for definite diagnosis. Histological analysis, on hematoxylin-eosin (HE) stain, shows tumor nests composed of small round to ovoid blue cells in the dermis that can invade the subcutis, fascia, and muscle. The tumor cells exhibit a high nuclear to cytoplasmic ratio and a dispersed nuclear chromatin pattern and indistinct nucleoli [49, 50]. Immunohistochemistry (IHC) is necessary to distinguish MMC from its mimics, such as basal cell carcinoma and other "small round blue cell" tumors: small cell carcinoma of the lung, melanoma, lymphoma, Ewing sarcoma, and so on. Characteristically, it expresses cytokeratin 20 (CK20—a paranuclear dot pattern of positivity is the norm), neuroendocrine markers (chromogranin A, synaptophysin, CD56), neurofilament (NF), and often MCPyV [50]. Once the diagnosis of MCC is confirmed, additional imaging exams may be necessary for staging the disease. Sentinel lymph node biopsy is considered for patients with localized disease and clinically negative lymph nodes [7].

There are no specific guidelines for treatment of MCC in SOTRs. Nevertheless, general treatment guidelines for MCC are pertinent for both SOTRs and non-SOTR MCC patients [45]. Complete surgical excision of the lesion with negative margins is currently the standard therapy. Patients that present regional and/or local tumors with high-risk features, such as rapid growth rate, size larger than 2 cm, and intravascular invasion are benefited with the association of radiotherapy [47]. Systemic chemotherapy—using cisplatin and etoposide or PD1-inhibitors—can be used in patients with advanced or metastatic disease [7]. Revision of the immunosuppressive regimen must be analyzed case to case [42, 43].

For the general population, follow-up visits of MCC patients should be done every 3–6 months for 3 years and every 6–12 months thereafter. Nevertheless, as immunosuppressed patients have higher risk of recurrence, more frequent follow-up visits are advisable. Complete skin and lymph node exam must be performed. Imaging studies are clinically indicated in high-risk patients [44, 48].

Melanoma

The incidence of melanoma in SOTRs is subject to debate. Some data report up to three- to eightfold increase in this tumor compared to the non-organ transplant population. Risk factors for melanoma in SOTRs are similar to those in the general population and include the presence of multiple nevi (also associated with immunosuppression) and fair complexion. It seems that immunosuppression favor melanocyte proliferation; however, its role in melanocyte biology remains of interest [4, 6].

The mean duration from posttransplant to the development of melanoma is 5 years. Regarding SOTRs with melanoma, there are three clinical scenarios of concern: transplant recipients with a history of melanoma pretransplant, transplant recipients developing melanoma as a result of transmission from the organ donor, and transplant recipients who develop de novo melanoma posttransplantation. SOTRs present similar outcomes of melanoma <2 mm Breslow thickness, but a worse outcome for melanoma >2 mm Breslow compared to general population [4, 6, 51].

For patients with a history of melanoma before transplantation, waiting periods have been proposed. For patients with in situ disease, no wait time is needed, while those with Breslow thickness of <1 mm or negative sentinel lymph node biopsy, a 2-year time is recommended. For patients with Breslow thickness of >2 mm, a 5-year wait is mandatory. Patients with lymph node involvement or metastatic disease should not receive a solid organ transplant [52].

Management

SOTRs with melanoma should be treated according to generally applicable guidelines. This entails wide local excision with margins based on Breslow thickness, as in non-immunosuppressed patients (0.5 cm for in situ disease up to 2 cm for deeper invasive tumor, i.e., 4 mm). Knowledge of lymph node status in this population is crucial for management decisions. For patients with positive lymph nodes, additional staging investigations in the form of PET, PET/CT, or directed CT or MRI should be undertaken [6, 52].

The benefit of reducing or switching immunosuppression in metastatic melanoma remains unclear and should be weighed on an individual basis [6, 51–53].

Atypical Fibroxanthoma (AF)

Atypical fibroxanthoma (AF) and a more-aggressive, deeper variant, undifferentiated pleomorphic sarcoma (UPS) is rare, spindle cell cutaneous malignancies. Malignant soft tissue tumors have been estimated to occur 7.3 times more frequently in SOTRs than in immunocompetent individuals [54]. Due to the rarity of AF and UPS, their incidence in SOTRs is unknown. However, these tumors seem to have a greater risk for recurrence, metastases, and mortality in SOTRs, which is likely a reflection of the immunosuppressive load and decrease immune surveillance [55].

AF most commonly presents as a solitary, pink to red, asymptomatic papule or nodule on the head and neck (Fig. 24.11). It may ulcerate or bleed. Predisposing factors include male gender, radiotherapy, trauma, and most importantly UV exposure. SOTRs tend to have large tumors [54, 55].

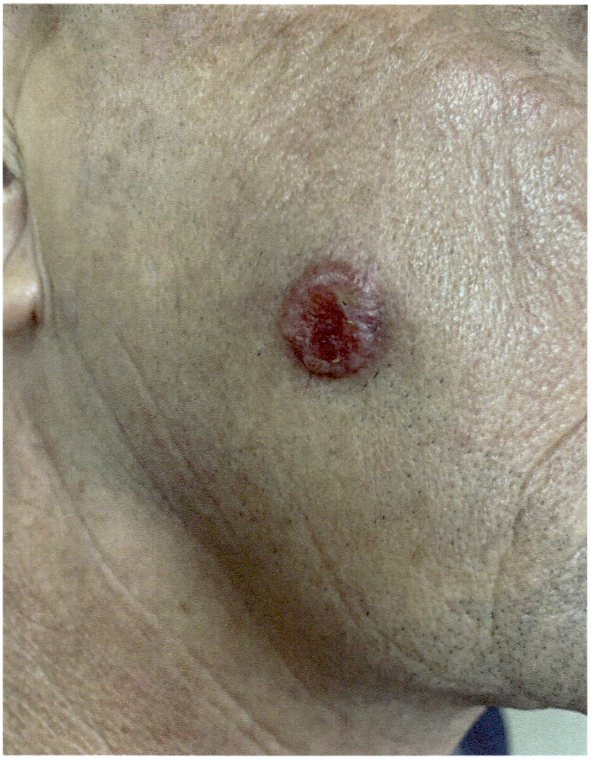

Fig. 24.11 Atypical fibroxanthoma: an erythematous ulcerated nodule on the face. (Courtesy of Walmar Roncalli Pereira de Oliveira, MD)

Immunohistochemical evaluation is recommended to exclude other spindle cell tumors. AF and UPS may be differentiated using clinical criteria, size of tumor, and depth of invasion to subcutaneous tissues [54–56].

SOTRs with AF or UPS may be treated aggressively in order to reduce the risk of local recurrence and metastasis. These tumors should be staged appropriately and treated using MMS or wide local excision, followed by field adjuvant radiotherapy. Reduction of immunosuppression should also be considered when possible [55, 56].

Lymphoproliferative Disorders

Posttransplant lymphoproliferative disorder (PTLD) rarely affects the skin. Most cases are B-cell neoplastic proliferation due to proliferation Epstein-Barr virus (EBV) and present within the first year after transplant. Gastrointestinal tract, liver, lymph nodes, lung, kidney, or the transplanted organ itself are the most commonly affected sites [57]. Primary cutaneous T-cell PTLD seem to have worse outcomes compared to CTCL in immunocompetent patients, contrasting with B-cell PTLD, which has better prognosis than CBCL in non-OTR patients. Skin biopsy is the gold standard for diagnosis [58, 59].

Risk factors for PTLD include pretransplant EBV seronegativity, very young recipient age, cytomegalovirus infection or mismatching (donor positive-recipient negative), aggressive immunosuppression, and type of organ transplanted. Immunosuppression regimen using calcineurin inhibitors has been found to promote the development of EBV-driven lymphoproliferation, by inhibiting the generation of EBV-specific cytotoxic cells [59].

Primary cutaneous T-cell posttransplant lymphoproliferative disorders can manifest as mycosis fungoides (classical, folliculotropic, or syringotropic), CD30+ lymphoproliferative disorders, such as cutaneous anaplastic large cell lymphoma (cALCL) and lymphomatoid papulosis, adult-type T-cell leukemia/lymphoma (ATLL), Sézary syndrome, or primary cutaneous peripheral T-cell lymphoma not otherwise specified (NOS). On the other hand, primary cutaneous B-cell posttransplant lymphoproliferative disorders include EBV-associated B-cell lymphoproliferations (plasmablastic lymphoma and lymphomatoid granulomatosis) and non-EBV-related B-cell lymphoma, such as large B-cell lymphoma [60].

Management and follow-up will be guided according to the type of PTLD. Measures to prevent the development of EBV+ PTLD include testing for primary EBV infection with PCR posttransplant. Monitoring EBV viral loads and modulating immunosuppression regimens can decrease the incidence of PTLD and related mortality [61]. Once PTLD are predominantly B-cell disorders, treatment of CD20+ PTLD with the response-dependent sequential use of reduction on immunosuppression, rituximab, and cytotoxic chemotherapy is recommended [62].

Cutaneous Malignancies and HIV Infection

Since antiretroviral therapy (ART) became common practice in the mid to late 1990s, there has been a significant improvement in morbidity, mortality, and life expectancy of patients infected with human immunodeficiency virus (HIV) [63]. The number of individuals living with AIDS, as well as the incidence of AIDS-defining illnesses, including AIDS-defining malignancies, has been on the decline.

On the other hand, conflicting evidence suggests that the incidence of the non-AIDS-defining cancers (NADCs) has been on the rise after the introduction of ART. Non-AIDS-defining cancers (NADCs) are cancers not previously associated with HIV and AIDS and include cancers of the lung, liver, kidney, anus, head and neck, and skin, Hodgkin's lymphoma, among others [63]. This may be due to the fact that HIV-infected patients are living longer on ART and, thus, are more likely to develop malignancies. However, in populations benefiting from ART, NADCs have a higher relative incidence compared with the same cancer rates seen in the general population, even after controlling for known cancer risk factors. The reasons for these increased cancer rates are poorly understood [63].

Multiple factors may contribute to the increased incidence of malignancy in patients infected with HIV. These include immunosuppression, direct effects of the HIV virus itself, coinfection with oncogenic viruses, environmental factors, and possibly the use of antiretroviral therapy [63].

Immunosuppression

The development of malignancies in HIV-infected patients is similar to that observed in solid organ transplant recipients who receive chronic immunosuppressive agents. Among people living with HIV, NADCs present as more aggressive cancers and with more advanced stages of the disease. They are also diagnosed at younger ages, possibly reflecting accelerated cancer progression or exposure to risk factors [63].

The Role of HIV

HIV infection may have a direct effect on a variety of cellular processes that contribute to the development of cancer. Postulated mechanisms include the activation of proto-oncogenes, alterations in cell cycle regulation, inhibition of tumor suppressor genes, including p53, and other genetic alterations that lead to oncogenesis. Additionally, infected tissues may be more sensitive to the effects of carcinogens from the environment, and HIV-related pro-angiogenesis signaling may enhance the development of tumor growth and metastasis [63].

Coinfection with Oncogenic Organisms

Patients infected with HIV have an increased risk of coinfection with other viruses that are known to cause cancer [63]. Furthermore, the natural history of these viral infections may be accelerated in these patients [63].

Kaposi Sarcoma and HIV Infection

KS is a low-grade soft tissue sarcoma of vascular origin associated with HHV-8 infection, also known as the KS-associated herpesvirus (KSHV). KSHV encodes several genes that induce proliferation, cytokine production, and angiogenesis and thereby contributes to pathogenesis [64].

AIDS-related or epidemic KS is the most common tumor arising in HIV-infected patients and is considered an AIDS-defining illness in the United States Centers for

Disease Control and Prevention (CDC) guidelines. Its incidence has declined substantially since the widespread use of potent antiretroviral therapy (ART) [63], yet the risk remains substantially elevated as compared with the risk in the general population, even among patients who receive effective combination ART for years, have normal CD4+ counts, or both [64].

In patients with AIDS-related KS, the CD4 count appears to be an important factor associated with the development of KS [64]. There is a high incidence immediately following ART initiation that may be attributable to the relatively severe immunosuppression that led to ART or to unmasking of KS by the immune reconstitution inflammatory syndrome.

Corticosteroid therapy has also been associated with the induction or exacerbation of KS in both HIV-infected and non-AIDS persons. This association is important because of the frequent use of these agents in HIV-infected patients with a variety of disorders. If this medication is responsible for the induction of KS or acts like a precipitating factor remains unknown, but in some cases, KS lesions may regress upon reduction or withdrawal of steroids [65].

AIDS-related KS has a variable clinical course, ranging from an asymptomatic incidental finding to explosive growth resulting in significant morbidity and mortality. Skin involvement is most common, but extracutaneous involvement can also occur, particularly on the oral cavity, lungs, and digestive tract.

Cutaneous KS

Although KS can involve any body site, cutaneous disease is the usual initial presentation for KS [64]. The cutaneous lesions appear most often on the lower extremities and face (especially the nose, eyelids, and ears).

The lesions are often elliptical and may be arranged in a linear fashion along skin tension lines and in a symmetric distribution [66]. Usually, there is no pain, pruritus, or necrosis of the overlying skin or underlying structures associated. As the disease progresses, the lesions evolve from macules to plaques and then to small nodules that may coalesce to involve large areas of the body surface (Fig. 24.12) [66]. The papular form is the most common presentation. Plaque-like lesions are seen on the soles of the feet and thigh. Occasionally, exophytic and fungating presentation with breakdown of the overlying skin may be observed.

The colors associated with these lesions are variable, due to their vascularity, and include pink, red, purple, and brown. A yellowish perilesional halo may occasionally be seen.

Lymphedema, particularly in the face, genitalia, and lower extremities may be out of proportion to the extent of the disease and may be related to both vascular obstruction by lymphadenopathy and the cytokines involved in the pathogenesis of KS.

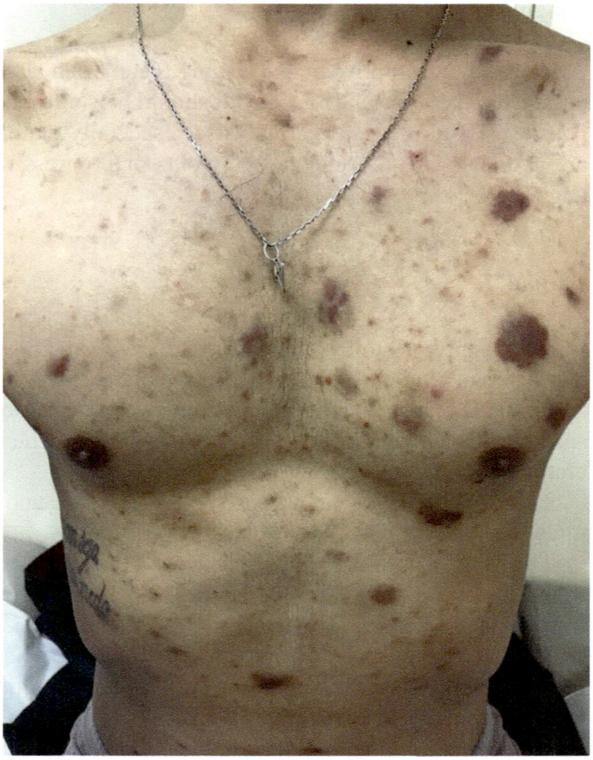

Fig. 24.12 Kaposi sarcoma: multiple violaceous plaques on the trunk of a HIV-infected patient. (Courtesy of Walmar Roncalli Pereira de Oliveira, MD, PhD)

Differential Diagnosis

Early lesions of KS can easily be mistaken as purpura, hematomas, stasis dermatitis, pyogenic granuloma, angiomas, angiosarcoma, dermatofibromas, or nevi [66].

Bacillary angiomatosis is the most important differential diagnosis. This disease is caused by Bartonella, a slow-growing gram-negative bacillus, that can be readily treated with antibiotic therapy. Cutaneous presentation of bacillary angiomatosis usually comprises numerous small red to purple papules that may expand into large pedunculated nodules and become friable. Symptoms such as fever, chills, malaise, headache, and anorexia may be associated.

It is of note that KS and bacillary angiomatosis can occur simultaneously in the same patient. Furthermore, bacillary angiomatosis lesions can be associated with neovascularization and solid areas of spindle cells that mimic KS. The diagnosis of bacillary angiomatosis is established by the identification of the causative organisms with Warthin-Starry silver staining.

Diagnosis

Although a presumptive diagnosis of KS can often be made based upon the characteristic appearance of the lesions, it should be confirmed by a skin biopsy whenever possible. Histopathological analysis is especially important for atypical lesions that are associated with systemic symptoms or progress rapidly, to rule out bacillary angiomatosis.

Pathology

There are three histologic features that are characteristic of KS, independently of the different epidemiologic groups: angiogenesis, inflammation, and proliferation. Additionally, the lesions generally show two major abnormalities: whorls of spindle-shaped cells with leukocytic infiltration and neovascularization with aberrant proliferation of small vessels.

These small vessels lack a basement membrane and display leaky behavior with microhemorrhages and hemosiderin deposition.

These histopathologic findings, however, may be variably pronounced according to the stage of development of the disease. Early patch-like lesions exhibit discrete histopathologic changes, with an increase in the number of dermal vessels, outlined by slightly irregular endothelial cells. These superficial vessels are parallel to skin surface and may form bizarre slits. The main differential diagnoses of this stage are lymphangioma and granulation tissue [66].

KS plaques, on the other hand, display more characteristic features, with extensive vascular proliferation throughout the entire dermis, with multiple dilated and angulated vascular spaces dissecting the collagen tissue [66].

KS papules present with solid cords of spindle cells arranged between jagged vascular channels. With progression of the disease, a more sarcomatous morphology is seen, with nodular KS consisting predominantly of spindle cells arranged in bundles, interlacing fascicles and interspersed irregular, slit-like vascular spaces without endothelial lining. Advanced lesions may display pronounced pleomorphism, nuclear atypia, and mitotic figs [66].

Visceral Disease

KS involvement has been observed in almost all visceral sites, with the most affected non-cutaneous areas being the oral cavity, gastrointestinal tract, lymph nodes, and respiratory system [66]. Visceral involvement as the initial manifestation of KS is relatively uncommon.

Involvement of the oral cavity as the first sign of KS occurs in about two-thirds of patients with the disease. On these cases, the dental practitioner might be the first healthcare professional to identify the lesions [67].

For intraoral KS, the most common clinical appearance is purple macular lesions, followed by mixed purple macular and nodular lesions. As to the most affected site, KS usually presents on the palate followed by the gingiva [67].

Furthermore, oral KS may be accompanied by pain, ulceration, bleeding, and secondary infection from trauma during chewing. Difficult nutrition and speech may result from growing of lesions [67].

KS may also involve the gastrointestinal tract with or without symptoms, such as weight loss, abdominal pain, nausea, gastrointestinal bleeding, malabsorption, intestinal obstruction, and diarrhea. An endoscopy might be indicated to investigate and perform biopsy of the suspected lesions, even though the lesions are underdiagnosed histologically because they are located on the submucosa and may escape the biopsy forceps. The stomach and duodenum are the most affected sites [66].

The respiratory system may also be affected, with patients presenting shortness of breath, fever, cough, hemoptysis, or chest pain. However, pulmonary involvement may be an asymptomatic finding first observed on chest radiograph. Bronchoscopy with transbronchial biopsy is helpful for diagnosing pulmonary KS [66].

Staging

Prior to commencement of treatment, it is important to stage the disease, as it correlates with prognosis. The initial evaluation of a patient with KS consists of a thorough physical examination with special attention paid to those areas typically affected by the disease. Evaluation for visceral involvement is guided by symptomatology and basic laboratory testing.

Testing the stool for occult blood as screening for gastrointestinal involvement is indicated. On cases which occult blood tests positive or there are gastrointestinal symptoms, endoscopy must be performed.

Chest X-ray is also useful to screen for pulmonary lesions. Bronchoscopy should be reserved for those with an abnormal radiograph and persistent respiratory symptoms in the absence of another cause.

CT scanning of the chest, abdomen, and pelvis is typically not necessary. The CD4 cell count and HIV viral load are important for staging and prognosis. A staging system for AIDS-related KS was developed by the AIDS Clinical Trial Group (ACTG) [64]. This system categorizes patients into good or poor risk prognostic categories, according to three parameters, akin to the tumor-node-metastasis (TNM) system used to stage other tumors [68].

It is important to note that this staging system is most frequently used in research. Clinically, patients may be grouped more generally by a clinician into either (a) sick patients needing an immediate fast-acting intervention (clinically severe Kaposi's sarcoma) or (b) those patients that can be treated with HAART alone (clinically mild to moderate Kaposi's sarcoma). There is continued debate in the literature as to the definition of the severity of KS that extremely requires immediate fast-acting intervention as compared to HAART alone [69].

- Extent of tumor (T)—A favorable prognosis is associated with disease limited to the skin or with minimal involvement of the oral cavity (T0). Associated lymphedema, more extensive oral cavity involvement, or other visceral disease are considered to have a poor prognosis (T1).
- Immune status (I)—Patients with a CD4 count greater than 200 cells/μL are considered to have a favorable prognosis (I0), while those with a lower CD4 count are classified as poor prognosis (I1).
- Severity of systemic illness (S)—Features associated with a poor risk included the following (S1): a history of opportunistic infection, thrush, B symptoms (fever, night sweats, significant weight loss, diarrhea for more than 2 weeks).

Management

The major goals of treatment for AIDS-related KS are symptom palliation, prevention of disease progression, and shrinkage of tumor to alleviate edema, organ compromise, and psychological stress.

ART is a cornerstone for the treatment of AIDS-related Kaposi's sarcoma. The introduction of ART has been associated with a substantial decrease in both morbidity and mortality of AIDS-associated KS [69]. Immune reconstitution due to control of the HIV infection is the most likely explanation for this change, rather than a direct effect on tumor.

Immune reconstitution inflammatory syndrome (IRIS) may be responsible for the progression of KS within 3–6 weeks after starting antiretroviral therapy [64].

The need for treatment beyond ART and the choice among the various options depend upon the extent and rate of tumor growth, the HIV-1 viral load, the CD4 cell count, and the patient's overall medical condition [70].

Locally directed therapy is often used for limited disease, to palliate symptoms caused by a specific tumor or to treat cosmetic disfigurement [66]. With high recurrence rates, local treatment usually adds little to ART [64]. They include the following:

- Surgical excision [66].
- Cryotherapy: The preconized regimen includes up to 60-s freeze cycles, with 2–3 freeze-thaw cycles and up to three sessions [66, 70].
- Intralesional chemotherapy: This treatment is preferred for small lesions. Vinblastine is the most widely used agent. It can be injected directly into a KS lesion as a 0.2–0.5 mg/mL solution with a volume of 0.1 mL per 0.5 cm^2 of lesion. Multiple injections may be necessary for larger lesions. Treated lesions will fade and regress although typically not resolve completely. Common side effects include hyperpigmentation and pain [67, 70–72].

- Radiation therapy: This therapeutic modality may be particularly useful to treat symptomatic disease that is too extensive to be treated with intralesional chemotherapy but is not extensive enough to require systemic therapy, or lesions at sites that are difficult to reach by other local approaches [66]. Because severe mucositis may develop even at relatively low radiation dosages (300 cGy) radiotherapy is usually reserved for lesions partially or totally obstructing the aerodigestive tract [67].
- Topical alitretinoin: Alitretinoin (9-*cis* retinoic acid) is available as a topical gel at 0.1% that the patient can apply twice daily for 12 weeks to treat cutaneous KS lesions. The most common adverse effect is local irritation. Undesirable skin lightening may also occur. Response is usually noted after 4–8 weeks of treatment [66, 71, 73].

Systemic therapy is required for more extensive or rapidly progressive disease and for visceral involvement. Other possible indications include unresponsiveness to local treatment, painful or ulcerated lesions, edema, Kaposi's sarcoma IRIS, or psychological withdrawal because of the stigma of visible lesions [64, 66]. Nonetheless, it must be considered that it may add injury to an immune system that is already severely compromised.

When chemotherapy is indicated, initial treatment should be performed with liposomal anthracyclines, such as pegylated liposomal doxorubicin or liposomal daunorubicin [64, 66, 70, 71]. A typical regimen consists of 20 mg/m^2 of the drug of choice intravenously every 2–4 weeks [66]. Paclitaxel is associated with more toxic effects and is generally used as second-line therapy [64]. Other more recent options include pomalidomide and lenalidomide. Bleomycin, vinblastine, vincristine, and etoposide have less favorable activity and side-effect profiles but are often administered when the high cost of liposomal doxorubicin or paclitaxel is not possible to afford [64, 70, 74].

It is of note, however, that small, randomized trials have demonstrated that although response rates are higher with the addition of chemotherapy to ART, it doesn't seem to reflect on a survival benefit [75–77].

The treatment should be stopped if an adequate response is achieved as a plateau. If not, consideration should be given to switching to a different therapy. Many patients achieve long-term control, especially with the immune reconstitution provided by ART. However, KSHV cannot be eradicated, and tumors may recur and require additional therapy [64].

Other systemic treatments for KS currently reported include immune checkpoint inhibitors. PD-1 is upregulated on CD8 T cells in HIV and has been shown to be associated with T-cell exhaustion during chronic viral infection. Blocking the PD-1/L1 interaction is, therefore, hypothesized to decrease viremia, decrease immunosuppression, and result in tumor regression due to increased immune surveillance of malignancy [70].

Non-AIDS-Defining Cancers

In persons with HIV, all cancers except Kaposi's sarcoma, aggressive B-cell lymphoma, and invasive cervical cancer are considered non-AIDS-defining cancers. These include HIV-associated tumors and incidental cancers. HIV increases the risk of several cancers, including SCC and MCC [64].

Early in the AIDS epidemic, patients with AIDS were often too fragile to receive standard cancer therapy. However, this situation has changed with the use of ART; non-AIDS-defining and incidental cancers should generally be managed according to the standard of care. In cases in which no good standard treatment options exist, referral of patients to enrollment in clinical trials should be considered. In the management of cancer, HIV should be treated as a chronic condition, and attention should be paid to potential drug interactions among HIV medications and cancer therapy, as well as to the prevention of opportunistic infections [64].

BCC, SCC, and HIV Infection

HIV-infected individuals have a two- to threefold increased risk of nonmelanoma skin cancer [78]. The observed increased incidence rate for SCCs among HIV subjects, however, is much lower than the more than 50-fold higher rates observed among transplant populations.

BCC is substantially more common than SCC in these individuals, in contrast with organ transplant recipients, where SCC is more frequent [79]. Increased incidence rate of BCC for HIV+ subjects, nevertheless, appears to be limited to men, whereas the increased incidence rate of SCCs was observed for women, HIV+ men who have sex with men (MSM), and other HIV-infected men [78].

General risk factors for BCC and SCC are similar to those in HIV-uninfected individuals, including increasing age, white ethnicity, sun exposure, and family history of skin cancer [79]. Higher census-based household income has also been associated with increased risk for BCC [78]. Lower recent CD4 counts appears to be related with a higher incidence rate for SCC but not for BCC [78].

As for clinical presentation, the most common clinical and histologic form of BCC is the superficial type, which appears on the trunk and may be multiple. In contrast, other immunosuppressed states have a statistically significant increase in infiltrative-type BCC [79].

SCC is clearly associated with infection with HPV in anogenital, cervical, and oral cancer, in SCC of the nail unit, and in epidermodysplasia verruciformis. HPV in these cases generally is of a high-risk or an unusual HPV type [79]. On other SCC presentations, HPV is not an oncogenic factor in the development of tumors [66].

Cutaneous SCCs may be dangerous in the context of HIV disease. HIV-infected patients with SCC tend to be younger, present a high risk for local recurrence, metastasis, and mortality [79].

HIV-infected persons need aggressive primary prevention with strong encouragement for sunscreen use and sun avoidance. Secondary prevention with regular careful examinations and early biopsy of suspicious lesions are imperative. It must be kept in mind that as in any immunocompromised state, the differential diagnosis is broadened for NMSC in HIV+ patients. After treatment, patients should undergo regular follow-up for local recurrence or nodal metastasis [79].

Multiple treatment options are available for BCC and SCC based upon patient-specific factors. BCCs and SCCs in HIV-infected persons should be treated as they would in their HIV-uninfected counterparts. However, some authors recommend that HIV patient with high-risk SCC should be considered for local or regional adjunctive radiation or chemotherapy, or both, and sentinel node procedures. There is no evidence that BCCs in HIV-infected persons require more aggressive therapy than those in HIV-negative persons [79].

Anal Cancer and HIV Infection

The term "anal cancer" usually refers to SCC of the anal canal, which represents most cancers arising in the anal region. However, SCCs can also arise in the perianal skin and in the rectum, and SCCs arising at these sites are generally treated in the same manner as anal canal SCCs. Even though infection with HIV is a risk factor for anal cancer, anal cancer is not a disease-defining condition for progression to AIDS.

Pathogenesis

HIV and anal co-infection with HPV are independent risk factors associated with an increased risk for anal neoplasia in males and females regardless of sexual orientation [66].

HPV-6 and 11 infect nonkeratinized epithelium, such as anogenital sites causing warts. HPV-16, 18, 31, and 33 cause precancerous lesions, low-grade squamous intraepithelial lesions (SIL), high-grade SIL, and invasive SCC [66, 79]. The precursor lesion of anal SCC has been called squamous intraepithelial lesion (SIL), analogous to that routinely used in cervical cytology. Anal intraepithelial neoplasia is used to describe and grade the histologic findings of dysplasia [79]. Risk factors for SIL include lower CD4 counts, the presence of dysplasia-associated high-risk HPV type, and infection with multiple different HPV types and are more prevalent in HIV-positive MSM than in women [64, 79].

HPV infection is thought to transform anal epithelia through low-grade SIL dysplasia to high-grade SIL. There is no apparent correlation between the relative risk of developing invasive anal cancer and the CD4 cell count, but trends with correlation with low CD4 counts have been observed [66, 71, 79].

The specific interaction between HIV and HPV has not been fully characterized [79]. Immune dysfunction and decreased immune surveillance may play a more important role on the pathogenesis of anal cancer than direct viral effect since there is a stronger association with declining CD4+ counts than with rising viral HIV RNA titers [66]. However, patients with successful immune reconstitution often do not show improvement of their dysplasia [79].

Clinical Features

Patients with anal intraepithelial neoplasia-SIL are largely asymptomatic and undergo diagnosis with cytologic or histologic examination.

Occasionally, the disease may be symptomatic and easily visible during physical examination [79]. In these cases, rectal bleeding is the most common initial symptom of anal cancer. Other symptoms include anorectal pain, sensation of a rectal mass, or change in bowel habits. Differential diagnosis with hemorrhoids or warts may delay the diagnosis [80]. Tumors of the perianal skin, especially Bowen's disease or Paget disease, may present with pruritus ani or a bleeding erythematous eczematoid plaque [80]. Invasive SCC arising on external anogenital area is usually detected earlier and is less aggressive than that arising on the anal canal [66].

Among the patients with anal squamous cell cancer (SCC), a history of previous anorectal condyloma may be present.

Management

Anal intraepithelial neoplasia may be treated with topical therapy, including imiquimod, podophyllotoxin, 80% trichloroacetic acid, or liquid nitrogen. Lesions may also be excised or treated with destructive modalities such as fulguration [66]. Unlike Kaposi's sarcoma and cervical intraepithelial neoplasia, where ART can lead to regression of lesions, it does not appear to lead to resolution of anal intraepithelial neoplasia [71].

For minimally invasive SCC arising on the anal verge, surgical excision with adequate borders is recommended [66]. For anal cancer, local control and sphincter preservation, as for immunocompetent individuals, remain the major challenges [71].

Patients for whom curative treatment is likely to be appropriate should have a computed tomography (CT) scan of the chest, abdomen, and pelvis or pelvic magnetic resonance imaging (MRI) [71].

HIV-associated anal SCC is potentially curable with combined modality therapy, and in general, HIV-positive patients are treated similarly to non-HIV-positive individuals, and most data suggest that response to therapy, local control, and survival are as good as in non-HIV-infected patients, particularly in the era of potent antiretroviral therapy.

Combined modality treatment includes radiation therapy and chemotherapy, using mitomycin C, 5-FU, and radiation, and is appropriate for most patients [66].

Other forms of treatment, such as surgical excision, may be considered by anal cancer multidisciplinary teams, but surgery is usually reserved for salvage [71]. Even though low CD4 count does not necessarily predict for greater treatment-related toxicity, patients with active HIV-/AIDS-related complications or a history of opportunistic infections, or other HIV-related malignancies, may not tolerate full-dose therapy, or may not tolerate mitomycin, and require either dose adjustment or treatment without mitomycin [78]. Prognosis in these cases seems to be better for patients with higher CD4+ counts at time of diagnosis [66].

Prevention

If HIV status is unknown, the National Comprehensive Cancer Network (NCCN) recommends HIV testing for all individuals with newly diagnosed anal squamous cell cancer (SCC).

Management of external anogenital HPV infection in HIV-infected individuals is directed at identifying high-grade SIL before progression to invasive SCC.

All HIV-infected individuals should be examined annually for evidence of HPV infection [66]. Screening for anal intraepithelial neoplasia can be done through anal cytology examination of the lower rectum, squamocolumnar junction, and anal canal (anal Pap test) [79]. Persons with abnormal Pap test results undergo examination with high-resolution anoscopy (the equivalent of colposcopy) and biopsy of visible lesions [66, 79]. Individuals with documented external anogenital SIL should undergo periodic follow-up examinations every 4–6 months, and biopsy of suspected new lesions is recommended [4].

Melanoma and HIV Infection

The incidence of melanoma in patients infected with HIV may be moderately increased compared with the general population. There is no evidence that atypical presentations are more common in the context of HIV disease. Melanomas in HIV-infected patients seem to be often multiple, frequently metastasize, and are associated with a poor prognosis, with the latter being associated with lower CD4 counts [79].

Merkel Cell Carcinoma and HIV Infection

Merkel cell carcinoma is a neuroendocrine carcinoma arising in the skin, which is etiologically linked with infection with the Merkel cell polyoma virus. The incidence of Merkel cell carcinoma is increased more than tenfold in persons with HIV infection.

References

1. Brin L, Zubair AS, Brewer JD. Optimal management of skin cancer in immunosuppressed patients. Am J Clin Dermatol. 2014;15(4):339–56.
2. Schulz TF. Cancer and viral infections in immunocompromised individuals. Int J Cancer. 2009;125(8):1755–63.
3. Califano J, Lydiatt WM, Nehal KS, et al. Cutaneous carcinoma of the head and neck. AJCC cancer staging manual. 8th ed. American Joint Committee on Cancer; 2017. p. 171–81.
4. O'Reilly Zwald F, Brown M. Skin cancer in solid organ transplant recipients: advances in therapy and management: Part I. Epidemiology of skin cancer in solid organ transplant recipients. J Am Acad Dermatol. 2011;65(2):263–79.
5. Bangash HK, Colegio OR. Management of non-melanoma skin cancer in immunocompromised solid organ transplant recipients. Curr Treat Options Oncol. 2012;13(3):354–76.
6. Hofbauer GFL, Anliker M, Arnold A, Binet I, Hunger R, Kempf W, et al. Swiss clinical practice guidelines for skin cancer in organ transplant recipients. Swiss Med Wkly. 2009;139(29–30):407–15.
7. Mittal A, Colegio OR. Skin cancers in organ transplant recipients. Am J Transplant. 2017;17(10):2509–30.
8. Jiyad Z, Marquart L, O'Rourke P, Green AC. The natural history of actinic keratoses in organ transplant recipients. J Am Acad Dermatol. 2017;76(1):162–4.
9. Willenbrink TJ, Ruiz ES, Cornejo CM, Schmults CD, Arron ST, Jambusaria-Pahlajani A. Field cancerization: definition, epidemiology, risk factors, and outcomes. J Am Acad Dermatol. 2020;83(3):709–17.
10. Heppt MV, Steeb T, Niesert AC, Zacher M, Leiter U, Garbe C, et al. Local interventions for actinic keratosis in organ transplant recipients: a systematic review. Br J Dermatol. 2019;180(1):43–50.
11. Wallingford SC, Russell SA, Vail A, Proby CM, Lear JT, Green AC. Actinic keratoses, actinic field change and associations with squamous cell carcinoma in renal transplant recipients in Manchester, UK. Acta Derm Venereol. 2015;95(7):830–4.
12. Collins L, Asfour L, Stephany M, Lear JT, Stasko T. Management of non-melanoma skin cancer in transplant recipients. Clin Oncol. 2019;31(11):779–88.
13. Trakatelli M, Katsanos G, Ulrich C, Kalabalikis D, Sotiriadis D, Stockfleth E. Efforts to counteract locally the effects of systemic immunosuppression: a review on the use of imiquimod, a topical immunostimulator in organ transplant recipients. Int J Immunopathol Pharmacol. 2010;23(2):387–96.
14. Ulrich C, Bichel J, Euvrard S, Guidi B, Proby CM, Van De Kerkhof PCM, et al. Topical immunomodulation under systemic immunosuppression: results of a multicentre, randomized, placebo-controlled safety and efficacy study of imiquimod 5% cream for the treatment of actinic keratoses in kidney, heart, and liver transplant patients. Br J Dermatol. 2007;157(Suppl 2):25–31.
15. Piaserico S, Belloni Fortina A, Rigotti P, Rossi B, Baldan N, Alaibac M, et al. Topical photodynamic therapy of actinic keratosis in renal transplant recipients. Transplant Proc. 2007;39(6):1847–50.
16. Wlodek C, Ali FR, Lear JT. Use of photodynamic therapy for treatment of actinic keratoses in organ transplant recipients. Biomed Res Int. 2013;2013:1.
17. Euvrard S, Kanitakis J, Cochat P, Cambazard F, Claudy A. Skin diseases in children with organ transplants. J Am Acad Dermatol. 2001;44(6):932–9.
18. Winkelhorst JT, Brokelman WJ, Tiggeler RG, Wobbes T. Incidence and clinical course of de-novo malignancies in renal allograft recipients. Eur J Surg Oncol. 2001;27(4):409–13.
19. Chockalingam R, Downing C, Tyring S. Cutaneous squamous cell carcinomas in organ transplant recipients. J Clin Med. 2015;4(6):1229–39.
20. Euvrard S, Morelon E, Rostaing L, Goffin E, Brocard A, Tromme I, et al. Sirolimus and secondary skin-cancer prevention in kidney transplantation. N Engl J Med. 2012;367(4):329–39.

21. Salgo R, Gossmann J, Schöfer H, Kachel HG, Kuck J, Geiger H, et al. Switch to a sirolimus-based immunosuppression in long-term renal transplant recipients: reduced rate of (pre-) malignancies and nonmelanoma skin cancer in a prospective, randomized, assessor-blinded, controlled clinical trial. Am J Transplant. 2010;10(6):1385–93.
22. Otley CC, Berg D, Ulrich C, Stasko T, Murphy GM, Salasche SJ, et al. Reduction of immunosuppression for transplant-associated skin cancer: expert consensus survey. Br J Dermatol. 2006;154(3):395–400.
23. Ilyas M, Colegio OR, Kaplan B. Cutaneous toxicities from transplantation-related medications. Am J Transplant. 2017;17:2782–9.
24. George R, Weightman W, Russ GR, Bannister KM, Mathew TH. Acitretin for chemoprevention of non-melanoma skin cancers in renal transplant recipients. Australas J Dermatol. 2002;43(4):269–73.
25. Harwood CA, Leedham-Green M. Low-dose retinoids in the prevention of cutaneous squamous cell carcinomas in organ transplant recipients. Arch Dermatol. 2005;141(5):3071–6.
26. Chen AC, Martin AJ, Choy B, Fernández-Peñas P, Dalziell RA, McKenzie CA, et al. A phase 3 randomized trial of nicotinamide for skin-cancer chemoprevention. N Engl J Med. 2015;373(17):1618–26.
27. Chen AC, Martin AJ, Dalziell RA, McKenzie CA, Lowe PM, Eris JM, et al. A phase II randomized controlled trial of nicotinamide for skin cancer chemoprevention in renal transplant recipients. Br J Dermatol. 2016;175(5):1073–5.
28. Tee LY, Sultana R, Tam SYC, Oh CC. Chemoprevention of keratinocyte carcinoma and actinic keratosis in solid-organ transplant recipients: systematic review and meta-analyses. J Am Acad Dermatol. 2021;84(2):528–30.
29. Boyd K, Shea SM, Patterson J. Cetuximab for treatment of advanced squamous cell carcinoma in solid organ transplant recipients. Wien Med Wochenschr. 2013;163(15–16):372–5.
30. Falchook GS, Leidner R, Stankevich E, Piening B, Bifulco C, Lowy I, et al. Responses of metastatic basal cell and cutaneous squamous cell carcinomas to anti-PD1 monoclonal antibody REGN2810. J Immunother Cancer. 2016;4(1):1–5.
31. Connolly K, Manders P, Earls P, Epstein RJ. Papillomavirus-associated squamous skin cancers following transplant immunosuppression: one notch closer to control. Cancer Treat Rev. 2014;40(2):205–14.
32. Nindl I, Gottschling M, Stockfleth E. Human papillomaviruses and non-melanoma skin cancer: basic virology and clinical manifestations. Dis Markers. 2007;23(4):247–59.
33. Boza JC, Peruzzo J, de Oliveira FB, Nazar FL, Bakos RM. Epidermodysplasia verruciformis-like skin eruption in an HIV-positive patient. Trop Med Health. 2014;42(4):185–6.
34. Papakostas D, Stockfleth E. Topical treatment of basal cell carcinoma with the immune response modifier imiquimod. Future Oncol. 2015;11(22):2985–90.
35. Krynitz B, Olsson H, Lundh Rozell B, Lindelöf B, Edgren G, Smedby KE. Risk of basal cell carcinoma in Swedish organ transplant recipients: a population-based study. Br J Dermatol. 2016;174(1):95–103.
36. Vidal D, Alomar A. Efficacy of imiquimod 5% cream for basal cell carcinoma in transplant patients. Clin Exp Dermatol. 2004;29(3):237–9.
37. Cusack CA, Nijhawan R, Miller B, Henien M, Malat G, Doyle A, et al. Vismodegib for locally advanced basal cell carcinoma in a heart transplant patient. JAMA Dermatol. 2015;151(1):70–2.
38. Raedemaeker J, Marot L, Camboni A, Kanaan N. Kaposi sarcoma after kidney transplantation. BMJ Case Rep. 2019;12(5):1–2.
39. Ercan Z, Demir ME, Merhametsiz O, Yayar O, Ulas T, Ayli MD. Kaposi's sarcoma in the early post-transplant period in a kidney transplant recipient. Nefrologia. 2013;33(6):861–2.
40. Delyon J, Rabate C, Euvrard S, Harwood CA, Proby C, Güleç AT, et al. Management of Kaposi sarcoma after solid organ transplantation: a European retrospective study. J Am Acad Dermatol. 2019;81(2):448–55.
41. Thivolet J. Skin cancers after organ transplants. Melanoma Res. 1996;6(Suppl 1):S18.

42. Euvrard S, Kanitakis J. Skin cancers after liver transplantation: what to do? J Hepatol. 2006;44(1):27–32.
43. Normann M. Metastatic Merkel cell carcinoma in a kidney transplant patient: experiences from treatment with a checkpoint inhibitor (avelumab) - a case report. Oncol Cancer Case Rep. 2021;07(1):1–5.
44. Coggshall K, Tello TL, North JP, Yu SS. Merkel cell carcinoma: an update and review: pathogenesis, diagnosis, and staging. J Am Acad Dermatol. 2018;78(3):433–42.
45. Koljonen V, Sahi H, Böhling T, Mäkisalo H. Post-transplant Merkel cell carcinoma. Acta Derm Venereol. 2016;96(4):442–7.
46. Clarke CA, Robbins HA, Tatalovich Z, Lynch CF, Pawlish KS, Finch JL, et al. Risk of Merkel cell carcinoma after solid organ transplantation. J Natl Cancer Inst. 2015;107(2):1–9.
47. Xin H, Wei R, Ma Q, Wang N, Li A, Li W. Merkel cell carcinoma after liver transplantation: a case report and review of the literature. Ann Palliat Med. 2021;10(7):8425–30.
48. Ma JE, Brewer JD. Merkel cell carcinoma in immunosuppressed patients. Cancers (Basel). 2014;6(3):1328–50.
49. Ogawa T, Donizy P, Wu CL, Cornejo KM, Ryś J, Hoang MP. Morphologic diversity of Merkel cell carcinoma. Am J Dermatopathol. 2020;42(9):629–40.
50. Walsh NM, Cerroni L. Merkel cell carcinoma: a review. J Cutan Pathol. 2021;48:411–21.
51. Matin RN, Mesher D, Proby CM, McGregor JM, Bouwes Bavinck JN, Del Marmol V, et al. Melanoma in organ transplant recipients: clinicopathological features and outcome in 100 cases. Am J Transplant. 2008;8(9):1891–900.
52. O'Reilly Zwald F, Brown M. Skin cancer in solid organ transplant recipients: advances in therapy and management: Part II. Management of skin cancer in solid organ transplant recipients. J Am Acad Dermatol. 2011;65(2):253–61.
53. Stasko T, Brown MD, Carucci JA, Euvrard S, Johnson TM, Sengelmann RD, et al. Guidelines for the management of squamous cell carcinoma in organ transplant recipients. Dermatol Surg. 2004;30(4 II):642–50.
54. Hafner J, Künzi W, Weinreich T. Malignant fibrous histiocytoma and atypical fibroxanthoma in renal transplant recipients. Dermatology. 1999;198(1):29–32.
55. McCoppin HH, Christiansen D, Stasko T, Washington C, Martinez JC, Brown MD, et al. Clinical spectrum of atypical fibroxanthoma and undifferentiated pleomorphic sarcoma in solid organ transplant recipients: a collective experience. Dermatol Surg. 2012;38(2):230–9.
56. Ang GC, Roenigk RK, Otley CC, Kim Phillips P, Weaver AL. More than 2 decades of treating atypical fibroxanthoma at mayo clinic: what have we learned from 91 patients? Dermatol Surg. 2009;35(5):765–72.
57. Samolitis NJ, Bharadwaj JS, Weis JR, Harris RM. Post-transplant lymphoproliferative disorder limited to the skin. J Cutan Pathol. 2004;31(6):453–7.
58. Beynet DP, Wee SA, Horwitz SS, Kohler S, Horning S, Hoppe R, et al. Clinical and pathological features of posttransplantation lymphoproliferative disorders presenting with skin involvement in 4 patients. Arch Dermatol. 2004;140(9):1140–6.
59. Ravat FE, Spittle MF, Russell-Jones R. Primary cutaneous T-cell lymphoma occurring after organ transplantation. J Am Acad Dermatol. 2006;54(4):668–75.
60. Seçkin D, Barete S, Euvrard S, Francès C, Kanitakis J, Geusau A, et al. Primary cutaneous posttransplant lymphoproliferative disorders in solid organ transplant recipients: a multicenter European case series. Am J Transplant. 2013;13(8):2146–53.
61. Allen UD, Preiksaitis JK. Post-transplant lymphoproliferative disorders, Epstein-Barr virus infection, and disease in solid organ transplantation: guidelines from the American Society of Transplantation Infectious Diseases Community of Practice. Clin Transpl. 2019;33(9):1–22.
62. Evens AM, Blum KA. Non-Hodgkin lymphoma. Pathology, imaging and current therapy. Cancer Treat Res. 2015;165:1–25.
63. Deeken JF, Tjen-A-Looi A, Rudek MA, Okuliar C, Young M, Little RF, Dezube BJ. The rising challenge of non-AIDS-defining cancers in HIV-infected patients. Clin Infect Dis.

2012;55(9):1228–35. https://doi.org/10.1093/cid/cis613. Epub 2012 Jul 9. PMID: 22776851; PMCID: PMC3529613
64. Yarchoan R, Uldrick TS. HIV-associated cancers and related diseases. N Engl J Med. 2018;378(22):2145. https://doi.org/10.1056/NEJMc1804812. PMID: 29847760
65. Trattner A, Hodak E, David M, Sandbank M. The appearance of Kaposi sarcoma during corticosteroid therapy. Cancer. 1993;72(5):1779–83.
66. Fitzpatrick TB, Freedberg IM. Fitzpatrick's dermatology in general medicine. New York: McGraw-Hill, Medical Pub. Division; 2003.
67. Nichols CM, Flaitz CM, Hicks MJ. Treating Kaposi's lesions in the HIV-infected patient. J Am Dent Assoc. 1993;124(11):78–84.
68. Krown SE, Metroka C, Wernz JC. Kaposi's sarcoma in the acquired immune deficiency syndrome: a proposal for uniform evaluation, response, and staging criteria. AIDS Clinical Trials Group Oncology Committee. J Clin Oncol. 1989;7(9):1201–7.
69. Gbabe OF, Okwundu CI, Dedicoat M, Freeman EE. Treatment of severe or progressive Kaposi's sarcoma in HIV-infected adults. Cochrane Database Syst Rev. 2014;8(8):CD003256.
70. Etemad SA, Dewan AK. Kaposi sarcoma updates. Dermatol Clin. 2019;37(4):505–17.
71. Bower M, Collins S, Cottrill C, Cwynarski K, Montoto S, Nelson M, Nwokolo N, Powles T, Stebbing J, Wales N, Webb A, AIDS Malignancy Subcommittee. British HIV Association guidelines for HIV-associated malignancies 2008. HIV Med. 2008;9(6):336–88.
72. Epstein JB. Treatment of oral Kaposi sarcoma with intralesional vinblastine. Cancer. 1993;71(5):1722–5.
73. Bodsworth NJ, Bloch M, Bower M, Donnell D, Yocum R, International Panretin Gel KS Study Group. Phase III vehicle-controlled, multi-centered study of topical alitretinoin gel 0.1% in cutaneous AIDS-related Kaposi's sarcoma. Am J Clin Dermatol. 2001;2(2):77–87.
74. Donato V, Guarnaccia R, Dognini J, de Pascalis G, Caruso C, Bellagamba R, Morrone A. Radiation therapy in the treatment of HIV-related Kaposi's sarcoma. Anticancer Res. 2013;33(5):2153–7.
75. Mosam A, Shaik F, Uldrick TS, Esterhuizen T, Friedland GH, Scadden DT, Aboobaker J, Coovadia HM. A randomized controlled trial of highly active antiretroviral therapy versus highly active antiretroviral therapy and chemotherapy in therapy-naive patients with HIV-associated Kaposi sarcoma in South Africa. J Acquir Immune Defic Syndr. 2012;60(2):150–7.
76. Hosseinipour MC, Kang M, Krown SE, Bukuru A, Umbleja T, Martin JN, Orem J, Godfrey C, Hoagland B, Mwelase N, Langat D, Nyirenda M, MacRae J, Borok M, Samaneka W, Moses A, Mngqbisa R, Busakhala N, Martínez-Maza O, Ambinder R, Dittmer DP, Nokta M, Campbell TB, A5264/AMC-067 REACT-KS Team. As-needed vs immediate etoposide chemotherapy in combination with antiretroviral therapy for mild-to-moderate AIDS-associated Kaposi sarcoma in resource-limited settings: A5264/AMC-067 randomized clinical trial. Clin Infect Dis. 2018;67(2):251–60.
77. Martin-Carbonero L, Barrios A, Saballs P, Sirera G, Santos J, Palacios R, Valencia ME, Alegre M, Podzamczer D, González-Lahoz J, Caelyx/KS Spanish Group. Pegylated liposomal doxorubicin plus highly active antiretroviral therapy versus highly active antiretroviral therapy alone in HIV patients with Kaposi's sarcoma. AIDS. 2004;18(12):1737–40.
78. Silverberg MJ, Leyden W, Warton EM, Quesenberry CP Jr, Engels EA, Asgari MM. HIV infection status, immunodeficiency, and the incidence of non-melanoma skin cancer. J Natl Cancer Inst. 2013;105(5):350–60.
79. Wilkins K, Turner R, Dolev JC, LeBoit PE, Berger TG, Maurer TA. Cutaneous malignancy and human immunodeficiency virus disease. J Am Acad Dermatol. 2006;54(2):189–206; quiz 207–10.
80. Singh R, Nime F, Mittelman A. Malignant epithelial tumors of the anal canal. Cancer. 1981;48(2):411–5.

Chapter 25
Palliative Care in Patients with Cutaneous Malignancies

Ana Cristina Pugliese de Castro and Ana Paula de Souza Borges

Key Points

- In advanced-stage skin malignancies, the demand to promote comfort and quality of life is necessary in different intensity and settings.
- Palliative care improves the quality of life of patients and their families through the prevention and relief of suffering
- Pain, nausea, dyspnea, and bleeding are frequent symptoms that should be properly addressed.
- Advanced care planning enables patients to make plans for their future healthcare and should address all domains of care.

Introduction

According to the WHO definition, palliative care is "an interprofessional approach that improves the quality of life of patients and their families facing the problem associated with life-threatening illness, through the prevention and relief of suffering by means of early identification and impeccable assessment and treatment of pain and other problems, physical, psychosocial, and spiritual." It should be applicable early in the course of the illness, in conjunction with other therapies that are intended to prolong life [1].

A. C. Pugliese de Castro (✉) · A. P. de Souza Borges
Hospital Sírio-Libanês, São Paulo, Brazil
e-mail: ana.cpcastro@hsl.org.br

C. M. Z. Abdalla et al. (eds.), *Oncodermatology*,
https://doi.org/10.1007/978-3-031-29277-4_25

WHO determines that palliative care practice must follow some principles:

- Provides relief from pain and other distressing symptoms
- Affirms life and regards dying as a normal process
- Intends neither to hasten nor to postpone death
- Integrates psychological and spiritual aspects of patient care
- Offers a support system to help patients live as actively as possible until death
- Offers a support system to help the family cope during the patient's illness and in their own bereavement
- Uses a team approach to address the needs of patients and their families, including bereavement counseling if indicated
- Will enhance quality of life and may also positively influence the course of illness
- Is applicable early in the course of illness, in tandem with other therapies that are intended to prolong life, such as chemotherapy or radiation therapy, and includes those investigations that are necessary to better understand and manage distressing clinical complications [1]

In advanced-stage skin malignancies, the demand to promote comfort and quality of life is necessary in different intensity and setting of suffering in the course of the disease. Melanoma treatments can be numerous debilitating physical and psychological effects to both patients and their caregivers. Treatment- or disease-related effects include reduced global health status and quality of life, pain, loss of appetite, fatigue, anxiety and depression, low self-esteem, poor work productivity, as well as relationship and family suffering. The absence of supportive or palliative care can lead to poor coping, emotional distress, burden symptoms, and a poor quality of life [2, 3].

An improvement of such a burden can be achieved by an integration of oncology and early palliative care centered by the patient's needs. As proposed by ASCO and ESMO [4–6], the goal of integration is to optimize patient access to early palliative care and, ultimately, to improve the quality of life of patients and caregivers. It is important to differentiate the levels of palliative care (Table 25.1), since this approach can be performed at different levels depending on the patient's needs and

Table 25.1 Levels of palliative care (Adapted from Ferrell BR et al. Integration of palliative care into standard oncology care: American Society of Clinical Oncology Clinical Practice Guideline Update. J Clin Oncol. 2017) [4]

Basic (Level A: undergraduate and postgraduate)
Integrate palliative care methods and procedures in general care, for all healthcare professionals
Advanced (Level B: postgraduate)
For professionals involved with palliative care, but not as their main occupation (e.g., oncologists)
Specialist (Level C: postgraduate)
For professionals working solely in palliative care whose main activity is complex problems requiring specialized skills and competencies. The main role of specialist palliative care is to manage patients and families with more complex and challenging needs while supporting and training generalist palliative care providers

the time of illness, as well as the availability of the service. In 2017, ASCO published a guideline with specific recommendations for integrating palliative care and oncological treatment, since the diagnosis (Fig. 25.1) listed in Table 25.2 [4–6, 8].

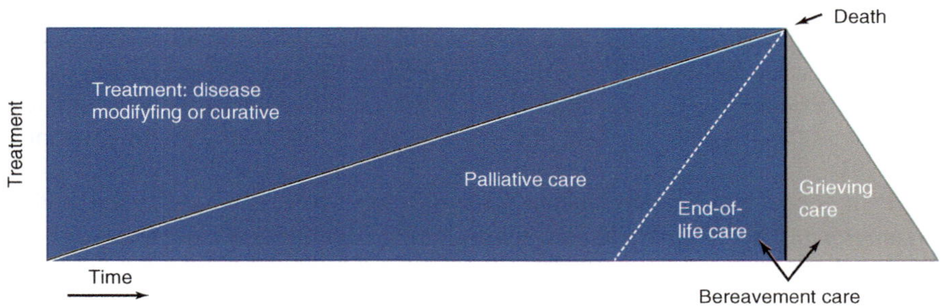

Fig. 25.1 When to start supportive and palliative care [7]

Table 25.2 Integration of palliative care into standard oncology care (Adapted from ASCO Clinical Practice Guideline) [4]

1	Patients with advanced cancer should be referred to interdisciplinary palliative care teams (consultation) that provide inpatient and outpatient care early in the course of disease, alongside active treatment of their cancer
2	Palliative care for patients with advanced cancer should be delivered through interdisciplinary palliative care teams with consultation available in both outpatient and inpatient settings
3	Patients with advanced cancer should receive palliative care services, which may include a referral to a palliative care provider. Essential components of palliative care include may include the following: • Rapport and relationship building with patient and family caregiver(s) • Symptom, distress, and functional status management (i.e., pain, dyspnea, fatigue, sleep disturbance, mood, nausea, or constipation) • Exploration of understanding and education about illness and prognosis • Clarification of treatment goals • Assessment and support of coping needs (i.e., provision of dignity therapy) • Assistance with medical decision-making • Coordination with other care providers • Provision of referrals to other care providers as indicated
4	For newly diagnosed patients, early palliative care involvement, within 8 weeks of diagnosis, is suggested
5	Among patients with cancer with high symptom burden, high expectant needs, or great anticipation of experiencing overlapping phases of care (diagnosis, staging, treatment, and end of life), outpatient programs of cancer care should provide and use dedicated resources (palliative care clinicians) to deliver palliative care services to complement existing program tools
6	For patients with early or advanced cancer for whom family caregivers will provide care in the outpatient setting, nurses, social workers, or other providers may initiate caregiver-tailored palliative care support, which could include telephone coaching, education, referrals, and face-to-face meetings. For family caregivers who may live in rural areas or be unable to travel to clinic, offering telephone support over face-to-face support may be offered

Symptom Management

Pain

According to the International Association for the Study of Pain, the definition of pain is "an unpleasant sensory and emotional experience associated with, or resembling that associated with, actual or potential tissue damage." Pain is always a personal experience that is influenced to varying degrees by biological, psychological, and social factors. Through their life experiences, individuals learn the concept of pain [9].

Pain is one of the most frequent symptoms in oncology. A skin lesion itself is symptomatic, and pain is also the most common symptom for patients with skin cancer. In addition, 43% of patients with unresectable skin cancer have bone metastasis, which can become one of the sources of pain. The presence of metastasis in the liver, pleura, and other sites of metastasis also causes of pain in metastatic melanoma [10].

Treatment: For cutaneous lesions, resection is the best choice for controlling pain. Surgery, radiotherapy, and appropriate tumoricidal treatments, as well as non-drug treatments, have an important role in some patients. For patients with bone metastasis, palliative radiation therapy is effective for improving pain and preventing bone fracture. Bisphosphonate can also be used for preventing pain and bone fracture due to bone metastasis. A combined approach can lead to optimum analgesia with minimum side effects. Analgesic drugs, however, remain the best choice in managing cancer pain. The choice of drug should be based on the severity of the pain, not the stage of disease. If a non-opioid or, in turn, an opioid for moderate pain is not sufficient, a strong opioid for severe pain should be used. The WHO analgesic ladder, as seen on Fig. 25.2, should be used for drugs of choice [10–14]. The best

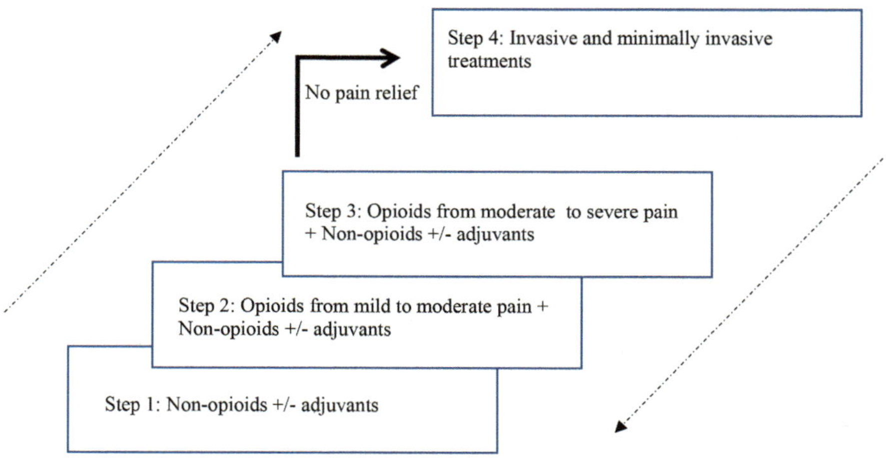

Fig. 25.2 The WHO analgesic ladder (adapted by the revised WHO analgesic ladder) [11, 12]

opioid depends on patient's features, and the knowledge of the doctor about the drug: evaluation of the diseases, age, side effects and route of administration, and choice according to intensity of the patient's pain. For dosages and routes of administration, see Table 25.3. Adjuvant analgesic drugs may be usefully added at any

Table 25.3 Prescription of opioids [14, 15]

Opioid	Route	Duration	Initial doses	Equivalence to morphine OR	Attention
Codeine	OR	6 h	30 mg every 6 h	30 mg morphine OR: 240 mg tramadol	≥360 mg/day not recommended
Tramadol	OR/IV	6 h	50 mg every 4–6 h	30 mg morphine OR: 120 mg tramadol	≥400 mg/day not recommended
Morphine	IV/SC	2–4 h	2–3 mg every 4 h	1:3	There is no dose ceiling; optimal dose is limited by side effects Be careful in renal failure
Morphine	OR	2–4 h or 12 h (extended-release)	5–10 mg every 4/4 h	1	
Methadone	IV/SC	7–59 h	2.5 mg each 12/12 h Dose adjustment every 4/4 h	Variable	There is no dose ceiling; optimal dose is limited by side effects Be careful in hepatic failure
Methadone	OR		5 mg every 12/12 h Dose adjustment every 4/4 h		
Fentanyl	IV	30–60 min	Bolus: 0.5–1 mcg/kg every 1–2 h Continue infusion: 0.5 mcg/kg/h	100:1	Be careful in hepatic failure
Fentanyl	TD	72 h	25 mcg every 72 h	100:1	
Fentanyl	Intranasal route	30–60 min	100 or 200 mcg/dose	100:1	
Oxycodone (extended-release)	OR	40 min and 4–6 h	10 mg each 12 h	1:1.5	Be careful in renal failure
Buprenorphine	TD	3.5–7 days	5 mcg/hora	75:1	Be careful in hepatic failure

Table 25.4 Adjuvant analgesics [16]

Common adjuvant analgesics for cancer pain	
Drugs	Indications
Nonsteroids anti-inflammatories	Bone pain, soft infiltration, hepatomegaly
Corticosteroids	Raised intracranial pressure, soft tissue infiltration, nerve compression, hepatomegaly
Antidepressants, anticonvulsivants, antiarrythmics	Neuropathic pain, nerve compression or infiltration, paraneoplastic neuropathies
Biphosphonates	Bone pain

stage. An adjuvant analgesic is a drug whose primary indication is for something other than pain but that has an analgesic effect in some painful conditions (Table 25.4) [11, 12, 14, 16].

Attention to details: Safe and effective control of cancer pain demands thorough knowledge of the pharmacokinetics and pharmacodynamics of opioids that guide dosing, titration, and rotation.

- Extended-release opioid regularly (oral or transdermal)
- Immediate-release opioid for breakthrough pain, orally (10% of the daily dose)

Prevention and management of adverse effects of opioids require careful assessment and knowledge regarding agents used to treat these complications.

- Laxative regularly and titrate to normal frequency before cancer (e.g., senna, polyethylene glycol).
- Antiemetic available for all patients upon initiation or dose increase (metoclopramide). Consider adjuvant drugs [14].

Gastrointestinal Symptoms

Nausea and vomiting: Nausea and vomiting are symptoms prevalent in 62% of advanced cancer patients; 34% present only nausea. Around 50% of chemotherapy or radiotherapy patients may present these symptoms even while using antiemetics. In patients with malignant skin tumors, nausea is present in most stages, be it as a side effect of treatment, associated with anorexia or cachexia syndrome, or associated with liver metastases, causing discomfort and worsening quality of life [10, 17–20].

Being aware of nausea and/or vomiting physiopathology allows for a better treatment by considering how different receptors are affected by the medication being used. Table 25.5 correlates receptors with causes of nausea/vomiting. The center of vomiting in the central nervous system is affected from four different pathways [17–20]:

Table 25.5 Causes of nausea and vomiting and action mechanisms with receptors (Receptors: 5-HT3, serotonin type; D2, dopamine type; NK1, NK type; M1, muscarinic type; H1, histamine type; GABA, γ-aminobutyric acid) [17–20]

Triggering mechanism	Site/receptor	Site/receptor
– Gastric stasis – Constipation, intestinal obstruction – Gastrointestinal irritation (candidiasis, other infections, chemotherapy, radiotherapy) – Extrinsic compression – Drugs (chemotherapy, opioids, antibiotics, nonsteroidal anti-inflammatory, iron)	– Intestinal wall receptors (5-HT3) – Vagal and sympathetic afferents (5-HT3, D2, NK1)	– Vomiting center (H1, M1): it receives input from cerebral areas, gastrointestinal tract via vagal afferents, chemoreceptor trigger zone, and vestibula system
– Movements	– Vestibular system (M1, H1)	
– Uremia – Hypercalcemia – Drugs (chemotherapy, opioids, digoxin)	– Chemoreceptor trigger zone (5-HT3, D2)	
– Anxiety and stress – Pain – Hyponatremia – Intracranial hypertension – CNS metastasis – Meningeal irritation	– Cerebral córtex (GABA, H1)	

- Peripheral route: vagal and splanchnic afferent fibers originating from gastrointestinal viscera.
- Vestibular system.
- Chemoreceptor trigger zone (CTZ) located at the area postrema in the brainstem. This area is involved by a permeable blood-brain barrier, which makes it sensible to emetogenic substances that are present in blood circulation.
- Cerebral cortex and vomit center.

It is necessary to evaluate when symptoms begin, vomit characteristics, triggering factors, improvement and worsening factors, relation with food and smells, difficulty swallowing, medications and treatments (chemotherapy, radiotherapy), disease worsening, and comorbidities. Reversible causes such as intestinal constipation, new medication or dose adjustment (antibiotics, digoxin, or opioids), and electrolytic disorders (hypercalcemia, dehydration, hyponatremia, uremia) should be treated.

Assessment of nauseas and vomiting should be multimodal:

- Nonpharmacologic management:
  - Diet adjustments: diet fractioning, small quantities, patient's choice of food, cold or frozen foods, clear liquids, ice chips; avoid greasy food, strong smells, and condiments; avoid recumbency for at least 1–2 h after meals
  - Acupuncture
  - Transcutaneous electrical nerve stimulation (TENS) may be of help
  - Hypnosis, relaxation, and visualization techniques
  - Psychotherapy for anticipatory or fear, anxiety-triggered nausea
- Pharmacologic management: The choice of treatment is based on mechanisms of symptom action and targets of drug receptors. It is common for the patient to present multifactorial nausea and vomiting, which demands the association of many medications that act on different receptors. See Table 25.6 for major antiemetics dosages and side effects [17–20].

Table 25.6 Major antiemetics, doses, indications, collateral effects, and action mechanisms [17, 18]

Drug	Dose	Recommendation	Side effects	Action mechanism
Metoclopramide Bromopride	10 mg PO, IV, SC 3–4×/day 10 mg PO, IV 3–4×/day	First choice for gastroparesis	Extrapyramidal symptoms, agitation, drowsiness Avoid in malignant intestinal obstruction	D2 antagonist
Haloperidol	0.5–1.5 mg PO, IM, SC 8/8h	First choice for opioids induced nausea and vomiting Malignant bowel obstruction Intracranial hypertension	Extrapyramidal symptoms, agitation, drowsiness, lowers seizure threshold	D2 antagonist
Chlorpromazine Promethazine	25–50 mg PO, IM 8/8h 15–25 mg PO 8/8h	Malignant bowel obstruction, nausea and vomiting of unknown cause, peritoneal irritation Intracranial hypertension	Drowsiness, arterial hypotension, constipation, urinary retention, dry mouth	D2, M1, H1 antagonist
Ondansetron Granisetron Palonosetron	8 mg PO, IV, SC 8/8h 3 mg IV 8/8h 250 mcg IV 1×/day	First choice for chemotherapy-induced nausea and vomiting, postoperative	Headache, constipation, dizziness	5HT3 antagonist

Table 25.6 (continued)

Drug	Dose	Recommendation	Side effects	Action mechanism
Dimenhydrinate	50–100 mg PO 6/6h 30 mg EV 6/6h or 4/4h	nausea and vomiting of unknown cause, peritoneal irritation, nausea of vestibular cause Intracranial hypertension	Dry mouth, drowsiness	H1 antagonists
Scopolamine	10–20 mg PO, IV, SC 8/8h or 6/6h	Malignant bowel obstruction, peritoneal irritation, and intracranial hypertension	Dry mouth, drowsiness, constipation, urinary retention, agitation	M1 antagonists
Olanzapine	5–10 mg PO per day	Nausea and vomiting of unknown cause, second choice for association to treatment refractory nausea	Drowsiness, lowers seizure threshold, dry mouth, constipation	5HT3, H1, M1 antagonist
Dexamethasone	4–20 mg PO, IV	Post-chemotherapy Intracranial hypertension	Agitation, edema	Unknown; reduces tumor edema
Octreotide	150–1500 μg SC	Pseudointestinal obstruction	Abdominal pain, headache, constipation	Reduces gastrointestinal secretions and mobility
Lorazepam	0.5–1 mg PO, SL 4×/day	Anticipatory nausea and vomiting	Drowsiness, *delirium*	benzodiazepine
Fosaprepitant	125 mg PO on day 1, 80 mg PO on days 2 and 3	Prevention of chemotherapy-induced nausea and vomiting	Hiccup, asthenia, fatigue, drowsiness, anxiety, anorexia	NK1 antagonist

Constipation: Intestinal constipation is common in patients with advanced cancer, causing discomfort and poor quality of life. Medication, bad performance status, and reduced mobility are causes for constipation or its worsening. Nausea, vomiting, hyporexia, and abdominal pain may be concomitant symptoms. In advanced cancer, 63% of patients need laxatives; for opioid-using patients, prevalence is 87%. Evidence shows that its treatment is (frequently) inadequate in oncological and palliative care units, leading to the suffering and the aggravation of other symptoms [21–24].

Opioids act on the gastrointestinal tract μ-receptors, delaying gastric emptying, increasing the pyloric sphincter's tonus, and slowing down traffic through the ileocecal valve and colon. Among the strong opioids, there is evidence that transdermal fentanyl and transdermal buprenorphine cause less constipation than morphine or oral oxycodone. The same goes for methadone, less constipating than morphine or hydromorphone, which is attributed to methadone action on NMDA receptors [23, 24]. The causes of constipation are shown in Table 25.7.

Table 25.7 Causes for intestinal constipation in palliative care (Adapted from Sykes NP. In: Cherny NI et al, editors. Oxford Textbook of Palliative Medicine) [22]

Medication	• Opioids • Anticholinergics: scopolamine, hyoscine, tricyclic drugs, antiparkinsonism drugs, neuroleptics (chlorpromazine and haloperidol), diuretics, anti-seizure drugs • Others: iron, drugs for hypertension, vincristine	
Cancer	• Intestinal obstruction • Cauda equina syndrome • Hypercalcemia • Poor intake, low-fiber diet • Dehydration • Somnolence • Mobility reduction • Confusion • Depression	
Comorbidities	• Diabetes mellitus • Hypothyroidism • Hypokalemia • Hernia • Diverticular disease	• Rectocele • Anal fissure or stenosis • Anal prolapse • Hemorrhoids • Colitis

Table 25.8 Laxatives and doses (Adapted from Consenso Brasileiro de Constipação Intestinal induzida por Opioides, 2009) [23]

Drug class	Drugs	Action time
Bulk-forming laxatives	Soluble and insoluble fibers Plantago Psyllium	
Irritating agents	Sene 10 g/200 mL PO Bisacodyl 10–20 mg PO Picosulfate 10 mg PO/nasoenteral tube Prucalopride 1–2 mg PO per day	6–12 h 6–12 h 6–12 h Once a day Average 2.5 h
Osmotic agents	Lactulose 15–30 mL PO 1 a 2×/day PEG/Macrogol 14–28 g/200 mL PO Magnesium citrate 15–60 mL PO per day	24–48 h 2–4 days 0.5–3 h
Emollients	Glycerin suppository 1 unit rectal route/per day Docusate 100–400 mg PO per day Mineral oil 30–60 mL PO per day Glycerin enema 500 mL rectal/SOS	15–60 min 24–72 h 6–8 h 5–60 min

Good control of other symptoms helps in preventing, alleviating, and better treating intestinal constipation. Dyspnea and pain relief improves mobility, and controlled nausea improves patient diet and hydration. It is necessary to correct metabolic alterations such as hypercalcemia and dehydration, to suspend medication that does not yield benefits, prescribing prophylactic laxatives for patients using opioids (see Table 25.8 for main laxatives and dosages), anticholinergics, and tricyclics [21, 25].

The World Health Organization recommends preventive measures for patients on palliative care and using opioids. Patients and caregivers must be educated on the necessity of ingesting liquids and, whenever possible, to the regular use of laxatives [23].

In the majority of advanced-stage cancer patients, it`s not possible to maintain good liquid ingestion and mobility, both of which assist intestinal motility. Moreover, the use of constipating drugs hinders the effect of medication that forms fecal cake. Therefore, the use of these drugs may lead to collateral effects such as pain, abdominal distention, flatulence, and fecal impaction. Osmotic agents like lactulose act by retaining fluids in the intestinal lumen, often taking up to 3 days to exert the desired effect. Its collateral effects are distention, flatulence, and colic. PEG is a nonabsorbable sugar that is not metabolized by colonic bacteria, thus reducing abdominal distention and flatulence. It may be used as prophylaxis and control of opioid-induced constipation. Irritating agents stimulate intestinal motility and augment intraluminal secretion of liquids and electrolytes in the distal ileum and colon. Patients using nasoenteral tube or gastrostomy warrant special attention; sodium picosulfate is the irritative of choice, given that bisacodyl tablets cannot be macerated. There is no evidence in literature that supports macerating prucalopride pills. Among emollients, mineral oil is to be avoided in patients with swallowing difficulties, dyspnea, or with lower levels of conscience due to the risk of bronchoaspiration. Docusate sodium aids the absorption of other laxatives and may be associated to an irritative; the most common association is bisacodyl with docusate sodium. In cases of impacted or hardened stool in the rectal ampulla, a suppository of glycerin, enema, or glycerin enema is to be used. Manual fecal "breaking" is painful and should be avoided, but if used must be preceded by analgesia. End-of-life patients, without oral ingestion and with poor responsiveness, may get uncomfortable or go into *delirium*. In such cases, glycerin enema is the recommended measure [21–25].

When prescribing analgesic opioids, a laxative of the stimulant/irritative type is to be implemented as prophylaxis. In opioid-related constipation, the first choice of treatment are stimulant/irritative laxatives; if symptoms do not improve within 2 days, a laxative agent of the osmotic type is to be associated. A third laxative may be used if necessary, preferably an emollient. It is important to maintain regular use of laxatives while opioids are being used. If opioid-related constipation does not improve with laxative use, opioid rotation is to be implemented [23, 24].

Dyspnea

Dyspnea is an important symptom because of its prevalence during the advanced stage of cutaneous malignancies [10] and because of the emotional burden that comes with it (involving feelings like anxiety, fear, abandonment). Being aware of diagnosis and treatment of conditions that lead to dyspnea is not always sufficient to managing the suffering it causes when it becomes refractory. Subjectivity, multidimensionality, and the paroxysm of advanced disease offer a dimension of the intense level of suffering it causes [26, 27]. It afflicts around 50% of patients on late stages of cancer and becomes more frequent and intense as it gets closer to the end of life [28].

The mechanisms involved in dyspnea are not entirely known. It is known that central and peripheral chemoreceptors, as well as sensorial receptors on respiratory, vagal, and pulmonary muscles, generate afferent signals related to a physiological status that lead to adjustments to the functions of respiratory muscles. Dyspnea occurs from a neuromechanical dissociation, in other words an incompatibility between the neural stimulus to breathe and the effectory (mechanic) response. Breathing becomes voluntary and the sensation of dyspnea appears. Sensorial information is processed on superior cerebral centers that account for the influence of cognitive, emotional, and behavioral factors. The term "dyspnea" encompasses qualitatively different sensations that are linked to distinct physiopathological mechanisms [26, 29, 30].

The essential basis of dyspnea measurement is patient complain. Instruments for quantification, such as numerical, analogical, or modified Borg scales [29] are unidimensional and rarely used in practice. Anamnesis consists of reporting the experience of respiratory discomfort, triggers, adaptive responses, and meanings and emotions attached to that experience [30]. It is vital to understand if it represents a new event or if it is an effect from deterioration of the base illness [26]. The findings from the physical examination will direct the diagnosis of the cause of dyspnea (see Table 25.9 for causes of dyspnea on patients with skin malignancies). The absence

Table 25.9 Causes for dyspnea on skin malignancy patients (*COPD: chronic obstructive pulmonary disease) (Adapted from Parshall MB et al. An official American Thoracic Society statement: update on the mechanisms, assessment, and management of dyspnea. Am J Respir Crit Care Med. 2012 and Kamal AH et al. Dyspnea review for the palliative care professional: treatment goals and therapeutic options. J Palliat Med. 2012) [26, 30]

Category	Causes
Tumor related	• Pleural, pericardiac effusion • Pulmonary mass or metastasis • Phrenic paralysis • Carcinomatous lymphangitis • Bronchial obstruction—atelectasis • Superior vena cava syndrome • Disease progression—final stages of life
Cardio pulmonary	• Pulmonary congestion • Pulmonary embolism • Pulmonary infection • Related illnesses, i.e. COPD*, cardiac insufficiency
Systemic	• Cachexia—sarcopenia • Anemia • Ascites • Abdominal distension—constipation, intestinal occlusion • Metabolic acidosis • Obesity • Critical patient myopathy
Oncological treatment related	• Pulmonary post-resection • Actinic pneumonitis • Drug-related pneumonitis

of clinical signs or hypoxemia does not disqualify the complaint of dyspnea. It is important to observe changes of vital signs, oximetry, respiratory pattern, and frequency; usage of accessory muscles, cyanosis, and pale skin; variations of pulmonary propaedeutic that indicate congestion, bronchospasm, consolidation, or atelectasis; and signals of conditions such as edemas, ascites, venous thrombosis, and abdominal distension [26]. Laboratory and imaging exams must be recommended according to clinical hypothesis and physical examinations. Laboratory exams may indicate anemia, infections, cardiac and/or renal dysfunctions, or cachexia. Imaging exams must have a clear objective and be proportional to the current stage of the disease and to therapeutic possibilities: simple thorax or abdomen radiographies, ultrasound, echocardiography, thorax tomography, bronchoscopy, angiographic studies, and functional proofs. Some exams contain therapeutic possibilities, such as bronchoscopy and interventionist radiology [26, 30].

The fundamental principle of dyspnea management is the treatment of base causes and aggravating factors [26, 31, 32]. When there is no consistent response or when the worsening of symptoms is related to tumor progression, we consider it as refractory dyspnea [31]. The management of refractory dyspnea involves pharmacological and nonpharmacological interventions and is summarized in Fig. 25.3.

Nonpharmacological interventions: When considered separately, interventions such as acupuncture, meditation, and yoga are not backed by evidence [26]. That being said, recent studies show that dyspnea support centers that coordinate nonpharmacological and pharmacological measures with a holistic and interdisciplinary approach (listed in Table 25.10) have been showing results like better dyspnea control and stress and depression and anxiety reduction and offering customized interventions and patient-centered care [27, 30, 32–34].

Oxygen therapy—noninvasive ventilation (NIV) and high-flow nasal cannula (HFNC): the use of supplementary oxygen (administered via catheter or masks) on oncological patients presents controversial evidence; it is argued whether the benefit comes from the oxygen itself or from wind blowing. Regardless, available evidence points favorably to the use of supplementary oxygen on hypoxemic patients. It must be discontinued if it does not alleviate dyspnea symptoms [26, 30].

Although the use of NIV is widespread on a number of clinical situations, its use for dyspnea symptom relief in advanced disease stages remains controversial. Many patients are uncomfortable with wearing masks, and the potential for extending the death process is a real danger. The recommendation for NIV use within palliative care is to be on a case-by-case basis and with clear objectives. It is necessary for the patient to have a high tolerance on NIV and that deadlines be set for reevaluation and revision of objectives. NIV should be suspended if the patient experience a decline of level of conscience or if no symptom alleviation is verified. Even though few studies have been made on the subject, in clinical practice, the HFNC has been used as an alternative to NIV; it is safe, is frequently met with high tolerance, and allows for interactions with family members [26, 30, 35–37].

Pharmacological treatment: Opioids are the only pharmacological class with evidence for alleviating dyspnea symptoms that are corroborated by clinical practice. Opioids reduce respiratory drive as well as anxiety and alter central perception

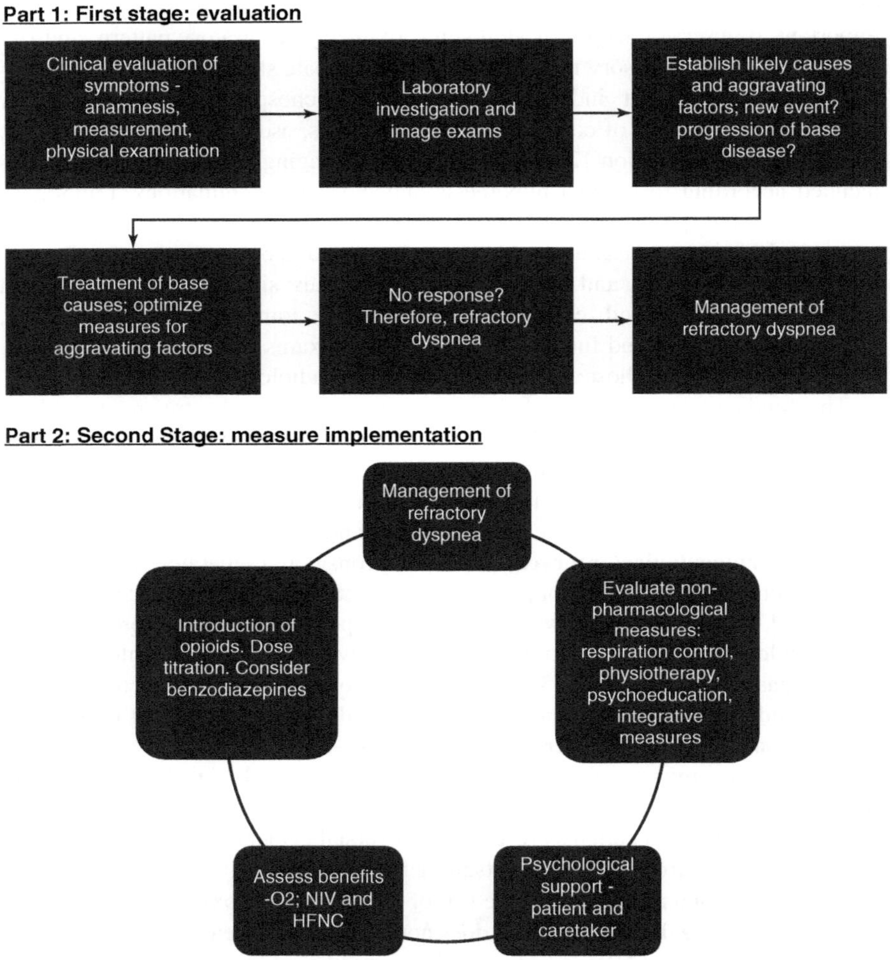

Fig. 25.3 Flowchart for the management of refractory dyspnea (prepared by the author) [26, 29–35]

Table 25.10 Nonpharmacological interventions coordinated within a multidisciplinary team (dyspnea support center) [30, 32–34]

Education for patients and caretakers (psych-education)
Psychological support (cognitive-behavioral therapy, group therapy)
Facial ventilator
Integrative therapy (music therapy, art therapy, relaxation techniques, mindfulness, meditation)
Forward lean positions
Breathing control techniques
Strategies for energy saving
Physiotherapy and physical exercise
Social—spiritual—family support

by connecting to μ-opioid receptors located on bronchiolar and alveolar walls. The action takes place via a central modulation process that disconnects the feeling of discomfort. Emotional states such as depression and anxiety, and individual pharmacogenetic variations may influence the physiological response. The best available evidence was obtained with the use of morphine on individuals with COPD. Studies with other opioids (especially fentanyl) failed to offer better results than morphine. The use of nebulized opioids is not recommended. Regular doses are smaller or equal to 30 mg of oral morphine within 24 h. Adverse effects are mild and include constipation and nausea, while respiratory depression is not common when recommended doses are used. Despite not being backed by evidence, buprenorphine has been used empirically with an equianalgesic-based dose, achieving satisfactory results. Table 25.11 displays main opioid dosages for dyspnea.

Table 25.11 Pharmacological management of dyspnea [26, 27, 30, 31, 33, 35, 38–40]

	Route of administration	Dose	Procedure/notes
Choice of drug for titration: **morphine**	Intravenous, oral, or subcutaneous	Initial dose: 30–50% analgesic dosage (opioid-naive patient). Patient already using opioids • Increase the dose by 25–50%	Start with 1–2 mg IV/SC or 5 mg PO (patient already using opioids: increase the usual dose by 25–50%) for dyspnea crisis, or by the clock (4/4h) • Titrate until dyspnea relief. Immediate-release opioid for crisis (10% daily dose). Consider continuous infusion if difficult to control or frequent crisis
After titration, switch opioids using same equianalgesic dose ratio	PO (morphine) or TD (fentanyl or buprenorphine)	Options for PO route (ratio IV:PO = 1:3) • Short-release pills 10–30 mg • Slow-release pills 30, 60, and 100 mg • Oral solution 10 mg/ml (1 mL = 32 drops)	• Transdermal opioids available: fentanyl or buprenorphine. Use equianalgesic dose ratio • Always leave rescue option for dyspnea crisis with oral or parenteral morphine—Rescue dose: 1/6 of the total opioid dose in 24 h
If relevant component of anxiety and/or poor response to opioids, consider associate benzodiazepines	• PO lorazepam or alprazolam • Sublingual medicine clonazepam • IV/SC midazolam	Initial doses: • Lorazepam 0.5 mg/dose • Alprazolam 0.25 mg/dose • Clonazepam 0.5 mg/dose • Midazolam 1 mg/dose	• Use during dyspnea crisis • Evaluate response • Titrate until dyspnea relief • Consider prescribe by the clock

Benzodiazepines are considered second-tier dyspnea control and are associated with opioids when there is a relevant component of anxiety. Though evidence is scarce, they are frequently prescribed in clinical practice, especially during the end of life. Literature suggest the usage of ultrashort or short half-life benzodiazepines such as midazolam, lorazepam, or alprazolam, although clonazepam is often used in palliative care owing to its simple sublingual presentation. Other drugs (diuretics, herbal medicines, antidepressants, cannabinoids) are not recommended due to lack of evidence. Corticosteroids are recommended only if a major pulmonary parenchyma involvement is present [30, 31, 35, 38–43]. If refractory dyspnea is still ongoing after the resources above have been used, the patient is likely in the last days of life, and a palliative sedation should be considered.

Bleeding

Skin cancer, especially unresectable tumors, may present local complications such as bleeding, exudate, or offensive odor, with a reported incident rate of about 30% which is higher than that in all types of cancer. The main implication of these symptoms is that quality of life is compromised [10].

For these symptoms, surgery and radiation are effective therapeutic options, such as cryotherapy. Invasive handling is often the only option to stop bleeding. However, extensive and mutilating resections are frequently contrary to the goals of care. Thus, procedures with a potential to cause impairment or excessive suffering need individualized analysis with regard to proportionality. In such cases, radiotherapy and cryotherapy (though this is a painful option) can be efficient resources for symptom control [10].

If using these resources is impossible, topical ointments and dressing materials are additional options for controlling the offensive odor of malignant wounds. Topical metronidazole, Mesalt® dressing, curcumin ointments, and activated carbon dressing were reported to be useful [10]. It is also important to remark that the use of dark blue linen and dressings reduces the visual impact of voluminous bleeding exteriorization for the patient and his family.

When dealing with voluminous bleeding, arteriography with vessel embolization can be useful for hemorrhage control. In some cases, embolization is the treatment of choice to avoid surgery or remains as an option if a surgical treatment is impossible. In that case, it must be possible to selectively catheterize the arterial supply of the tumor. Due to the procedure's technical complexity and the risk of complications, patient selection must be made with caution and a prudent assessment of the risks and benefits involved in the proposed intervention [44]. Consultation with an interventional radiologist with expertise in this kind of procedure is mandatory.

Delirium

Delirium is a clinical syndrome caused by cerebral inefficiency and presents the following characteristics: acute confusion with varying levels of consciousness, attention, and cognition, with inattention, disorientation, thought disorganization, hallucinations, sleep cycle alterations, torpor, somnolence, and often psychomotor agitation. It is common on advanced-stage cancer patients, with prevalence of 90% on the last days of life, of which 70% also display disquiet, agitation, or aggressive behavior [45–48].

Delirium can be reversed when its cause is identified and corrected or mitigated. Causes of *delirium* are listed in Table 25.12. On late-stage cancer, it is generally multifactorial and may be irreversible and an indication of the imminence of the end of life. It is a risk factor for prolonged hospitalization, complications such as falls and pressure ulcers, difficulty in evaluating other symptoms, and higher hospital mortality and a cause for suffering for the patient and family members [44, 49, 50].

Delirium diagnosis is based on clinical history and physical examinations. Resources such as CAM (Confusion Assessment Method) are used for screening—see Table 25.13 [47]. Previous performance status, stage of the disease, and cognitive level are important for the differential diagnosis and the outlining of an investigation of identifiable and potentially reversible causes or if the *delirium* represents an indication of the evolution toward the end of life. Investigation with complementary exams must be individualized [45–47].

Table 25.12 Causes of *delirium* in patients with advanced-stage skin cancer (Adapted from Caraceni A et al. Neurological problems in advanced cancer. In: Cherny NI et al., editors. Oxford textbook of Palliative Medicine, 2015) [45]

Direct central nervous system causes	Metastatic spreads to brain Seizures (including nonepileptiform status epilepticus)
Indirect causes	Metabolic encephalopathy due to major organ failure Electrolyte imbalance
	Treatment side effects from chemotherapeutic agents, corticosteroids, radiation therapy, opioids, anticholinergics, antiemetics, antivirals, and other medications and therapeutic modalities
	Infections
	Hematological abnormalities
	Nutritional deficiencies
	Paraneoplastic syndromes
	Terminal *delirium*

Table 25.13 CAM (Confusion Assessment Method) (Adapted from Inouye SK. The dilemma of Delirium: clinical and research controversies regarding diagnosis and evaluation of delirium in hospitalized elderly medical patients. Am J Med 1994) [47]

A) Acute onset and fluctuating course
B) Inattention, distractibility
C) Disorganized thinking, illogical or nuclear ideas
D) Alteration in consciousness
The diagnosis of delirium required the presence of both features A and B, plus either feature C or D

Table 25.14 Summary of nonpharmacological interventions used in the prevention and treatment of *delirium* (Adapted from Breitbart W, Alici Y. Agitation and delirium at the end of life. "We couldn't manage him". JAMA 2008) [50]

Reducing polypharmacy
Control of pain
Sleep hygiene
Monitor for dehydration and fluid-electrolyte disturbances
Monitor nutrition
Monitor for sensory deficits (provide visual and hearing aids)
Encourage early mobilization
Minimize the use of immobilizing catheters, IV lines, and physical restraints
Monitor bowel and bladder functioning
Reorient the patient frequently
Place an orientation board, clock, or familiar objects in patient room
Encourage cognitively stimulating activities

Delirium can be hyperactive, predominance of disquiet and agitated behavior; hypoactive, predominance of somnolence and inactivity; or mixed, with components from both hyperactive and hypoactive *delirium*. Identifying the type of *delirium* is important for its recognition and better clinical management [48, 51].

The objective of treatment is managing reversible causes and controlling associated symptoms. During end-of-life *delirium*, focus should be kept in good symptom control and seeking comfort for the patient. Treatment for existing symptoms such as pain is to be maintained. Opioids should be kept in prescription for patients with previous usage. Opioid intoxication is to be treated with dosage reduction, opioid rotation, and hydration if recommended. Review and pay close attention to nonpharmacologic management (see Table 25.14), which can be both therapeutic and prophylactic for *delirium*. Good communication and orientation for family members and caregivers are essential in managing *delirium* and achieving greater understanding to better mitigate the suffering caused by *delirium* [45, 46, 48–50, 52, 53].

Pharmacological management: Symptom treatment with psychotropic medications is necessary to control *delirium*. In palliative care settings, evidence supports short-term low-dose use of antipsychotics in the control of symptoms of *delirium* with close monitoring for possible side effects [53]. Haloperidol is the choice antipsychotic for *delirium* treatment in patients with advanced diseases. It presents high efficacy and tolerability with few anticholinergics effects. For patients with fluctuation tending to hyperactivity, haloperidol is to be considered due to its very low antihistamine effect, which thereby reduces the chance of sedating the patient. It can be administered oral, intravenous, or subcutaneous routes. Most patients can take haloperidol by oral route, but in cases of agitation or oral unavailability, usual palliative care practice is resorting to subcutaneous or intravenous administration, in that order of preference. The IM administration, though safe and effective, is painful and uncomfortable for patients. Intravenous administration is to be used with caution as it often causes extrapyramidal collateral effects and QT interval enlargement. A common strategy is the association of parenteral lorazepam with haloperidol in order to handle hyperactive *delirium* with sedative action without extrapyramidal effects associated with antipsychotics. Patients with significant hyperactive *delirium*, with aggressiveness, elevated psychomotricity, risk of fall, or previous necessity of mechanic restriction can benefit from typical antipsychotics with greater antihistaminergic power such as chlorpromazine, which can be administered orally or venously. Atypical neuroleptics (risperidone, quetiapine, olanzapine, ziprasidone, and aripiprazole) are used to mitigate extrapyramidal adverse effects. For dosages and side effects, refer to Table 25.15 [53–59].

Table 25.15 Antipsychotic medications used in the treatment of *delirium* [53–60]

Medication Dose range Routes of administration	Side effects
Haloperidol 0.5–2 mg every 2–12 h PO, IV, IM, SC	Extrapyramidal adverse effects can occur at higher doses Monitor QT interval on electrocardiogram (EKG) **Remains the gold standard therapy for delirium. May add lorazepam (0.5–1 mg every 2–4 h) for agitated patients
Chlorpromazine 12.5–50 mg every 4–6 h PO, IV, IM	More sedating and anticholinergic compared with haloperidol Monitor blood pressure for hypotension More suitable for use in intensive care unit settings for closer blood pressure monitoring **May be preferred in agitated patients due to its sedative effect
Olanzapine 2.5–5 mg every 12–24 h PO, IM	Sedation is the main dose-limiting adverse effect in short-term use Older age, preexisting dementia, and hypoactive subtype of delirium have been associated with poor response
Risperidone 0.25–1 mg every 12–24 h PO	Extrapyramidal adverse effects can occur with doses of >6 mg/day Orthostatic hypotension
Quetiapine 12.5–100 mg every 12–24 h PO	Sedation, orthostatic hypotension Sedating effects may be helpful in patients with sleep-wake cycle disturbance
Ziprasidone 10–40 mg every 12–24 h PO, IM	Monitor QT interval on EKG
Aripiprazole 5–30 mg every 24 h PO, IM	Monitor for akathisia

End-of-life *delirium*: Approximately 30% of dying patients with delirium do not have their symptoms adequately controlled with antipsychotic medications. Processes causing delirium may be ongoing and irreversible during the active dying phase. In such cases, a reasonable choice is the use of sedative agents such as benzodiazepines (e.g., midazolam and lorazepam) to achieve a state of quiet sedation. Delirium has, in fact, been identified as the main indication for the use of palliative sedation in up to 82% of cases in symptom control studies among the terminally ill [61, 62].

Empathetic Communication, Family Support, and Grief Support

Interdisciplinary support in palliative care seeks the management of biopsychosocial and spiritual symptoms as well as the process for decision-making throughout the sickness, through the elaboration of goals of care and advanced care planning that respects values, wishes, and the patient's biography. Such skills are based on abilities of clear, empathetic, and assertive communication [4, 6].

Communication must be guided by protocols that verifiably foment the formation of rapport, as well as the patient's and family's comprehension of cancer diagnosis and prognosis, even when considering the high degree of uncertainty in some situations, keeping in mind the growing possibilities of new treatments that make possible results of survival with much greater quality than those seen until a few years ago. Such protocols also have the goal of helping the healthcare team in the comprehension of patient wishes and needs, leading to a care that is effectively patient centered [6, 63].

Take the SPIKES Protocol as an example. Its principles can be used in breaking bad news as well and communicating prognosis. It is necessary for empathetic communication that the supply of information be preceded by the listener's permission to start that conversation at that point in time, and of the active listening to comprehend what the patient already knows, and what are their expectations and concerns. The success of these conversations is directly linked to the capacity of healthcare professionals to respond adequately to emotions provoked by unpleasant news with a welcoming, supportive, and judgment-free approach [64, 65].

These conversations frequently take place in many stages, in which the prognostic is communicated clearly and assertively, doubts are addressed, and aims of care are defined. Sequential meetings make time for the patient and family to process information and elaborate questionings to reach the consensus of a shared decision-making [4, 6, 65, 66].

Efficient communication is especially important because the patient, family, and medical team may have multiple objectives at the same time, which may be conflicting and may complicate decision-making. Only the empathetic listening of necessities, doubts, and possible conflicts can help all involved parties to clarify their understanding of the situation as well as define objectives of care and elaborate a planning that reflects the medical reality and the priorities of the patient. The patient's understanding of the perspectives of prognostic must be well evaluated because incorrect assumptions about its comprehension, especially during a single conversation, may create confusion and anguish. The process of communication and rapport for decision-making requires experience, empathy, and concentration, as well as the knowledge of the tools and protocols at hand [4, 66, 67].

The medical team's comprehension of the grief process, according to the dual model of Stroebe and Schut that postulates that the breaking of the presumed world leads to a process of oscillating between extremes of loss and restoration, is fundamental to adequately deal with different styles of coping. This enables the healthcare professionals to be well prepared to deal with resistance and ambivalence to such conversations, allowing to access the comprehension of patient in a stepwise manner and scaling necessary information according to the more urgent clinical necessities [68, 69].

It is important to remark that family members and caregivers of advanced care and reserved prognostic patients are also grieving, and studies show that this leads to high rates of depression and anxiety. Thus, the multidisciplinary team must be attentive to address the needs of family members separately. Caring for the caretaker is often caring for the patient himself [70].

The role of the palliative care team does not end with the patient's death; going forward to support for family member's grief and referencing them for psychological attention when the existence or effective risk of a complicated grief process is verified [70].

Advanced Care Planning

Advanced care planning (ACP) enables patients to make plans for their future healthcare, mainly in the event of a potentially fatal disease and when there is risk of losing decisional capacity, and should address all domains of care. The original concept of ACP comprehends an advanced care directive and the designation of a surrogate if the patient becomes unable to make decisions [71, 72].

The barriers for ACP discussions are not only systemic, such as focus at treatment and cure and lack of coordination and structured approach to ACP, but can also be patient related (insufficient knowledge about their own health situation, unpredictable disease course, and difficult prognostication) or health professional related (hesitance to discuss end of life with patients, fear to take away patients' hope, lack of training and skills) [71, 72].

Doubts about the correct moment to begin such conversations are another barrier. They may occur at any moment during the course of the disease, but they are in general more objective when the disease worsens and when faced with milestones like disease progression and relapses. It is recommended that ACP conversations begin during periods of stability and not when faced with acute decompensations or terminality, because during stability, the patient will be at his/her best period for exerting autonomy. It is also recommended that decisions and documents should be updated regularly, as values and preferences may change overtime [66, 71].

A Delphi panel published in 2017 provides recommendations for oncological ACP implementation [73]. Table 25.16 summarizes its main points.

The process of decision-making usually begins with comprehending the patient's biography, wishes, preferences, and values. It is vital for health professionals to clarify the patient on his/her prognostic and expected outcomes, while keeping in mind the set of appropriate medical conducts and the set of patient values and wishes and establishing a shared objective of care that will orient the entire ACP. Depending on each case's peculiarities, a decision may be made in a short span of time, requiring only one or two meetings, or may be the result of a prolonged and dramatic process spanning months of difficult and challenging conversations. The main point of the challenge is to deal with people that display a variety of

Table 25.16 Main recommendations for oncological ACP (Adapted from Rietjens JAC et al.; European Association for Palliative Care. Definition and recommendations for advance care planning: an international consensus supported by the European Association for Palliative Care. Lancet Oncol. 2017) [73]

1	ACP should be adapted to the individual's readiness to engage in the ACP process
2	Healthcare professionals should adopt a person-centered approach when engaging in ACP conversations with individuals and, if the individual prefers so, their family. This requires tailoring the ACP conversation to the individual's health literacy, style of communication, and personal values
3	Healthcare professionals need to have the necessary skills and display an openness to talk about diagnosis, prognosis, death, and dying with individuals and their family
4	Healthcare professionals should provide individuals and their family with clear and coherent information concerning ACP
5	A trained non-physician facilitator can support an individual in the ACP process
6	The initiation of ACP (that is, the exploration of the individual's experiences, knowledge, personal values, and concerns) can occur in healthcare settings or non-healthcare settings
7	Where appropriate, ACP includes information about diagnosis, disease course, prognosis, advantages and disadvantages of possible treatment, and care options
8	Appropriate healthcare providers are needed for clinical elements of ACP, such as discussing diagnosis, prognosis, treatment, and care options, exploring the extent to which goals and preferences for future medical treatment and care are realistic, and documenting the discussion in the medical file
9	ACP might include the appointment of a personal representative and documentation thereof
10	ACP might include the completion of an advance care directive
11	Depending on the study or project aims, the following constructs should be assessed: • Knowledge of ACP • Self-efficacy to engage in ACP • Identification of goals and preferences • Communication about goals and preferences with family • Communication about goals and preferences with healthcare professionals • Identification of a personal representative • Documentation of goals and preferences • Revision of ACP discussions and documents over time

responses when faced with life-threatening situations, responses that are determined by biographical, cultural, and religious/spiritual factors that need to find a balance between hope and realistic objectives when facing dark prognostics. Conversations about ACP frequently arouse intense and contradictory emotions on patients and their family members, such as anxiety, denial, anger, frustration, sadness, and grief. This requires a training of the healthcare team to respond adequately to such emotions in a way that they do not become an obstacle for the best decisions of care. The participation of all members of the multidisciplinary team—nurses, chaplains, psychologists, counselors, and others—is essential. It is imperative that educational programs be available for multidisciplinary team professionals to instruct them on how to conduct and participate in these conversations while contemplating all the dimensions of care [4, 6, 63, 65, 66, 69].

Researchers have been recently analyzing the impact of ACP on care and questioning its benefits. The main points presented are the difficulty of suiting decision based on hypothetical scenarios to real life and the fact that the main point of ACP is not the production of medical records and filled forms and should not be restricted to something like a checklist. ACP is about talking, listening, comprehending without judgements what really matters to patients, informing prognostic scenarios empathically and realistically, and helping patients so that treatment decisions are adequate to their values [74].

End-of-Life Care

The early identification of palliative care needs in patients with advanced-stage cancer is critical to prevent and relieve distressing symptoms and to provide emotional and social support. It also allows for the healthcare team to initiate advance care planning and to discuss the continuation (or not) of life-prolonging treatments. Considering the relatively young age of melanoma patients and the introduction of innovative treatments for the advanced stage of the disease, a French study published in 2016 [75] showed that a large proportion of patients dying from advanced melanoma is exposed to aggressive cancer care near the end of life: more than 50% received chemotherapy in the last 3 months before death and 7.6% in the last week. During the final month before death, 12% of patients received radiation therapy, and 12.1% were transferred into the ICU. Only 17% of all patients died in palliative care inpatient units [75]. Although generalizability and comparability of these results may be restricted, the aggressiveness of cancer care for advanced melanoma patients raises serious concerns. The transition from predominantly curative to mostly palliative goals of care allows anticipating potential adverse events near the end of life, to ensure the adequate management of distressing symptoms, to properly address the patients' preferences regarding the goals of care, and to avoid futile treatments—thus, making end-of-life care centered in patient's needs.

End-of-life care can take place in many different settings, such as at the patient's home or at hospice facilities. It is recommended that the place of death and the necessary resources for care are included in advance care planning [73].

Regardless of the place of choice, the priority of end-of-life care is to improve symptoms, reduce patient and caregiver distress, promote and allow for greater interaction of the patient with his loved ones, and improve the chances of dying where one wishes, which is usually at home [76]. Studies show that end-of-life-care patients at home or at hospices show significantly lower rates of hospital readmission [77, 78].

End-of-life care must be delivered by multidisciplinary teams and be based on key elements such as psychological support, palliative support, educational-counseling support, spiritual support, preferential support, and supportive interactions [79]. Palliative support must prioritize rigorous symptom control through coordinating pharmacological and nonpharmacological interventions. The presence of nurses, counselors, psychologists, and chaplaincy is indispensable, given that the last moments of life are a trigger for emotional and spiritual questions [76, 79]. It is the time to confront the 4 Rs—remembering, reassessing, reconciling, reunion—to give resolution to pending matters, to express the meaning of the life that is coming to an end, to elaborate a legacy, say the last goodbyes, and express the wishes concerning the burial and memorial service [80].

With regard to management of symptoms during the end of life, we add those presented above, and the possibility of palliative sedation when faced with intolerable suffering caused by refractory symptoms. It is also necessary to be watchful for noisy respiratory secretions, usually associated with the patient being deeply unconscious. As no pharmacological or nonpharmacological intervention has been shown to be of predictable benefit in changing the clinical course of secretions, it is important to orient and give emotional shelter to the family. The entire care, monitorization, and medication planning must aim at promoting comfort and avoid distressing symptoms. Thus, the construction of a holistic and value-oriented care centered on patient necessities contributes toward a dignified and peaceful death, with support to distressing situations that derive from multidimensional suffering for the patient and his family. Studies show measurable benefits for family members of patients that pass away under such care, such as lower depression rates and adequate grieving [76, 79].

Palliative Sedation

Palliative sedation (PS) is a precious resource in oncological patient care during the final moments of life [81–85]. Although sedative prescription is a medical procedure, PS is considered a multidisciplinary intervention: End-of-life suffering demands the coordination of efforts from a highly trained multidisciplinary team [86]. Palliative sedation is defined as an intentional and monitored reduction of the patient's conscience level in order to relieve *intolerable* suffering that stems from *refractory* symptoms in end-of-life stage patients (with a life expectancy equal or shorter than 2 weeks, i.e., *the imminence of death*) [81–85]. With regard to terminology, the use of "palliative sedation" or "palliative sedation therapy" is widely accepted in literature. The expression "terminal sedation" has been abolished. The term "continuous deep sedation" refers to a specific modality of palliative sedation and should also be avoided [86, 87].

Strategies for PS implementation vary in depth and continuity. Its depth can be superficial, moderated, or deep. The timing can be intermittent, continuous, or transitory. The principle of proportionality is thus observed with sedatives dosed to the smallest dose necessary for symptom control. Palliative sedation frequently begins superficially and/or intermittently and progresses gradually according to the patient's need [81–85, 88, 89].

Prevalence of palliative sedation is variable and depends on the sort of institutions, ranging from 5 to 10% at hospices to over 60% in general hospitals [81–85, 88, 89].

Indication and criteria: The only indication for PS is the occurrence of refractory symptoms that cause intolerable suffering *for the patient* [81–85]. A symptom is defined as refractory when its available treatments are not effective in a reasonable term and/or there are unacceptable adverse effects [88]. The most frequent indications for palliative sedation are delirium, dyspnea, and pain, albeit any symptom can become refractory [81–85, 88].

The indication of palliative sedation for existential suffering is complex and controversial, although it is currently well accepted. It is recommended that the decision for palliative sedation for existential suffering is to be taken collectively, with the participation of mental health professionals. In such cases, intermittent or transitory palliative sedation is advised [90–92].

The previous definition of prioritizing comfort over artificial life-sustaining support as a goal of care is an indispensable criterion for PS implementation, and documentation of a DNR order in medical records is highly advised [93]. Table 25.17 lists situations where the use of PS is considered inappropriate or unacceptable.

Technical aspects: PS is to be implemented when one or more refractory symptoms are verified to be leading the patient to intolerable suffering. A survival estimate of around 2 weeks is required. It is desirable that the case be amply revised and

Table 25.17 Situations where the use of SP is considered inappropriate or unacceptable [85, 86, 88, 94]

Inadequate clinical circumstances: symptoms that are wrongly classified as refractory
Omission: delay of PS prescription due to fear of adverse effects or not wanting to deal with the communication and decision-making process
Inadequate process: poor communication; lack of informed consent; inappropriate drugs (such as opioid sedation); inadequate monitoring; deficiency in end-of-life care; lack of support for the family and assistance team
Abuse: PS prescription with the primary intent to rush death through dosages higher than needed for symptom control or deep palliative sedation when there are no refractory symptoms. Such practices are ethically unacceptable and illegal in most countries, including Brazil

discussed by the multidisciplinary team, assuring that all reasonable treatments have been unsuccessfully attempted and that the procedure is in accordance with the patient's values and desires [94]. The discussion concerning the option of palliative sedation is ideally to be held before the patient's condition aggravates. Topics that should be emphasized are the following: irreversibility of the clinical condition; the use of PS as a last resort, when all other possible treatments fail; how the monitorization and end-of-life care will take place; and the risks and effects of sedation. Inherent aspects of palliative sedation, such as the possibility of abolishing mental capacity, autonomy, and communication, are to be considered before implementation. If the patient does not wish to engage in this discussion, or does not have the clinical condition to do so, it must be made with the surrogate, who will decide through substitute judgement, free from pressures and conflicts of interest. If the patient's or the surrogate's informed consent is impossible, the decision is to be technical and based on the patient's best interest [83, 93–95].

Palliative sedation prescription: Benzodiazepines, neuroleptics, and barbiturates are the recommended drugs [81–85, 87, 88, 94]. Opioids are not good sedatives and not indicated for PS, although they can be used concomitantly for pain and dyspnea control. Midazolam is the drug of choice, followed by levomepromazine (its parenteral presentation is unavailable in Brazil), chlorpromazine, haloperidol, and phenobarbital. Other sedatives, such as propofol, dexmedetomidine, and pentobarbital can be prescribed under specific conditions or when facing refractoriness [81–85, 87, 88, 94]. Table 25.18 summarizes commonly used dosages. The usual routes of administration are intravenous and subcutaneous by hypodermoclysis. Monitorization should be focused on the level of sedation, pain/symptom control, and adverse effect detection. The deterioration of vital signs is expected in the death process; therefore, its systematic measurement is not recommended, while controls that concern comfort should be preserved [88]. The decision-making procedure,

Table 25.18 Drugs used for adult palliative sedation [88, 94]

Drug	Initial dosage	Usual effective dosage
Midazolam[a]	0.5–1 mg/h IV or SC (continuous)	1–20 mg/h IV or SC (continuous)
Chlorpromazine	12.5 mg IV every 4–12 h or 3–5 mg/h IV (continuous)	37.5–150 mg/day IV (continuous)
Levomepromazine[a, b]	12.5–25 mg IV every 8 h (+rescue treatment up to 1 h) or 50–75 mg/day IV or SC (continuous)	12.5–25 mg IV or SC every 8 h (+rescue treatment to 1 h) or until 300 mg/day IV or SC (continuous)
Fenobarbital[a]	Bolus 1–3 mg/kg followed by continuous infusion 0.5 mg/kg/h IV or SC	50–100 mg/h IV or SC (continuous)
Pentobarbital	Bolus IV slowly 2–3 mg/kg (do not exceed 50 mg/min) followed by continuous infusion 1 to 2 mg/kg/h IV	Titrate to the desired level of sedation
Propofol	0.5 mg/kg/h IV (continuous)	1– 4 mg/kg/h IV (continuous)

[a] Can be administered through hypodermoclysis

[b] Intravenous presentation unavailable in Brazil

conduct of plan, and monitorization process must be registered on medical records, as well as the non-resuscitation order.

The average survival after PS is implemented ranges from 1 to 6 days, and 96% of patients die within a week. Observational studies show that technically adequate palliative sedation does not reduce survival and does not rush death [83–85, 94].

Ethical aspects: Palliative care is based on the respect for patient values and dignity, within the principles defined by the WHO [1]. In that regard, it is essential to establish if palliative sedation is irreprehensible from an ethical viewpoint. The EAPC Ethical Task Force [94] compared euthanasia and palliative sedation with respect to three fundamental topics: intention, process, and result. Regarding intention, palliative sedation seeks to relieve intolerable suffering, while euthanasia aims at death. Concerning the process, sedation involves individualized, titled, and monitored sedative administration (usually benzodiazepines) to mitigate refractory symptoms; euthanasia is made with fixed, standardized doses of lethal drugs (barbiturates). Finally, the desired outcome in sedation is the relief of suffering, and in euthanasia, it is death. Therefore, the distinction is very clear [85, 96]. Palliative sedation is an intervention consensually accepted as a useful tool in the management of refractory symptoms during the end of life. It should be used as the last resort in the relief of intolerable suffering. Its implementation should follow a rigorous decision-making procedure, with informed consent, and take place within recommended technical precepts. Oncologists should develop basic skills for the management of palliative sedation. Within this framework, palliative sedation is both ethical and legal and conforms with the palliative care principles espoused by the WHO.

References

1. WHO. World Health Organization. WHO definition of palliative care. [Internet] 2002 [cited 2022 March 01]. http://www.who.int/cancer/palliative/definition/en/.
2. Fu H, Teleni L, Crichton M, et al. Supportive care and unmet needs in patients with melanoma: a mixed-methods systematic review. Support Care Cancer. 2020;28:3489–501. https://doi.org/10.1007/s00520-020-05464-3.
3. Fitch MI. Supportive care framework. Can Oncol Nurs J. 2008;18(1):6–24. English, French. https://doi.org/10.5737/1181912x181614.
4. Ferrell BR, Temel JS, Temin S, Alesi ER, Balboni TA, Basch EM, Firn JI, Paice JA, Peppercorn JM, Phillips T, Stovall EL, Zimmermann C, Smith TJ. Integration of palliative care into standard oncology care: American Society of Clinical Oncology clinical practice guideline update. J Clin Oncol. 2017;35(1):96–112. https://doi.org/10.1200/JCO.2016.70.1474.
5. Schrijvers D, Cherny NI, ESMO Guidelines Working Group. ESMO clinical practice guidelines on palliative care: advanced care planning. Ann Oncol. 2014;25 Suppl 3:iii138–42. https://doi.org/10.1093/annonc/mdu241.
6. Kaasa S, Loge JH, Aapro M, Albreht T, Anderson R, Bruera E, Brunelli C, Caraceni A, Cervantes A, Currow DC, Deliens L, Fallon M, Gómez-Batiste X, Grotmol KS, Hannon B, Haugen DF, Higginson IJ, Hjermstad MJ, Hui D, Jordan K, Kurita GP, Larkin PJ, Miccinesi G, Nauck F, Pribakovic R, Rodin G, Sjøgren P, Stone P, Zimmermann C, Lundeby

T. Integration of oncology and palliative care: a Lancet Oncology Commission. Lancet Oncol. 2018;19(11):e588–653. https://doi.org/10.1016/S1470-2045(18)30415-7.
7. Murray SA, Kendall M, Boyd K, Sheikh A. Illness trajectories and palliative care. BMJ. 2005;330(7498):1007–11. https://doi.org/10.1136/bmj.330.7498.1007.
8. Smith CB, Phillips T, Smith TJ. Using the new ASCO clinical practice guideline for palliative care concurrent with oncology care using the TEAM approach. Am Soc Clin Oncol Educ Book. 2017;37:714–23. https://doi.org/10.1200/EDBK_175474.
9. IASP. International Association for the Study of Pain. [Internet] 2020 [cited 2022 May 25]. https://www.iasp-pain.org/publications/iasp-news/iasp-announces-revised-definition-of-pain/.
10. Goto H, Yoshikawa S, Otsuka M, Omodaka T, Yoshimi K, Yoshida Y, Yamamoto O, Kiyohara Y. Symptom prevalence in patients with advanced skin cancer. J Dermatol. 2017;44(2):123–6. https://doi.org/10.1111/1346-8138.13527.
11. WHO. World Health Organization. WHO revision of pain management guidelines. [Internet] 2019 [cited 2022 April 26]. https://www.who.int/news/item/27-08-2019-who-revision-of-pain-management-guidelines.
12. Anekar AA, Cascella M. WHO analgesic ladder. 2022. In: StatPearls [Internet]. Treasure Island: StatPearls Publishing; 2022. https://www.ncbi.nlm.nih.gov/books/NBK554435/.
13. Barnes EA, Breen D, Culleton S, Zhang L, Kamra J, Tsao M, Balogh J. Palliative radiotherapy for non-melanoma skin cancer. Clin Oncol (R Coll Radiol). 2010;22(10):844–9. https://doi.org/10.1016/j.clon.2010.07.014.
14. Bruera E, Paice JA. Cancer pain management: safe and effective use of opioids. Am Soc Clin Oncol Educ Book. 2015:e593–9. https://doi.org/10.14694/EdBook_AM.2015.35.e593
15. Braun LM, Martins IS, Vigna ABD, Motta TMV. Uso de opióides na dor no câncer. In: Fonseca PRB, Barros CM, Lima ACB et al., editors. Tratado de dor oncológica. Rio de Janeiro: Atheneu; 2019. p. 395–420
16. Mitra R, Jones S. Adjuvant analgesics in cancer pain: a review. Am J Hosp Palliat Care. 2012;29(1):70–9. https://doi.org/10.1177/1049909111413256.
17. Hardy JR, Glare P, Yates P, Mannix KA. Palliation of nausea and vomiting. In: Cherny NI, Fallon MT, Kaasa S, Portenoy RK, Currow DC, editors. Oxford textbook of palliative medicine. Oxford: Oxford University Press; 2015. p. 661–674
18. Associação brasileira de cuidados paliativos. Consenso brasileiro de náusea e vômito. Revista Brasileira de Cuidados Paliativos. 3 (3) - Suplemento 2 (2011) https://nutritotal.com.br/pro/wp-content/uploads/sites/3/2011/08/222-ConsensoNauseaVomito.pdf. Accessed 2 Mar 2022.
19. Collis E, Mather H. Nausea and vomiting in palliative care. BMJ. 2015;351:h6249. https://doi.org/10.1136/bmj.h6249.
20. Leach C. Nausea and vomiting in palliative care. Clin Med (Lond). 2019;19(4):299–301. https://doi.org/10.7861/clinmedicine.19-4-299.
21. Ministério da saúde, Instituto do Câncer—INCA. Constipação intestinal no câncer avançado. Série cuidados paliativos. 2009. https://bvsms.saude.gov.br/bvs/publicacoes/inca/constipacao.pdf.
22. Sykes NP. Constipation and diarrhoea. In: Cherny NI, Fallon MT, Kaasa S, Portenoy RK, Currow DC, editors. Oxford textbook of palliative medicine. Oxford: Oxford University Press; 2015. p. 674–685
23. Associação brasileira de cuidados paliativos. Consenso Brasileiro de Constipação Intestinal induzida por Opioides. Revista Brasileira de Cuidados Paliativos, 2 (3) - Suplemento 1. 2009. https://wp.ufpel.edu.br/francielefrc/files/2019/06/consenso-brasileiro-de-constipa%C3%A7%C3%A3o-por-opi%C3%B3ides.pdf.
24. Farmer AD, Holt CB, Downes TJ, Ruggeri E, Del Vecchio S, De Giorgio R. Pathophysiology, diagnosis, and management of opioid-induced constipation. Lancet Gastroenterol Hepatol. 2018;3(3):203–12. https://doi.org/10.1016/S2468-1253(18)30008-6.
25. Longstreth GF, Thompson WG, Chey WD, Houghton LA, Mearin F, Spiller RC. Functional bowel disorders. Gastroenterology. 2006;130(5):1480–91. https://doi.org/10.1053/j.gastro.2005.11.061.

26. Parshall MB, Schwartzstein RM, Adams L, Banzett RB, Manning HL, Bourbeau J, Calverley PM, Gift AG, Harver A, Lareau SC, Mahler DA, Meek PM, O'Donnell DE, American Thoracic Society Committee on Dyspnea. An official American Thoracic Society statement: update on the mechanisms, assessment, and management of dyspnea. Am J Respir Crit Care Med. 2012;185(4):435–52. https://doi.org/10.1164/rccm.201111-2042ST.
27. Mularski RA, Reinke LF, Carrieri-Kohlman V, Fischer MD, Campbell ML, Rocker G, Schneidman A, Jacobs SS, Arnold R, Benditt JO, Booth S, Byock I, Chan GK, Curtis JR, Donesky D, Hansen-Flaschen J, Heffner J, Klein R, Limberg TM, Manning HL, Morrison RS, Ries AL, Schmidt GA, Selecky PA, Truog RD, Wang AC, White DB, ATS Ad Hoc Committee on Palliative Management of Dyspnea Crisis. An official American Thoracic Society workshop report: assessment and palliative management of dyspnea crisis. Ann Am Thorac Soc. 2013;10(5):S98–S106. https://doi.org/10.1513/AnnalsATS.201306-169ST.
28. Kelley AS, Morrison RS. Palliative care for the seriously ill. N Engl J Med. 2015;373:747–55. https://doi.org/10.1056/NEJMra1404684.
29. Kamal AH, Maguire JM, Wheeler JL, Currow DC, Abernethy AP. Dyspnea review for the palliative care professional: treatment goals and therapeutic options. J Palliat Med. 2012;15(1):106–14. https://doi.org/10.1089/jpm.2011.0110.
30. Pisani L, Hill NS, Pacilli AMG, Polastri M, Nava S. Management of dyspnea in the terminally ill. Chest. 2018;154(4):925–34. https://doi.org/10.1016/j.chest.2018.04.003.
31. Johnson MJ, Currow DC. Opioids for breathlessness: a narrative review. BMJ Support Palliat Care. 2020;10(3):287–95. https://doi.org/10.1136/bmjspcare-2020-002314.
32. Higginson IJ, Bausewein C, Reilly CC, Gao W, Gysels M, Dzingina M, McCrone P, Booth S, Jolley CJ, Moxham J. An integrated palliative and respiratory care service for patients with advanced disease and refractory breathlessness: a randomised controlled trial. Lancet Respir Med. 2014;2(12):979–87. https://doi.org/10.1016/S2213-2600(14)70226-7.
33. The Cambridge BIS manual; building a breathlessness intervention service [manual]. Cambridge: Cambridge University Hospitals NHS Foundation Trust; 2011.
34. Brighton LJ, Miller S, Farquhar M, Booth S, Yi D, Gao W, et al. Holistic services for people with advanced disease and chronic breathlessness: a systematic review and meta-analysis. Thorax. 2019;74(3):270–81. https://doi.org/10.1136/thoraxjnl-2018-211589.
35. Ambrosino N, Fracchia C. Strategies to relieve dyspnoea in patients with advanced chronic respiratory diseases: a narrative review. Pulmonology. 2019;25(5):289–98. https://doi.org/10.1016/j.pulmoe.2019.04.002.
36. Wilson ME, Mittal A, Dobler CC, Randall Curtis J, Majzoub AM, Soleimani J, et al. High-flow nasal cannula oxygen in patients with acute respiratory failure and do-not-intubate or do-not-resuscitate orders: a systematic review. J Hosp Med. 2020;2:101–6. https://doi.org/10.12788/jhm.3329.
37. Ruangsomboon O, Dorongthom T, Chakorn T, Monsomboon A, Praphruetkit N, Limsuwat C, Surabenjawong U, Riyapan S, Nakornchai T, Chaisirin W. High-flow nasal cannula versus conventional oxygen therapy in relieving dyspnea in emergency palliative patients with do-not-intubate status: a randomized crossover study. Ann Emerg Med. 2020;75(5):615–26. https://doi.org/10.1016/j.annemergmed.2019.09.009.
38. Abdallah SJ, Jensen D, Lewthwaite H. Updates in opioid and nonopioid treatment for chronic breathlessness. Curr Opin Support Palliat Care. 2019;13(3):167–73. https://doi.org/10.1097/SPC.0000000000000449.
39. Blumenfeld-Kouchner F, Bullis L, Koch K. Transmucosal buprenorphine in the treatment of dyspnea: case series and review of the literature. Palliat Med Rep. 2021;2(1):21–4. https://doi.org/10.1089/pmr.2020.0091.
40. Barnes H, McDonald J, Smallwood N, Manser R. Opioids for the palliation of refractory breathlessness in adults with advanced disease and terminal illness. Cochrane Database Syst Rev. 2016;3(3):CD011008. https://doi.org/10.1002/14651858.CD011008.pub2.
41. Mahler DA. Opioids for refractory dyspnea. Expert Rev Respir Med. 2013;7(2):123–34; quiz 135. https://doi.org/10.1586/ers.13.5.

42. Henson LA, Maddocks M, Evans C, Davidson M, Hicks S, Higginson IJ. Palliative care and the management of common distressing symptoms in advanced cancer: pain, breathlessness, nausea and vomiting, and fatigue. J Clin Oncol. 2020;38(9):905–14. https://doi.org/10.1200/JCO.19.00470.
43. Haywood A, Duc J, Good P, Khan S, Rickett K, Vayne-Bossert P, Hardy JR. Systemic corticosteroids for the management of cancer-related breathlessness (dyspnoea) in adults. Cochrane Database Syst Rev. 2019;2(2):CD012704. https://doi.org/10.1002/14651858.CD012704.pub2.
44. Hulme B, Wilcox S, Ashwood P, Deacon L, Gilkes H, Montgomry V. Assessment and management of bleeding complications in the medically ill. In: Cherny NI, Fallon MT, Kaasa S, Portenoy RK, Currow DC, editors. Oxford textbook of Palliative Medicine, Oxford: Oxford University Press; 2021. p. 727–738.
45. Caraceni A, Martini C, Simonetti F. Neurological problems in advanced cancer. In: Cherny NI, Fallon MT, Kaasa S, Portenoy RK, Currow DC, editors. Oxford textbook of Palliative medicine. Oxford: Oxford University Press; 2015. p. 885–905.
46. Agar M, Alici Y, Breitbart WS. Delirium. In: Cherny NI, Fallon MT, Kaasa S, Portenoy RK, Currow DC, editors. Oxford textbook of palliative medicine. Oxford: Oxford University Press; 2015. p. 1092–1100.
47. Inouye SK. The dilemma of delirium: clinical and research controversies regarding diagnosis and evaluation of delirium in hospitalized elderly medical patients. Am J Med. 1994;97(3):278–88. https://doi.org/10.1016/0002-9343(94)90011-6.
48. Bush SH, Kanji S, Pereira JL, Davis DHJ, Currow DC, Meagher D, Rabheru K, Wright D, Bruera E, Hartwick M, Gagnon PR, Gagnon B, Breitbart W, Regnier L, Lawlor PG. Treating an established episode of delirium in palliative care: expert opinion and review of the current evidence base with recommendations for future development. J Pain Symptom Manage. 2014;48(2):231–48. https://doi.org/10.1016/j.jpainsymman.2013.07.018.
49. Bruera E, Bush SH, Willey J, Paraskevopoulos T, Li Z, Palmer JL, Cohen MZ, Sivesind D, Elsayem A. Impact of delirium and recall on the level of distress in patients with advanced cancer and their family caregivers. Cancer. 2009;115(9):2004–12. http://doi.prg/10.1002/cncr.24215.
50. Breitbart W, Alici Y. Agitation and delirium at the end of life: "We couldn't manage him". JAMA. 2008;300(24):2898–910, E1. https://doi.org/10.1001/jama.2008.885.
51. Leonard MM, Agar M, Spiller JA, Davis B, Mohamad MM, Meagher DJ, Lawlor PG. Delirium diagnostic and classification challenges in palliative care: subsyndromal delirium, comorbid delirium-dementia, and psychomotor subtypes. J Pain Symptom Manage. 2014;48(2):199–214. https://doi.org/10.1016/j.jpainsymman.2014.03.012.
52. Yennurajalingam S, Braiteh F, Bruera E. Pain and terminal delirium research in the elderly. Clin Geriatr Med. 2005;21(1):93–119, viii. https://doi.org/10.1016/j.cger.2004.09.002.
53. Bush SH, Tierney S, Lawlor PG. Clinical assessment and management of delirium in the palliative care setting. Drugs. 2017;77(15):1623–43. https://doi.org/10.1007/s40265-017-0804-3.
54. Seitz DP, Gill SS, van Zyl LT. Antipsychotics in the treatment of delirium: a systematic review. J Clin Psychiatry. 2007;68(1):11–21. https://doi.org/10.4088/jcp.v68n0102.
55. Oliveira IR. Antipsicóticos atípicos: farmacologia e uso clínico. Rev Bras Psiquiatr. 2000;22(Suppl 1):38–40.
56. Hui D, Reddy A, Palla S, Bruera E. Neuroleptic prescription pattern for delirium in patients with advanced cancer. J Palliat Care. 2011;27(2):141–7.
57. Leonard MM, Nekolaichuk C, Meagher DJ, Barnes C, Gaudreau JD, Watanabe S, Agar M, Bush SH, Lawlor PG. Practical assessment of delirium in palliative care. J Pain Symptom Manage. 2014;48(2):176–90. https://doi.org/10.1016/j.jpainsymman.2013.10.024.
58. Bush SH, Bruera E, Lawlor PG, Kanji S, Davis DH, Agar M, Wright DK, Hartwick M, Currow DC, Gagnon B, Simon J, Pereira JL. Clinical practice guidelines for delirium management: potential application in palliative care. J Pain Symptom Manage. 2014;48(2):249–58. https://doi.org/10.1016/j.jpainsymman.2013.09.023.
59. Hui D, Dev R, Bruera E. Neuroleptics in the management of delirium in patients with advanced cancer. Curr Opin Support Palliat Care. 2016;10(4):316–23. https://doi.org/10.1097/SPC.0000000000000236.

60. Guia práctica de farmacologia del SNC. 11.ed. 2009. p. 195–263.
61. Hui D, De La Rosa A, Wilson A, Nguyen T, Wu J, Delgado-Guay M, Azhar A, Arthur J, Epner D, Haider A, De La Cruz M, Heung Y, Tanco K, Dalal S, Reddy A, Williams J, Amin S, Armstrong TS, Breitbart W, Bruera E. Neuroleptic strategies for terminal agitation in patients with cancer and delirium at an acute palliative care unit: a single-centre, double-blind, parallel-group, randomised trial. Lancet Oncol. 2020;21(7):989–98. https://doi.org/10.1016/S1470-2045(20)30307-7.
62. Hosker CM, Bennett MI. Delirium and agitation at the end of life. BMJ. 2016;353:i3085. https://doi.org/10.1136/bmj.i3085.
63. Gilligan T, Coyle N, Frankel RM, Berry DL, Bohlke K, Epstein RM, Finlay E, Jackson VA, Lathan CS, Loprinzi CL, Nguyen LH, Seigel C, Baile WF. Patient-clinician communication: American Society of Clinical Oncology consensus guideline. J Clin Oncol. 2017;35(31):3618–32. https://doi.org/10.1200/JCO.2017.75.2311.
64. Baile WF, Buckman R, Lenzi R, Glober G, Beale EA, Kudelka AP. SPIKES-A six-step protocol for delivering bad news: application to the patient with cancer. Oncologist. 2000;5(4):302–11. https://doi.org/10.1634/theoncologist.5-4-302.
65. Hagerty RG, Butow PN, Ellis PM, Dimitry S, Tattersall MH. Communicating prognosis in cancer care: a systematic review of the literature. Ann Oncol. 2005;16(7):1005–53. https://doi.org/10.1093/annonc/mdi211.
66. Bernacki RE, Block SD, American College of Physicians High Value Care Task Force. Communication about serious illness care goals: a review and synthesis of best practices. JAMA Intern Med. 2014;174(12):1994–2003. https://doi.org/10.1001/jamainternmed.2014.5271.
67. Greer JA, Applebaum AJ, Jacobsen JC, Temel JS, Jackson VA. Understanding and addressing the role of coping in palliative care for patients with advanced cancer. J Clin Oncol. 2020;38(9):915–25. https://doi.org/10.1200/JCO.19.00013.
68. Stroebe M, Schut H. The dual process model of coping with bereavement: rationale and description. Death Stud. 1999;23(3):197–224. https://doi.org/10.1080/074811899201046.
69. Jackson VA, Jacobsen J, Greer JA, Pirl WF, Temel JS, Back AL. The cultivation of prognostic awareness through the provision of early palliative care in the ambulatory setting: a communication guide. J Palliat Med. 2013;16(8):894–900. https://doi.org/10.1089/jpm.2012.0547.
70. El-Jawahri A, Greer JA, Park ER, Jackson VA, Kamdar M, Rinaldi SP, Gallagher ER, Jagielo AD, Topping CEW, Elyze M, Jones B, Temel JS. Psychological distress in bereaved caregivers of patients with advanced cancer. J Pain Symptom Manage. 2021;61(3):488–94. https://doi.org/10.1016/j.jpainsymman.2020.08.028.
71. Block SD. Practical considerations including difficult conversations. In: Cherny NI, Fallon MT, Kaasa S, Portenoy RK, Currow DC, editors. Oxford textbook of palliative medicine. Oxford: Oxford University Press; 2021. p. 277–285.
72. Rietjens J, Korfage I, Seymour J. Advance care planning. In: Cherny NI, Fallon MT, Kaasa S, Portenoy RK, Currow DC, editors. Oxford textbook of palliative medicine. Oxford: Oxford University Press; 2021. p. 286–294.
73. Rietjens JAC, Sudore RL, Connolly M, van Delden JJ, Drickamer MA, Droger M, van der Heide A, Heyland DK, Houttekier D, Janssen DJA, Orsi L, Payne S, Seymour J, Jox RJ, Korfage IJ, European Association for Palliative Care. Definition and recommendations for advance care planning: an international consensus supported by the European Association for Palliative Care. Lancet Oncol. 2017;18(9):e543–51. https://doi.org/10.1016/S1470-2045(17)30582-X.
74. Morrison RS, Meier DE, Arnold RM. What's wrong with advance care planning? JAMA. 2021;326(16):1575–6. https://doi.org/10.1001/jama.2021.16430.
75. Gallais Sérézal I, Beaussant Y, Rochigneux P, Tournigand C, Aubry R, Lindelöf B, Morin L. End-of-life care for hospitalized patients with metastatic melanoma in France: a nationwide, register-based study. Br J Dermatol. 2016;175(3):583–92. https://doi.org/10.1111/bjd.14631.
76. Currow DC, Agar MR, Phillips JL. Role of hospice care at the end of life for people with cancer. J Clin Oncol. 2020;38(9):937–43. https://doi.org/10.1200/JCO.18.02235.
77. Enguidanos S, Vesper E, Lorenz K. 30-day readmissions among seriously ill older adults. J Palliat Med. 2012;15:1356–61.

78. O'Connor NR, Moyer ME, Behta M, et al. The impact of inpatient palliative care consultations on 30-day hospital readmissions. J Palliat Med. 2015;18:956–61.
79. Ghezelsefli Z, Ahmadi F, Mohammadi E. End-of-life care provided for cancer patients: a metasynthesis study. Holist Nurs Pract. 2020;34(4):210–20. https://doi.org/10.1097/HNP.0000000000000391.
80. Derrickson BS. The spiritual work of the dying: a framework and case studies. Hosp J. 1996;11(2):11–30. https://doi.org/10.1080/0742-969x.1996.11882818.
81. Kirk TW, Mahon MM, Palliative Sedation Task Force of the National Hospice and Palliative Care Organization Ethics Committee. National Hospice and Palliative Care Organization (NHPCO) position statement and commentary on the use of palliative sedation in imminently dying terminally ill patients. J Pain Symptom Manage. 2010;39(5):914–23. https://doi.org/10.1016/j.jpainsymman.2010.01.009.
82. Maltoni M, Scarpi E, Rosati M, et al. Palliative sedation in end-of-life care and survival: a systematic review. J Clin Oncol. 2012;30(12):1378–83. Erratum for: J Clin Oncol. 2012;30(27):3429. https://doi.org/10.1200/JCO.2011.37.3795.
83. Claessens P, Menten J, Schotsmans P, et al. Palliative sedation: a review of the research literature. J Pain Symptom Manage. 2008;36(3):310–33. https://doi.org/10.1016/j.jpainsymman.2007.10.004.
84. Verkerk M, van Wijlick E, Legemaate J, et al. A national guideline for palliative sedation in the Netherlands. J Pain Symptom Manage. 2007;34(6):666–70.
85. Maltoni M, Scarpi E, Nanni O. Palliative sedation in end-of-life care. Curr Opin Oncol. 2013;25(4):360–7. https://doi.org/10.1097/CCO.0b013e3283622c47.
86. Taboada P. Sedation at the end of life. Clinical realities, trends and current debate. In: Taboada P, editor. Sedation at the end-of-life: an interdisciplinary approach. Dordrecht: Springer; 2015.
87. Abarshi E, Rietjens J, Robijn L, et al. International variations in clinical practice guidelines for palliative sedation: a systematic review. BMJ Support Palliat Care. 2017;7(3):223–9. https://doi.org/10.1136/bmjspcare-2016-001159.
88. Walker PW. Clinical aspects of palliative sedation for refractory symptoms. In: Taboada P, editor. Sedation at the end-of-life: an interdisciplinary approach. Dordrecht: Springer; 2015.
89. Seymour JE, Janssens R, Broeckaert B. Relieving suffering at the end of life: practitioners' perspectives on palliative sedation from three European countries. Soc Sci Med. 2007;64(8):1679–91. https://doi.org/10.1016/j.socscimed.2006.11.030.
90. Rodrigues P, Crokaert J, Gastmans C. Palliative sedation for existential suffering: a systematic review of argument-based ethics literature. J Pain Symptom Manage. 2018;55(6):1577–90. https://doi.org/10.1016/j.jpainsymman.2018.01.013.
91. Morita T. Palliative sedation to relieve psycho-existential suffering of terminally ill cancer patients. J Pain Symptom Manage. 2004;28(5):445–50. https://doi.org/10.1016/j.jpainsymman.2004.02.017.
92. Portnoy A, Rana P, Zimmermann C, et al. The use of palliative sedation to treat existencial suffering: a reconsideration. In: Taboada P, editor. Sedation at the end-of-life: an interdisciplinary approach. Dordrecht: Springer; 2015.
93. Sullivan WF. Palliative sedation and the goals of care. In: Taboada P, editor. Sedation at the end-of-life: an interdisciplinary approach. Dordrecht: Springer; 2015.
94. Cherny NI, Radbruch L, Board of the European Association for Palliative Care. European Association for Palliative Care (EAPC) recommended framework for the use of sedation in palliative care. Palliat Med. 2009;23(7):581–93. https://doi.org/10.1177/0269216309107024.
95. Robijn L, Seymour J, Deliens L, et al. The involvement of cancer patients in the four stages of decision-making preceding continuous sedation until death: a qualitative study. Palliat Med. 2018;32(7):1198–207. https://doi.org/10.1177/0269216318770342.
96. Materstvedt LJ, Clark D, Ellershaw J, et al. Euthanasia and physician-assisted suicide: a view from an EAPC Ethics Task Force. Palliat Med. 2003;17(2):97–101; discussion 102–79. https://doi.org/10.1191/0269216303pm673oa.

Index

C. M. Z. Abdalla et al. (eds.), *Oncodermatology*,
https://doi.org/10.1007/978-3-031-29277-4

GPSR Compliance

The European Union's (EU) General Product Safety Regulation (GPSR) is a set of rules that requires consumer products to be safe and our obligations to ensure this.

If you have any concerns about our products, you can contact us on ProductSafety@springernature.com

In case Publisher is established outside the EU, the EU authorized representative is:

Springer Nature Customer Service Center GmbH
Europaplatz 3
69115 Heidelberg, Germany

Batch number: 10732632

Printed by Printforce, the Netherlands